T0332743

BIOSTATISTICS FOR MEDICAL AND BIOMEDICAL PRACTITIONERS

BIOSTATISTICS FOR MEDICAL AND BIOMEDICAL PRACTITIONERS

JULIEN I. E. HOFFMAN

Tiburon, California, USA

Amsterdam • Boston • Heidelberg • London • New York • Oxford
Paris • San Diego • San Francisco • Singapore • Sydney • Tokyo

Academic Press is an imprint of Elsevier

Academic Press is an imprint of Elsevier
125 London Wall, London EC2Y 5AS, UK
525 B Street, Suite 1800, San Diego, CA 92101-4495, USA
225 Wyman Street, Waltham, MA 02451, USA
The Boulevard, Langford Lane, Kidlington, Oxford OX5 1GB, UK

Notices
Knowledge and best practice in this field are constantly changing. As new research and experience broaden our
understanding, changes in research methods, professional practices, or medical treatment may become necessary.

Practitioners and researchers must always rely on their own experience and knowledge in evaluating and using any
information, methods, compounds, or experiments described herein. In using such information or methods they
should be mindful of their own safety and the safety of others, including parties for whom they have a professional
responsibility.

To the fullest extent of the law, neither the Publisher nor the authors, contributors, or editors, assume any liability
for any injury and/or damage to persons or property as a matter of products liability, negligence or otherwise,
or from any use or operation of any methods, products, instructions, or ideas contained in the material herein.

ISBN: 978-0-12-802387-7

British Library Cataloguing-in-Publication Data
A catalogue record for this book is available from the British Library

Library of Congress Cataloging-in-Publication Data
A catalog record for this book is available from the Library of Congress

For information on all Academic Press publications
visit our website at http://store.elsevier.com/

Working together
to grow libraries in
developing countries

www.elsevier.com • www.bookaid.org

Publisher: Mica Haley
Acquisition Editor: Rafael Teixeira
Editorial Project Manager: Mariana Kuhl
Production Project Manager: Julia Haynes
Designer: Victoria Pearson

Typeset by TNQ Books and Journals
www.tnq.co.in

Printed and bound in the United States of America

CONTENTS

See the companion website: www.booksite.elsevier.com/9780128023877 for additional content for this title.

ABOUT THE AUTHOR

Julien I. E. Hoffman was born and educated in Salisbury (now named Harare) in Southern Rhodesia (now named Zimbabwe) in 1925. He entered the Faculty of Medicine at the University of the Witwatersrand in Johannesburg, South Africa, and obtained a BSc Hons in Anatomy and Physiology in 1945 and a medical degree (MB, BCh) in 1949. After working for almost 3 years at the Central Middlesex Hospital in London, England, as a house officer and registrar in Medicine, he returned to Johannesburg as a senior registrar in the Department of Medicine for 18 months, and then returned to England to work for the Medical Research Council. In 1957, he went to Boston Children's Hospital to study congenital heart disease, and this was followed by 15 months as a Fellow in the Cardiovascular Research Institute at the University of California in San Francisco.

In 1962, he joined the faculty at the Albert Einstein College of Medicine in New York City as an Assistant Professor of Pediatrics and Internal Medicine, and in 1966, returned to the University of California in San Francisco as Associate Professor of Pediatrics and member of the Cardiovascular Research Institute. He was a clinical pediatric cardiologist, taking care of children with heart disease, but spent about 50% time running a research laboratory to study the pathophysiology of the coronary circulation.

His interest in statistics began while taking his Science degree. After going to England, he took short courses in Biostatistics from Bradford Hill and his colleagues. On returning to South Africa, as the only department member to know anything about statistics, he was assigned to perform statistical analyses for other members of the department. This was a period of learning by trial and error, helped by Dr J Kerrich, head of the University's Division of Statistics.

When he went to San Francisco as a Fellow, he was assigned to give statistics lectures to the Fellows and Residents, and when returned to San Francisco in 1966, he gave an officially sanctioned course in Biostatistics to research Fellows and Residents. These lectures were given annually for over 30 years. He was a member of the Biostatistics group, a semiformal group that supervised statistical teaching and consultation. He also was a statistical consultant to the journal *Circulation Research*, and was often assigned manuscripts by other journals, mostly from the *American Heart Association*, to check on the statistical procedures used.

PREFACE

In my 40 years experience of advising medical research workers about how to analyze their studies, certain problems arose frequently. For examples, many investigators wanted to compare two Poisson distributions, yet some introductory books on Biostatistics give little attention to the Poisson distribution, even though it is an important distribution that answers the question about how often a rare event occurs, such as the number of deliveries per hour in a delivery room. Few people can navigate the minefield of multiple comparisons, involved when several different groups are compared, often done incorrectly by performing multiple t-tests, yet most elementary texts do not deal with this problem adequately. Problems of repeated measures analysis in which several measurements are made in each member of the group and thus are not independent occur frequently in medical research but are not often discussed. Tolerance tests are often needed to set ranges of normal values so that a single measurement can be assessed as likely to be normal or abnormal (such as a single fasting blood glucose concentration). Because most basic books do not discuss this problem, most people incorrectly set confidence limits that should apply only to mean values. In fact, one of the incentives for this book was the lack of books in introductory Biostatistics that could be understood relatively easily, but nevertheless were advanced enough that most investigators would not need to buy additional books or hunt through unfamiliar journals for appropriate tests.

The book is intended to help physicians and biologists who might have had a short course on Statistics several years ago, but have forgotten all but a few of the terms and concepts and have not used their knowledge of statistics for reading the literature critically or for designing experiments. The general aim is to extend their knowledge of statistics, to indicate when various tests are applicable, what their requirements are, and what can happen when they are used inappropriately.

This book has four components.

1. It covers the standard statistical approaches for making descriptions and inferences—for example, mean and standard deviation, confidence limits, hypothesis testing, t-tests, chi-square tests, binomial, Poisson, and normal distributions, analysis of variance, linear regression and correlation, logistic regression, and life tables—to help readers understand how the tests are constructed, how to look for and avoid using inappropriate tests, and how to interpret the results. Examples of injudicious use of these tests are given. Although some basic formulas are presented, these are not essential for understanding what the tests do and how they should be interpreted.

2. Some chapters include a section on advanced methods that should be ignored on a first reading but provide information when needed, and others have an appendix where

some simple algebraic proofs are given. As this is not intended to be a mathematically rigorous book, most mathematical proofs are omitted, but a few are important teaching tools in their own right and should be studied. However, knowledge of mathematics (and differential calculus in particular) beyond elementary algebra is not required to use the material provided in this book. The equations indicate what the tests are doing.

3. Scattered throughout the chapters are variations on tests that are often needed but not frequently found in basic texts. These sections are often labeled "Alternative Methods," and they should be read and understood because they often provide simpler and more effective ways of approaching statistical inference. These include:

   a. Robust statistics for dealing with grossly abnormal distributions, both univariate and bivariate.

   b. Extending McNemar's test, a test for comparing paired counts, to more than two categories; for example, if matched pairs of patients are given one of two treatments and the results recorded as improved, the same, or worse, how should these be analyzed?

   c. Equivalence or noninferiority testing, to determine if a new drug or vaccine is equivalent to or not inferior to those in standard use.

   d. Finding the break point between two regression lines. For example, if the lactate:pyruvate ratio remains unchanged when systemic oxygen delivery is reduced below normal until some critical point is reached when the ratio starts to rise, how do we determine the critical oxygen delivery value?

   e. Competing risks analysis used when following the survival of a group of patients after some treatment, say replacement of the mitral valve, and allowing for deaths from noncardiac causes.

   f. Tolerance testing to determine if a single new measurement is compatible with a normative group.

   g. Crossover tests, in which for a group of subjects each person receives two treatments, thus acting as his or her own control.

   h. Use of weighted kappa statistics for evaluating how much two observers agree on a diagnosis.

   Some of these analyses can be found only in journals or advanced texts, and collecting them here may save investigators from having to search in unfamiliar sources to find them.

4. Some chapters describe more complex inferences and their associated tests. The average investigator is not likely to use any of these tests without consultation with a statistician, but does need to know that these techniques exist and, if even vaguely, what to look for and how to interpret the results of these tests when they appear in publications. These subjects include:

   a. Poisson regression (Chapter 34), in which a predicted count, for example, the number of carious teeth, is determined by how many subjects have zero, 1, 2, etc., carious teeth.

b. Resampling methods (Chapter 37), in which computer-intensive calculations allow the determination of the distributions and confidence limits for mean, median, standard deviations, correlation coefficients, and many other parameters without needing to assume a particular distribution.

c. The negative binomial distribution (Chapter 19) that allows investigation of distributions that are not random but in which the data are aggregated. If we took samples of seawater and counted the plankton in each sample, a random distribution of plankton would allow us to fit a standard distribution such as a binomial or Poisson distribution. If, however, some samples had excessive numbers of plankton and others had very few, a negative binomial distribution may be the way to evaluate the distribution.

d. Meta-analysis (Chapter 36), in which the results of several small studies are aggregated to provide a larger sample, for example, combining several small studies of the effects of beta-adrenergic blockers on the incidence of a second myocardial infarction, is often used. The pitfalls of doing such an analysis are seldom made clear in basic statistics texts.

e. Every investigator should be aware of multiple and nonlinear regression techniques (Chapter 30) because they may be important in planning experiments. They are also used frequently in publications, but usually without mentioning their drawbacks.

With the general availability of personal computers and statistical software, it is no longer necessary to detail computations that should be done by computer programs. There are many simple free online programs that calculate most of the commonly used statistical descriptions (mean, median, standard deviation, skewness, interquartile distance, slope, correlation, etc.) as well as commonly used inferential tests (*t*-test, chi-square, ANOVA, Poisson probabilities, binomial probabilities, life tables, etc.), along with their associated graphics. More complex tests require commercial programs. There are free online programs for almost all the tests described in this book, and hyperlinks are provided for these.

Problems are given in appropriate chapters. They are placed after a procedure is described so that the reader can immediately practice what has been studied to make sure that the message is understood; the procedures are those that should be able to be performed by the average reader without statistical consultation. Although the problems are simple and could be done by hand, it is better to use one of the recommended online calculators because they save time and do not make arithmetic errors. This frees up time for the reader to consider what the results mean.

The simpler arithmetic techniques, however, are still described in this book because they lead to better understanding of statistical methods, and show the reader where various components of the calculation come from, and how the components are used and interpreted. In place of tedious instructions for doing the more complex arithmetic procedures, there is a greater concentration on the prerequisites for doing each test and for interpreting the results. It is easier than ever for the student to think about what the statistical tests are doing and how they contribute to solving the problem. On the other hand, we need to resist the temptation to give a cookbook approach to solving problems without giving some understanding of their bases, even though this may involve some elementary algebra. As Good and Hardin (2009) wrote: "Don't be too quick to turn on the computer. Bypassing the brain to compute by reflex is a sure recipe for disaster."

Many people who learn statistics devise and carry out their own experiments, and for them a good knowledge of statistics is essential. There are many excellent statistical consultants, but not enough of them to advise every investigator who is designing an experiment. An investigator should be able to develop efficient experiments in most fields, and should reserve consultation only for the more complex of these. But more numerous and important are those who do not intend to do their own research. Even if the person is not a research worker, he or she is still responsible for assessing the merit of the articles that they are reading to gain new knowledge. It is no longer good enough for such a reader to know only technical information about the drugs used, the techniques for measuring pressure and flow, or to understand the physiologic and biochemical changes that take place in the disease in question. It is as essential for the reader to learn to read critically, and to know how to evaluate the statistical tests used. Who has not been impressed by the argument that because Fisher's exact test showed a probability of 0.003, the two groups were different, or that because the probability was 0.08 the two groups were not different? Who has heard of Fisher's exact test? Of McNemar's test? Of the Kolmogorov—Smirnov two group test? Of Poisson regression? And if the reader has not heard of them, how can he or she know if they should have been used, or have been used and interpreted correctly? With the pace at which new knowledge is appearing and being incorporated into medical practice, everyone engaged in medical research or practice needs to be well grounded in Statistics. Statistical thinking is not an addendum to the scientific method, but is an integral component of it.

What can you expect to achieve after studying this book?

1. A better appreciation of the role of variation in determining average values, and how to take account of this variation in assessing the importance of measured values or the difference between these values in two or more groups.

2. A better understanding of the role of chance in producing unexpected results, and how to make decisions about what the next steps should be.

3. An appreciation of Bayes' theorem, that is, how to improve estimates of probability by adding in potential explanatory variables, and the importance of the population prevalence in making clinical predictions.

4. An ability to perform simple statistical tests (e.g., t-tests, chi-square, linear regression and correlation, McNemar's test, simple analysis of variance, calculate odds ratios and their confidence limits, and calculate simple life tables), as well as understanding their limitations.

5. Appreciate that there are many statistical techniques that can be used to address specific problems, such as meta-analysis, bioassay methods, nonlinear and multiple regression, negative binomial distributions, Poisson regression, and time series analysis. It is unlikely that after studying this book you will be able to perform these analyses on your own, but you should know that such methods exist and that a statistical consultant can help you to choose the right analytic method.

Statistical procedures are technologies to help investigators interpret their data, and are not ends in themselves. Like most technologies, Statistics is a good servant but a bad master. Francis Galton (1889) wrote: "Some people hate the very name of statistics, but I find them full of beauty and interest. Whenever they are not brutalized but delicately handled by the higher methods, and are warily interpreted, their power of dealing with complicated phenomena is extraordinary."

REFERENCES

Galton, F.I., 1889. Natural Inheritance. Macmillan and Company, London, p. 62.

Good, P.I., Hardin, J.W., 2009. Common Errors in Statistics (and How to Avoid Them). John Wiley & Sons, Hoboken, NJ, p. 274.

ACKNOWLEDGMENTS

Many people have helped me eradicate errors and clumsy phrasing. I owe a debt of gratitude to Joseph P. Archie, Jr, Raul Domenech, Stanton Glantz, Gus Vlahakes, and Calvin Zippin. My special thanks to my wife for help with editing.

I also wish to thank the staff of Elsevier for their hard work, with particular thanks to Rafael Teixeira, Mariana Kühl Leme, and Julia Haynes.

## PART 1

Basic Aspects of Statistics

CHAPTER 1

Basic Concepts

Contents

INTRODUCTION

Statistics is a crucial part of scientific method for testing theories derived from empirical studies. In most scientific studies the investigator starts with an idea, examines the literature to determine what is known and not known about the subject, formulates a hypothesis, decides what and how measurements should be made, collects and analyzes the results, and draws conclusions from them. Excellent introductions to these processes are provided by Altman (1992) and Hulley et al. (2007).

One of the main aims of scientific study is to elucidate causal relationships between a stimulus and a response: if A, then B. Because responses to a given stimulus usually vary, we need to deal with variation and the associated uncertainty. In thinking about the height of adult males in the USA, there is some typical number that characterizes height, for example, 70 in or 178 cm, but there is variation around that typical value. Although fasting normal blood glucose is about 100 mg/dl, not every normal person will have this exact blood sugar concentration. If we measure the length of 2-in long 20-gauge needles with great accuracy, there will be variation in length from needle to needle. It is an essential role of statistical thought to deal with the uncertainty caused by variability. One of the major ways to assess uncertainty is by doing an appropriate statistical test, but the test is merely the instrument that produces a result that needs to be interpreted. Performing a statistical test without the correct interpretation may lead to incorrect conclusions.

For a list of all websites referred to in this chapter, as clickable links, see the book companion website: www.booksite.elsevier.com/9780128023877.

Biostatistics for Medical and Biomedical Practitioners
http://dx.doi.org/10.1016/B978-0-12-802387-7.00001-9

Populations and Samples

It is essential to distinguish between measurements in an entire group with a given characteristic, known as a *population*, and those in a subset known as a *sample* drawn from the larger population. A population consists of all the possible measurements for a given variable; for examples, heights of all present and future 10-year-old children in Iowa, weights of all adult white males in California in 2011, or all fasting blood sugars in children aged 5–7 years. Because it may be impossible or impractical to make all the measurements in a population, we usually take a sample of a larger population, make the measurements, and then make certain inferences about the population from which the sample came. Almost all population symbols are Greek letters, and almost all sample symbols are in our usual Roman alphabet. For examples, the population mean is symbolized by μ whereas the sample mean is symbolized by $\overline{X}$. The slope of a straight line (for example, relating height to blood pressure in a population of children) is symbolized by β, but in a sample from that population is symbolized by b.

The Effects of Variability

How does variability interfere with drawing valid conclusions from the data obtained in a study? A recent article described that in the year 2000, adult Dutch males were 4.9 cm taller than their US counterparts (Komlos and Lauderdale, 2007). Several questions can be asked about this result. First, how the measurements were made and with what accuracy; this is not a statistical question, but one that requires knowledge of the field of study; second, how likely is that difference in height in the samples to be a true measure of the height differences.

One way to answer this question would be to measure the whole *population*. All the adult males in the Netherlands constitute one population, and all adult males in the USA form another population. In theory, heights could be measured in the whole population of adult males in both countries, but this would be an enormous undertaking in time, resources, and money. It is much easier to select a sample (a subset of the population) of adult males from each country and use the resultant measurements to make inferences about national heights. We need a precise definition of the population being studied. For example, national heights depend on the year of measurement: In 1935, adult males in the Netherlands and the USA had equal average heights that were both less than those measured in the year 2000. Population 1935 and Population 2000 are two different populations.

If the measurements were made in the whole population, the results would be unambiguous, and no statistical inference is needed—all adult males in the Netherlands in year 2000 would be on average 4.9 cm taller than their US counterparts. But if the measurements are actually made in a sample from each country, another question arises. How well does the difference in the averages of the two samples reflect the true difference in the averages of the two populations? Is it possible that the sample from the Netherlands contained a disproportionate number of tall subjects, and that the two population average heights differ by less than 4.9 cm? Indeed, it is possible, either because of bias in selecting subjects or even at random. The term *random* means "governed by chance," so that any member of the population has an equal chance of being included in the sample; if the sample taken was of basketball players, then their heights clearly do not represent the heights in the general population. Issues of randomization and selection bias are dealt with in detail in Chapter 38. What statistical analysis can do is to allow us to infer from the samples to the population, and in this instance to indicate, based on our samples, the likely values for the population averages.

The same considerations apply to experiments. In a population of people with diabetes mellitus, their fasting blood glucose concentrations might range from 110 to 275 mg/dl. If we select two samples of 10 patients each from this population, it is unlikely that the two samples will have the same concentrations; almost certainly, one group will have some concentrations higher or lower than any concentrations in the other group, and the mean concentrations in the two groups are unlikely to be the same. If the group with the lower mean blood glucose concentration had been given a drug that in reality had no effect on fasting blood glucose concentration, not knowing that both were from the same population would lead to the false conclusion that the drug had caused fasting blood glucose concentration to decrease. It is to guard against this type of error (and many other types) that we need to think about statistical inference.

Variables and Parameters

A characteristic that has different values in different people, times, or things is a *variable*. Variables such as weight, height, age, or blood pressure can be measured in appropriate units. Others, such as eye color, gender, or presence or absence of illness, are *attributes*, and typically we count the number of items possessing each attribute. Sometimes we deal with one variable at a time, for example, weight gain of groups of young rats on different diets; these lead to univariate statistical descriptions and testing. At other times we try to relate one variable to another, such as age and height in growing children, and then we are dealing with bivariate statistics. Finally, many different variables might be involved.

Measured variables have several components. If we measure the heights of different people, there will be differences due to individual genetic and environmental (nutritional) influences. These differences are due to the biological processes that control height and may be the signals that we are examining. On the other hand, if we measured the height of one particular person several times, we might get variations that are due to the degree to which the subject stretches. The person's true height is not changing over a few seconds, but there is variability of the measurement process itself. This source of variability is sometimes known as *noise*, and we usually do our best to eradicate or minimize it. Finally, the signal might not represent the true value. For example, if each person measured wore shoes with 1-in heels, their heights would all be 1-in greater than they should be. This represents a consistent *bias*, and as far as possible such biases should be detected and eliminated. These ideas produce a model:

$$\text{Measured value} = \text{True value} \pm \text{Bias} \pm \text{Noise.}$$

We get this   We want this   We do not want these

The more we can reduce the second and third sources of error (bias and noise), the closer will be the measured and true values. Statistics is therefore a method for separating the signal from the noise in which it is embedded. Statistical tests help to allow for noise, but do not eliminate bias unless special steps are taken.

"Noise" includes not only measurement error, but also legitimate variation. Thus in the example of adult male heights, the true value sought is the average in each country. Any one person can be above or below that average for reasons of genetics or nutrition, so that the model is slightly different. It is:

Measured height in subject A = Average national height $\pm$ individual difference between the height of subject A and the average. This individual difference from the average is known as "error," often symbolized by ε.

This is a form of noise that is biological, not due to measurement error, but it plays the same role in making it difficult to determine the true value of the desired signal.

The term "parameter" has different meanings in different fields of study. In statistics, it is generally used to indicate the numerical characteristic of a population, such as the mean μ (average), slope of a relationship β, and proportion of positive results π. The individual sample values from the population are variables, the characteristic number is the parameter.

BASIC USES OF STATISTICS

Description

The first use is *descriptive*: how many people survived therapy A? What was the average length of the femur at any given age in children with growth hormone deficiency with and without treatment? How close is the relation of height to blood pressure? There are many ways of making these descriptions, most of them relatively simple. The results obtained are termed *point estimates*.

These descriptions concern a specific set of observations, and are unlikely to be identical for another similar set of data. What is important is how much other similar sets of data from the same population might vary from that data set. One way of determining this is to draw many samples from the population and determine how their means vary, but there is a simpler way to obtain the same answer. Elementary statistical theory provides limits within which 99%, 95%, 90% (or any other percentage desired) of the means of all future sets of similar data will fall. Thus the sample average (or mean) height of 97 children of a particular age may be 39 in and the standard deviation (a measure of variability) may be 1.2 in. This point estimate of the mean and the observed standard deviation then are used to predict that 95% of all similar sized groups of children of that age will have mean heights varying between 37.3 and 40.7 in; these are referred to as 95% *confidence limits* or *intervals*. (A confidence interval is a range of values based on the sample observations that allows us to predict with a given probability (usually 95%) where the true characteristic value of the population is likely to occur. The interval is determined by using information from the size of the sample—a small sample is less reliable than a large one and gives a bigger interval—and the variability of the sample data as indicated by the standard deviation.) Therefore an estimate of mean height in a single sample (the point estimate) allows us to predict the limits within which the means of other samples of the same size are likely to lie, and therefore within what range the population mean is likely to be. Setting these confidence limits is an essential extension of descriptive analysis. How to estimate the population mean from the sample mean will be discussed in later chapters.

Point estimates are specific for a particular sample and are as accurate as measurement and calculation can make them. They give a specific answer, just as an assayer testing an ore sample can tell how much gold is present. However, the confidence limits not only depend on the model used but also convey the degree of uncertainty that exists. Given the data, there is a 95% probability of being right in setting the limits for that mean value in other samples from the same population, but that goes along with a 5% chance of being wrong. Limits may be widened to 99%, or 99.5%, or 99.9999%, but certainty is never achieved. Could the randomly chosen sample of adult males have by chance selected the tallest members of the population so that the estimate of mean height, instead of being 175 cm, was 185 cm? Yes, indeed such an aberrant sample could have been chosen, even if it is very unlikely, and if it had been chosen our estimates of the mean population height would be seriously in error. That is the uncertainty that we have to live with.

Statistical Inference

When we ask whether the mean heights of treated and untreated children with growth hormone deficiency are different, we invoke the second use of statistics—*statistical inference* that is done with the aid of *hypothesis tests*. In general, we generate hypotheses about the possible effects of treatment, and then deploy statistical techniques to test the appropriateness of these hypotheses. Often the null hypothesis is selected, that is, we test the possibility that the differences between the groups (taking growth hormone) have not caused a change in an outcome (mean height). If the tests indicate that the differences observed would be unlikely to occur by chance, then we may decide to reject the null hypothesis. One of the advantages of the statistical method is that it can give an approximate probability of correctly rejecting the null hypothesis. It does so by calculating a P value that may be defined as the probability of finding an observed difference or even more extreme differences (say in mean heights) if the null hypothesis is true. This subject is dealt with in depth in Chapter 8.

Statistical methods also allow us to investigate *relationships* among variables that may be thought of as either causative (*independent*) or responsive (*dependent*). Thus if we give a drug to patients and observe a fall in blood pressure, we believe that the drug (independent cause) produced the fall in pressure (dependent response).

We investigate relationships in two main ways. In the *survey method*, we collect examples from one or more populations and determine if the independent and dependent variables are related. In the survey there may or may not be a comparison group. Without comparison groups it is a *descriptive* study. With comparison groups it is an *analytical* study (Grimes and Schulz, 2002). For example, the role of fluoride in preventing dental caries was examined in cities that did or did not supplement their water supplies with fluoride; the amount of caries was much lower in people living in the cities with higher water fluoride concentrations (Grimes and Schulz, 2002). The advantages of an observational study are that large populations can be studied and that individuals do not have to be manipulated and assigned to groups; the disadvantage is that factors other than the fluoride might have caused the observed differences in the incidence of dental caries. Factors extraneous to but related to the factors being studied are termed *confounding* factors. For example, the incidence of dental caries might really be due to deficiency of another factor (X) that is inversely correlated with fluoride. If we do not know about X, or do not measure it, then we would rightly conclude that increased fluoride in the water was associated with decreased incidence of caries, but would be incorrect in stating that the increased amount of fluoride *caused* the decreased incidence of caries because that decrease was really caused by a deficiency of substance X. X is the confounding factor. Confounding variables are not necessarily unimportant, but they confuse the relationship that is being examined.

Had subjects been allocated at random to a high- or a low-fluoride group, there would have been fewer possible confounding factors, but there would have been far fewer people examined (because of the cost), and the investigators would have had to make sure that no other sources of fluoride were introduced.

There are three main types of analytical studies. One is the *cohort* study, in which people exposed to an agent are compared with people who are not so exposed. For example, a survey might compare a large group of people who took aspirin regularly with another group (matched for age, gender, and anything else that seems to be important) that did not take aspirin (exposed vs nonexposed), and after some years the investigators determine how many in each group had had a myocardial infarction (outcome). This might be a prospective study, but could also be retrospective if the outcomes were examined from a database started 10 years ago. A second type of study, *case-control* study, starts with the outcome and then looks back at exposure; for example, taking 100 patients who had a myocardial infarction and another 100 with no infarction (appropriately matched for age and gender) and looking back to see how many in each group had taken regular aspirin. The case-control study is often used when investigating rare diseases or outcomes. The third type of study is the *cross-sectional* study in which exposure and outcome are determined at the same time in the study population. For example, in a group of hospitalized patients, high-density lipoprotein (HDL) concentrations are measured in those who have had a myocardial infarction and a comparable group who have not. If the first group has low HDL concentrations on average and the second group does not, then there is an association between HDL concentration and myocardial infarction. This type of study is relatively easy and cheap to do, but it does not determine if having a low HDL is a cause of a myocardial infarction.

The other type of relationship is that determined by *experiment* in which the independent variable is deliberately manipulated. For example, two groups of people with normal blood pressures are selected, and one group is deliberately exposed to increased stress or a high-salt diet. If the blood pressures increase in this group but not in the control group, then it is possible that stress or the salt content of the diet is a cause of hypertension, and the mechanisms by which this occurs can then be investigated.

These statistical inferences indicate the probability that the differences observed could occur due to chance alone. Frequently, statistical procedures begin with the assumption of the *null hypothesis*, for example, that the means of two populations are identical, and then tests to determine if observed sample differences could easily have occurred by chance. If differences of the magnitude observed could easily have occurred by chance, then the null hypothesis should not be rejected and there is no good reason to postulate a causative effect.

Setting confidence limits and making statistical inferences can be done efficiently only after an effective description of the data. Therefore the initial part of this book is devoted to descriptive methods on which all subsequent developments are based.

DATA

Statistics involves thinking about numbers, but sometimes these are not what they seem. For example, a university proudly announces that its ranking has improved because last year it accepted only 5% of all applicants. This might mean that it is indeed a prestigious university so that many candidates apply, but it might also mean that the university indulges in misleading advertising so that many who have no chance of admission are persuaded to apply. A university department might assert that it has greatly improved its teaching because 97% of the class passed with flying colors, but that might conceal the fact that several students who were not doing well were advised to withdraw from the course. Therefore whether the university or the department has improved depends not on the numbers provided (often by people who have a stake in the impression given) but on what the data actually mean. This is true of all data, and it is as well to consider what the numbers mean before beginning to analyze them.

Models

All statistical tests are based on a particular mathematical model. A model is a representation of reality, but it should never be mistaken for the reality that underlies it. As Box and Draper wrote "Essentially, all models are wrong, but some are useful" (Box and Draper, 1987).

All statistical tests use models, either explicitly or implicitly. For example, consider the heights of a group of people in the USA and a group of Central African pygmies. In each group the heights will vary, but on average the pygmies will be much shorter than the Americans. The model that we use is to regard the pygmies as having an average height of μ_P cm and the Americans as having an average height of μ_A cm. Any one pygmy may differ from the pygmy average by a difference ε_i, and any one American may differ from the American average by difference ε_j. An assumption is that each of these sets of differences is normally distributed (Chapter 6). To compare the two sets of heights to determine if they really are different from each other, a test such as the t-test is used in which this model is required. If the population distributions fit the model and are indeed normally distributed, then the t-test is an efficient way of comparing the two sets of heights. If, on the other hand, the population heights are far from normally distributed, then using a test that demands a statistical model with normal distributions can produce misleading conclusions. Therefore whenever a statistical test is used, the model being invoked must be considered and the data must be evaluated to find out if they reasonably fit the model. If the model chosen is incorrect, then the test based on that model may give incorrect results.

GENERAL APPROACH TO STUDY DESIGN

After studying this book, the reader should be able to design simple studies and tell if someone else's studies have been correctly designed. The following discussion summarizes what should be done, and gives some guidance about selecting the appropriate analyses.

The first requisite for any study is to ask a focused question. It is of little use to ask "What happens if we place a normal human adult in a temperature of 35 °C (95 °F) for 3 weeks?" Many hundreds of anatomic, physiologic, neurologic, biochemical, and molecular biologic changes probably occur. You may be able to measure only some of these, and for all you know have not measured the most important changes. Furthermore, if you could measure all the possible changes, the mass of results would be very difficult to interpret. That is not to state that the effects of persistent high-ambient temperatures are not important and should not be studied, but rather that the study be designed to answer specific questions. For example, asking what mechanisms achieve adequate heat loss under these circumstances, and looking at possible factors such as changes in blood volume, renal function, and heat exchange through the skin are valid and important questions.

This requisite applies to any study. The study might be a laboratory experiment of norepinephrine concentrations in rats fed with different diets, a clinical trial of two treatments for a specific form of cancer, a retrospective search of population records for the relation between smoking and bladder cancer, or the relationship between prospective votes for Democrats, Republicans, and Independents related to race and gender.

The next decision is what population to sample. If the question is whether a new antihypertensive drug is better than previous agents, decide what the target population will be. All hypertensives or only severe hypertensives? Males and females, or only one gender? All ages or only over 65 years? All races or only Afro-Americans? With or without diabetes mellitus? With or without prior coronary artery disease? And so on, depending on the subject to be studied. These are not statistical questions, but they influence the statistical analysis and interpretation of the data. Therefore inclusion and exclusion criteria must be unambiguously defined, and the investigator and those who read the results must be clear that the results apply at best only to a comparable group.

Define what will be measured, and how. Will it be a random blood pressure, or one taken at 8 am every day, or a daily average? Will you use a standard sphygmomanometer or one with a zero-muddling device? Will you measure peripheral blood pressure or measure central blood pressure by using one of the newer applanation devices? Again these are not statistical questions, but they will affect the final calculations and interpretation. The number of possible variables in this comparatively simple study is large, and this explains in part why different studies with different variables often reach different conclusions.

Consider how to deal with confounders. It is rare to find a perfect one-to-one relationship between two variables in a biomedical study, and there is always the possibility that other factors will affect the results. These other factors are confounders. If we know about them, our study might be made more efficient by allowing for them; for example, including patients with diabetes mellitus when examining the outcome of stenting a stenosed coronary artery. Therefore in planning to study the outcome of stent implantation, we might want to incorporate potential confounders in the study; for example, diabetes mellitus, hypertension, obesity, elevated LDL concentrations, renal function, racial group, and age distribution. If we can arrange our study so that each group has subgroups each with an identical pattern of confounders, analysis will be easier and more effective. On the other hand, with too many subgroups, either the total numbers will be huge or else each subgroup may have insufficient numbers to allow for secure interpretation. If for practical reasons such balancing of confounders cannot be done, an approach such as Cox regression (Chapter 35) or propensity analysis (Chapter 38) might allow for the influence of each of these other factors. Either approach would be better than not considering these confounders at all. Finally, there are likely to be confounders that we do not know about. The only way to try to allow for these is to make sure that the various groups are chosen at random, so that it is likely that unknown confounders will be equally represented in all the groups.

The term "simple random sampling" means that each member of the target population has an equal chance of being selected, and that selection of one member has no effect on the selection of any other member. "Randomization" is the process of taking a given sample and dividing it into subgroups by random selection. As stated by Armitage and Remington (1970): "Randomization may be thought of as a way of dealing with all the unrecognized factors that may influence responses, once the recognizable factors, if any, have been allowed for by some sort of systematic balancing. It does not ensure that groups are absolutely alike in all relevant aspects; nothing can do that. It does ensure that they are all unlikely to differ on the average by more than a moderate amount in any given characteristic, and it enables the statistician to assess the extent to which an observed difference in response to different treatments can be explained by the hazards of random allocation." The hope is that any unrecognized but relevant factors will be equalized among the groups and therefore not confound the results. More details about randomization are given in Chapter 38.

When making these decisions, the type of statistical analysis that will be used needs to be specified before starting the study. Will there be two groups, one given the new drug A and one a standard drug B? Will there be a crossover experiment, giving group 1 drug A first and drug B second, whereas group 2 gets drug B first and drug A second? Is there to be one group, giving drug A first and drug B second? The answer to these questions will in part determine how to design the details of the study, how to select subjects, and what form of analysis to use. The more effective the design, the more informed will be the final interpretation.

In deciding about the statistical approach to be used, define what will be measured and how it will be done. If the outcomes are dichotomous ("yes" if the pressure falls >10 mm Hg, "no" if it does not) versus outcomes that are continuous ratio numbers, then different approaches will be needed. Decide what to do if any subject cannot complete the study.

Although the outcomes are not yet available, make some guesses as to what to expect, because this leads to the calculations of sample size. For a new antihypertensive drug there will be some prior information from animal or anecdotal human studies, and the important question to ask is what magnitude of result to expect. No one would do a study to find a decrease of 1 mm Hg blood pressure, but what are you going to do if you expected a 15 mm Hg decrease and the preliminary results showed a decrease of ≤ 5 mm Hg? Do you have a stopping rule? Did you factor this possibility into your calculation of sample size?

Begin analysis of any data set with simple preliminary exploration and description before plunging into hypothesis testing.

A BRIEF HISTORY OF STATISTICS

For centuries, governments collected demographic data about manpower, births and deaths, taxes, and other details. Early examples of this were a Chinese census in AD2 by the Han dynasty that found 57.67 million people in 12.36 million households, and the tabulation in 1085 by William the Conqueror of details of all the properties in England, as collected in the *Domesday Book*. Other than a large collected list, however, no manipulation of data was done until John Graunt (1620—1674) published his "Natural History and Political Observations on the London Bills of Mortality" in 1662, perhaps the first major systematic contribution in the field of what was termed "political arithmetic." Graunt not only collected data systematically, but also analyzed them.

In 1631 (Lewin, 2010) the term "statist" was used to describe a person interested in political arithmetic who "desires to look through a Kingdome," perhaps the first time this term was used. However, the term "statistics" seems to have been used first by a professor of politics in Gottingen in 1749, when he wanted a term to describe numerical information about the *state*: number of kilometers of roads, number of people, number of births and deaths, number of bushels of wheat grown, and so on (Yule and Kendall, 1937). (Kaplan and Kaplan (2006) attribute the term to a professor in Breslau in Prussia.) Today these are termed economic and vital statistics. The items in a group are often referred to as statistics, but there is usually no difficulty deciding whether the term statistics refers to items in a group or to the field of study.

One of the origins of statistics concerns *probability theory*. Even before the Roman empire, people were interested in the odds that occur in games of chance, and these were systematized by Cardano (1501—1576) in *Liber de Ludo Aleae* (Book of Dice Games) published in 1663 but written in 1560 (as described in delightful books by Weaver (1963) and Kaplan and Kaplan (2006)). However, the first specific mathematical theory of probability originated in 1654 with a gambling problem that puzzled Antoine Gombaud, Chevalier de Méré, Sieur de Baussay. There is a game of chance in which the house (the gambling establishment) offers to bet even money that a player will throw at least one 6 in four throws of a die. On the average, the player will win 671 times for every 625 times he loses. What concerned Chevalier de Méré, however, was that it was not favorable to the player to bet on throwing at least one double 6 in 24 throws of a pair of dice. After solving this problem (try it yourself, then see Chapter 5), he checked his solution with Blaise Pascal (1623—1662), the great French mathematician. Pascal confirmed his answer, and then went on to investigate other probabilities related to gambling. He exchanged letters with Pierre de Fermat (1601–1665), and then other mathematicians were drawn into the field that grew rapidly. Although the problem above was a real problem, it was probably known well before Pascal was involved, and the story may be apocryphal (Ore, 1960).

Egon Pearson (1973) (1895–1980) emphasized that big advances in statistics were nearly always made by a combination of a real problem to be solved and people with the imagination and technical ability to solve the problem. For example, about 100 years after Pascal, mathematicians were concerned about the accuracy with which astronomical observations could be made. At this time, Newton's theories were well known, and astronomers were making accurate measurements of the heavenly bodies. This was not just for curiosity, but because navigation, commerce, and military actions depended critically on accurate knowledge of time and position, including the errors of making these measurements (Stigler, 1986). Many of the developments were made in response to specific practical questions about the orbits of celestial objects or the best estimates of length and weight. In the first half of the eighteenth century, mathematicians began to investigate the theory of errors (or variability), with a major contribution from Gauss (1777–1855). This phase culminated when Legendre (1752–1833) introduced the *method of least squares* in 1805.

The introduction of statistical methods into nonphysical sciences came relatively late, and began with data collection and analyses, many performed by those we now term epidemiologists. Adolphe Quetelet (1796–1874), an astronomer, studied populations (births, deaths, and crime rates). Although he did not invent the method of least squares for assessing errors (variability), he used it in his work. In 1852, William Farr (1807–1883) studied cholera fatalities during the cholera epidemic of 1848/1849 and demonstrated that the fatality rate was inversely related to the elevation above sea level. He published a revealing figure that plotted fatality rate against elevation, and showed a conical figure with a wide base and narrow top. Florence Nightingale (1820–1920) analyzed deaths in the Crimean campaign, and in 1858 published what might have the first modified pie chart (called a coxcomb chart) to demonstrate that most deaths were due to preventable diseases rather than to battle injuries (Joyce, 2008). Because of her revolutionary work, in 1858 she was the first woman to be elected a Fellow of the Statistical Society of London.

Gustav Theodor Fechner (1801–1887) was apparently the first to use statistical methods in experimental biology, published in his book on experimental psychology (*Elemente der Psychophysik*) in 1860. Then Francis Galton (1822–1911) began his famous studies on heredity with the publication in 1869 of his book *Hereditary Genius*. He not only analyzed people in innumerable ways, but also did experiments on plants. He appears to have been the first person to take an interest in variability, his predecessors being interested mainly in mean values (Pearson, 1973). In 1889 he published a book, *Natural Inheritance*, which influenced mathematicians such as Francis Ysidro Edgeworth

(1845–1926) and Karl Pearson (1857–1936) to develop better methods of dealing with the variable data and peculiar distributions so often found in biology.

A notable advance was made when William Sealy Gosset (1876–1937) published his article "The Probable Error of a Mean" (Student, 1908). Gosset, who studied mathematics and chemistry at Oxford, was employed by Guinness brewery to analyze data about the brewing of beer. Up to that time all statistical tests dealt with data sets with over 1000 measurements, and Gosset realized that tests were necessary to analyze more practical problems that involved small numbers of measurements (Boland, 1984). He worked on this in 1906 while on sabbatical leave, where he was closely associated with Karl Pearson. His publication in 1908 of what became called the t-test was a landmark. Because at that time the Guinness Company did not allow its employees to publish the results of any studies done (for fear of leakage of industrial secrets), Gosset published his study under the pseudonym of "Student" to avoid association with his employer.

One final root of modern statistics deserves special mention. In agricultural experiments efficient experimental design has particular importance. Most crops have one growing season per year, and their growth can be influenced by minor variations in the composition, environment, and drainage of the soil in which they grow. Thus experiments concerning different cultivars or fertilizers have to be designed carefully so that the greatest amount of information can be extracted from the results. It would be inefficient to test one fertilizer one year, another the next year, and so on. It was this impetus that lead to the extensive developments of statistical design and analysis in agriculture. As early as 1771 Arthur Young (1741–1820) published his *Course of Experimental Agriculture* that laid out a very modern approach to experiments (Young, 1771), and in 1849 James Johnson published his book *Experimental Agriculture* to emphasize the importance of experimental design (Owen, 1976). In 1843 John Lawes, an entrepreneur and scientist, founded an agricultural research institute at his estate Rothamsted Manor to investigate the effect of fertilizers on crop yield. Ronald Aylmer Fisher (1890–1962) joined what was then known as the Rothamsted Experimental Station in 1919 to develop the objective methods of evaluating the results, and in doing so made Rothamsted a major center for statistics and genetics. Since that time, many of the world's major statisticians have been based where there is agricultural research, and many of the best-known textbooks reflect this experience. In parallel with Fisher's work at Rothamsted, L.H.C. Tippett (1902–1985) in 1925 worked with the British Cotton Institute where his statistical insights produced industrially important improvements in the cotton mills, then a major economic force in Great Britain. Also in 1925, Walter Shewhart (1891–1967) began his studies at the Bell Telephone Laboratories that revolutionized the field of industrial quality control and standardization. When he joined the laboratories, the telephone industry was beginning an unprecedented expansion, and large quantities of precision equipment with a high standard of performance and uniform quality were needed. One of his disciples was W. Edwards Deming (1900—1993) who was asked by the US Government to help rehabilitate Japan's industry after the World War II. He was so successful in introducing notions of effective management, statistical analysis, and quality control that he was in part responsible for Japan's renown in high-quality innovative products.

A detailed history of the development of medical statistics was provided by Armitage (1985).

REFERENCES

Altman, D.G., 1992. Practical Statistics for Medical Research.

Armitage, P., 1985. Biometry and medical statistics. Biometrics 41, 823—833.

Armitage, P., Remington, R.D., 1970. Experimental design. In: Statistic in Endocrinology, pp. 3—31.

Boland, P.J., 1984. A biographical glimpse of William Sealy Gosset. Am. Stat. 38, 179—183.

Box, G.E.P., Draper, N.R., 1987. Empirical Model-Building and Response Surfaces. Wiley, New York.

Grimes, D.A., Schulz, K.F., 2002. An overview of clinical research: the lay of the land. Lancet 359, 57—61.

Hulley, S.B., Cummings, S.R., Browner, W.S., et al., 2007. Designing Clinical Research. Lippincott Williams & Wilkins, Philadelphia.

Joyce, H., 2008. Florence Nightingale: a lady with more than a lamp. Significance 5, 181—182.

Kaplan, M., Kaplan, E., 2006. Chances Are: Adventures in Probability. Viking Penguin, New York.

Komlos, J., Lauderdale, B.E., 2007. The mysterious trend in American heights in the 20th century. Ann. Hum. Biol. 34, 206—215.

Lewin, C., 2010. The Politick Survey of a Kingdome: the first statistical template? Significance 7, 36—39.

Ore, O., 1960. Pascal and the invention of probability theory. Am. Math. Mon. 67, 409—419.

Owen, D.B., 1976. On the History of Probability and Statistics. Marcel Dekker, Inc., New York.

Pearson, E.S., 1973. Some historical reflections on the introduction of statistical methods in industry. The Statistician 22, 165—179.

Stigler, S.M., 1986. The History of Statistics. Harvard University Press, Cambridge, MA.

Student, 1908. The probable error of a mean. Biometrika 6, 1—25.

Weaver, W., 1963. Lady Luck. The Theory of Probability. Dover Publications, Inc., New York.

Young, A., 1771. In: Fenwick, J. (Ed.), A Course of Experimental Agriculture.

Yule, G.U., Kendall, M.G., 1937. An Introduction to the Theory of Statistics. Charles Griffin & Co., London.

CHAPTER 2

Statistical Use and Misuse in Scientific Publications

Contents

EARLY USE OF STATISTICS

How well is statistical thought incorporated into existing scientific publications? Do reviewers and editors guarantee that the statistical interpretations of the data are correct?

In the early twentieth century, most scientific reports were descriptive and numerical analysis was rudimentary. Gradually elementary statistical analysis began to appear in publications. A landmark publication with a major effect on the perception and practice of medical statistics occurred with the publication in 1937 by A. Bradford Hill. The first edition of his book *Principles of Medical Statistics*, was based on a series of articles that he had written for *The Lancet*; it is now in its 12th edition (Hill and Hill, 1991). In the United States, an equally important book that can still be read with pleasure and profit is "Elementary Medical Statistics," published in 1952 by Donald Mainland (1963). A third influential publication was "Clinical Biostatistics" by Alvin Feinstein (1977). Published in 1977, this book consolidated a series of articles written by Feinstein between 1970 and 1976 published in the journal *Clinical Pharmacology and Therapeutics*.

After 1952, statistical analysis in medical research became more common. Hayden (1983) reviewed the articles published in the journal *Pediatrics* for 1952, 1962, 1972, and 1982, and observed that the proportion of articles using interpretive statistical techniques increased from 13% in 1952 to 48% in 1982. Furthermore, whereas in 1952 knowledge of the basic *t*-test, chi-square test, and Pearson's correlation coefficient sufficed to understand 97% of the articles that used statistics, by 1982 only 65% of the articles used these tests, and the others used more sophisticated tests. Hayden pointed out that the increasing use of sophisticated tests often puts the reader at a disadvantage. In 2007,

For a list of all websites referred to in this chapter, as clickable links, see the book companion website: www.booksite.elsevier.com/9780128023877.

Biostatistics for Medical and Biomedical Practitioners
http://dx.doi.org/10.1016/B978-0-12-802387-7.00002-0

Hayden and his colleagues (Hellems et al., 2007) surveyed the same journal for 2005. They noted that the proportion of articles that used any inferential statistics increased from 48% in 1982 to 89% in 2005. The most commonly encountered statistical procedures were "…descriptive statistics, tests of proportions, measures of risk, logistic regression, *t*-tests, nonparametric tests, analysis of variance, multiple linear regression, sample size and power calculation, and tests of correlation." They went on to remark that a reader familiar only with these tests would understand the analyses used in only 47% of these articles. Horton and Switzer reached a similar conclusion based on a study of the *New England Journal of Medicine* from 1978 to 2005 (Horton and Switzer, 2005). In another study of surgical publications between 1985 and 2003, the percentage of articles with no statistics declined from 35% to 10%, nonparametric tests increased from 0–12% (depending on the journal) to 33–49%, and the use of more complex tests increased (Kurichi and Sonnad, 2006).

Today, with computers ubiquitous and software statistical packages freely available, the most complex statistical analyses are within the grasp of the nonstatistician. However, this does not mean that investigators necessarily choose the appropriate analyses or perform them correctly. As Hofacker (1983) stated "The good news is that statistical analysis is becoming easier and cheaper. The bad news is that statistical analysis is becoming easier and cheaper."

CURRENT TESTS IN COMMON USE

The statistical tests most often used (80–90%) between 1978 and 2010 in several major medical journals, in a wide variety of medical fields are shown in Table 2.1 (Altman, 1991; Baer et al., 2010; du Prel et al., 2010; Emerson and Colditz, 1983; Greenfield et al., 2009; Hellems et al., 2007; Lee et al., 2004; Oliver and Hall, 1989; Pilcik, 2003; Reed et al., 2003).

Table 2.1 List of commonly used statistical procedures

1. Descriptive measures of position, dispersion and shape, confidence interval
2. *t*-test
3. Contingency tables (chi-square) and other tests of proportions
4. Nonparametric tests
5. Transformations, e.g., from linear to logarithmic
6. Correlation and regression, including multiple and logistic regression
7. Analysis of variance
8. Multiple comparisons
9. Life tables
10. Epidemiology statistics (e.g., odds ratios, attributable risk)
11. Sample size and power calculations, but only in a minority of publications

STATISTICAL MISUSE

Many investigators have examined the use of statistics in both clinical and basic science biomedical publications. Altman reviewed the use and misuse of statistics up to the 1980s (Altman, 1991); more recent studies as summarized by Glantz (2005), Good and Hardin (2009), and Kilkenny et al. (2009) are discussed below. The results have been fairly uniform. Of the published articles in which statistical analyses were used, from 50% to 78% used incorrect tests; this figure has varied little over the past 60 years (Badgley, 1961; Emerson and Colditz, 1983; Freiman et al., 1978; Glantz, 1980; Gore et al., 1977; Kilkenny et al., 2009; Pocock et al., 1987; Reed and Slaichert, 1981; Ross, 1951; Schoolman et al., 1968; Schor and Karten, 1966; Sheehan, 1980; Sheps and Schechter, 1984; Williams et al., 1997). Some investigators reported that recently statistical usage, especially associated with clinical trials, showed slight improvement (Altman and Dore, 1990; Altman, 1991; Dar et al., 1994; Greenfield et al., 2009; Kober et al., 2006). In some articles the misuse of statistical analyses did not alter the conclusions drawn by the investigators, but in others the incorrect choice of analysis caused the investigators to draw incorrect conclusions, based on their own data and a subsequent correct analysis. As Norman and Streiner (1994) put it "…doing statistics really is easier now than doing plumbing, but unfortunately errors are much better hidden—there is no statistical equivalent of a leaky pipe. Also, there is no building inspector or building code in statistics,…"

Good statistical practice is still uncommon, even in high-quality journals. For example, Curran-Everett and Benos (2007) surveyed articles published in three high-quality journals: *American Journal of Physiology*, *Journal of Applied Physiology*, and the *Journal of Neurophysiology* for the years 1996, 2003, and 2006. There was slight improvement over time, but even in 2006 only 0—6% of the articles described confidence intervals, and only 13—38% gave exact P values; both of these omissions indicate poor statistical practice. In 2011, Drummond et al. on behalf of the Physiological and Pharmacological Societies of the UK, began a series of short articles on statistical procedures to remedy the fact that the quality of data reporting and statistical analysis was still poor. It seems that little improvement has occurred (Drummond et al., 2011).

Many types of errors found in the literature, with some representative references, are set out in Table 2.2. The first five are the most important, but any one of them can vitiate a potentially useful study.

The failure to use and interpret statistical tests correctly in such a large number of research enterprises, despite the ready availability of programs that will do the tests, is serious. Chalmers and Glasziou (2009), who included in their list of errors the failure to take cognizance of preexisting studies of a problem, concluded that all these errors might account for 80% wastage of the US $100 billion spent annually worldwide on biomedical research.

Table 2.2 List of some important statistical errors in biomedical publications

1. Failure to state clearly the hypothesis to be tested (Drummond et al., 2010; Harris et al., 2009; Ludbrook, 2008)
2. Failure to check the accuracy of data used for analysis
3. Failure to describe the statistical tests and software used (innumerable)
4. Failure to understand the prerequisites of statistical tests, leading frequently to serious misinterpretation of the results (Badgley, 1961; Glantz, 1980; Gore et al., 1977; Hayden, 1983; Pocock et al., 1987; Schoolman et al., 1968; Schor and Karten, 1966; Sheehan, 1980; Sheps and Schechter, 1984); failure to use control groups, or adequate control groups (Badgley, 1961; Ross, 1951; Schor and Karten, 1966); and failure to indicate whether the data are normally distributed or not, with consequent complications of analysis and interpretation (Gore et al., 1977; Kurichi and Sonnad, 2006)
5. Failure to assess effect size or to use a large enough sample size to give adequate power (Freiman et al., 1978; George, 1985; Hokanson et al., 1986; Huang et al., 2002; Kurichi and Sonnad, 2006; Murphy, 1979; Sackett, 1981b; Sheps and Schechter, 1984; Williams et al., 1997; Yates, 1983)
6. Confusion between standard deviation and standard error (Bunce et al., 1980; Gardner, 1975; Glantz, 1980; Oliver and Hall, 1989; Reed et al., 2003; Weiss and Bunce, 1980) and absence or misuse of confidence limits (Harris et al., 2009; Hayden, 1983; Hokanson et al., 1986; Huang et al., 2002)
7. Use of multiple *t*-tests without appropriate correction or failure to use techniques such as analysis of variance designed for comparisons of more than two groups (Glantz, 1980; Kurichi and Sonnad, 2006; Kusuoka and Hoffman, 2002; Pocock et al., 1987; Schor and Karten, 1966; Williams et al., 1997)
8. Incorrect use or definition of sensitivity and specificity (Schor and Karten, 1966; Sheps and Schechter, 1984) and failure to understand when the odds ratio is an unreliable guide to relative risk (Feinstein, 1986; Holcomb et al., 2001; Katz, 2006; Schwartz et al., 1999)
9. Failure to understand how P values should be interpreted (Dar et al., 1994; Oliver and Hall, 1989)
10. A number of the above errors are common in clinical trials, which may also show failure of or inadequate randomization, failure to describe how patients are included in the trial, failure to use double blind procedures, failure to define when a trial should be stopped early (Harris et al., 2009; Hayden, 1983; Hokanson et al., 1986; Huang et al., 2002)

Schoolman et al. (1968) observed: "Current practices have created an extraordinary and indeterminate risk to the reader if he accepts the authors' conclusions based on statistical tests of significance." This statement is still true today. The readers of these journals, who for the most part are not statistically sophisticated, frequently cannot tell if the statistical tests have been correctly performed and interpreted (Berwick et al., 1981). An important article emphasizing serious misuse of statistical tests was published by Motulsky (2015).

Some editorial boards of medical journals address these issues by having statistical consultants. There is, however, no general policy about which submitted manuscripts receive statistical analysis. Although over the years more and more submitted manuscripts are inspected by statistical reviewers (Gardner and Bond, 1990; George, 1985; Goodman et al., 1998), there are differences among journals that correlate roughly with the size of their circulations (Goodman et al., 1998). Journals in lowest quartile of circulation numbers had about 31% probability of having a statistical consultant on the staff as compared to 82% in journals in the upper quartile. In the lower three quartiles, only 15% of articles were submitted to statistical review, whereas 40% were reviewed in the highest quartile. The reader cannot assume that statistical adequacy of the study has been verified before publication. This is not to discount the value of statistical consultation by the journals. Gardner and Bond (1990) in a small study in the *British Medical Journal* for 1988 observed that only 5/45 relevant articles were statistically acceptable on submission, but this had increased to 38/45 after consultation and revision. Having statistical consultants on Biomedical journals, however, does nothing to prevent major errors of planning and analysis by the investigators before the manuscript is submitted for review.

Erroneous conclusions from faulty statistical tests not only produce incorrect information but lead to major ethical consequences. If more animals or people are used than are needed to establish a statistically valid conclusion, or if the numbers are too few to establish that a real difference between treatments exists, then time, money, and animals are wasted, and some subjects are treated ineffectively when they might have been switched to a more effective treatment (Altman, 1980; Chalmers and Glasziou, 2009; Freiman et al., 1978; Gore et al., 1977; Mann et al., 1991; Williams et al., 1997; Yates, 1983). It is incumbent on the investigator to plan the study and analyze its results effectively. As Altman and Simera wrote: "Complete, accurate and transparent reporting should be regarded as an integral part of responsible research conduct. Researchers who fail to document their research study according to accepted standards should be held responsible for wasting money invested in their research project. In addition, researchers have a moral and ethical responsibility to research participants, funders and society at large" (Altman and Simera, 2010). Recently a study of 635 NIH funded completed clinical trials found that only 46% were published in peer-reviewed journals within 30 months of trial completion; about one-third were still not reported after a median of 51 months after completion (Ross et al., 2012). This indicates serious deficiencies of the research system, and is not only harmful to the research enterprise but is also unethical and wasteful of public funds.

In addition to problems stemming from unconscious incorrect use of statistical tests, there is a more pervasive problem of bias in reporting. There is a tendency not to submit or publish negative reports. Turner et al. (2008) examined the results of 74 trials of antidepressants submitted, as required by law, to the FDA. Of 38 studies with positive results, 37 were published. Of 36 with negative or equivocal results, 22 were not published and 11 were published in a way that suggested better results than were obtained. Other studies support these conclusions (Chalmers and Glasziou, 2009; Dwan et al., 2008; Easterbrook et al., 1991; Hopewell et al., 2009). There is also evidence of conscious bias in that an unduly high proportion of published studies have found results favoring a given company's product when that company has sponsored the research (Bero et al., 2007; Catala-Lopez et al., 2013; Chalmers and Glasziou, 2009; Montori et al., 2004; Ross et al., 2012).

The reader should be aware that even the correct use of a statistical test can lead to incorrect conclusions if simple arithmetical or typographical errors are made. One might think that with computer programs the calculations would be correct. That is probably true, but unfortunately people who transcribe the results can misplace decimal points or minus signs. Vickers (2006) reported a brief litany of such disasters. Recently major flaws were uncovered in an important study of the sensitivity of various cell lines to drugs at Duke University (Baggerly and Coombes, 2009). Errors occurred, for example, because of failure to check the numbers used in the various tests, incorrect labeling of samples, and poor documentation. When the authors of this critical report reexamined data from their own institution (M.D. Anderson Cancer Institute) they found similar examples that needed to be corrected. Both these institutions are sophisticated and have access to experienced statistical consultants, yet serious errors were made.

It is clear from this litany of potential errors that the reader must be able to assess statistical techniques and interpret results with the greatest of care, and must be aware of likely problems.

Finally, and perhaps most important of all, the study must be worthwhile and well designed. As Schoolman et al. (1968) emphasized "Good answers come from good questions not from esoteric analysis." Even the best statistical analysis cannot produce useful conclusions from a poorly conceived and poorly executed study.

BASIC GUIDES TO STATISTICS

There are many articles in the literature that can help the reader evaluate important aspects of an experiment or study. One very readable article is by Finney (1982). The Department of Clinical Epidemiology and Biostatistics at McMaster University Health Sciences Center at Hamilton, Ontario, Canada has published a useful and detailed series to help the average reader ask the right questions (Haynes, 1981; Sackett, 1981a,b; Trout, 1981; Tugwell, 1981, 1984). Recently guidelines for statistical use and reporting for animal experiments (Drummond, Paterson and McGrath, 2010; Kusuoka and Hoffman, 2002) and randomized trials (Montori et al., 2004; Ross et al., 2012) have been published, and the EQUATOR (Enhancing the QUAlity and Transparency Of health Research) program published a catalog of reporting guidelines for health research (Simera et al., 2010).

Why is it that despite innumerable articles, books, and exhortations about the correct use of statistics there are still so many errors made? One plausible reason is that Statistics is regarded as peripheral to Science, rather than an integral part of it. A physician who would not consider treating a patient for a given ailment without thorough knowledge of the advantages and disadvantages of different treatments usually has no compunction about doing a research project without knowing anything about statistical analysis and interpretation. No one is allowed to practice Medicine without a license to show that a standard of competence has been attained, yet anyone may spend millions of dollars doing research without having the requisite credentials.

One of the difficulties that we face as nonmathematicians is that we are uncomfortable with the language of mathematics so that even fairly simple reports about statistics appear to be hard to read. Nevertheless we should try to understand what they are telling us. We should avoid "…The tendency for clinicians to respond to the advances of the mathematician with one of two extremes, truculent skepticism or obsequious docility" (Murphy, 1979). It is the responsibility of all of us to familiarize ourselves with the role of statistics in designing and evaluating the results of research.

REFERENCES

Altman, D.G., 1980. Statistics and ethics in medical research. III. How large a sample? BMJ 281, 1336−1338.

Altman, D.G., Dore, C.J., 1990. Randomisation and baseline comparisons in clinical trials. Lancet 335, 149−153.

Altman, D.G., 1991. Statistics in medical journals: developments in the 1980s. Stat. Med. 10, 1897−1913.

Altman, D.G., Simera, I., 2010. Responsible reporting of health research studies: transparent, complete, accurate and timely. J. Antimicrob. Chemother. 65, 1−3.

Baer, H.J., Tworoger, S.S., Hankinson, S.E., et al., 2010. Body fatness at young ages and risk of breast cancer throughout life. Am. J. Epidemiol. 171, 1183−1194.

Baggerly, K.A., Coombes, K.R., 2009. Deriving chemosensitivity from cell lines: forensic bioinformatics and reproducible research in high-throughput biology. Ann. Appl. Stat. 3, 1309−1334.

Bero, L., Oostvogel, F., Bacchetti, P., et al., 2007. Factors associated with findings of published trials of drug-drug comparisons: why some statins appear more efficacious than others. PLoS Med. 4, e184.

Berwick, D.M., Fineberg, H.V., Weinstein, M.C., 1981. When doctors meet numbers. Am. J. Med. 71, 991−998.

Bunce III, H., Hokanson, J.A., Weiss, G.B., 1980. Avoiding ambiguity when reporting variability in biomedical data. Am. J. Med. 69, 8−9.

Badgley, Robin F., 1961. An assessment of research methods reported in 103 scientific articles from two Canadian medical journals. Can. Med. Assoc. J. 85, 246−250.

Catala-Lopez, F., Sanfelix-Gimeno, G., Ridao, M., et al., 2013. When are statins cost-effective in cardiovascular prevention? A systematic review of sponsorship bias and conclusions in economic evaluations of statins. PLoS One 8, e69462.

Chalmers, I., Glasziou, P., 2009. Avoidable waste in the production and reporting of research evidence. Obstet. Gynecol. 114, 1341−1345.

Curran-Everett, D., Benos, D.J., 2007. Guidelines for reporting statistics in journals published by the American Physiological Society: the sequel. Adv. Physiol. Educ. 31, 295−298.

Dar, R., Serlin, R.C., Omer, H., 1994. Misuse of statistical test in three decades of psychotherapy research. J. Consult Clin. Psychol. 62, 75−82.

Drummond, G.B., Paterson, D.J., Mcgrath, J.C., 2010. ARRIVE: new guidelines for reporting animal research. J. Physiol. 588, 2517.

Drummond, G.B., Paterson, D.J., Mcloughlin, P., et al., 2011. Statistics: all together now, one step at a time. Exp. Physiol. 96, 481−482.

Dwan, K., Altman, D.G., Arnaiz, J.A., et al., 2008. Systematic review of the empirical evidence of study publication bias and outcome reporting bias. PLoS One 3, e3081.

Easterbrook, P.J., Berlin, J.A., Gopalan, R., et al., 1991. Publication bias in clinical research. Lancet 337, 867–872.

Emerson, J.D., Colditz, G.A., 1983. Use of Statistical Analysis in the New England Journal of Medicine. N. Engl. J. Med. 309, 709–713.

Feinstein, A.R., 1977. Clinical Biostatistics. C.V. Mosby, Co.

Feinstein, A.R., 1986. The bias caused by high values of incidence for p1 in the odds ratio assumption that 1-p1 approximately equal to 1. J. Chronic Dis. 39, 485–487.

Finney, D.J., 1982. The questioning statistician. Stat. Med. 1, 5–13.

Freiman, J.A., Chalmers, T.C., Smith Jr., H., et al., 1978. The importance of beta, the type II error and sample size in the design and interpretation of the randomized control trial. N. Engl. J. Med. 299, 690–694.

Gardner, M.J., 1975. Understanding and presenting variation. Lancet 1, 230–231.

Gardner, M.J., Bond, J., 1990. An exploratory study of statistical assessment of papers published in the British Medical Journal. JAMA 263, 1355–1357.

George, S.L., 1985. Statistics in medical journals: a survey of current policies and proposals for editors. Med. Pediatr. Oncol. 13, 109–112.

Glantz, S.A., 2005. Primer of Biostatistics. McGraw-Hill.

Glantz, S.A., 1980. Biostatistics: how to detect, correct, and prevent errors in the medical literature. Circulation 61, 1–7.

Good, P.I., Hardin, J.W., 2009. Common Errors in Statistics (And How to Avoid Them). John Wiley & Sons.

Goodman, S.N., Altman, D.G., George, S.L., 1998. Statistical reviewing policies of medical journals: caveat lector? J. Gen. Intern. Med. 13, 753–756.

Gore, S.M., Jones, I.G., Rytter, E.C., 1977. Misuse of statistical methods: critical assessment of articles in BMJ from January to March 1976. BMJ 1, 85–87.

Greenfield, M.L., Mhyre, J.M., Mashour, G.A., et al., 2009. Improvement in the quality of randomized controlled trials among general anesthesiology journals 2000 to 2006: a 6-year follow-up. Anesth. Analg. 108, 1916–1921.

Harris, A.H., Reeder, R., Hyun, J.K., 2009. Common statistical and research design problems in manuscripts submitted to high-impact psychiatry journals: what editors and reviewers want authors to know. J. Psychiatr. Res. 43, 1231–1234.

Hayden, G.F., 1983. Biostatistical trends in *Pediatrics*: implications for the future. Pediatrics 72, 84–87.

Haynes, R.B., 1981. How to read clinical journals. II. To learn about a diagnostic test. Can. Med. Assoc. J. 124, 703–710.

Hellems, M.A., Gurka, M.J., Hayden, G.F., 2007. Statistical literacy for readers of Pediatrics: a moving target. Pediatrics 119, 1083–1088.

Hill, A.B., Hill, I.D., 1991. Bradford Hill's Principles of Medical Statistics. Hodder Education Publishers.

Hofacker, C.F., 1983. Abuse of statistical packages: the case of the general linear model. Am. J. Physiol. 245, R299–R302.

Hokanson, J.A., Luttman, D.J., Weiss, G.B., 1986. Frequency and diversity of use of statistical techniques in oncology journals. Cancer Treat. Rep. 70, 589–594.

Holcomb Jr., W.L., Chaiworapongsa, T., Luke, D.A., et al., 2001. An odd measure of risk: use and misuse of the odds ratio. Obstet. Gynecol. 98, 685–688.

Hopewell, S., Loudon, K., Clarke, M.J., et al., 2009. Publication bias in clinical trials due to statistical significance or direction of trial results. Cochrane Database Syst. Rev. MR000006.

Horton, N.J., Switzer, S.S., 2005. Statistical methods in the journal. N. Engl. J. Med. 353, 1977–1979.

Huang, W., Laberge, J.M., Lu, Y., et al., 2002. Research publications in vascular and interventional radiology: research topics, study designs, and statistical methods. J. Vasc. Interv. Radiol. 13, 247–255.

Katz, K.A., 2006. The (relative) risks of using odds ratios. Arch. Dermatol. 142, 761–764.

Kilkenny, C., Parsons, N., Kadyszewski, E., et al., 2009. Survey of the quality of experimental design, statistical analysis and reporting of research using animals. PLoS One 4, e7824.

Kober, T., Trelle, S., Engert, A., 2006. Reporting of randomized controlled trials in Hodgkin lymphoma in biomedical journals. J. Natl. Cancer Inst. 98, 620–625.

Kurichi, J.E., Sonnad, S.S., 2006. Statistical methods in the surgical literature. J. Am. Coll. Surg. 202, 476–484.

Kusuoka, H., Hoffman, J.I., 2002. Advice on statistical analysis for circulation research. Circ. Res. 91, 662–671.

Lee, C.M., Soin, H.K., Einarson, T.R., 2004. Statistics in the pharmacy literature. Ann. Pharmacother. 38, 1412–1418.

Ludbrook, J., 2008. The presentation of statistics in Clinical and Experimental Pharmacology and Physiology. Clin. Exp. Pharmacol. Physiol. 35, 1271–1274 author reply 4.

Mainland, D., 1963. Elementary Medical Statistics. W.B. Saunders Company.

Mann, M.D., Crouse, D.A., Prentice, E.D., 1991. Appropriate animal numbers in biomedical research in light of animal welfare considerations. Lab. Anim. Sci. 41, 6–14.

Montori, V.M., Jaeschke, R., Schunemann, H.J., et al., 2004. Users' guide to detecting misleading claims in clinical research reports. BMJ 329, 1093–1096.

Motulsky, H.J., 2015. Common misconceptions about data analysis and statistics. Br. J. Pharmacol. 172, 2126–2132.

Murphy, E.A., 1979. Probability in Medicine. Johns Hopkins University Press.

Norman, G.R., Streiner, D.L., 1994. Biostatistics. The Bare Essentials. Mosby.

Oliver, D., Hall, J.C., 1989. Usage of statistics in the surgical literature and the 'orphan P' phenomenon. Aust. N. Z. J. Surg. 59, 449–451.

du Prel, J.B., Rohrig, B., Hommel, G., et al., 2010. Choosing statistical tests: part 12 of a series on evaluation of scientific publications. Dtsch. Arzteblatt Int. 107, 343–348.

Pilcik, T., 2003. Statistics in three biomedical journals. Physiol. Res./Acad. Sci. Bohemoslovaca 52, 39–43.

Pocock, S.J., Hughes, M.D., Lee, R.J., 1987. Statistical problems in the reporting of clinical trials. N. Engl. J. Med. 317, 426–432.

Reed 3rd, J.F., Salen, P., Bagher, P., 2003. Methodological and statistical techniques: what do residents really need to know about statistics? J. Med. Syst. 27, 233–238.

Reed III, J.F., Slaichert, W., 1981. Statistical proof in inconclusive 'negative' trials. Arch. Intern. Med. 141, 1307–1310.

Ross, J.S., Tse, T., Zarin, D.A., et al., 2012. Publication of NIH funded trials registered in ClinicalTrials.gov: cross sectional analysis. BMJ (Clinical Research ed.) 344, d7292.

Ross Jr., O.B., 1951. Use of controls in medical research. J. Am. Med. Assoc. 145, 72–75.

Sackett, D.L., 1981a. How to read clinical journals. V. To distinguish useful from useless or even harmful therapy. Can. Med. Assoc. J. 124, 1156–1162.

Sackett, D.L., 1981b. How to read clinical journals. I. Why to read them and how to start reading them critically. Can. Med. Assoc. J. 124, 555–558.

Schoolman, H.M., Becktel, J.M., Best, W.R., et al., 1968. Statistics in medical research: principles versus practices. J. Lab. Clin. Med. 71, 357–367.

Schor, S., Karten, I., 1966. Statistical evaluation of medical journal manuscripts. J. Am. Med. Assoc. 195, 145–150.

Schwartz, L.M., Woloshin, S., Welch, H.G., 1999. Misunderstandings about the effects of race and sex on physicians' referrals for cardiac catheterization. N. Engl. J. Med. 341, 279–283 discussion 86–7.

Sheehan, T.J., 1980. The medical literature. Let the reader beware. Arch. Intern. Med. 140, 472–474.

Sheps, S.B., Schechter, M.T., 1984. The assessment of diagnostic tests: a survey of current medical research. J. Am. Med. Assoc. 252, 2418–2422.

Simera, I., Moher, D., Hoey, J., et al., 2010. A catalogue of reporting guidelines for health research. Eur. J. Clin. Invest. 40, 35–53.

Trout, K.S., 1981. How to read clinical journals. IV. To determine etiology or causation. Can. Med. Assoc. J. 124, 985–990.

Tugwell, P.X., 1981. How to read clinical journals. III to learn the clinical course and prognosis of disease. Can. Med. Assoc. J. 124, 869–872.

Tugwell, P.X., 1984. How to read clinical journals. Can. Med. Assoc. J. 130, 377–381.

Turner, E.H., Matthews, A.M., Linardatos, E., et al., 2008. Selective publication of antidepressant trials and its influence on apparent efficacy. N. Engl. J. Med. 358, 252—260.

Vickers, A.J., 2006. Look at Your Garbage Bin: It May Be the Only Thing You Need to Know about Statistics (Online). Available: http://www.medscape.com/viewarticle/546515.

Weiss, G.B., Bunce III, H., 1980. Statistics and biomedical literature. Circulation 62, 915 (letter).

Williams, J.L., Hathaway, C.A., Kloster, K.L., et al., 1997. Low power, type II errors, and other statistical problems in recent cardiovascular research. Am. J. Physiol. 273, H487—H493 (Heart and Circulation Physiology 42).

Yates, F.E., 1983. Contributions of statistics to the ethics of science. Am. J. Physiol. 244, R3—R5 (Regulatory and Integrative Comparative Physiology 13).

CHAPTER 3

Some Practical Aspects

Contents

STATISTICS PROGRAMS

There are many statistics programs that not only avoid the drudgery of computation but also allow the investigator to explore the data. Some of these extensive programs, costing from ~$300 to ~$1000, (some with academic discounts) are JMP, Minitab, PolyStat, Prism, SAS, SigmaStat, SPSS, S-Plus, Stata, Systat; the list is incomplete. In addition, there are highly specialized programs such as Cytel and PASS. One extensive free program developed by Daniel Stricker is called BrightStat (http://www.brightstat.com/index.php?option=com_frontpage&Itemid=1). It runs on Windows systems or any system running Adobe Macromedia Flash. An extensive free program for Macintosh computers called SOFA (Statistics Open For All) can be downloaded at http://www.sofastatistics.com/home.php. There are some inexpensive programs such as AcaStat (http://www.acastat.com/StatisticalProcs.htm) that for $29.95 perform a large number of statistical procedures for both Macintosh and Windows operating systems. Some programs work only with Windows operating systems, others with Macintosh operating systems, and some with both. Many programs have quite long learning curves and are better suited to professionals than amateurs.

In addition, there are numerous free interactive programs on the Internet. One free YouTube course that covers basic statistical thought and tests is provided by the Khan

For a list of all websites referred to in this chapter, as clickable links, see the book companion website: www.booksite.elsevier.com/9780128023877.

Biostatistics for Medical and Biomedical Practitioners
http://dx.doi.org/10.1016/B978-0-12-802387-7.00003-2
27

Academy, and can be accessed at http://www.saylor.org/courses/ma121/ or http://www.khanacademy.org/math/statistics. The talks are easily followed and useful. An outstanding interactive program was developed by W. Douglas Stirling of Massey University in Australia, and can be obtained free at http://cast.massey.ac.nz/init/public_ebooks.html.

A large range of free online offerings for performing statistical tests is available. Some are complete programs that cover a vast range of statistical tests, and others are designed for one specific test. General programs include the following:

1. Vassar College VassarStats: http://www.vassarstats.net
2. A wide range of tests by Web-enabled scientific services & applications can be found at http://www.wessa.net/test.wasp
3. John C. Pezzullo's interactive statistics http://statpages.org/index.html
4. Martindale's Calculators On-Line: http://www.martindalecenter.com/Calculators2A_2_AZ.html
5. SISA interactive statistical analysis: http://www.quantitativeskills.com/sisa/
6. Statistics Online Computational Resource (SOCR) from UCLA http://www.socr.ucla.edu/htmls/SOCR_About.html
7. http://easycalculation.com/statistics/statistics.php
8. A wide range of programs is available from Daniel Soper at danielsoper.com/statcalc3/default.aspx
9. A set of programs (Windows) by Bill Miller http://statpages.info/miller/OpenStatMain.htm
10. There is a free Excel add-on named Merlin at http://www.heckgrammar.co.uk/index.php?p=10310, and many Excel type calculators can be found online. In addition, Excel performs a wide range of statistical tests.
11. Although Microsoft Office 2011 does not have a statistical package, it does work with a free online program called StatPlus:mac LE 2009 that carries out many statistical programs based on data in Excel spreadsheets.
12. A very powerful program called R is available free at http://www.uni-koeln.de/themen/statistik/software/s/index.e.html and https://launchpad.net/ubuntu/+source/r-base/2.8.1-1
13. The Department of Obstetrics and Gynecology of Hong Kong University provides an extensive set of statistical procedures in a program called StatsToDo at http://www.statstodo.com/index.php

A review of a large number of free and extensive programs for Windows and/or Macintosh computers can be found at http://www.freestatistics.info/stat.php and at http://statpages.org/javasta2.html#General.

Many of the cited programs provide graphs. Free graphics programs with a range of simple graphs are found at http://www.onlinecharttool.com/ and http://www.printfreegraphpaper.com

These programs include a large variety of statistical tests, often with a simple explanation of the basis for the test. There are also many specific tests mentioned in the appropriate chapters. Where possible, several hyperlinked Web sites are provided for each test because different sites often offer different additional information, and some give examples or instructional details. Some programs are easy to use and merely involve filling in data values in a table by hand or sometimes by copying and pasting from a data file. These often cannot handle large data files. Other programs are more difficult to use and need some practice.

Warning: some websites may not be maintained forever.

If the listed web sites are not available, search the internet for alternatives.

VARIABLES

Variables are discrete or continuous. A *discrete variable* is one with gaps between its measured values. The number of people in the hospital cafeteria is counted in whole numbers; we do not recognize 63.36 people. The number of missing teeth per mouth is a whole number, and is a discrete variable. There can even be discrete variables that are not whole numbers; for example, spin quantum numbers take on half-integer values but never intermediate values. On the other hand, *continuous* variables allow interpolation of another value between any two adjacent values. Thus although one person may weigh 64.5678 kg and another person may weigh 64.5679 kg, it is possible to have many people with weights intermediate between these two boundaries, even though there may not be tools to measure with this degree of accuracy. The distinction between discrete and continuous data is not absolute. For example, although age is a continuous measurement, we often record ages to the nearest year, or the last birthday. Furthermore, for convenience we often group continuous data into discrete groups; for example, systolic blood pressure from 90 to 100 mm Hg, 100 to 110 mm Hg, and so on.

Data are termed *censored* if they cannot be measured accurately but are known to be beyond some limit. For example, there may be a lower limit of detection for endothelin that in one assay has a lower detectable limit of 0.025 pmol/L. There is always some endothelin in the blood, but if it is less than the threshold of measurement we cannot measure it. The value is *censored* at the lower limit of detectability—*left censored*, because the lower values usually occur on the left side of a distribution. As another example, when analyzing the survival of groups of patients on one or more treatments for a particular illness, some patients in each group will be dead, so we know how long they survived after the treatment started. On the other hand, we do not know how long those who are still alive at the end of the trial will live; these patients are said to be *right censored*, that is, we do not know the upper limit of their survival. Censored values require special types of analysis.

MEASUREMENT SCALES

A number such as 4 may mean different things under different measurement scales. A classification of such scales was first proposed by Stevens (1946). Most numbers in daily use are measured in the *ratio scale*: 4 mg is twice the mass of 2 mg, 15 cm is three times the length of 5 cm, and so on. Furthermore, the difference between 4 and 2 mg is the same as the difference between 6 and 4 mg. A similar scale is the *interval scale*, in which the distance between any two values can be measured, but in which the two numbers are not ratio numbers. The classical example of this is the centigrade temperature scale, inasmuch as the numerical difference between 30 and 20 °C is the same as the difference between 20 and 10 °C; however, 20 °C is not twice as hot as 10 °C, because zero on this scale is arbitrary and does not indicate the absence of the factor (molecular movement) responsible for creating the temperature. If measured in degrees Kelvin, then temperatures would be ratio numbers. In general, numbers generated in ratio or interval scales can be handled statistically in the same way. This is, however, not true for interval scales found in circular repeated measurements such as time (0–24 h) and direction (0°–360°). Although intervals such as 4–2 pm and 6–4 pm are equal, as are intervals from 60° to 30° and 90° to 60°, it makes no sense to take ratios of 1 am–11 pm, or +10° to −30°. These circular intervals require specific methods of analysis (Zar, 2010). Not all numbers are ratio numbers—for example, telephone numbers or area codes.

By contrast, consider grading the amount of aortic atheroma as +, ++, +++, or ++++. Now ++++ is not twice ++, and the difference between +++ and ++ is not necessarily the same as the difference between ++ and +. All that we can state is that +++ is more than ++, but not necessarily in an exact ratio or by an exact interval. The scale from + to ++++ is a ranking or *ordinal scale*; it gives the order of magnitude and ranking of the variable in that one plaque is bigger than another, but does not give exact amounts. If, on the other hand, we measured the surface area of the atheromatous plaques, or extracted and quantitated the amount of cholesterol in them, then we would produce ratio numbers. Numbers on the ordinal scale require their own special statistical treatment.

Ordinal scales, although inexact, have considerable value. Consider assessing the degree of shortness of breath (Stulbarg and Adams, 1994) in evaluating patients with lung or heart disease. The American Thoracic Society has a scale with grades 0–4 (Table 3.1).

Even though grade 2 is not twice as bad as grade 1, a person with grade 2 is worse off than someone with grade 1, and a change from grade 2 to grade 1 is an improvement.

Table 3.1 American Thoracic Society scale of breathlessness

Description	Grade	Degree
No shortness of breath hurrying on level or walking up a short hill	0	None
Troubled by shortness of breath hurrying on level or walking up a short hill	1	Mild
Walks on level slower than peers or may have to stop to rest	2	Moderate
Stops after walking 100 yards or a few minutes on the level	3	Severe
Breathless on dressing or undressing; cannot leave house	4	Very severe

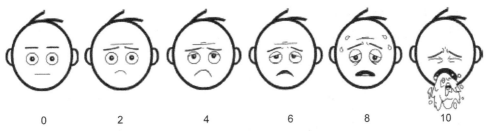

Figure 3.1 Nausea scale.

There are ordinal scales used in many other fields; for example, a somatotype drawing to represent different degrees of body fat, with a high correlation between this visual scale and the measured body mass index, (Must et al., 1993) or a set of facial expressions to indicate the degree of nausea (Figure 3.1) (Baxter et al., 2011).

Respiratory Medicine distinguishes shortness of breath from the sensation of discomfort on breathing, and the latter is even harder to quantify because it is subjective. One way of quantifying this is to use a visual analog scale. To create this scale, draw a line (Figure 3.2) with the left end indicating no sensation of breathlessness and the right end indicating severe breathlessness.

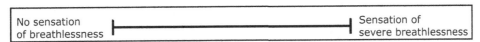

Figure 3.2 Visual analog scale for the sensation of breathlessness.

A subject being tested is then asked where on this line his or her sensation should be placed. A scale of this type is frequently used in evaluating pain. Such a scale needs to have its ends defined carefully. It is particularly useful for following changes from time to time in the same person.

In psychosocial research Likert scales are often used. A typical Likert item is the well-known approval rating system: strongly disagree, disagree, neither agree nor disagree, agree, strongly agree. The scale is designed so that the central value is neutral and the intervals between adjacent values approximately equal. Sometimes seven or nine choices are given. A useful discussion of Likert scales is provided by Uebersax (2006).

Ordinal scales are often combined to produce scores. For example, the well-known Apgar score (Apgar, 1953) taken at 1 and 5 min after birth is useful in assessing the status of a newborn infant (Table 3.2).

The higher the score is, the better the infant's health and prognosis (Table 3.3).

Each score is given the same weight. However, a score of 7 can be obtained in several ways, and they may not be equivalent.

Scoring systems are used in all branches of medicine. For example, Brody et al. (2006) described for bronchiectasis a scoring system based on the extent of bronchiectasis in central and peripheral lung lobes, peribronchial thickening, mucous plugging, cysts, opacities, and air trapping. This scoring system was subsequently used by Sanders et al.

Table 3.2 Apgar score

Score	0	1	2
Heart rate	Absent	<100/min	>100/min
Respiration	Absent	Slow, irregular	Good, crying
Muscle tone	Limp	Some flexion	Active motion
Reflex irritability (nasal catheter)	No response	Grimace	Cough, sneeze, cry
Color	Blue or pale	Body pink, limbs blue	All pink

Table 3.3 Original Apgar results for 1 and 5 min scores

Score	Infants	Deaths in group (%)
0, 1, or 2	65	9 or 14
3, 4, 5, 6, or 7	182	2 or 1.1
8, 9, or 10	772	1 or 0.13

(2011) for prognosis in patients with cystic fibrosis. Scoring systems may also include a historical component such as that developed by Shaper et al. (1986) for identifying the risk of coronary heart disease in men. In addition to some continuous variables such as blood pressure and cholesterol concentration, this score also included recall of diagnosis of ischemic heart disease, presence of angina pectoris, diabetes mellitus, or death of a parent from heart disease. These scores were included in the final prediction equation:

7 × years of smoking cigarettes + 6.5 × mean blood pressure (mm Hg) + 270 for recall of heart disease + 150 for history of angina + 85 if either parent died of heart disease + 150 if diabetic. A score >1000 put the patient in the highest quintile for risk.

Finally, there is the *nominal scale*, derived from naming observations (attributes), classifying them into categories, and counting how many observations are in each category; there is no implied order among the categories. The categories may be binary—for examples, men and women, or yes and no—or there may be several categories, for example, blue, green, and brown eyes; single, married, widowed, divorced. Nominal scales have their own forms of statistical analysis.

Many statistics programs have developed specific procedures for dealing with each class of numbers. There is, however, disagreement about the usefulness and even the discreteness of these four types of number scales (Velleman and Wilkinson, 1993). The number of years of education is not made strictly of interval numbers, because we do not know if the educational gain from year 2 to year 3 is the same as that from year 3 to year 4. Nevertheless, these numbers are not pure ordinal numbers in which the interval between 3 and 4 can be any multiple of the interval between 2 and 3. Such a scale falls between two of Steven's categories. The same reasoning applies to scores that are derived from sets of scales (Gardner, 1975). For example, consider a scale of dyspnea (Table 3.1), and scales for chest discomfort and degree of muscle fatigue. In each scale, despite no specified fixed interval, subjects are likely to space out the scale marks fairly evenly. It is highly unlikely that a subject would judge the difference between 9 and 10 as greater than the distance from 0 to 9; there may be an unconscious attempt to keep intervals fairly constant. If the results from each scale are combined into a score, this score will be more than an ordinal but less than true interval scale. Furthermore, there are sets of numbers that fit none or two of the criteria, or that might change from one type to another depending on the circumstances; at times several types seem to be involved (Velleman and Wilkinson, 1993). In a technique known as Winsorization (Chapter 4) the extreme values at each end of a set of numbers are replaced with less extreme numbers. If this is done, the part of the set between these extremes contains ratio numbers, and the replaced extremes are ordinal numbers. Thus although there is concern about how one analyzes ordinal numbers vis-à-vis ratio numbers, the actual technique used depends on more than Stevens' classification.

An ordinal scale is often assigned numerical values and then treated as a ratio scale. For example, course grades of A, B, C, D, and F are assigned numerical values of 4, 3, 2, 1, and 0, and from these grade point averages are calculated, despite the fact that these are not ratio numbers. Labovitz (1967) showed that a monotonic transformation of these ordinal numbers with or without constant intervals causes only small differences in statistics such as correlation coefficient and t-test. (A monotonic function is one that preserves a given order; e.g., always increasing or always decreasing with time, but not necessarily linearly.)

Most computer programs require the type of scale to be assigned before they allow data entry. Although many of the assignments are standard, for example, ratio numbers are entered as numeric and continuous, whereas names are entered as character and nominal, sometimes the defaults for programs are not obvious. It pays to read the instructions!

Problem 3.1

Can you allocate the following scales correctly?
a. Annual dates, such as 1936, 1937, 1955, etc.
b. Results of a horse race win, place, lose
c. Grading peaches as fresh, free from blemishes, soft, sweet, good value
d. Grading the appearance of peaches as excellent, good, fair, or bad
e. Mohs scale for the hardness of minerals 1, 2,...10

DISPLAYING DATA SETS

The different types of scales are often combined in data sets (Table 3.4).

Typically, the table has one row for each subject, and one column for each variable. The first column is an identifier column, and may contain the subject's name, initials, or

Table 3.4 A typical data set

Name	Age (years)	Gender	Height (cm)	Weight (kg)	Pacemaker life (months)	Censored	NYHA class	Comments
JD	33	M	180	60	36	1	2	
AA	45	M	186	77	13	1	2	
LM	47	F	165	72	22	0	1	
KH	22	F	168	77	56	1	3	
RR	67	F	160	81	5	0	2	
SR	44	M	169	72	16	0	3	
TW	39	F	171	66	16	1	3	
EA	26	F	164	70	23	0	1	
KL	52	M	165	85	28	1	1	

NYHA, New York Heart Association.

an identifying number. The second column contains a continuous ratio number (age) that, for convenience, has been put down as discrete intervals of 1 year. The third column is a nominal or categorical variable, denoting male or female. Sometimes these are turned into numerical indicators by listing one gender as a 0, and the other as a 1. The fourth to fifth columns are ratio numbers, height and weight; these are continuous variables. The sixth column is a ratio number, the duration of life of an implanted pacemaker. It is given in discrete units of months, but could have been given in weeks or days. The seventh column is again a nominal, categorical, or indicator variable that tells us whether the pacemaker was still functioning at the indicated time. A 1 for subject JD indicates that the pacemaker did not function after 36 months, and a 0 for subject LM indicates that the pacemaker was still functioning at 22 months. Finally, in the last column, the New York Heart Association class is an assessment of the degree of disability and discomfort, with 1 indicating mild discomfort and 4 being very severe. This is in the ordinal scale, with 4 being more severe than 2, but not necessarily twice as severe. The final column labeled "Comments" allows the investigator to insert any nonnumerical comments.

Practical Issues of Data Sets

Because statistical programs are designed to handle numbers or symbols, descriptive comments should be reserved for a separate column. To show whether patients did or did not receive an inotropic agent, one can put Yes or No, but statistical computer programs, however, prefer to deal with numbers rather than letters, so that there may be an advantage in defining 0 for no agent and 1 for its presence (or the other way around; it is immaterial). If information about inotrope usage is unavailable for a particular patient, leave the space blank rather than put n/a or an equivalent term; once again, the computer is looking for numbers or defined symbols, not letters. If most patients received dobutamine but a few were given milrinone, then note this in the Comments column; do not put 1 (milrinone) because the program will see this as something different from 1. If the issue about the type of inotrope is important, it is simple to use a numerical scale of 0 for no inotrope, 1 for dobutamine, 2 for milrinone, and so on. This ensures that the column to be analyzed has the data in appropriate form.

Frequently, data are collected for two or more groups, each set out in its own column; for example, glucose concentrations in males in one column and in females in the second column. These are termed split columns. Many statistics programs, however, prefer to have all the glucose concentrations in one column, and the second column to indicate whether the concentration is from a male or a female. An example of this is shown in Table 3.4 where the third column shows gender and the fourth column shows weight. These are termed stacked columns, and most programs allow automatic conversion from split to stacked columns or the reverse.

ACCURACY OF MEASUREMENT

Sometimes simple crude measurements suffice, but at other times great accuracy is needed, even to several decimal places. The greater the accuracy needed, however, the higher the price to be paid for the measuring equipment.

The number of decimal places used in recording the measurement has a specific meaning. If a weight is recorded as 2.634 g, the first three numbers are correct and the fourth number is between 0.0035 and 0.0045 (Dwyer, 1951). Therefore, a weight of 2.634 g represents a weight range between 2.6335 and 2.6345 g. If the accuracy of the third figure is uncertain, do not add the fourth figure. Note that 2.634 g is the same as 0.002634 kg. The accuracy of the two measurements is obviously the same, which means that we are indicating the accuracy only of the figures beyond the zeros; it is still the fourth place figure that has some inaccuracy. We speak of significant figures when restricting the indication of accuracy to those digits that carry meaning about its precision, excluding leading zeros after a decimal point that merely indicate scale.

Similarly, if the weight is 2,634,000 ng, we do not imply that the weight is correct to the seventh figure. With four significant figures, the first, second and third figures are accurate, and the fourth could be from 3.5 to 4.5. In measurements, do not give results to more significant figures than we can be sure of.

A way of making the number of digits equal to the number of significant figures is to use scientific notation, that is, to multiply by powers of 10. Any number can be written as a number between 1 and 10 multiplied by a power of 10. Thus 2,634,000 ng with four significant figures can be written as 2.634×10^6 ng; in this form it is clear that there are four significant figures. Because computers may not always recognize or depict super-scripted components such as 10^6, an alternative format is to write E6 or e6, where the E or e substitutes for the number 10 and the number represents the exponent. This e has nothing to do with the exponential constant or function.

There is some difference when calculating. Even though we may record weights to the nearest kilogram, the average weight of a set of weights might not be a whole number such as 50 kg but rather 50.32 kg. Furthermore, if we then proceed to do a series of computations with those values, it is necessary to keep a large string of decimal places and not round off until the end to avoid computational errors (see below).

Rounding off and Truncation

The output of calculators and computers often appears with many more decimal places than are needed. For example, weights may be measured in kilograms to two decimal places, but the computer may give a mean value of 53.2769925 kg. If we want four significant figures, *round off* the value to the next highest value of 53.28 that meets the requirement that the value be between 53.275 and 53.285. Had the mean value been 53.2748217, round off to the next lower number of 53.27. What if the mean value came out as 53.275000? By convention, most people round off to the closest even number, that is, to 53.28.

Rounding off is not the same as truncation. Truncation means that the value is shortened to the desired number of figures, no matter how large or small the excess figures may be, and without any adjustment to the final figure. Thus to truncate the mean weight to four figures, both 53.2769925 and 53.2748217 become 53.27. Truncation is used in computer programs, often to set a value at a whole number that is used as an indicator rather than as a number. Truncation also occurs when in a table, for example, in Excel, the column is too narrow to hold the needed number of figures. The program automatically truncates the number rather than rounding it off.

Both truncation and premature rounding off can lead to errors if a long sequence of calculations is done: squaring a series of numbers, summing them, squaring and summing another set of numbers, and then subtracting the two totals can lead to large errors (Table 3.5).

For the complete numbers with four decimal places the difference between the sums of the squares of the A set and the B set is 0.9553, and the difference for the rounded off numbers is 0.64. Consider how much more error might occur for a longer series of numbers submitted to a more complex set of additions, subtractions, and divisions.

Table 3.5 Sets of numbers for squaring and addition

	Group A		Group B	
	Complete	Rounded	Complete	Rounded
	3.9726	3.97	5.0019	5.00
	4.6177	4.62	6.7444	6.74
	8.9311	8.93	7.8735	7.87
	9.5503	9.55	7.5849	7.58
	7.9130	7.91	8.9281	8.93
Sums of squares	270.6931	270.2058	269.7378	269.5658

Accuracy and Precision

Accuracy indicates how close to the true value the measured value is, and *precision* indicates how reproducible the measurement is. Great precision indicates that all the measurements on a single subject or object are close to each other, but tells nothing about how close to the true value they are (Figure 3.3).

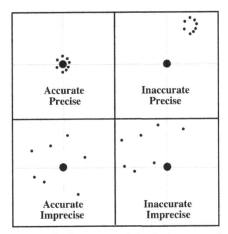

Figure 3.3 Accuracy and precision. The large central dot is the true value to be estimated, and the smaller dots represent measured values.

In the upper left panel all measurements are near the true value, so that the measurements are accurate (similar to the true value) and precise (showing good reproducibility). In the upper right panel the measurements are reproducible and close to each other (precise) but are far from the true value (inaccurate). The lower left panel shows that the measurements vary markedly from one to the other (imprecise) but they cluster around the true value so that averaging them gives a value near the true value (accurate). In the lower right panel reproducibility is poor (imprecise) and none of the measurements are close to the true measurement (inaccurate); averaging these imprecise values does not improve accuracy.

NOTATION

Variables such as weight (in grams), intelligence quotient (in points), or glucose concentrations (mMol/L) are usually symbolized by letters near the end of the alphabet such as X, Y, and Z. In most but not all texts, these are the upper case (capital) letters. Letters near the beginning of the alphabet such as A, B, and C are usually reserved for *constants*. N or n symbolizes the total number of measurements in an array. In order to indicate which member of a group is referred to, put a subscript next to the letter that denotes the variable. The first member of a group of numbers is X_1, the second is X_2, and the last value is X_n. To refer to any member of the group, it is customary to refer to X_i or X_j or X_k.

In some texts, the lower case letter is used to indicate the difference between the value of an individual measurement and the mean of the group. This convention simplifies the formulas, but is not universal, so that the reader must verify what the writer means by any given symbol. In the texts that use this convention:

$$x_i = \overline{X} \pm \text{difference between the mean and the individual value,}$$

where $\overline{X}$ refers to the typical average measurement in the group, and the variation may be positive or negative. This concept leads to a model for these measurements:

Individual measurement = typical value + variation about that value,

= typical value + deviation between individual and typical values,

= typical value + *error*.

The term "error" does not mean a mistake, but is used in the sense of random individual variation. It is what was referred to as "noise" as in Chapter 1. To put this as a formula, write:

$$x_i = \overline{X} \pm \varepsilon_i,$$

where $\overline{X}$ is the typical value and ε_i is the error or random deviation for that individual measurement; the error may be positive or negative.

OPERATORS

An operator is a symbol that instructs users to do something with the variables or numbers that follow it. What follows the operator is termed the argument. The two commonly used operators in statistics are the summation sign Σ (upper case letter sigma) and the multiplication sign Π (upper case letter pi).

The expression $\sum_{i=1}^{n} X_i$ tells the reader to add up all the X variables, beginning with the first value of X ($i = 1$) and then adding in all the other X variables sequentially (X_2, X_3, X_4,...) until the last member of the series, namely X_n. Therefore,

$$\sum_{i=1}^{n} X_i = X_1 + X_2 + X_3 + ...X_n.$$

The information above and below the summation sign tells us how much of the series to include. Thus the expression $\sum_{i=3}^{n-2} X_i$ is the instruction: "Start with the third value of X from the beginning of the series, and add each subsequent value of X until the third last value of the X array is reached"; in other words, add up all the values of X except for the first two and the last two values. Therefore,

$$\sum_{i=3}^{n-2} X_i = X_3 + X_4 + X_5 + ...X_{n-2}.$$

Usually we begin with the first of the series and continue adding until the end of the series is reached, so that some authors leave out the qualifying beginning and terminating instructions with the understanding that summation starts with the first member of the series and ends with the last member of the series: $\sum X_i$ indicates $\sum\limits_{i=1}^{n} X_i$.

There is a similar operator that instructs us to multiply all the values in the array together. This is the Π operator, and it indicates the limits of the operation in the same way.

These operators can be manipulated in various ways. For example,

$$\sum_{i=1}^{n} (X_i + 1) = (X_1 + 1) + (X_2 + 1) + (X_3 + 1) + \ldots\ldots(X_n + 1)$$

$$= (X_1 + X_2 + X_3 + X_n) + (1_1 + 1_2 + 1_3 + \ldots 1_n)$$

$$= \sum_{i=1}^{n} X_i + \sum_{i=1}^{n} 1_i$$

What does the expression $\sum\limits_{i=1}^{n} 1_i$ mean? The instruction is to add up all the values of the argument, starting with the first member and continuing until the last member. But this is the same as $1 + 1 + 1 + \ldots n$ times, so that $\sum\limits_{i=1}^{n} 1_i = n$ (or N). Therefore,

$$\sum_{i=1}^{n} (X_i + 1) = \sum_{i=1}^{n} X_i + n.$$

Similarly, the expression

$$\sum_{i=1}^{n} (X_i + A) = \sum_{i=1}^{n} X_i + nA,$$

where A is a constant value.

The expression

$$\sum_{i=1}^{n} 2X_i = (X_1 + X_1) + (X_2 + X_2) + \ldots(X_n + X_n)$$

$$= (X_1 + X_2 + \ldots X_n) + (X_1 + X_2 + \ldots X_n)$$

$$= \sum_{i=1}^{n} X_i + \sum_{i=1}^{n} X_i$$

$$= 2\sum_{i=1}^{n} X_i.$$

A constant multiplier of the argument can be taken outside the summation sign, and indicates that the sum is to be multiplied by the constant: $\sum\limits_{i=1}^{n} AX_i = A \sum\limits_{i=1}^{n} X_i$.

There is no reason that summation has to be applied to only one variable. $\sum\limits_{i=1}^{n} X_i Y_i$ is the same as $(X_1 Y_1 + X_2 Y_2 + \ldots X_n Y_n)$; multiply the first X by the first Y, add the product to the product of the second X and the second Y, and so on up to the product of the last X and the last Y.

If an operation is to be carried out on the values of X before or after the summation, then indicate this by parentheses or some other form of mathematical punctuation. For example, $\sum_{i=1}^{n} (X_i^2) = (X_1^2 + X_2^2 + ...X_n^2)$. This is different from $\left(\sum_{i-1}^{n} X_i\right)^2$, which is $(X_1 + X_2 + ...X_n)^2$. The former is the sum of n squares, the latter is the square of a single sum.

Problem 3.2

What does $\sum_{i=3}^{n-1} X_i$ mean?

WEIGHTS

Frequently we need to assess the reliability of some information. For example, we need to do some outdoor work tomorrow, but must be reasonably sure that it will not rain. We check the weather forecasts on two television programs, A and B. Station A predicts that it will rain tomorrow, whereas station B predicts that it will not rain until the day after tomorrow. From past experience, we know that station B is much more reliable at forecasting the weather than is station A, so we decide to do our outdoor work in the belief that it will not rain tomorrow. We give more *weight* to the information given by B than by A.

Consider another example. Some small airplanes have an upper limit to the mass of passengers plus cargo that they can carry, and so need to know the mass of the passengers exactly. There are two women and eight men to go on the plane. We do not know their individual masses, but do know that the mean mass of the women is 50 kg, and the mean mass of the men is 80 kg. If we averaged the two means to get 65 kg, we imply that the total mass for all 10 people would be 65 kg × 10 = 650 kg. This would be wrong, because the masses of the two women add up to 100 kg, the masses of the eight men add up to 640 kg, so the total mass is 740 kg and the mean mass of all 10 people is 740/10 = 74 kg. The error in the first calculation lies in not allowing for the different numbers of people in each group from which the means were calculated. To be correct, *weight* each mean by the number of observations from which it was derived. In general, if group 1 has mean $\overline{X_1}$ for N_1 observations, and group 2 has mean $\overline{X_2}$ with N_2 observations, then the *weighted mean* is:

$$\frac{N_1\overline{X_1} + N_2\overline{X_2}}{N_1 + N_2}.$$

Another form of weighting is required in regression statistics. Figure 3.4 shows data relating the value of a variable Y to the corresponding value of variable X.

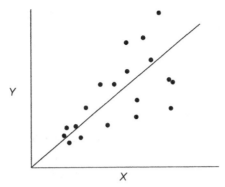

Figure 3.4 Scattergram or scatter plot.

The scatter plot and the line of best fit are shown. It is clear that Y is much more closely related to X when X is small than when X is big; we can put more weight (=reliability) on small values of X than on large values of X when trying to predict what the value of Y might be. It does not seem reasonable to give as much weight in the calculations to big values of X as to small values of X, and so some correction for the unreliability of the larger values of X is needed. One way of doing this would be to give more weight to smaller values of X, as discussed in Chapter 27.

STATISTICS BOOKS

There are many books on preliminary statistics available for biologists and physicians, all with advantages and disadvantages. Those that I have found to be most useful in describing and illustrating concepts are given below:

Altman, D.G., Gore S.M., 1982. Statistics in Practice. British Medical Association, London, pp. 100. (Selected notes, not a full text).

Altman, D.G., 1992. Practical Statistics for Medical Research. Chapman & Hall, London, pp. 611.

*Armitage, P., Berry G., Matthews, J.N.S., 2002. Statistical Methods in Medical Research, fourth ed. Blackwell Scientific Publications, Oxford, pp. 817.

Bland, M., 2000. An Introduction to Medical Statistics, third ed. Oxford University Press, Oxford, pp. 405.

Freedman, D., Pisani, R., Purves, R., 2007. Statistics, fourth ed. W. W. Norton & Co., New York, pp. 513 + appendix. (A very different way of explaining basic concepts that can be very useful.)

Glantz, S.A., 2011. Primer of Biostatistics, seventh ed. McGraw-Hill, New York, pp. 312.

*Glantz, S.A., Slinker, B.K., 2001. Primer of Applied Regression and Analysis of Variance. McGraw-Hill, Inc., New York, pp. 947.

Goldstein, A., 1964. Biostatistics, an Introductory Course. Macmillan Company, New York, pp. 272.

Ingelfinger, J.A., Mosteller, F., Thibodeau, L.A., Ware, J.H., 1994. Biostatistics in Clinical Medicine. McGraw-Hill, Inc., New York, pp. 418. (An excellent book that uses clinical problems to illuminate statistics rather than the other way around.)

Koopmans, L.H., 1987. Introduction to Contemporary Statistical Methods. Duxbury Press, Boston, pp. 683.

Pagano, M., Gauvreau, K., 2000. Principles of Biostatistics, second ed. Duxbury Press, Belmont, CA, pp. 524.

Sokal, R.R., Rohlf, F.J., 1995. Biometry. The Principles and Practice of Statistics in Biological Research. W.H. Freeman and Company, New York, pp. 887.

Zar, J.H., 2010. Biostatistical Analysis. Upper Saddle River, Prentice Hall, NJ, pp. 944.

The two books marked with asterisks are more rigorous and mathematical than the others, and the last two on the list are the most comprehensive, with a wealth of detailed examples. The books by Altman, Glantz, and Pagano and Gauvreau are the easiest to read, making learning of statistics (almost) painless!

I also highly recommend a series of free interactive statistics texts written by W. Douglas Stirling of Massey University in Australia, available from http://cast.massey.ac.nz/collection_public.html. These texts allow you to use sliders and other devices to change graphs in order to gain further understanding of statistical processes, and the experience is invaluable.

REFERENCES

Apgar, V., 1953. A proposal for a new method of evaluation of the newborn infant. Curr. Res. Anesth. Analg. 32, 260–267.

Baxter, A.L., Watcha, M.F., Baxter, W.V., et al., 2011. Development and validation of a pictorial nausea rating scale for children. Pediatrics 127, e1542–e1549.

Brody, A.S., Kosorok, M.R., Li, Z., et al., 2006. Reproducibility of a scoring system for computed tomography scanning in cystic fibrosis. J. Thorac. Imaging 21, 14–21.

Dwyer, P.S., 1951. Linear Computations. John Wiley & Sons, Inc.

Gardner, P.L., 1975. Scales and statistics. Rev. Educ. Res. 45, 43–57.

Labovitz, S., 1967. Some observations on measurement and statistics. Soc. Forces 46, 151–160.

Must, A., Willett, W.C., Dietz, W.H., 1993. Remote recall of childhood height, weight, and body build by elderly subjects. Am. J. Epidemiol. 138, 56–64.

Sanders, D.B., Li, Z., Brody, A.S., et al., 2011. Chest computed tomography scores of severity are associated with future lung disease progression in children with cystic fibrosis. Am. J. Respir. Crit. Care Med. 184, 816–821.

Shaper, A.G., Pocock, S.J., Phillips, A.N., et al., 1986. Identifying men at high risk of heart attacks: strategy for use in general practice. Br. Med. J. (Clin. Res. Ed.) 293, 474–479.

Stevens, S.S., 1946. On the theory of scales of measurement. Science 103, 677–680.

Stulbarg, M.S., Adams, L., 1994. Dyspnea. In: Murray, J.F., Nadel, J.A. (Eds.), Textbook of Respiratory Medicine. W.B. Saunders Company.

Uebersax, J., 2006. Likert Scales: Dispelling the Confusion (Online). http://john-uebersax.com/stat/agree.htm.

Velleman, P.F., Wilkinson, L., 1993. Nominal, ordinal, interval, and ratio typologies are misleading. Am. Stat. 47, 65–72.

Zar, J.H., 2010. Biostatistical Analysis. Prentice Hall.

CHAPTER 4

Exploratory Descriptive Analysis

Contents

For a list of all websites referred to in this chapter, as clickable links, see the book companion website: www.booksite.elsevier.com/9780128023877.

Biostatistics for Medical and Biomedical Practitioners
http://dx.doi.org/10.1016/B978-0-12-802387-7.00004-4

BASIC CONCEPTS

Counting

When counting items, a common technique is to put a vertical stroke opposite the group into which the item falls (Figure 4.1).

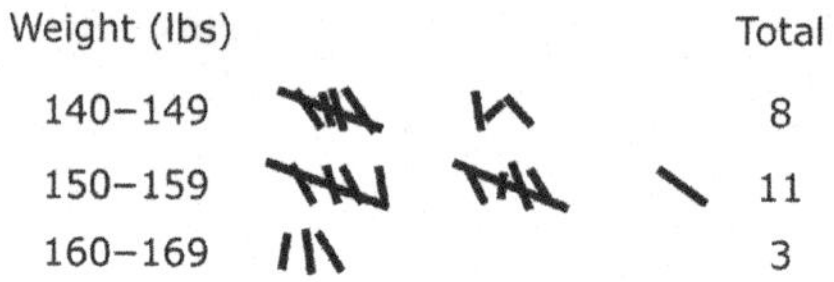

Weight (lbs)			Total
140–149	☰	☰	8
150–159	☰	☰	☰ 11
160–169	/I\		3

Figure 4.1 Tallying in fives.

After four vertical strokes, a diagonal line is added to make a cluster of five. After all the items are recorded, the totals for each subgroup are obtained. This method is prone to error. When counting rapidly and putting down the lines carelessly, it is easy to put a fifth vertical line on top of the fourth, and then the oblique line demarcates a group of six, not five. For this reason, John Tukey (1977) introduced a safer counting method (Figure 4.2).

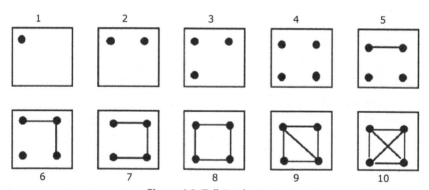

Figure 4.2 Tallying by tens.

A square is drawn. For the first four counts, one dot is placed in each corner of the square. For the next four counts, lines join pairs of dots. For the ninth count, a diagonal line joins two dots, and for the tenth count the other diagonal line is drawn. Thus each completed square registers 10 counts. Not only is it marginally easier to count in tens than in fives, but the separation of the points makes it less easy to mistake the number of counts.

Distribution

Fasting blood sugar concentrations in nondiabetic people varies from 80 to 130 mg/dl, so that the values are *distributed* over a range. This is true of all variables. One definition of a distribution is a set of values that a variable can assume, and how often each value occurs. Before analyzing a distribution, we need answers to certain questions:

How symmetrical is the distribution?

How variable are the data?

Are there some unusually small or big values?

Are there clumps of data, with big gaps between subsets of data?

Could the data have come from a normal (Gaussian) distribution?

The questions apply equally to relations among two or more variables.

A Sorting Experiment

There are three boxes, one red, one green, and one blue, and a crate with a mixture of red, green, and blue balls. A blindfolded assistant picks out balls one at a time from the crate and gives them to you. You put each ball into the bin with the same color as the ball. After 20 picks, there are 4 red balls, 11 green balls, and 5 blue balls. Therefore, the sample of 20 balls drawn from the population has been sorted or *distributed* into three groups or classes based on the color of the balls. The results—4 red, 11 green, and 5 blue balls—may therefore be called the distribution of the sample, and they makeup a frequency distribution. Sometimes the results are given as proportions rather than as absolute numbers; in the sample of 20 balls, 20% are red, 55% are green, and 25% are blue. Often, the sample size is called 1, and the proportions of 1 made up by each color (the relative frequency distribution) are determined; here they are 0.2, 0.55, and 0.25. These data are displayed in Figure 4.3, a bar graph designed to display nominal or ordinal data in which each bar represents a category or ordinal value and has a height proportional to the counts or relative frequencies.

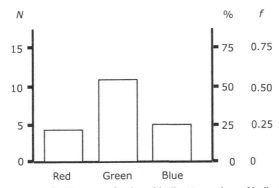

Figure 4.3 Discrete frequency distribution of colored balls. *N*, number of balls; %, percentage of each color; *f*, fraction or proportion of each color.

The classes make up a probability density distribution. The boxes into which the balls are put are often called *bins*, and may contain real or abstract entities; for example, one bin may contain odd numbers and another bin may contain even numbers.

Histograms and Frequency Polygons

The classes in the colored ball experiment are discrete categories, but they need not be. Consider sampling the weights of 2000 people from a larger population. Rather than list all 2000 weights, group them into a *grouped* frequency distribution: <50 kg, 50−100 kg, and 100−150 kg. Suppose that there were 400 people <50 kg, 1100 people between 50 and 100 kg, and 500 people between 100 and 150 kg. Then the bins represent the three weight groups or classes, and show a distribution of weights from that population. This graph resembles that for the distribution of colored balls, but with the difference that the columns touch each other because the range of weights represents continuous ratio numbers (Figure 4.4, upper panel). This figure is termed a histogram and the distribution is termed a frequency distribution or, when the areas are taken as proportions of 1, a probability density distribution. A histogram can be used also for interval numbers, but never for ordinal or nominal data.

With continuous distributions what is done about measurements that fall on a boundary, for example, 100 kg? One solution is to weigh with greater accuracy, so that a weight of 100.1 kg goes into the highest class, and one of 99.9 kg goes into the middle class. If that cannot be done, the convention is for one half to go into one class and one half into the adjacent class.

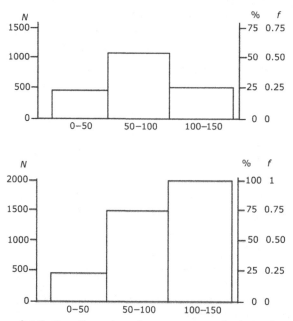

Figure 4.4 Continuous distribution. *N*, number of measurements; *f*, relative frequency or proportion.

It is possible to calculate a cumulative frequency or probability density distribution by adding successive results. Thus for the cumulative frequency distribution, there are 400 <50 kg, $400 + 1100 = 1500$ <100 kg, and $400 + 1100 + 500 = 2000$ <150 kg. For the cumulative probability density distribution, there are 0.20 <50 kg, $0.20 + 0.55 = 0.75$ <100 kg, and $0.20 + 0.55 + 0.25 = 1.00$ <150 kg (Figure 4.4, lower panel).

When grouping measurements into classes, such as those in the above figure, giving the beginning and ending values of the class makes it impossible to do further calculations. It is easier to define each class by a single number. To do this, take the midpoint of the range of values in each class, so that the class 0–50 becomes 25, the class 50–100 becomes 75, and so on. Assuming that the values are evenly distributed throughout the range in each class, then the average represents them all. This assumption is reasonable if there are large numbers of measurements in many classes and the distribution is not severely asymmetrical.

We can draw Figure 4.4 in another way. Take the midpoint of each column, and join these points up to get Figure 4.5.

This is a frequency polygon, and it gives the same information as in Figure 4.4. Cumulative distribution polygons are termed ogives. The frequency polygon may be easier to interpret than the histogram when several groups are being compared (Scott, 1985).

When drawing a histogram to show a grouped frequency distribution, the convention is to make the area under the column proportional to the frequency. If the base width (the class interval) is constant for all the columns, then the heights are proportional to the frequencies. (The probability of being in any one group is the area under the rectangle. Dividing the area by the class size, that is, the width of the base, gives

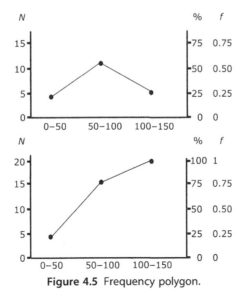

Figure 4.5 Frequency polygon.

the height; this height is termed the probability density. Therefore probability = probability density × class interval, just as mass = density × volume (Box et al., 1978)). In the example above, each group (or class) interval is 50 kg, but it could be 5, 8, 15 kg, or whatever is useful, as long as it is constant.

Histograms can be produced using online programs: www.wessa.net/rwasp_varia1. wasp, http://easycalculation.com/graphs/create-histogram.php.

Histograms can be misleading. A change in the class interval (bin size) or the origin of the figure can greatly alter the apparent distribution that is indicated by the outline of the columns. This is shown in Figure 4.6 of the same data formatted in three different ways.

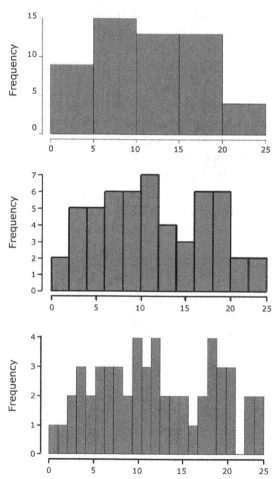

Figure 4.6 Three histograms drawn with the same data but different starting points and bin sizes. Because the starting points were different, some data were included in a lower rather than a higher class, with large changes in shape of the histogram.

Striking examples of these distortions are given by Scott (2010) who demonstrated that these distortions can be minimized by using an averaged shifted histogram; the method is available in some specialized programs. In principle, the method estimates an optimal bin width, then produces a number of histograms with different starting points, and averages them (Mohamed). The optimal bin width can be estimated from $3.5 \times$ standard deviation $\times n^{-1/3}$.

The online programs listed above allow the user to change the number of columns (bin width) and examine the result.

Sometimes two histograms can be placed back to back so that two distributions can be compared (Figure 4.7).

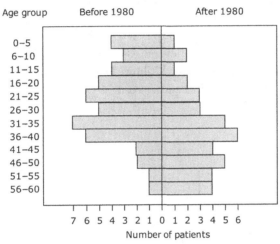

Figure 4.7 Hypothetical data of age distribution in two time periods at a clinic. The shift to older subjects after 1980 is well shown. This type of histogram can be drawn with the online program http://www.wessa.net/rwasp_backtobackhist.wasp#output.

Problem 4.1
The following data are the smiling times in seconds of an 8-week-old baby observed over several hours (Dean and Illowsky, 2012).

10.4	19.6	18.8	13.9	17.8	16.8	21.6	17.9	12.5	11.1	4.9
12.8	14.8	22.8	20.0	15.9	16.3	13.4	17.1	14.5	19.0	22.8
1.3	0.7	8.9	11.9	10.9	7.3	5.9	3.7	17.9	19.2	9.8
5.8	6.9	2.6	5.8	21.7	11.8	3.4	2.1	4.5	6.3	10.7
8.9	9.4	9.4	7.6	10.0	3.3	6.7	7.8	11.6	13.8	18.6

Smiling times (seconds).
Create histograms using different bin widths or numbers of bins.

Shapes of Distributions
Transformations

Certain shapes are common. One shape, discussed in Chapter 6, is the symmetrical bell-shaped, normal, or Gaussian curve that has great theoretical significance. More often, the distribution is asymmetrical and pulled (or skewed) to the right or left by a few unusually high or low values respectively. Sometimes the skewing is so marked that the greatest frequency is observed at one end of the scale (Figure 4.8, upper panel) With marked skewing, some type of transformation such as a logarithmic transformation may make the distribution less skewed (Figure 4.8, lower panel).

Other transformations may be used, for example, square roots, reciprocals, and power functions. All of these can be done on almost any handheld calculator, but usually for only one number at a time. On-line programs for logarithmic transformation to any base can be performed online at http://www.1728.org/logrithm.htm and www.calculators.org/math/algebra.php. They can also be performed for batches of numbers at http://vassarstats.net/index.html (see Utilities, Data Transformation) that allows other transformations such as reciprocal or square root.

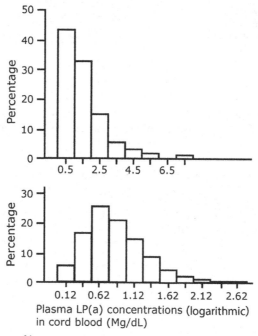

Figure 4.8 Distribution of lipoprotein(a) in men in Singapore. *(Adapted from Low et al. (1996).)*

Stem-and-Leaf Diagrams

Listing all the data in a set preserves the details but makes it difficult to picture the distribution. Consider the data set out as hypothetical consecutive measurements in Table 4.1.

Table 4.1 Consecutive measurements

1.65	**0.93**	1.30	1.40	1.30	1.12
2.05	1.05	1.25	1.25	1.17	1.19
1.80	1.20	1.11	1.29	0.95	1.66
1.10	1.17	1.26	1.39	0.95	1.18
1.12	1.45	1.14	1.20	1.20	1.35
1.10	1.28	1.12	1.16	1.25	1.16
1.12	1.25	1.86	1.16	1.40	1.17
1.23	1.32	1.85	1.50	1.18	1.53
1.20	1.50	1.30	1.32	1.50	

The smallest and the largest measurements are displayed in bold type. It is difficult to envision the form of this distribution by inspecting the data.

The next maneuver is to arrange the data in order from smallest to biggest value (Table 4.2).

Table 4.2 Ordered measurements

0.93	0.95	0.95	1.05	1.10	1.10
1.11	1.12	1.12	1.12	1.12	1.14
1.16	1.16	1.16	1.17	1.17	1.17
1.18	1.18	1.19	1.20	1.20	1.20
1.20	1.23	1.25	1.25	1.25	1.25
1.25	1.26	1.29	1.30	1.30	1.30
1.32	1.32	1.35	1.39	1.40	1.40
1.45	1.50	1.50	1.50	1.53	1.65
1.66	1.80	1.85	1.86	**2.05**	

This gives a better idea of the distribution, but it is still not easy to perceive its shape. Therefore go one further stage, and produce a histogram (Figure 4.9).

The distribution is skewed to the right; the peak is at a low X value, and there is a long tail at higher X values. However, some detail is lost. In the 17 measurements between 1.1 and 1.2, we do not know if the measurements are evenly distributed throughout the

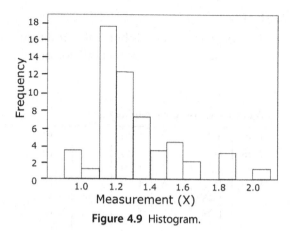

Figure 4.9 Histogram.

interval, or are clustered at the low or the high end. If we characterize this column by the average of 1.15, we have lost detail.

There is, however, a way to have the best of both worlds, and that is to create a stem-and-leaf diagram, as shown in Figure 4.10.

To apply this principle to the data set of Table 4.2, examine the data that ranges from 0.93 to 2.05. Arbitrarily call the numbers up to the first decimal place the stems, and the

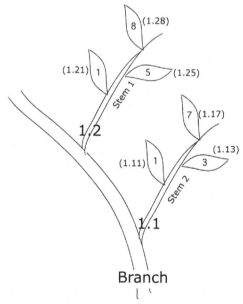

Figure 4.10 This branch has two stems, each with three leaves. The lower stem is labeled 1.1, and the three leaves attached to it have the numbers 1, 3, and 7. These leaves represent the full numbers shown in parentheses beside them. Thus the leaf with 3 on stem 1.1 represents 1.13.

second decimal place numbers the leaves to get 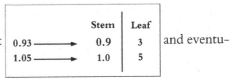 and eventu-

ally produce a display as shown below in Table 4.3:

Table 4.3 Stem-and-leaf diagram

Sum	Stem	Leaf
3	0.9	3, 5, 5
1	1.0	5
17	1.1	0, 0, 1,2, 2, 2, 2, 4, 6, 6, 6, 7, 7, 7, 8, 8, 9
12	1.2	0, 0, 0, 0, 3, 5, 5, 5, 5, 5, 6, **9**
7	1.3	0, 0, 0, 2, 2, 5, 9
3	1.4	0, 0, 5
4	1.5	0, 0, 0, 3
2	1.6	5, **6**
0	1.7	
3	1.8	0, 5, 6
0	1.9	
1	2.0	5

Take the first stem of 0.9. The leaves represent the second decimal place. Thus stem 0.9, leaf 3 represents 0.93; stem 1.2, leaf 9 represents 1.29; stem 1.6, leaf 6 represents 1.66; and so on. The column labeled "Sum" indicates the number of measurements on each stem.

In this diagram all the information has been preserved, and it is possible to see the shape of the distribution. In fact, the outline of the numbers is like a histogram on its side, as shown in Figure 4.11.

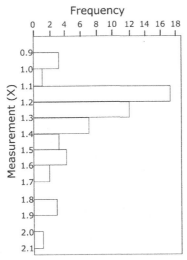

Figure 4.11 Histogram of Figure 4.9 rotated 90°.

In the stem-and-leaf diagram, the order of the measurements has been preserved, and each measurement is separated from the next by a comma for reasons discussed below.

Stem-and-leaf diagrams can be created online at http://www.calculatorsoup.com/calculators/statistics/stemleaf.php, www.wessa.net/rwasp_stem.wasp, and at http://easycalculation.com/statistics/stem-leaf-plot.php.

A common question is how many classes (bins) to have in a histogram or stems in a stem-and-leaf diagram. One class or stem for each number does not give enough data to represent the shape of the distribution accurately (Table 4.4):

On the other hand, dividing the data into too few classes also is inefficient (Table 4.5).

There is some guidance to an effective number of classes (Emerson and Hoaglin, 1983). The upper limit of the number of lines for a stem-and-leaf display or the number of intervals for a histogram can be estimated from either $10\log_{10}n$ or $4\sqrt[3]{n}$, where n is the number of observations; these rules work well for n between 20 and 300. Therefore if n is 53, as in the example above, the recommended upper number of classes is 17 by the first rule and 15 by the second rule.

Table 4.4 Too many classes

Sum	Stem	Sum	Stem
1	0.93	1	1.29
2	0.95	3	1.30
1	1.05	2	1.32
2	1.10	1	1.35
1	1.11	1	1.39
4	1.12	2	1.40
1	1.14	1	1.45
3	1.16	3	1.50
3	1.17	1	1.53
2	1.18	1	1.65
1	1.19	1	1.66
4	1.20	1	1.80
1	1.23	1	1.85
5	1.25	1	1.86
1	1.26	1	2.05

Table 4.5 Too few classes

Sum	Class/stem	
3	<1.0	0.93, 0.95, 0.95
49	1.0–1.99	1.05, 1.10, 1.10, 1.11, 1.12, 1.12, 1.12, 1.12, 1.14, 1.16, 1.16, 1.16, 1.17, 1.17, 1.17, 1.18, 1.18, 1.19, 1.20, 1.20, 1.20, 1.20, 1.23, 1.25, 1.25, 1.25, 1.25, 1.25, 1.26, 1.29, 1.30, 1.30, 1.30, 1.32, 1.32, 1.35, 1.39, 1.40, 1.40, 1.45, 1.50, 1.50, 1.50, 1.53, 1.65, 1.66, 1.80, 1.85, 1.86
1	≥2.0	2.05

The next question is what stems to use. As the diagram is intended for ease of use, select a convenient stem such as 0.1. This matches the "natural" classification that gave 12 intervals, close enough to the recommended upper limit. There were 30 intervals in Table 4.4 and 3 intervals in Table 4.5; both of these are of little use.

Sometimes the stem-and-leaf classification must be adapted when the natural numbering system by ones or tens does not give a reasonable number of classes. Consider, for example, having 32 measurements with stems of 1, 2, 3, and 4. Using these stems, one to a line, will not give a good idea of the distribution, because there will be too many leaves on any one line, as in Table 4.6A. To get more lines, divide each line into two, each with the same stem, but with leaves 0—4 going on the first line and leaves 5—9 going on the second line, and distinguish the two sets by putting a star (*) next to the stem on the first line and a dot (•) next to the stem on the second line. As an example, consider the hypothetical data in Table 4.6B.

Table 4.6A Artificial data set

1.1, 1.1, 1.3, 1.5, 1.7, 1.7, 1.7, 1.9
2.0, 2.0, 2.2, 2.2, 2.2, 2.5, 2.6, 2.6, 2.8, 2.8, 2.9
3.1, 3.1, 3.3, 3.3, 3.5, 3.6, 3.9
4.2, 4.2, 4.6, 4.7, 4.7, 4.9

Table 4.6B Doubled stem display

Sum	Stem	Leaf
3	1*	1, 1, 3,
5	1•	5, 7, 7, 7, 9
5	2*	0, 0, 2, 2, 2
6	2•	5, 6, 6, 8, 8, 9
4	3*	1, 1, 3, 3
3	3•	5, 6, 9
2	4*	2, 2
4	4•	6, 7, 7, 9

Splitting the stems has converted 4 lines into 8, and this might be enough.

If there still are not enough lines, split each unit into 5 lines per stem by taking two subunits at a time, as follows:

Stem * represents 0,1.

T represents 2, 3 (both terms begin with T).

F represents 4, 5 (both terms begin with F).

S represents 6, 7 (both terms begin with S).

• represents 8, 9.

Consider the data set of 73 values shown in Table 4.7A:

The upper number of lines needed is $\sim 10\log_{10}73 = 18.6$, or 19 to the nearest whole number. Select 0.2 as a useful unit for the stem, and get the modified stem-and-leaf diagram shown in Table 4.7B.

Table 4.7A Hypothetical data set

0.1, 0.1, 0.1, 0.1, 0.1, 0.1, 0.2, 0.2, 0.2, 0.2,
0.3, 0.3, 0.3, 0.3, 0.3, 0.3, 0.3, 0.3, 0.4, 0.4,
0.4, 0.4, 0.4, 0.4, 0.4, 0.4, 0.5, 0.5, 0.5, 0.5,
0.6, 0.6, 0.6, 0.6, 0.7, 0.7, 0.7, 0.8, 0.8, 0.8,
0.9, 0.9, 0.9, 0.9, 0.9, 0.9, 0.9, 0.9, 0.9, 1.0,
1.0, 1.0, 1.0, 1.0, 1.1, 1.1, 1.1, 1.2, 1.3, 1.3,
1.3, 1.3, 1.4, 1.4, 1.5, 1.5, 1.5, 1.6, 1.6, 1.7,
    1.8, 2.0, 2.5

Table 4.7B Five lines per unit stem

Sum	Stem	Leaf
6	0*	1, 1, 1, 1, 1, 1
12	T	2, 2, 2, 2, 3, 3, 3, 3, 3, 3, 3, 3,
12	F	4, 4, 4, 4, 4, 4, 4, 4, 5, 5, 5, 5
7	S	6, 6, 6, 6, 7, 7, 7
12	0•	8, 8, 8, 9, 9, 9, 9, 9, 9, 9, 9, 9
8	1*	0, 0, 0, 0, 0, 1, 1, 1
6	T	2, 3, 3, 3, 3, 3,
5	F	4, 4, 5, 5, 5
3	S	6, 6, 7
1	1•	8
1	2*	0
0	T	
1	F	5
	S	
	2•	

The choice of the number of stems to use in a stem-and-leaf diagram depends on the number of data values and the range to be covered, but should always be guided by convenience. There is no single way to do a stem-and-leaf diagram, and more than one diagram can provide information.

If the distribution of measurements is badly skewed so that, for example, the highest number is a million times as big as the smallest number, there would be enormous gaps between the stems. It would be more useful to take logarithms of the numbers, so that a range from 1 to 1,000,000 becomes a range from 0 to 6 (Mosteller et al., 1983). On the other hand, if the distribution has most of its measurements within a given range, and a few measurements very far from the rest, it would be inappropriate to use logarithms, and unwieldy to use a conventional stem-and-leaf diagram with dozens of empty stems. Under these circumstances, use a conventional stem-and-leaf diagram without the extreme observations, and put these extremes as numbers at the bottom of the graph.

Stem-and-leaf diagrams are impractical with huge databases, and should be replaced by histograms or box plots.

Problem 4.2

Use the data set from Problem 4.1 to create stem-and-leaf diagrams. Compare these with the histograms that you created from the same data set.

Measures of Central Tendency (Location)

In any set of data, it is useful to have a single number to summarize the data set. For example, a value of 7 lbs characterizes the weights of healthy, full-term newborn human infants. Some infants are lighter and some are heavier than 7 lbs, but the value of 7 lbs conveys information to someone who did not know what the characteristic weight of a term human infant is. As with other summarizing numbers, what we gain by compactness we lose by ignoring details. Summary numbers require prior attention to the whole distribution.

Arithmetic Mean

What properties should this summarizing number have? It should be near the middle of the distribution, with many measurements below it and many above it. The measure most often used is the arithmetic mean of the data set. To calculate this number, add up all the measurements and divide the total by the number of measurements to give the *arithmetic* mean. In formal terms,

$$\overline{X} = \frac{\sum\limits_{i=1}^{n} X_i}{N},$$

where $\overline{X}$ is the mean, X_i stands for any member of the data set, and N is the number of observations. There are also harmonic means (seldom used) and geometric means that have specific uses to be discussed below. Unless one of these is specified, the term "mean" implies the arithmetic mean.

As an example, take the data set in Table 4.8:

Table 4.8 Data set for mean

2, 4, 6, 8, 10, 12

The mean is $(2 + 4 + 6 + 8 + 10 + 12)/6 = 7$. This is indeed in the middle of this data set. If these were the weights in pounds of newborn human infants, each infant has a weight that differs from the weight typical of the group (7 lbs) by some individual deviation from that mean, be it negative or positive.

If the values are plotted on a line (Figure 4.12), the mean is the point at which the line with its points balances, just as a seesaw balances with equal weights on the two ends.

The sum of deviations from the mean is always zero.

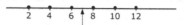

Figure 4.12 Line diagram of points and their mean. There is no requirement that the mean be an observed value.

What other properties should the measure of central tendency have? Instead of considering deviations of individual measurements from the mean, important statistical methodology has revolved around measuring the square of these deviations. One criterion is termed the *Principle of Least Squares*,[1] which states that the sum of the squared deviations of the individual measurements from some number will be the least if that number is the mean. This is exemplified in Table 4.9.

Table 4.9 Principle of least squares

1	2	3
X_i	$(X_i - 7)^2$	$(X_i - 5)^2$
2	25	9
4	9	1
6	1	1
8	1	9
10	9	25
12	25	49
$\sum_{n=1}^{\infty} X_i = 42$	$\sum_{i=1}^{N} (X_i - \overline{X})^2 = 70$	$\sum_{n=1}^{\infty} (X_i - X_k)^2 = 94$
$\overline{X}_i = 7$		Let $X_k = 5$

The data set in column 1 has a mean of 7, and the sum of squared deviations from the mean of 7 is 70 (Column 2). Deviations from another value, such as 5 (shown in column 3) give a larger sum of squared deviations: 94. This will be true for any value that is not the mean.

Formal proofs of the least squares principle are given in the Appendix.

Thus the mean is easily calculated, and conforms to the Principle of Least Squares. However, the mean has one major disadvantage—it is not a resistant statistic. Statisticians use the term *resistant* to mean that the statistic used is not much affected by unusually large or unusually small observations. Unfortunately, the mean is definitely not a resistant statistic. Consider what happens to the mean by changing the last value in the data set from 12 to 20 lbs (Table 4.10). (According to the Guinness Book of World Records, the biggest human infant to survive weighed 22.5 lbs at birth.)

---

[1] Most statistical tests evaluate a difference between two or more groups by relating that difference to a measure of variability. The less the variability, the more likely is it that a given difference is not due to chance selection. Therefore, all other things being equal, any test that minimizes variability makes it easier to make statistical inferences. That is why the Principle of Least Squares is used so often in Statistics.

Table 4.10 Data set for altered mean

2, 4, 6, 8, 10, 20

Then the mean becomes 8.33 lbs, not 7 lbs. A change in a single value has increased the mean that no longer serves to provide a reasonable indication of where the middle of the distribution is. A line diagram (Figure 4.13) shows how the balance point has shifted from the center.

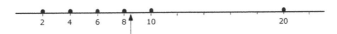

Figure 4.13 Line diagram for points and their mean.

Median and Quantiles

To deal with the lack of resistance, use another measure of central tendency that is resistant, the *median*. This is the value of the measurement that splits the data set into two equal halves, so that 50% of the values are *below or equal to* the median and 50% are *above or equal* to it. In Table 4.11 the median is 7 because two of the measurements are below it and two are above it.

Table 4.11 Data set for median

2, 4, **7**, 8, 10

Change the last X value from 10 to 50 and, applying this definition of the median, the median remains 7; the median has been resistant to the huge change in the final measurement. The median has to be used in place of the mean with censored observations, and can also be used for ordinal values.

The definition includes the words "equal to." This is to meet the contingency shown in Table 4.12.

Table 4.12 Data set for altered median

2, 4, 6, 6, 6, 8, 10

Here the median is 6, because half of the measurements (2, 4, 6) are below or equal to 6, and half of the measurements (6, 8, 10) are equal to or >6.

What happens to the median with an even number of measurements in the data set? In Table 4.10 above no one of these numbers satisfies the definition. The median cannot be 6, because then two measurements will be below it and three above, nor can it be 8 that produces three smaller and two larger measurements. By convention, the median is taken as the average of the two middle measurements, that is, $(6 + 8)/2 = 7$. Even though this is not one of the measurements, it satisfies the requirement that half of the six measurements are below it and half are above it. Values such as 6.3 and 7.8 also fit the definition of the median, but by convention are not so designated. Care is needed in using the values for the median, because if the two numbers used to form the median are far apart, their average might not be a good estimate of the population median.

To make the definition more general, the median is the value of the $(N + 1)/2$nd measurement. If N is 5, then the median is the value of the $(5 + 1)/2 = 3$rd measurement, and if N is 6 then the median is the value of the $(6 + 1)/2 = 3.5$th measurement. Distinguish between measurements and ranks. If the measured values are ordered from smallest to largest, the smallest measurement is rank 1. The next smallest is rank 2, and so on. The rank gives the position of the measured value in the array. Thus the median is the measured value corresponding to the $(N + 1)/2$nd rank.

In a grouped frequency distribution the median is calculated in a different way. Table 4.13 shows heights of adult males grouped in class intervals of 2 in.

Table 4.13 Grouped frequency distribution

Heights (in)	f	Cf
55	3	3
57	8	11
59	53	64
61	215	279
63	346	625
65	278	903
67	119	1022
69	23	1045
71 and over	7	1052
Total	1052	

f, frequency; Cf, cumulative frequency.

The median is the value of the observation with rank $(1052 + 1)/2 = 526.5$th rank. By examining the cumulative frequencies, this rank lies within the group labeled with a height of 63 in. The class interval is 2 in, so that this group contains 346 people with heights from 62 to 64 in. The cumulative rank frequency up to that group is 279, so another $526.5 - 279 = 247.5$ ranks are required to reach the median value. If the measurements of height in this group are distributed evenly throughout the group, then the median value occurs 247.5/346th ($=0.715$) of the way through that group from its beginning at 62 in. This value is therefore $62 + 0.715 \times 2 = 63.43$ in.

The median is one of the ways in which a set of ordered data can be divided. In general, dividing an ordered set into equal parts produces *quantiles* (or fractiles). Division of the set into 4, 5, 8, 10, or 100 equal parts, produces quartiles, quintiles, octiles, deciles, and percentiles (or centiles) respectively. $X_{(i)}$, the ith percentile, is estimated as $100\left(\frac{i-0.5}{N}\right)$. By rearrangement, this becomes

$$i\text{th percentile} = \frac{iN}{100} + 0.5$$

Therefore, to find the rank of the 50th percentile (the median) calculate

$$\text{Median (50th percentile)} = \frac{50N}{100} + 0.5 = \frac{N}{2} + 0.5 = \frac{N+1}{2}$$

Each half of the data set (one below and one above the median) can be further sub-divided into halves in the same way, so that the total data set can be divided into *quartiles*. The lower quartile (the 25th percentile) is the value of the measurement such that 25% of the measurements are below or equal to it and 75% are above or equal to it. The upper quartile (75th percentile) is the value of the measurement such that 75% of the measurements are below or equal to it and 25% are above or equal to it (Table 4.14).

Table 4.14 Data set for quartiles

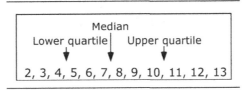

The lower quartile is 4.5, because 3 of the 12 measurements are below or equal to it. The median is 7.5, because half the measurements are below (or equal) to it, and half are above it. The upper quartile is 10.5, because 9 of the 12 measurements are below or equal to it, and 3 are equal to or above it.

Similarly, the 10th centile is the value of a measurement in an ordered array that has 10% of the measurements smaller and 90% of the measurements larger than it is. The value may be one of the measurements in the array, or may be interpolated.

The calculation of any quantile in a grouped frequency distribution is similar to that for calculating the median.

The stem-and-leaf diagram is particularly well suited to defining the median and the quartiles (Table 4.15, based on Table 4.4).

Table 4.15 Complete stem and leaf diagram

Cumulative total	Sum	Stem	Leaf	
53	3	3	0.9	3, 5, 5
50	4	1	1.0	5
49	21	17	1.1	0, 0, 1, 2, 2, 2, **2**, 4, 6, **6**, 6, 7, 7, 7, 8, 8, 9
32	33	12	1.2	0, 0, 0, 0, 3, **5**, 5, 5, 5, 5, 6, 9
20	40	7	1.3	0, 0, 0, 2, 2, 5, *9*
13	43	3	1.4	0, 0, 5
10	47	4	1.5	0, 0, 0, 3
6	49	2	1.6	5, 6
4	49	0	1.7	
4	52	3	1.8	0, 5, 6
1	52	0	1.9	
1	53	1	2.0	5

Bold and italic numbers described in text.

Two new left-hand columns are added. The second column next to the column labeled sum is the cumulative total starting from the first line. Thus there are 3 measurements in the first line, 4 in the first two lines, 21 in the first three lines, and so on. The left-hand column is the cumulative sum starting from the last line and working up. The median is the value of the (53 + 1)/2nd measurement, that is, the 27th measurement. The number 27 is the *rank* of the measurement. Because the first three lines cumulate to 21 measurements, to reach the 27th rank add another 6 to get to the number 5 in the fourth line. This is indicated in bold and enlarged type. If the 27th measurement is the median, then the lower fourth (or quartile) is the (27 + 1)/2nd = 14th measurement from the lowest one, namely the 6 on the third line indicated by the enlarged number in bold italics. Similarly, the upper fourth or quartile is the 14th measurement back from the highest measurement, or the 9 on the fifth line; it is the 9 and not the 0 on that line, because we are counting backward from higher to lower numbers. These quartiles can be calculated online at http://easycalculation.com/statistics/inter-quartile-range.php and http://www.alcula.com/calculators/statistics/dispersion/.

Mode

Another measure of central tendency is the measurement with the highest frequency—the *mode*. In a symmetrical distribution, the mean, median, and mode are identical. In an asymmetrical distribution, the median is toward the long-tailed side of the mode, and the mean is further away from the mode, being pulled toward one end by the larger measurements in the longer tail (Figure 4.14).

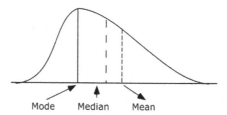

Mode   Median   Mean

Figure 4.14 Mode, median, and mean.

The Geometric Mean

For some data the arithmetic mean should be replaced by the geometric mean. Figure 4.15 is a graph relating pH to hydrogen ion concentration.

The pH scale is linear, but because pH is the negative logarithm of hydrogen ion concentration, the line relating the two sets of values is curved. For a mean pH of 5.5, the corresponding hydrogen ion concentration is $10^{-3.16}$, but averaging the hydrogen ion concentrations gives a mean hydrogen ion concentration of $10^{-3.90}$, an incorrect value. To avoid this error, calculate the geometric mean. By definition, this is

$$\text{Geometric Mean} = \sqrt[n]{\prod_{i=1}^{n} X_i}.$$

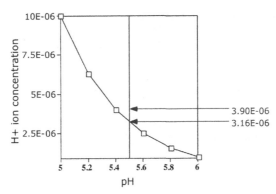

Figure 4.15 Hydrogen ion concentration versus pH.

That is, the *n*th root of the products of all the *n* values. In the pH example, Geometric Mean $= \sqrt[6]{10 \times 6.31 \times 3.98 \times 2.51 \times 1.58 \times 1}$, where the values are the arguments with exponents 10^{-6}. This comes out to be 3.16, a correct value as shown from Figure 4.15. Another way of calculating the geometric mean is

$$\text{Geometric Mean} = \text{antilog}\frac{1}{n}\sum_{i=1}^{n}\log X_i.$$

Therefore, taking the (negative) logarithms of the hydrogen ion concentrations produces the pH values; adding up these and dividing by 6 provides the true mean value. The geometric mean of raw data is the same as the arithmetic mean of the logarithm of the data.

Geometric means are used when data fit a logarithmic or an exponential function. One common application is when titers are measured with serial dilutions, for example, $1, \frac{1}{2}, \frac{1}{4}, \frac{1}{8}...$ (Chapter 31). They can also be used with badly skewed distributions, which can often be made reasonably symmetrical by taking the logarithms of the measurements.

Geometric means may be calculated online at http://www.calculator.tutorvista.com/math/444/geometric-mean, http://www.easycalculation.com/statistics/geometric-mean.php, and http://www.calculatewhat.com/math/average/geometric-mean-calculator/.

Harmonic Mean
This is the reciprocal of the arithmetic mean of reciprocals of individual values, and is written as $H = \frac{1}{N}\sum X_1^{-1}$, or alternatively as

$$\frac{1}{H} = \frac{\frac{1}{X_1} + \frac{1}{X_2} + ... \frac{1}{X_N}}{N} \quad \text{so that} \quad H = \frac{N}{\frac{1}{X_1} + \frac{1}{X_2} + ... \frac{1}{X_N}}.$$

It is used occasionally when rates of change are involved. Thus if a leukocyte moves 3 cm/min for 5 min, 5 cm/min for 5 min, and 7 cm/min for 5 min, its average speed of movement is not 5 cm/min but rather 4.44 cm/min (Table 4.16).

Table 4.16 Calculation of harmonic mean

$$\frac{1}{H} = \frac{\frac{1}{3} + \frac{1}{5} + \frac{1}{7}}{3} = 0.2254, \text{ and } H = 4.44 \text{ cm/min}.$$

To see why it is wrong to average the speeds, examine Table 4.17.

Table 4.17 Derivation of harmonic mean

Speed (cm/min)	Distance (cm)	Time (min)
3	5	1.67
5	5	1.00
7	5	0.71
	15	3.38
	Average = 15/3.38	
	= 4.44 cm/min	

As another example, if a car travels half the distance from A to B at 30 mph and the other half at 60 mph, what is the average speed? It cannot be 45 mph because the car has spent twice as much time in the first half than the second half. The harmonic mean by the above formula is 40 mph and is a weighted mean.

In harmonic means every value is weighted by its reciprocal, and these means are used in certain multiple comparison calculations (Chapter 24).

This mean can be calculated online at http://easycalculation.com/statistics/harmonic-mean.php and http://www.ncalculators.com/statistics/harmonic-mean-calculator.htm.

Measures of Variability

Figure 4.16 shows two distributions with the same mean but different variability. The terms variability, dispersion, and spread are often used interchangeably, but the term spread that has at least 25 different definitions should not be used.

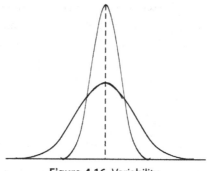

Figure 4.16 Variability.

Early in the history of statistics in biology attention was concentrated on averages, and it was Francis Galton who emphasized the importance of variation. In his book "Natural Inheritance" (Galton, 1889) he wrote: "It is difficult to understand why statisticians commonly limit their inquiries to Averages and do not revel in more comprehensive views. Their souls seem as dull to the charm of variety as that of the native of one of our flat English counties, whose retrospect of Switzerland was that, if its mountains could be thrown into its lakes, two nuisances would be got rid of at once. An Average is but a solitary fact, whereas if a single other fact be added to it, an entire Normal Scheme, which nearly corresponds to the observed one, starts potentially into existence."

Range

The simplest measure of variability is the *range*, the difference between the highest and the lowest measurements. For the data in Table 4.15, the range is $2.05 - 0.93 = 1.12$. However, although the range is simple to calculate, it is not a resistant number. One unusually large or small value at either end of the distribution greatly alters the range, even if the variability of the remaining measurements does not change.

Standard Deviation

Another approach to summarizing the variability is to take the deviations of each measurement from the mean, and average them:

$$\frac{\sum \left[X_i - \overline{X} \right]}{N}.$$

Unfortunately this is useless, because

$$\sum \frac{X_i - \overline{X}}{N} = \sum \frac{X_i}{N} - \sum \frac{\overline{X}}{N}.$$

But $\sum \frac{X_i}{N} = \overline{X}$, and $\sum \frac{\overline{X}}{N} = \frac{N\overline{X}}{N} = \overline{X}$, because $\overline{X}$ is a constant for this data set.

Therefore $\frac{\sum [X_i - \overline{X}]}{N} = \overline{X} - \overline{X} = 0$, and this is always true.

It is possible to avoid this problem by summing the deviations without regard to sign, and average them to give a mean absolute deviation. This is used with robust statistics (see below).

Another way of removing negative signs is to square the deviations. Calculate each deviation, square it, add up all the squared deviations, and divide by the number of deviations to get an average squared deviation that also gives a measure of variability known as the *variance* or *mean square*. However, the result gives squared units that may have no physical meaning. What possible meaning, for example, could square pounds have? Therefore, the estimate of variability and restoration of the original units is completed by taking the square root to give the *standard deviation*:

$$\text{Variance} = \frac{\sum (X_i - \overline{X})^2}{N}, \text{ and standard deviation} = \sqrt{\frac{\sum (X_i - \overline{X})^2}{N}}.$$

In a population, the standard deviation is σ, and the variance is σ^2. In a sample, the corresponding symbols are s and s^2.

As an example, consider Table 4.18.

Table 4.18 Calculation of standard deviation (1)

X_i	$X_i - \overline{X}$	$(X_i - \overline{X})^2$
2	$2 - 6 = -4$	16
4	$4 - 6 = -2$	4
6	$6 - 6 = 0$	0
8	$8 - 6 = 2$	4
10	$10 - 6 = 4$	16
$\sum X_i = 30$	$\sum (X_i - \overline{X}) = 0$	$\sum (X_i - \overline{X})^2 = 40$
$\overline{X} = 30/5 = 6$		

Variance $= 40/5 = 8$, standard deviation $= \sqrt{8} = 2.83$.

Mean and standard deviation can be calculated online at http://easycalculation.com/statistics/standard-deviation.php, http://www.alcula.com/calculators/statistics/dispersion/, http://www.calculator.net/standard-deviation-calculator.html, and http://vassarstats.net/ (see Miscellaneous, Basic Sample Stats).

The standard deviation has three problems.

1. It is not a resistant statistic. Change one value in Table 4.18, for example, 10−50, and the standard deviation changes drastically (Table 4.19).

Table 4.19 Calculation of standard deviation (2)

X_i	$X_i - \overline{X}$	$(X_i - \overline{X})^2$
2	$2 - 14 = -12$	144
4	$4 - 14 = -10$	100
6	$6 - 14 = -8$	64
8	$8 - 14 = -6$	36
50	$50 - 14 = 36$	1296
$\sum X_i = 70$	$\sum (X_i - \overline{X}) = 0$	$\sum (X_i - \overline{X})^2 = 1640$
$\overline{X} = 70/5 = 14$		

Variance $= 1640/5 = 328$, standard deviation $= \sqrt{328} = 18.11$.

The calculations of the mean and population standard deviation are correct, but no longer give good estimates of the center of the distribution or the average variability.

2. For the standard deviation of a whole population, dividing by N is correct. Usually, though, we determine the standard deviation of a sample. Statisticians refer to unbiased statistics, by which they mean that in the long run with more and more samples the statistic approaches the population parameter. If the long-run value of the statistic does not approach the population parameter, they refer to a biased statistic. Dividing the sum of the squared deviations from the mean by N to get variance of a sample and then taking the square root to get standard deviation provides a biased statistic. Intuitively a sample will usually not have the biggest and smallest measurements of the population, and is likely to have a little less variability than would the whole population. Furthermore, because in general the sample and population means will not be the same, the average deviations will be smaller about the sample mean than the population mean. To correct for this, divide the sum of squared deviations from the mean by some value less than N to compensate for this difference.

What we divide by depends on the *degrees of freedom*. Consider the following problem. I give you a number, say 110, and ask you to find three numbers that add up to 110. Then you can select any number as the first one, any number as the second one, but now the third number is fixed because when added to the other two it has to come to 110. Therefore, although there are three numbers to find, you have only two degrees of freedom of choice. Thus, $N = 3$ leads to $N - 1 = 2$ df. Dividing the sum of squares of the deviations from the mean by the degrees of freedom yields an unbiased estimate of the standard deviation. In the above example, because there is one data set (or, to put it another way, one mean or one total sum of all the measurements), the degrees of freedom are $N - 1$. Therefore the sample variance is $1640/4 = 410$, and the sample standard deviation is $\sqrt{410} = 20.25$, a little bigger than that calculated above. Another way of thinking about this is that when calculating N deviations from the mean, there are only $N - 1$ independent observations because all the deviations sum to zero, so that any one deviation can be determined by the remaining deviations. Consider the second column in Table 4.19. The sum of the first four deviations is -36, which but for the sign is the same as the fifth deviation. Therefore the fifth deviation is not an independent measurement. Thus the sum of squared deviations from the mean is the sum of one dependent and four independent deviations from the mean, so that it is more appropriate to take an average by dividing by 4 rather than by 5.

The degrees of freedom are not always $N - 1$. In general, they are $N - k$, where k is the number of sample means that are being investigated. Thus in the relationship between height and weight, each data set contributes one mean value, and so the total degrees of freedom are $N - 2$.

3. Calculating accuracy. In the example used above, with a small set of simple whole numbers, it is easy to calculate the sum of squares of deviations from the mean.

It would not be as easy, however, with 169 measurements, each to two decimal places, the mean also having two decimal places after rounding off. Then each subtraction risks an arithmetic error. Furthermore, because the mean might not be an exact number, every subtraction results in a small error (due to rounding off) that is exaggerated by squaring it. For these reasons, we need a calculation that avoids the mean, minimizes errors, and is quicker to perform. Such a method is found by considering the following identity.

$$\sum (X_i - \overline{X})^2 = \sum \left(X_i^2 - 2X_i\overline{X} + \overline{X^2} \right) = \sum X_i^2 - 2 \sum X_i\overline{X} + \sum \overline{X^2}.$$

Substitute $\frac{\sum X_i}{N}$ for $\overline{X}$. Then the expression becomes

$$\sum X_i^2 - 2 \sum X_i\frac{\sum X_i}{N} + \sum \left(\frac{\sum X_i}{N} \right)^2 = \sum X_i^2 - \frac{2(\sum X_i)^2}{N} + \frac{N(\sum X_i)^2}{N^2},$$

and collecting like terms gives

$$\sum (X_i - \overline{X})^2 = \sum X_i^2 - \frac{(\sum X_i)^2}{N}.$$

This is an identity that holds no matter what X_i and N may be. By using it, we have avoided using the mean. The first part of the equation, $\sum_{n=1}^{\infty} X_i^2$ tells us to square each of the X values and then add up all the squares. The second part tells us to subtract what we get by squaring the sum of the X values, and dividing that squared sum, a single number, by N. This method is accurate and time saving. You still have to divide by the degrees of freedom to get the variance. That step is not included in the identity.

The mean and standard deviation are often listed as $\overline{X}\pm s$; for example, 6 ± 1.5. Although there is no confusion about this format, it is strictly speaking incorrect, because a standard deviation can never be negative. It makes more sense to write $\overline{X}(s)$ or $\overline{X}(sd)$, and mention in the text that this is the format being used. Many books and journals are now turning to the latter format.

Interquartile Distance

If the standard deviation is not a resistant statistic, what can replace it? Because the extremes of the distribution are more likely to be unrepresentative of the distribution than the central values, it is useful to replace the standard deviation by a number based on the middle 50% of the measurements, namely, the distance between the lower and the upper quartiles—the *interquartile distance* (IQD). The IQD is not affected by alterations in the outermost 25% of measurements in each tail of the distribution, and represents well the variability of the bulk of the measurements. In a statement attributed to the statistician Charles Winsor (1895–1951) by Tukey "all distributions are normal in the middle."

Thus in Table 4.15, the IQD is $1.39 - 1.16 = 0.23$. The IQD also replaces the standard deviation when some values at one or both ends of the scale are censored (indeterminate) if, for example, the lowest values were listed as "<0.5 ng/ml," or the upper values were listed as ">200 kg."

IQDs can be determined online at http://www.alcula.com/calculators/statistics/dispersion/, http://easycalculation.com/statistics/inter-quartile-range.php, http://www.easycalculation.com/statistics/inter-quartile-range.php, and http://www.miniwebtool.com/interquartile-range-calculator/.

There are rough relationships among the range, standard deviation, and IQD if the distribution is approximately normal. The IQD is theoretically 1.349 times the standard deviation (Chapter 6). The ratio of the IQD to 1.349 is termed the pseudostandard deviation or PSD (Hamilton, 1990).

There is a relationship between range and standard deviation that depends on sample size. Dividing range by factor d from Figure 4.17 approximates the standard deviation.

This relationship is a check to see if the calculated standard deviation is approximately correct, and it allows an investigator to estimate the standard deviation for use in power analysis (see later) by using range data obtained in previous investigations. If the

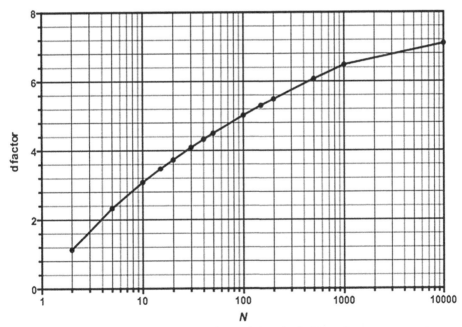

Figure 4.17 Using sample size *N* to obtain a factor d that divided into the range approximates the standard deviation. Based on Table 4. A-18 in Mosteller and Rourke (1973). These are the same as the Hartley constants used for control charts.

distribution is not normal, these divisors overestimate standard deviation, especially for sample sizes >100 (Browne, 2001).

Coefficient of Variation

The *coefficient of variation* is a dimensionless unit used for comparing variabilities. If three mice had weights 48, 50, and 52 g, their mean weight is 50 g and their standard deviation is 2 g. If three dogs had weights 48, 50, and 52 kg, their mean weight is 50 kg, and their standard deviation is 2 kg. The question "Which group has the greater variability?" is meaningless, because small light objects cannot vary as much as large heavy objects; a standard deviation of 2 kg is much more variable than a standard deviation of 2 g. But change the question and ask "Which of the two groups shows more variability relative to its average size?" Then a variability of 2 g out of 50 g is the same variability as 2 kg out of 50 kg. Therefore, to determine relative variability, compute the coefficient of variation as

$$\frac{\text{Standard deviation}}{\text{Mean}},$$

and convert this to a percentage by multiplying by 100. This is a useful measurement. Workers in any field soon get familiar with the coefficients of variation that they have to deal with, and if some group has more than the expected variability it needs further examination. The coefficient is also useful when determining sample sizes.

Tables and Graphs

One object of any publication is to present data clearly. In the publication there will be references to numerical data, and figures to illustrate the numbers. Although there are many ways of presenting numbers and figures, there are some do's and don'ts that often are neglected.

Tables

It is acceptable to include a few numbers in the text, for example, the mean and standard deviation of group A versus group B. If, however, the means and standard deviations of many groups are to be compared, writing them out in two or three lines makes it difficult for the reader to grasp the information without having to read the numbers several times. It is better to place the data in a simple table. The more the data, the more the need for a table. Compare two ways of presenting the following data:

1. "In group A the mean and standard deviation were 17.3 and 2.7 mg, in group B they were 19.2 and 5.1 mg, in group C they were 16.0 and 1.1 mg, in group D they were 20.2 and 3.9 mg, and in group E they were 18.8 and 4.4 mg respectively."
2. Table 4.20.

Table 4.20 Summary of data

Group (age)	Mean (mg)	Standard deviation (mg)
A (0–10)	17.3	2.7
B (11–20)	19.2	5.1
C (21–30)	16.0	1.1
D (31–40)	20.2	3.9
E (41–50)	18.8	4.4

There are many possibilities for such a table. Separation of subgroups by judicious use of space, for example, sets off groups A, B, and C from groups D and E. The publisher determines the exact display to reflect the style of the book or journal, but the way in which the authors set out the data can affect its readability. Where possible, use subheadings, and try to give the groups meaningful descriptions, such as 10–19 years, 20–29 years, and so on, rather than force the reader to find out what A, B, C, D, and E are by looking at the legend.

Larger data sets with more possible comparisons demand a table (Table 4.21).

Table 4.21 Section of table

	Diet alone $N = 30$ (%)	Statins $N = 30$ (%)	Placebo $N = 30$ (%)
Age (years)	62.1	64.6	59.3
Gender (male)	24 (80%)	27 (90%)	25 (83%)
High blood pressure	20 (67%)	24 (80%)	22 (74%)
Diabetes mellitus	0 (0%)	3 (10%)	2 (7%)
Smoking history	17 (57%)	14 (47%)	17 (57%)

Examples of effective tabulation are well shown by Ehrenberg (1975) and by Tufte (1997).

Figures and Graphs

The books by Tufte (1983, 1990, 1997) are masterpieces to show good and bad graphic examples, covering almost all fields of human endeavor. It was Tukey (1977) and Cleveland (1984, 1985) who initiated studies of what makes an effective scientific graph. Other excellent references include chapters by Spence and Lewandowsky (1990), Meyer (1975), and Good and Hardin (2009) and articles by Wainer (1984, 1992), Fienberg (1979), and Moses (1987). In general, graphs are used to display data in a more convenient form than the data from which they are derived, and often serve to emphasize and clarify relationships that would be difficult to obtain by examining the original data.

Many people (Cleveland, 1985; Tufte, 1983; van Belle, 2002) do not regard pie charts as useful in scientific articles. It is difficult to compare the areas of individual sectors without referring to the associated numbers that might just as well have been given without the chart. Almost always, data in a pie chart can be plotted on a linear scale, and it is easier to compare distances on a linear scale than angles in a pie chart. The pie chart has low data density, and may not show subsets readily. Historically, however, one of the most influential charts ever published was the coxcomb type of pie chart developed by Florence Nightingale (Joyce, 2008).

Plain bar graphs, although ubiquitous, are of doubtful value. As usually used in scientific publications they seldom give more information than could be put more accurately in a simple table. Box plots (see below) are more useful, and incorporate a mass of data in a small area. Stacked bar graphs are also not favored. Although they do show more information, with an attempt to display relationships, it is often difficult to extract details that could usually be better conveyed by line graphs (van Belle, 2002). Three-dimensional bar graphs are poor because it is often difficult to tell the exact height of the bars from the scale, and because the eye is diverted from the essential data by the third dimension. The vertical scale in any of these plots should indicate units clearly, and as a rule the lower limit should be zero. If it is not, for example, to emphasize small differences, there should be a break in the axis to indicate that the axis does not start at zero (Figure 4.18).

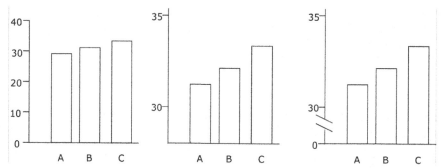

Figure 4.18 Left: full scale. Middle: expanded vertical scale, no zero. Right: expanded vertical scale with zero and break indicator.

The middle diagram can be misleading because it gives the appearance of large differences without warning the reader that zero has been suppressed and the scale changed. This warning is given in the right diagram. Other problems with bar charts are discussed by Reese (2007).

XY plots are very useful for showing relationships, and Cleveland (1985) gives a wealth of information about graph construction: the use of symbols, tick marks, color, fonts, spacing of numbers on the scale, and so on. The general advice is to use a rectangular graph with the width about 50–70% greater than the height, but this may need to be changed so that emphasis is correctly placed on the *X* variate or the *Y* variate. Just as in Figure 4.18, zero should be included or else its absence specified. Examples of how changes in the aspect ratio (vertical axis length/horizontal axis length) influence the reader's impression of the data are shown by Cook and Weisberg (1994).

A plot of two sets of data against time allows useful comparisons. Figure 4.19 shows the age distribution of population in two countries—one poor and one rich.

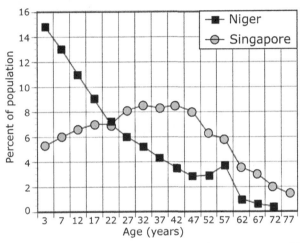

Figure 4.19 In the poor country (Niger) the bulk of the population are young (due to a high fertility rate), so that the burden of supporting the population falls on a small number of elders. In the rich country (Singapore) the age distribution is more even so that many people from 22 to 57 years who are wage earners contribute to the welfare of the country.

Multivariable graphs can be made to display five variables as a moving bubble graph (Figure 4.20). Two numeric variables are on the *X* and *Y* axes, bubble size represents another variable such as population, the bubbles are colored in various ways to represent different groups (e.g., countries and continents), and then a time variable can be added to give a moving representation of changes in the variables with time.

These bubble graphs, developed by Hans Rosling's GapMinder Foundation, are now available at Google under the name of TrendAnalyzer. This is described online at http://www.gapminder.org/world that shows where the software can be obtained. An outstanding talk by Rosling in which these moving bubble graphs are used can be seen at http://www.ted.com/talks/hans_rosling_shows_the_best_stats_you_ve_ever_seen.html.

Figure 4.20 Bubble graph to show relationship between infant mortality rate and fertility rate or income per capita and major world countries. The size of the bubble represents the relative population of a country; the two largest are China and India. The continents are color coded, and it is possible to label countries. The figure shows a static graph at a given time, but sequential figures to show the effects of time can be incorporated.

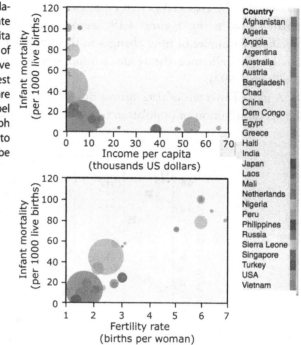

Box Plots

The data in Table 4.15 can also be set out in the form of a diagram known as a box plot, attributed to Tukey (1977) (Figure 4.21).

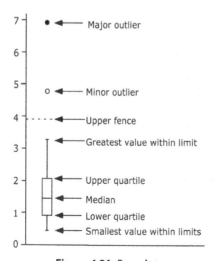

Figure 4.21 Box plot.

Figure 4.21 shows some of the summarizing numbers discussed above. The rectangular box (hence the name, box plot) has for ends the values corresponding to the upper and lower quartiles. The line across the middle of the box is the median. (Some programs also put in a symbol to indicate the mean.) Vertical lines ending in small crossbars are termed "whiskers," and they end with the largest and smallest measurements in the data set, providing that these values fall within normal limits. These limits are determined by taking the IQD (upper minus lower quartile) and multiplying this difference by 1.5 to obtain what is termed a "step." In this example, the IQD is $2.1 - 0.9 = 1.2$, and $1.2 \times 1.5 = 1.8$, so that the step is 1.8. The normal limits extend from the upper quartile plus the step (to give the upper "fence") down to the lower quartile minus the step (to give the lower fence); that is, from $2.1 + 1.8 = 3.9$ to $0.9 - 1.8$; because in this example the measurements cannot be less than zero, the lower fence is zero. The dashed line in Figure 4.21 shows the upper fence; it does not normally appear in box plots. Any value above the upper fence or below the lower fence is an outlier, and each of these is put into the plot; minor outliers lie between one and two steps beyond the quartiles, and major outliers are greater than two steps from the quartiles. The reason for selecting these values for minor and major outliers is that, with a normal distribution, only 0.35% of the observations will lie beyond the first fences (i.e., one step beyond the quartiles), and only 0.00012% will lie beyond the outer fences (i.e., more than two steps) beyond the quartiles.

Box plots and their associated numbers can be produced online at http://www.alcula.com/calculators/statistics/box-plot/, http://illuminations.nctm.org/activitydetail.aspx?id=77, and https://www.easycalculation.com/statistics/box-plot-grapher.php.

Box plots are useful for summarizing a lot of data in one figure, especially when two or more groups are compared. These plots are easier to read and label displayed horizontally rather than vertically (Reese, 2005). Some programs make the box width proportional to the size of the group or its square root. Others place a notch around the median such that if two notches do not overlap the medians are significantly different. Single box plots may be produced online at http://www.alcula.com/calculators/statistics/box-plot/, http://easycalculation.com/statistics/box-plot-grapher.php.

Comparison box plots can be produced online at http://www.wessa.net/rwasp_notchedbox1.wasp#output, which produces notched plots.

Box plots may be misleading if the data come from a bimodal distribution in which two clumps of data at high and low values are separated by a region with sparse intermediate data.

ADVANCED AND ALTERNATIVE CONCEPTS

Classical versus Robust Methods

General Aspects

The mean and standard deviation are the best-known and most often calculated summary statistics. Summary, however, is not their main purpose, and a box plot is a more extensive and useful summary of the needed information. The value of the mean and standard deviation is that they allow an estimation of the population values from which they were derived. However, they should not be used mechanically, but thought must be given to when they are or are not useful. If the sample is approximately normal (Gaussian, symmetrical—Chapter 6) then the mean and standard deviation lead to excellent estimates of those values in the population. Unfortunately many sample distributions are ill-behaved—asymmetrical, or having one or more unusually small or large measurements—and when this happens both the mean and standard deviation can be misleading. When this occurs, alternative measures of location and dispersion are needed.

The first line of defense is to use the median and the IQD as measures of location and dispersion. The median, however, has both advantages and disadvantages. Imagine an array of X values with a given median value of X_{med}. We could change all the values above the median 10-fold, and leave X_{med} unaltered. Clearly, to use the median alone as an indicator of the distribution would be inefficient. Further, consider the following array of numbers:

10, 20, 30, 70, 80, 90.

Conventionally, the median of this array is 50, but this might be an inefficient estimator of the location of the distribution, because any value from 31 to 69 could be the median, so that our judgment of the true population location could be greatly in error. The two examples given are bizarre, but they can occur and illustrate the need to consider the distribution before deciding how to use and analyze it.

A number of other measures have been used to improve our ability to deal with ill-behaved distributions.

Trimean

The trimean is defined as

$$TRI = \frac{q_l + 2\text{Med} + q_u}{4},$$

where q_l and q_u are the lower and upper quartiles, and Med is the median. These values correspond to the central rectangle in the box plot, and use its three most important numbers to give a single statistic. The trimean is a resistant value that adds information beyond that provided by the median, and gets rid of any difficulties resulting from using a single value.

The trimean can be calculated using http://www.had2know.com/academics/descriptive-statistics-calculator.html.

Trimming and Winsorization

Although the mean and standard deviation are not resistant statistics, they may be made more useful if some of the extreme outlying observations were modified. An example that most people are familiar with occurs in diving competitions. After each dive a panel of judges gives a score from 1 to 10. The highest and lowest scores are discarded, and the remaining scores are averaged. The idea is that extreme scores suggest poor adherence to the standards and should not play any further part. The method also guards in part against bias for or against a particular diver.

In statistics this technique is known as trimming (Koopmans, 1987; Mosteller and Rourke, 1973). A fraction of the data between 5% and 25% is discarded from *each* end of the distribution, and the trimmed mean is calculated. For $x\%$ trimming, calculate $x\%$ of N, the number in the array, and truncate it. Thus if N is 14, 10% gives 1.4 and this is converted into 1 number dropped at each end. For 20% trimming, then 20% of 14 is 2.8, truncate this to 2, and drop off 2 numbers at each end. For example, the data set might be 3, 4, 5, 8, 9, 10, 11, 12, 18, 23, 39. The underlined measurements are regarded as extremes (for more on outlying values, see Chapter 9), and we can discard 1 or 2 values at each end, for trimming percentages of $2/11 = 18\%$ and $4/11 = 36\%$ (Table 4.22).

Table 4.22 Effect of trimming

Statistic	All data	1-Trim	2-Trim
Mean	12.91	11.11	10.43
Upper quartile	18	15	12
Median	10	10	10
Lower quartile	5	6.5	8
IQD	13	8.5	4
Standard deviation	10.49	6.06	4.04
s_W		6.95	5.19
s_T		7.77	6.70
Trimean	10.75		

IQD, interquartile distance; s_W, Winsorized standard deviation; s_T, trimmed standard deviation.

Trimming differs from Winsorization which replaces the discarded numbers by the nearest retained values; for example, after trimming 2 values at each end the new array becomes 5, 5, 5, 8, 9, 10, 11, 12, 18, 18, 18. Now calculate the variance of this Winsorized sample, s_W^2, and calculate the trimmed standard deviation s_T as

$$s_T = \sqrt{\frac{(N-1)s_W^2}{N_T - 1}} \text{ or } s_W \sqrt{\frac{N-1}{N_T - 1}}$$

where N is the original sample size and N_T is the size of the trimmed sample.

As shown in Table 4.22, trimming brings the mean closer to the median, the biggest incremental change coming from trimming one value at each end of the array. Trimming has also markedly reduced the standard deviation. Thus trimming has given a sample mean and standard deviation that are more representative of the central part of the distribution. The choice between trimming 1 or 2 numbers from each end of the array depends in part on how discrepant the extreme numbers are, and is subjective. Either trimming, however, is better than the mean of the original data set. The trimean is closer to the trimmed means than the original mean. A variant of the trimmed mean is the *mid-mean*, the arithmetic mean of the middle 50% of the values; this is equivalent to a 25% trimming fraction. The free online program http://www.wessa.net/ct.wasp makes it easy to calculate these various measures of central tendency.

Two issues about trimming must be considered. One is that trimming does not work with very asymmetrical distributions. The second is that trimming comes dangerously near to selecting data. It might be more advantageous to ask why some data points are so far from the main mass of data and whether they are really part of that distribution, or even to retain the data but transform the whole data set into a more normal distribution. If trimming is done, the procedure should be accompanied by an adequate justification, and the original data should be given. Finally, think back to the original example of rating divers. Would the average mark be much affected if both the upper and lower values were retained?

Order Statistics
Median Absolute Deviation

A large set of estimators based on order statistics have been used. One of the most useful is based on the median absolute deviation (MAD)—the median of the absolute deviations of each value X_i from the median. It is the median of $|X_1 - \text{median}|$, $|X_2 - \text{median}|, \ldots |X_N - \text{median}|$ (Be careful. Some authors use MAD for mean absolute deviation that has different properties.).

Example: Data set is 2,4,6,8,50. The median is 6. Therefore, the absolute deviations are $|2 - 6| = 4$; $|4 - 6| = 2$; $|6 - 6| = 0$; $|8 - 6| = 2$; and $|50 - 6| = 44$. These deviations in order are 0, 2, 2, 4, 44 so that their median is 2. This is the value of MAD. It may be calculated online using http://www.miniwebtool.com/median-absolute-deviation-calculator/.

There are close relationships between MAD, standard deviation, and the IQD if the distribution is normal:

$$\text{MAD} \approx 0.6745\sigma$$
$$\sigma \approx 1.4826 \text{ MAD}$$
$$\text{IQD} \approx 2 \times \text{MAD}$$

Therefore if the distribution is normal, any value beyond $9 \times \text{MAD}$ is more than 6 standard deviations from the mean, and a factor of $6 \times \text{MAD}$ excludes residuals above 4 standard deviations from the mean (Mosteller and Tukey, 1977).

Many statisticians, including Tukey, recommend that when calculating location and dispersion, the mean and standard deviation should be accompanied by one of these resistant statistics. Large differences between the classical and robust statistics should lead the investigator to reconsider whether using classical statistics is the best way of proceeding. As an example, the height of American men in one study of 1052 adults had a mean of 62.49 in, a standard deviation of 2.435 in, and the interval of 57.72–67.26 in included 95% of the sample population. To determine how this compared with the heights of adult Chinese males in China, we could go to China, and by some random selection technique, perhaps based on the Census, select a sample of 30 adult males. Now in Shanghai there is a basketball player named Yao Ming (who played in the US) who is 90-in tall. This is an extremely rare height, but the fact remains that in a random selection, Yao Ming has as much chance of being selected as any other adult male. If our sample then included 29 people with heights of 57–68 in (and the same mean and standard deviation as found in the US) and one man of 90 in, and if we went ahead and calculated means and standard deviations by classical methods, the mean height would be about 63.41 in and the standard deviation about 5.17 in. These results imply that adult Chinese males are about 1-in taller with much greater variability in height than we observed in the US. Any robust method dealing with the one abnormal observation will give us better estimates.

Propagation of Errors

Sometimes we wish to know the standard deviation of the product when two numbers are added, subtracted, multiplied, or divided. If there are two or more sets of measurements made on the same population with the same methods, we can pool the sets and recalculate the mean and standard deviation from the larger pooled set. On the other hand, the measurements might have been made on samples from the same population but with different degrees of precision. The problem then becomes how to combine the data sets with due attention to the differences in variability. There are different approaches to this problem (Barford, 1967; Bevington and Robinson, 1992; Taylor, 1982) but all give similar results.

Combining Experiments (Addition)

Chapter 3 discussed weighting the data, in one example to take account of different numbers in the two samples by taking a weighted average, and in the other to account for differences in variance by dividing by a measure of variability. When combining two or more groups, both of these functions are involved by using the standard error (Chapter 7). It bears the same relationship to the variability of sample means drawn from the same population as standard deviation does to the variability of measurements in a sample, and is estimated by $s/\sqrt{N}$, the square of which is s^2/N.

This statistic when used to weight means includes both the number of items and their variability in one.

To add two sets of independent measurements of the same variable, n measurements of X_A and m measurements of X_B, the precision of each data set being different as assessed by their respective standard errors, then their sum Z will have mean estimated by (Barford, 1967).

$$Z = \frac{1}{se_A^{-2} + se_B^{-2}} \left(\frac{\overline{X_A}}{se_A^2} + \frac{\overline{X_B}}{se_B^2} \right)$$

and their combined standard error is

$$se_{AB}^2 = \frac{se_A^2 se_B^2}{se_A^2 + se_B^2}.$$

This formula can be extended to more than two data sets.

As an example, consider three sets of measurements of serum cholesterol from the same population with mean (and standard error) in milligram/liter being 141(10), 151(12), 161(41).

It would be unreasonable just to average them because we do not know the number in each group, and because the variability of the third group is so much higher than that of the other two groups. Plain averaging gives mean and standard deviation of 151(21).

On the other hand, their weighted averages are $\left(\frac{1}{10^{-2}+12^{-2}+41^{-2}} \right) \left(\frac{141}{10^2} + \frac{151}{12^2} + \frac{161}{41^2} \right) =$ $\frac{1.41+1.05+0.096}{\frac{1}{0.01+0.0069+0.00059}} \frac{2.56}{0.0175} = 146.29$ for the mean and 57.01 for the standard deviation.

The weighted average gives less prominence to the highest group with the largest standard error, as shown by the smallest terms derived from this third set of data.

Simple Multiplication (Scale Factor)

Consider a scale factor "a," for example, the distances between cities (X_i) on a map in which 1 in represents 10 miles. Then the measured and actual distances are related by $X_1 = az_1$, $X_2 = az_2$, etc., where z is the actual measurement.

Then $\overline{X_i} = \dfrac{X_1 + X_2 + \ldots X_n}{N} = \dfrac{az_1 + az_2 \ldots az_n}{N} = \dfrac{a(z_1 + z_2 \ldots z_n)}{N} = a\overline{z_i}$

By similar reasoning, that the population variance is $a^2 \sigma^2$, and the sample variance is $a^2 s^2$.

Multiplying Means (Taylor, 1982)

Assume that quantity Q is the product of two sets of simultaneous measurements of flow rate (F) and time (T), both measured with some error.

Define the fractional error se_f of flow as $\frac{se_F}{\overline{F}}$ and the fractional error se_t of time as $\frac{se_T}{\overline{T}}$. Then the variability of flow and time can be written as

$$\overline{F}\left(1 \pm \frac{se_F}{\overline{F}}\right) \ \text{and} \ \overline{T}\left(1 \pm \frac{se_T}{\overline{T}}\right) \ \text{respectively.}$$

Therefore the variability of $\overline{Q} = \overline{FT}$ is

$$\overline{FT}\left(1 \pm \frac{se_T}{\overline{T}}\right)\left(1 \pm \frac{se_F}{\overline{F}}\right) = \overline{FT}\left[1 \pm \left(\frac{se_T}{\overline{T}} + \frac{se_F}{\overline{F}} + \frac{se_T se_F}{\overline{TF}}\right)\right].$$

However, because the product of two small fractions is smaller still, neglect the final term to get

$$\overline{Q} = \overline{F}\,\overline{T}\left(1 \pm \frac{se_t}{\overline{T}}\right)\left(1 \pm \frac{se_f}{\overline{F}}\right) = \overline{F}\,\overline{T}\left(1 \pm \left[\frac{se_t}{\overline{T}} + \frac{se_f}{\overline{F}}\right]\right)$$

Example: Let mean flow in l/min be 3 with standard error 0.3, and let mean time in minutes be 5 with standard error 0.1, then the mean quantity in liters is estimated as $3 \times 5 = 15$, with standard error 0.12.

Dividing Means (Taylor, 1982)

By similar reasoning the best estimate of a value obtained by dividing two means $\overline{A}$ and $\overline{B}$ is

$$\overline{Q} = \frac{\overline{A}}{\overline{B}}\left[1 \pm \left(\frac{se_A}{\overline{A}} + \frac{se_B}{\overline{B}}\right)\right].$$

Three Useful Applications of the Variance

1. If each value of X_i is multiplied by a constant k, the variance of kX is
$$\text{Var } kX = \frac{\sum (kX_i - \overline{kX})^2}{N-1} = \frac{\sum [k(X_i - \overline{X})]^2}{N-1} = \frac{k^2 \sum [(X_i - \overline{X})]^2}{N-1}.$$

2. If there are two groups X_i and Y_i with equal sample sizes, what is the variance of $X_i + Y_i$?
By definition, variance is $\frac{\sum [(X_i - \overline{X})]^2}{N-1}$. Therefore the variance of $X_i + Y_i$ is

$$\text{Var } (X_i + Y_i) = \frac{\sum \left[(X_i + Y_i) - (\overline{X + Y})\right]^2}{N-1}.$$

This can be rearranged to give

$$\text{Var } (X_i + Y_i) = \frac{\sum \left[(X_i + \overline{X}) - (Y_i + \overline{Y})\right]^2}{N - 1}$$

$$= \frac{\sum \left[(X_i + \overline{X})^2 - 2(X_i - \overline{X})(Y_i - \overline{Y}) + (Y_i - \overline{Y})^2\right]}{N - 1}$$

$$= \frac{\sum (X_i + \overline{X})^2}{N - 1} - \frac{2(X_i - \overline{X})(Y_i - \overline{Y})}{N - 1} + \frac{\sum (Y_i - \overline{Y})^2}{N - 1}$$

However, if the two sets of data are independent, the term $\frac{2(X_i - \overline{X})(Y_i - \overline{Y})}{N-1}$ equals zero, involving as it does the sum of deviations from the mean. Therefore, the variance of the sum of two variables is the sum of the variances of each variable. This is true if there are more variables than two.

3. By similar argument, the variance of the difference between two variables is also the sum of the variances of each variable.

APPENDIX

Least Squares Principle

1. We wish to show that the expression $\sum [X_i - k]^2$ is a minimum when k is the mean. Take this expression and add to and subtract from it the mean, $\overline{X}$

$$\sum (X_i - k)^2 = \sum (X_i - k + \overline{X} - \overline{X})^2 = \sum \left[(X_i - \overline{X}) + (\overline{X} - k)\right]^2$$

$$= \sum \left[(X_i - \overline{X})^2 + 2(X_i - \overline{X})(\overline{X} - k) + (\overline{X} - k)^2\right]$$

$$= \sum (X_i - \overline{X})^2 + 2 \sum (X_i - \overline{X})(\overline{X} - k) + \sum (\overline{X} - k)^2$$

Now the sum of deviations from the mean, $\sum_{n=1}^{\infty} [X_i - \overline{X}]$, always equals zero (see above). Therefore,

$$\sum (X_i - k)^2 = \sum (X_i - \overline{X})^2 + \sum (\overline{X} - k)^2.$$

Therefore, the expression $\sum (X_i - k)^2$ will be a minimum when the last term in the right-hand side equals zero, that is, when $\overline{X} = k$.

REFERENCES

Barford, N.C., 1967. Experimental Measurements: Precision, Error and Truth. Addison-Wesley Publishing Co.
Bevington, P.R., Robinson, D.K., 1992. Data Reduction and Error Analysis for the Physical Sciences. McGraw-Hill, Inc.
Box, G.E.P., Hunter, W.G., Hunter, J.S., 1978. Statistics for Experimenters. An Introduction to Design, Data Analysis, and Model Building. John Wiley & Sons.

Browne, R.H., 2001. Using the sample range as a basis for calculating sample size in power calculations. Am. Stat. 55, 293−298.

Cleveland, W.S., 1984. Graphs in scientific publications. Am. Stat. 38, 261.

Cleveland, W.S., 1985. The Elements of Graphing Data. Wadsworth.

Cook, R.D., Weisberg, S., 1994. An Introduction to Regression Graphics. John Wiley & Sons.

Dean, S., Illowsky, B., May 25, 2012. Continuous Random Variables: The Uniform Distribution [Online]. Connexions. Available: http://cnx.org/contents/130e078d-6f27-4bde-8648-a67eae701805@17.

Ehrenberg, A.S.C., 1975. Data Reduction. Analysing and Interpreting Statistical Data. John Wiley and Sons.

Emerson, J.D., Hoaglin, D.C., 1983. Stem-and-Leaf displays. In: Hoaglin, D.C., Mosteller, F., Tukey, J.W. (Eds.), Understanding Robust and Exploratory Data Analysis. John Wiley & Sons, Inc.

Fienberg, S.E., 1979. Graphical methods in statistics. Am. Stat. 33, 165−179.

Galton, F.I., 1889. Natural Inheritance. Macmillan and Company.

Good, P.I., Hardin, J.W., 2009. Common Errors in Statistics (And How to Avoid Them). John Wiley & Sons.

Hamilton, L.C., 1990. Modern Data Analysis. A First Course in Applied Statistics. Brooks/Cole Publishing Co.

Joyce, H., 2008. Florence Nightingale: a lady with more than a lamp. Significance 5, 181−182.

Koopmans, L.H., 1987. Introduction to Contemporary Statistical Methods. Duxbury Press.

Low, P.S., Heng, C.K., Saha, N., et al., 1996. Racial variation of cord plasma lipoprotein(a) levels in relation to coronary risk level: a study in three ethnic groups in Singapore. Pediatr. Res. 40, 718−722.

Meyer, S.L., 1975. Data Analysis for Scientists and Engineers. John Wiley and Sons, Inc.

Mohamed, N.S. Introduction to Probability Density Estimation [Online]. Available: http://urrg.eng.usm.my/index.php?option=com_content&view=article&id=79:introduction-to-probability-density-estimation&catid=31:articles&Itemid=70.

Moses, L.E., 1987. Graphical methods in statistical analysis. Annu. Rev. Public Health 8, 309−353.

Mosteller, F., Rourke, R.E.K., 1973. Sturdy Statistics. Nonparametrics and Order Statistics. Addison-Wesley Publishing Company.

Mosteller, F., Tukey, J.W., 1977. Data Analysis and Regression. A Second Course in Statistics. Addison-Wesley.

Mosteller, F., Fienberg, S.E., Rourke, R.E.K., 1983. Beginning Statistics with Data Analysis. Addison-Wesley Publishing Company.

Reese, R.A., 2005. Boxplots. Significance 2, 134−135.

Reese, R.A., 2007. Bah! Bar charts. Significance 4, 41−44.

Scott, D.W., 1985. Frequency polygons: theory and application. J. Am. Stat. Assoc. 80, 348−354.

Scott, D.W., 2010. Averaged shifted histogram. WIREs Comp. Stat. 2, 160−164.

Spence, I., Lewandowsky, S., 1990. Graphical perception. In: Fox, J., Long, J.S. (Eds.), Modern Methods of Data Analysis. Sage Publications, Inc.

Taylor, J.R., 1982. An Introduction to Error Analysis. University Science Books.

Tufte, E.R., 1983. The Visual Display of Quantitative Information. Graphics Press.

Tufte, E.R., 1990. Envisioning Information. Graphics Press.

Tufte, E.R., 1997. Visual Explanation. Graphics Press.

Tukey, J.W., 1977. Exploratory Data Analysis. Addison-Wesley Publishing Co.

van Belle, G., 2002. Statistical Rules of Thumb. Wiley Interscience.

Wainer, H., 1984. How to display data badly. Am. Stat. 38, 137−147.

Wainer, H., 1992. Understanding graphs and tables. Educ. Res. 21, 14−23.

CHAPTER 5

Basic Probability

Contents

INTRODUCTION

We use concepts of probability almost every day. The weatherman states that there is a 40% probability of rain. We talk about the likelihood that interest rates will go down still further, and wonder about the chances of our favorite team winning the next game. People ask about the chances that changing our diet will prevent cancer of the colon.

TYPES OF PROBABILITY

Probability is often divided into two forms—objective and subjective. Objective probability is subdivided into classical or a priori probability and empirical or a posteriori probability. A priori probability is based on theory. For example, when tossing a coin we do not know whether the result will be a head or a tail, but believe that in the long run both heads and tails will occur half the time; this can be expressed symbolically as,

$$P(head) = P(tail) = 0.5, \text{ where P stands for probability.}$$

This hypothesis has been verified experimentally (Kerrich, 1964).

For another example, when tossing a six-sided die (one cube is a die, and the plural is dice) each of the numbers of dots from one to six should appear one-sixth of the time. This can be written symbolically as,

$$P(1) = P(2) = P(3) = P(4) = P(5) = P(6) = 1/6,$$

where the numbers in parentheses indicate the number of dots.

For a list of all websites referred to in this chapter, as clickable links, see the book companion website: www.booksite.elsevier.com/9780128023877.

Biostatistics for Medical and Biomedical Practitioners
http://dx.doi.org/10.1016/B978-0-12-802387-7.00005-6

These expectations apply only if the coin is a normal coin and the die is not loaded on one side.

On the other hand, there is no theoretical value for the probability of dying from a heart attack in a given year. Instead, make a ratio out of the number of people who die from heart attacks to the total number of people who are alive (frequently subdivided into subgroups based on age, sex, race, etc.); then the probability of dying from a heart attack in that subgroup is, for example, 250 out of 10,000. This can be expressed as,

$$P(dying) = \frac{Number\ dying\ of\ heart\ attack\ in\ 1\ year}{Number\ alive\ during\ that\ year}$$

More generally, empirical probability is derived from the relative frequency of a certain outcome. If an experiment is performed N times, and if m of these result in outcome E_i, then the relative frequency of E_i is $\frac{m}{N}$ and the probability of the occurrence of E_i is defined as,

$$P(E_i) = \text{limit}\left(\frac{m}{N}\right)\ \text{as}\ N \to \infty.$$

This ratio should be obtained when N is infinitely large, but in practice as long as N is reasonably large, the estimated probability approximates the true value.

Subjective probability is more vague. Consider the statement that the probability of finding a cure for AIDS in the next 5 years is 50%. There is no theory that will provide this information, and no numbers with which to make an empirical ratio. Instead, the statement provides a measure of confidence that indicates how advances in the field are going and thus the likelihood of a cure. There is more to subjective probability than in this simplified example, and Section 3.5 of the book by Barnett (1973) discusses subjective probability in more detail.

BASIC PRINCIPLES AND DEFINITIONS

An experiment is a process that produces a definite outcome, for examples, a head after tossing a coin, a five on throwing a die, a cure after a given treatment. The outcomes must be unique and mutually exclusive, that is, in a single experiment one outcome precludes any others being present. Thus if we throw a die, the outcome can be any one of six numbers of dots, but no two numbers can occur in a single throw. The sample space [S] for an experiment is the set of all the possible experimental outcomes. A set is a collection of objects that are termed elements or members of the set.

For coin tossing, S = [head, tail], and for rolling a die, S = [1,2,3,4,5,6]; the rectangle below (Figure 5.1A) indicates the sample space and the set of outcomes for S = [1,2,3,4,5,6]. The sample space for tossing two coins is S = [head, head; head tail; tail,

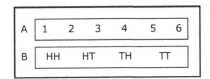

Figure 5.1 Sample spaces.

head; tail, tail], and the rectangle in Figure 5.1B indicates the sample space for these outcomes. The sample space for a pack of cards (not illustrated) is the 52 cards in the pack.

The three major axioms of probability (attributed to Andrey Kolmogorov (1903−1987)) are as follows:

1. If an experiment has n possible mutually exclusive outcomes, namely E_1, E_2,..., E_n, then the probability, P, of any given outcome E_i is a non-negative number: $P(E_i) \geq 0$. It is impossible to conceive of a negative probability.
2. The sum of the probabilities of all mutually exclusive outcomes is 1.

$$P(E_1) + P(E_2) + ... + P(E_n) = 1.$$

Thus in Figure 5.1A the sample space indicates a probability of 1, and each outcome has its own individual probability of 1/6; the sum of all these probabilities is 1. Furthermore, consider n occurrences of outcome E_i in m experiments. If all the outcomes of the experiment were E_i, then

$$P(E_i) = \frac{m}{m} = 1, \text{ in conformity with axiom 2.}$$

From these axioms, $0 \leq P(E_i) \leq 1$; the probability of any outcome must range from 0 (never occurring) to 1 (always occurring); usually an intermediate fraction occurs.

3. The probability of occurrence of either of two mutually exclusive outcomes E_i and E_j is the sum of their individual probabilities:

$$P(E_i \text{ or } E_j) = P(E_i) + P(E_j).$$

The probability of getting a 1 or a 3 on a throw of a die is 1/6 for a 1 and 1/6 for a 3. Therefore, the probability of getting one or the other is $1/6 + 1/6 = 1/3$ (the shaded area in Figure 5.2).

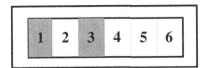

Figure 5.2 Adding probabilities.

This argument can be extended to more outcomes.

$$P(E_i \text{ or } E_j \text{ or } E_k) = P(E_i) + P(E_j) + P(E_k).$$

4. Two sets are equal only if they contain the same elements.
5. If set A has one or more elements from set B, and every element of set A is also an element of set B, then set A is termed a subset of set B; this is written $A \subset B$. For example, the shaded set [1,3,5] is a subset of the universal set $\mathbb{U}$ [1,2,3,4,5,6] (Figure 5.3).

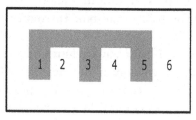

Figure 5.3 Subsets.

6. A collection of elements from a set or sample space is a subset or an event. Consider that the number of patients admitted with a myocardial infarction to an emergency room in 24 h may be 0,1,2,3,4, or 5. Then

$$\mathbb{U} = [0, 1, 2, 3, 4, 5]$$

$2 =$ the event that two or less patients are admitted with myocardial infarction

$= [0, 1, 2].$ This is a subset of the universal set $\mathbb{U}$.

Additional Definitions

1. The multiplication rule
   The probability of getting outcomes E_i and E_j in two experiments is

$$P(E_i \text{ and } E_j) = P(E_i) \times P(E_j).$$

What is the probability of getting a 2 and a 4 in two throws of a die (or one throw of two dice)? For each throw of the first die, there are six possible outcomes, each with a probability of 1/6. Each of these possible outcomes can be associated with six possible outcomes from the second throw as long as the two throws are independent, and each of these throws has a probability of 1/6. Therefore there are 36 possible combinations of outcomes involved in two throws of a die, so that any pair of outcomes has a probability of $1/6 \times 1/6 = 1/36$. Because the two dice are identical, a 2 on one die and a 4 on the other can occur in two ways: 2 on die 1 and 4 on die 2, with a probability of 1/36, and a 2 on die 2 with a 4, also with a probability of 1/36. Therefore, if the order of throwing the dice is irrelevant, the probability of one 2 and one 4 is $1/36 + 1/36 = 1/18$.

Notice the difference between the addition and multiplication rules. If you bet that horse A or horse B will win a race, then your chances of winning are the sum of each probability; you have doubled your chances of success. If you bet that horse A will win one race and horse B will win the next race, then your chances of winning both races is the product of each individual probability and is less than either.

2. The *union* of two subsets A and B, symbolized by ∪, is another set that consists of all the elements belonging to A or B, or both A and B. This is termed the *inclusive or* (Ash, 1993).

   Figure 5.4 shows a Venn diagram, in which the sample space is represented by a rectangle and the probabilities of various subsets are represented by geometric forms with different areas. (John Venn (1824−1923) was an eminent logician and student of probability. He did not invent this type of diagram, but his publication in 1880 popularized it.)

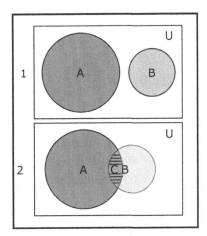

Figure 5.4 Venn diagrams.

The letter $\mathbb{U}$ in the sample space represents all the outcomes. The probabilities of the two subsets of outcomes, A and B, are represented by the areas in the circles. In panel 1, the union of A and B includes all the outcomes in A plus all the outcomes in B.

In panel 2, the union of A and B is not the same as the sum of the two areas because some outcomes are common to both, as shown by the cross-hatched area C; the total shaded area in panel 2 is less than that in panel 1. In panel 1, the two subsets are *disjoint*, because they have no elements in common, whereas in panel 2 the two subsets are *conjoint* because they have at least one element in common.

3. The intersection (symbolized by ∩) of two subsets A and B is another subset that consists of all the elements common to both A and B. In panel 2 above, the area C represents the intersection of A and B. Two events are mutually exclusive if A∩B = 0. This is the *exclusive or* (1).

4. If subset A is part of the universal set $\mathbb{U}$, then the complement of A consists of the elements in $\mathbb{U}$ that are not part of A. They form another subset that can be symbolized by $\overline{A}$ or A^c.

$$\mathbb{U} - A = \overline{A} \text{ and } P(A) = 1 - P(\overline{A})$$

Example 5.1

Two dice are thrown. What is the probability that (a) both dice have an uneven number or (b) one even and one uneven number?

(a) Die 1 can have an uneven number in 3/6 ways (1,3,5), and so can die 2. Therefore by the multiplication rule both will be uneven in $3/6 \times 3/6 = 9/36$ ways.

(b) Die 1 has a $\frac{1}{2}$ chance of having an even number, and die 2 has a $\frac{1}{2}$ chance of having an odd number. Therefore the combined probability is $\frac{1}{2} \times \frac{1}{2} = 1/4$. But this is also true if die 1 has the odd numbers and die 2 has the even numbers, so that the total probability is $\frac{1}{2}$.

---

5. In a disjoint pair of subsets, as in Figure 5.4 panel 1, the probability of the union of A and B is the sum of their two probabilities:

$$P(A \cup B) = P(A) + P(B).$$

If this relationship is correct, it means that the two subsets are independent of each other, and that the events in A and B are mutually exclusive.

In a conjoint pair of subsets, as in Figure 5.4 panel two, the probability of the union of A and B is the probability of A (the area in circle A) plus the probability of B (the area in circle B) minus the area of overlap (cross-hatched area C) that otherwise would be counted twice. Therefore

$$P(A \cup B) = P(A) + P(B) - P(A \cap B).$$

This is a more general form of expression than the previous one because it allows for the possibility of an intersection of the two subsets. If there is no intersection, then the term $P(A \cap B)$ is zero, and the two expressions are the same.

In a school with 100 students: 80 are athletes (A), 60 play basketball (B), and 50 play chess (C). Then the probability that a student plays basketball is $P(B) = \frac{60}{100} = 0.6$; the probability of a student being an athlete is $P(A) = \frac{80}{100} = 0.8$, and the probability of a student playing chess is $P(C) = \frac{50}{100} = 0.5$. The probability of a student playing basketball or chess or both is $P(B \cup C) = P(B) + P(C) - P(B \cap C) = 0.6 + 0.5 - P(B \cap C)$, the last term being unknown. It would be wrong to omit the last term, because then the probability would be 1.1, an impossibility.

Problem 5.1

What is the probability of drawing a king from a pack of cards?

Example 5.2

(a) What is the probability of drawing a heart (H) from a deck of cards, replacing it, and then drawing another heart?

Each probability is $13/52 = 1/4$, so that having both occur has a probability of $\frac{1}{4} \times \frac{1}{4} = 1/16$.

(b) What is the probability that at least one of the two cards is a spade? This can be symbolized by

$$P(S_1 \cup S_2) = P(S_1) + P(S_2) - P(S_1 \cap S_2)$$
$$= 1/4 + 1/4 - 1/16 = 7/16.$$

CONDITIONAL PROBABILITY

Table 5.1 shows the relationship between age and three different bacterial causes of fevers in patients with cyanotic heart disease: brain abscess (BA), infective endocarditis (IE), and other bacterial infections (OB).

Table 5.1 Age and causes of fever

<	<2 years	2–10 years	>10 years	Total
Other bacterial infections (OB)	40	15	5	60
Brain abscess (BA)	2	8	25	35
Infective endocarditis (IE)	1	3	7	11
Total	43	26	37	106

From this table, many probabilities can be determined. For example, what are the chances that a febrile patient will be under 2 years of age? There are 43 patients under 2 years of age out of a total of 106 patients, so that

$$P(BA) = \frac{n(BA)}{n(\mathbb{U})} = \frac{43}{106} = 0.4057.$$

However, there are more narrowly defined questions. What is the probability of a patient under 2 years of age having a brain abscess? This probability, from the definitions given above, is the intersection of being under 2 years of age and having a brain abscess. There are two patients in this category, so that the probability becomes

$$P(BA \cap < 2) = \frac{n[BA \cap < 2]}{n(\mathbb{U})} = \frac{2}{106} = 0.0189.$$

In these probabilities, the denominator is the total number of observations. Frequently, however, we may wish to determine a probability of the occurrence of an outcome in a subset of the total, that is, we wish to calculate the conditional probability, one that is conditional on the numbers in the marginal total. For example, we may want to ask the question: Among febrile patients with cyanotic heart disease, what is the probability of being under 2 years of age *and* having brain abscess?

This probability is symbolized by P(A|B), where the vertical line indicates that the probability of A is to be determined conditional on B being present. In the example above, we can write

$$P(BA|<2) = \frac{n[BA|<2]}{n(<2)} = \frac{2}{43} = 0.0465.$$

Divide the numerator and the denominator of this fraction by $n(\mathbb{U})$ to get

$$P(BA|<2) = \frac{\frac{n(BA\cap<2)}{n(\mathbb{U})}}{\frac{n(<2)}{n(\mathbb{U})}} = \frac{\frac{2}{106}}{\frac{43}{106}} = 0.0465.$$

From this way of expressing the fraction, it is clear that

$$P(BA|<2) = \frac{P(BA\cap<2)}{P(<2)}.$$

More generally,

$$P(A|B) = \frac{P(A\cap B)}{P(B)}, \quad \text{providing that } P(B) \neq 0.$$

What is the probability of selecting the king of spades from a pack of cards? Because it is one of 52 cards, the probability is obviously $\frac{1}{52}$. However, work this out on the basis of conditional probability. Let P(B) be the probability of drawing a king, and let P(A) be the probability of drawing a spade. Then the probability of drawing the king of spades is

$$P(B\cap A) = P(A) \times P(B|A)$$
$$= \frac{13}{52} \times \frac{1}{13} = \frac{1}{52}.$$

This relationship can be extended to three or more events.

$$P(A\cap B\cap C) = P([A\cap B]\cap C) = P(A\cap B) \times P(C|[A\cap B])$$
$$= P(A) \times P(B|A) \times P(C|[B]).$$

or

$$P(A\cap B\cap C) = P(A\cap[B\cap C]) = P(B\cap C) \times P(A|[B\cap C]).$$

The way in which multiple intersections can be combined is arbitrary, and does not affect the outcome.

Problem 5.2

What is the probability of drawing a king, a queen, and a jack in three successive draws from a pack of cards?

BAYES' THEOREM

Thomas Bayes (1701−1761) was an English Nonconformist clergyman who was skilled in mathematics, so much so that in 1742 he was elected a Fellow of the Royal Society (Bellhouse, 2004). He became interested in solutions to problems of scientific inference, but his publications were obscure and were delayed by some doubts that he had about his conclusions. His classical work was first presented to the Royal Society 2 years after his death by his friend Richard Price who probably contributed to its completion, (Hooper, 2013) and its importance was not recognized for more than 100 years. In medicine, the theorem is used to determine if adding new evidence to existing knowledge increases the probability of a disease being present. For example, the incidence of chest pain due to coronary artery disease in the total population is $\sim 2\%$, but if we add information that the subject is a 50-year-old obese male with diabetes then the probability of coronary artery disease becomes much higher. A simplified version of his theorem appears below.

Consider the equation that shows how to calculate $P(A|B)$ and the comparable equation for calculating $P(B|A)$, that is, the probability of B conditional on A being present

$$P(A|B) = \frac{P(A \cap B)}{P(B)} \ \text{ and } \ P(B|A) = \frac{P(B \cap A)}{P(A)}.$$

Multiply the first equation by $P(B)$ and the second equation by $P(A)$

$$P(A|B) \times P(B) = P(A \cap B) \ \text{ and } \ P(B|A) \times P(A) = P(B \cap A).$$

Because $P(B \cap A) = P(A \cap B)$, that is, the intersection of A with B is the same as the intersection of B with A, the right-hand sides of these two equations are equal. Therefore the two left-hand sides are also equal, and

$$P(B|A) \times P(A) = P(A|B) \times P(B)$$

$$\text{Therefore } \ P(B|A) = \frac{P(A|B) \times P(B)}{P(A)}.$$

In words, the conditional probability of B given A equals the conditional probability of A given B multiplied by the probability of B divided by the probability of A.

This relationship appears trivial, but consider what happens by replacing A by T+, standing for a positive result in a diagnostic test for a particular disease, and replacing B by D+, that particular disease. Then $P(D+|T+)$ is the conditional probability of having a certain disease if there is a positive test, and $P(T+|D+)$ is the conditional probability of having a positive test, given that the patient has the disease. In clinical practice we often do a diagnostic test, and if it is positive then ask how likely is it that the patient has a certain disease. Because tests are subject to false positives and false negatives, it is customary to take a number of patients with a given disease that is proven by some "gold standard," be it a biopsy, the results of surgery, an autopsy, or some other definitive test. This information yields $P(T+|D+)$. Then, if we want to know $P(D+|T+)$, the probability that the patient has the disease if the test is positive, we use Bayes' theorem:

$$P(D+|T+) = \frac{P(T+|D+)}{P(T+)}.$$

Returning to Table 5.1, the rows indicate the numbers associated with different diseases (D+) and the columns show the numbers associated with a category that can be regarded as a test outcome (T+). These data are used to estimate $P(T+|D+)$. Without knowledge about the marginal totals, the probability of a patient under 2 years of age having a brain abscess $[P(BA \cap <2)]$ is $2/106 = 0.0189$. This basic probability is referred to as the prior or pretest probability—the probability prior to having more information. Once we restrict the age group to <2 years (equivalent to a positive test result) and then ask about the probability of having a brain abscess, calculate

$$P(D+|T+) = \frac{P(T+|D+) \times P(D+)}{P(T+)}$$

$$\text{Thus } P(BA|<2) = \frac{P(<2|BA) \times P(BA)}{P(<2)}$$

$$= \frac{0.0572 \times 0.3302}{0.4057} = 0.0466.$$

Therefore by including knowledge of the outcome of some pertinent test the prior probability of 0.0189 has been increased to 0.0466; this latter probability is known as the posterior or posttest probability—the probability obtained after more information utilized. All that is required is knowledge of the particular $P(T+|D+)$ involved; this is usually determined empirically.

Excellent books for further reading are by Ash (1993), Hogg and Tanis (1977), Murphy (1979), Mosteller et al. (1970), and Ross (1984). They give large numbers of examples, some complex, which can be used as templates for specific problems. There is an easy self-teaching guide by Koosis (10).

The clinical application of diagnostic tests is described in detail in Chapters 20 and 21.

Examples

Many probability problems are related to gambling.

Consider two problems posed by the Chevalier de Méré to Blaise Pascal.

Example 1. What is the probability of throwing at least one six in four throws of a die?

With one throw, $P(6) = 1/6$ and the probability of a number not $6 = 5/6$.

Probability of a number not 6 in 4 throws $= (5/6)^4 = 0.48225$.

Probability of at least one 6 in 4 throws $= 1 - 0.48225 = 0.51775$.

Therefore in the long run the player beats the house, as long as the house is willing to play this game with even odds.

Example 2. What is the probability of throwing two 6s in 24 throws?

With 2 throws, the probability $P(6,6) = (1/6)^2 = 1/36$, and the probability of not having two 6s = 35/36.

With 24 throws, the probability of having at least two 6s is $1 - (35/36)^{24} = 0.49140$.

Therefore in the long run the player loses to the house.

Note that if the player has one more throw, the probability of having at least two 6s is $1 - (35/36)^{25} = 0.5055$. Evidently the gambling houses knew how to come out ahead.

Example 3. Perhaps the most famous modern probability problem is the Monty Hall door problem. On his guest show, Lets Make a Deal, Monty Hall would show the contestant three closed doors, (e.g., one red, one blue, and one green) and state that behind one was a new automobile and behind each of the other two was a goat. The contestant was asked to pick a door. After this was done, Monty Hall then opened one of the two remaining doors to reveal a goat. The contestant was then asked to decide whether or not to change the original choice. The point at issue is whether changing the choice improves the chances of winning after knowing that one of the three choices has been removed.

This problem caused enormous interest, with vast numbers of people advocating changing the choice and others advocating no change. Mathematical proofs of the wisdom of both recommendations were supplied, some by university professors. The correct answer is to switch, but this seemed counter-intuitive to many people.

There are numerous ways of describing the correct answer. One simple approach is to point out that initially the contestant has 1/3 chance of picking the car, and 2/3 chance of picking a goat. Switching is bad if the contestant initially picked the door with the car (1/3 of the time) but is good if the contestant had picked the goat that happens 2/3 of the time. Therefore the chances of winning have doubled by switching choices (Shermer, 2009). A short video clip by Clarke at http://www.youtube.com/watch?v=mhlc7peGlGg illustrates this approach.

Another way of explaining the answer is to point out that with the contestant's first pick (e.g., door 2), there is a 1/3 chance that the car is behind that door, and a 2/3 chance that it is behind one of the two remaining doors, 1 and 3. Once one door (say, 1) is opened to reveal a goat, the probability is still 2/3 that the car is behind door 1 or door 3, but because 1 has now been ruled out there is a 2/3 chance that the car is behind door 3.

(Continued)

Examples—cont'd

Another way of tackling this problem is to set out a table, often helpful in solving probability problems. (Based on solutions presented by vos Savant (1990/1991) and by Everitt (1999).)

No switch

Prize	First choice	Host opens door	No switch
Door 1	Door 1	2 or 3	Win
Door 2	Door 1	3	Lose
Door 3	Door 1	2	Lose

Switch

Prize	First choice	Host opens door	Switch to
Door 1	Door 1	2	3 Lose
Door 2	Door 1	3	2 Win
Door 3	Door 1	2	3 Win

To begin, there are three possible winning choices (doors 1, 2 or 3) There is a one in three chance of being right with any of the doors picked, and that does not change after the host opens a door because the choice has already been made. On the other hand, switching after added information has been given (i.e., which door does not conceal the prize) doubles the chances of winning.

Finally, we can apply Bayes' theorem:

Car is behind door 1, goat is behind door 2, goat is behind door 3.

Without knowing this information, the probability of picking the door with the car is 1/3 for each door.

$$P(1) = 1/3; \ P(2) = 1/3; \ P(3) = 1/3.$$

The contestant chooses door 1 (Car_1).

Monty Hall opens door 2 to show a goat (G_2), so the contestant can remain with door 1 or switch to door 3. These choices can be written:

$$P(Car_1|G_2) = \frac{P(G_2|Car_1)P(Car_1)}{P(G_2)} \ \text{ and } \ P(Car_3|G_2) = \frac{P(G_2|Car_3)P(Car_3)}{P(G_2)}.$$

Evaluate the conditional expressions $P(G_2|Car_1)$, $P(G_2|Car_2)$, $P(G_2|Car_3)$, $P(G_2|Car_1) = \frac{1}{2}$, because Monty Hall can choose only door 2 or door 3; door 1 has already been chosen by the contestant.

$P(G_2|Car_2) = 0$, because Monty Hall cannot open door 2 which hides the car, and $P(G_2|Car_3) = 1$, because if the car is behind 3, Monty Hall can only open door 2.

Now evaluate $P(G_2)$.

$P(G_2) = P(G_2|Car_1) + P(G_2|Car_2) + P(G_2|Car_3)$ because these are mutually exclusive events whose probabilities must add up to 1.

$$\text{Therefore } P(G_2) = \frac{1}{3} \times \frac{1}{2} + \frac{1}{3} \times 0 + \frac{1}{3} \times 1 = \frac{1}{2}$$

Examples—cont'd

Then by Bayes' theorem,

If do not switch

$$P\left(Car_1\middle|G_2\right) = \frac{P(G_2|Car_1) \times P(Car_1)}{P(G_2)} = \frac{\frac{1}{2} \times \frac{1}{3}}{\frac{1}{2}} = \frac{1}{3}$$

If switch

$$P(Car_3|G_2) = \frac{P(G_2|Car_3) \times P(Car_3)}{P(G_2)} = \frac{1 \times \frac{1}{3}}{\frac{1}{2}} = \frac{2}{3}$$

Another way of deciding whether or not to switch is divide $P(Car_3|G_2)$ by $P(Car_1|G_2)$

$\frac{P(Car_3|G_2)}{P(Car_1|G_2)} = \frac{P(G_2|Car_3) \times P(Car_3)}{P(G_2|Car_1) \times P(Car_1)} = \frac{1 \times \frac{1}{3}}{\frac{1}{2} \times \frac{1}{3}} = 2$. This shows that the contestant is twice as likely to

win by switching.

The problem has an extensive history, summarized in a comprehensive article in Wikipedia Monty Hall (2009). It has recently been reexamined at length but simply by Gill (2011).

Example 5.3 The birthday problem

There are 30 people in a room. What is the probability that at least two of them will have the same birthday (day and month, not year)? At first sight it appears to be low.

Start with calculating how many times none will have the same birthday. Person 1 could have a birthday on any one of 365/365 days (excluding leap years). Then if person 2 has a different birthday, his or her birthday must be on one of the remaining 364 days available. That is,

P(Person 1 and Person 2 have different birthdays) = P(Person 1 has a birthday on one of the 365 days in the year) $\times$ P(Person 2 has a birthday on any of the 364 remaining days)

$$= (365/365) \times (364/365)$$

Continuing this approach for all 30 persons, all with different birthdays, leads to P(no birthdays in common) = (365/365) $\times$ (364/365) $\times$ (363/365) $\times$ ...(336/365)

$$= \frac{365 \times 364 \times 363 \times ...336}{365^{30}} = \frac{365!}{365^{30}(365 - 30)!} = 0.2937.$$

Therefore the probability of not having all different birthdays is $1 - 0.2937 = 0.7063$.

This approach assumes that the chances of having a birthday are the same for each day in the year. This is incorrect, but differences from ignoring this assumption are small (Borja and Haigh, 2007).

Aplets for running repeated trials of this problem can be found at <mste.illinois.edu/reese/birthday/> and http://statweb.stanford.edu/~susan/surprise/Birthday.html.

Problem 5.3

Use the logic of the birthday problem to solve the following problem.

A group of 20 people are asked to choose at random any number between 1 and 100. What is the probability that two of them will have chosen the same number?

(a) <10%, (b) 10−25%, (c) 25−50%, (d) 50−75%, or (e) >75%

REFERENCES

Ash, C., 1993. The Probability Tutoring Book. An Intuitive Course for Engineers and Scientists, p. 470.

Barnett, V., 1973. Comparative Statistical Inference. John Wiley & Sons.

Bellhouse, D.R., 2004. The Reverend Thomas Bayes, FRS: a biography to celebrate the tercentenary of his birth. Stat. Sci. 1, 3−43.

Borja, M.C., Haigh, J., 2007. The birthday problem. Significance 4, 124−127.

Everitt, B.S., 1999. Chance Rules. An Informal Guide to Probability, Risk, and Statistics. Springer-Verlag.

Gill, R.D., 2011. The Monty Hall problem is not a probability puzzle. (It's a challenge in mathematical modelling.) Stat. Neerl. 65, 58−71.

Hogg, R.V., Tanis, E.A., 1977. Probability & Statistical Inference. Macmillan Publishing Company, Inc.

Hooper, M., 2013. Richard Price, Bayes' theorem, and God. Significance 10, 36−39.

Kerrich, J.E., 1964. An Experimental Introduction to the Theory of Probability. Belgisk Import Co.

Mosteller, F., Rourke, R.E.K., Thomas Jr., G.B., 1970. Probability with Statistical Applications. Addison-Wesley Publishing Company.

Murphy, E.A., 1979. Probability in Medicine. Johns Hopkins University Press.

Ross, S., 1984. A First Course in Probability. Macmillan Publishing Company.

Shermer, M., 2009. Prize probabilities. Sci. Am. 12.

vos Savant, M., 1990/1991. Game Show Problem (Online). Available. http://marilynvossavant.com/game-show-problem/.

Wikipedia Monty Hall, 2009. Available. http://en.wikipedia.org/wiki/Monty_Hall_problem.

PART 2

Continuous Distributions

CHAPTER 6

Normal Distribution

Contents

INTRODUCTION

What is a normal distribution, and why is it important? The term "normal" means different things in everyday conversation and in statistics. In conversation, it implies something that is usual and, if appropriate, healthy.

To determine the "normal" resting blood pressure in healthy 10-year-old girls, take about 1000 healthy girls and measure resting blood pressure accurately. Then set the results out as percentiles, just as in the well-known growth charts for children. One percent of these children will have pressures >99th percentile, 5% of them will have pressures >95th percentile, 10% of them will have pressures >90th percentile, and so on. This percentile distribution is not statistically normal (see below), although it might be fairly close to it. Although these measurements are made in healthy children, it is not clear that those at the extremes of the distribution are necessarily healthy. Children with resting blood pressures in the upper part of the percentile chart may have essential hypertension when they are adults. If this is true, then being above the 95th percentile, for example, may mean illness in the future, even if there is no illness now. This dilemma has been emphasized in relation to the standard growth charts for children (Cole, 2010). Because children are heavier now than they were 20 years ago, growth charts for the weights of "healthy" children at any age have a higher value for a given percentile now than they did

For a list of all websites referred to in this chapter, as clickable links, see the book companion website: www.booksite.elsevier.com/9780128023877.

Biostatistics for Medical and Biomedical Practitioners
http://dx.doi.org/10.1016/B978-0-12-802387-7.00006-8

earlier. Thus, a child overweight on a 1990 chart is in the normal range on a 2010 chart, but possibly destined to a variety of diseases in early adult life. The World Health Organization (WHO) distinguishes between a *normal* chart and a *standard* chart, the latter involving only children whose weights indicate future health (not an easy task).

NORMAL OR GAUSSIAN CURVE

In statistical usage, the term "normal" is applied to a distribution specified by the equation

$$f_i = \frac{1}{\sigma\sqrt{2\pi}} \cdot e^{-\frac{(X_i - \mu)^2}{2\sigma^2}}$$

f_i is the height of the curve at value X_i, μ is the mean of the distribution, and σ is its standard deviation; π and e are constants, μ and σ are parameters, and X_i is a variable. All normal distribution curves have the same bell shape (Figure 6.1), but differ in their means and standard deviations. The whole expression defines the Gaussian curve. Changing the values of the parameters changes the position and width of the curve, but not its bell shape. The value of X_i gives an estimate of the function of the expression at that value.

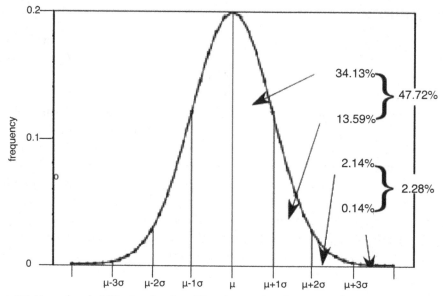

Figure 6.1 Normal probability density plot of X variate against frequency. The areas under the curve as related to deviations from the mean (μ) in units of standard deviation (σ) are shown. 2.28% of the area under the curve is greater than two standard deviations from the mean, and 0.14% of the area is greater than three standard deviations from the mean. 2.5% of the area under the curve is beyond 1.96 standard deviations from the mean. Such a normal curve is often described as $\mathcal{N}(0, 1)$ where the $\mathcal{N}$ refers to the normal distribution, not sample size, 0 is the mean, and 1 is the variance.

The first description of the normal distribution was given in 1733 by Abraham de Moivre (1667–1754), an Anglo-French mathematician who left France for England after the persecution of the Huguenots. He started with probability theory, in particular the binomial theorem (see Chapter 11) and developed the formula so that it would be possible to compute the binomial distribution when the number of binary events (e.g., coin tosses) was very large (Gridgeman, 1966). Later, scientists, particularly astronomers, began to be concerned about how to allow for measurement errors in celestial mechanics, and Laplace, Gauss, and others began to associate the distribution of these errors with the normal curve; the "true" value was the mean, and the errors distributed around the mean produced a normal curve.

This distribution produces the well-known bell-shaped or Gaussian curve (Figure 6.1).

Why is the X-axis labeled in standard deviation units? Different Gaussian curves have different means and standard deviations (Figure 6.2).

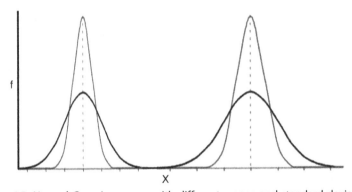

Figure 6.2 Normal Gaussian curves with different means and standard deviations.

Between any two points on the X-axis, expressed in terms of number of standard deviations from the mean, the area under the curve is the same for all normal curves. Therefore, subtracting the mean μ from each value of X_i and then dividing by the standard deviation σ produces *standard deviates* symbolized by z. Thus

$$z_i = \frac{X_i - \mu}{\sigma}$$

This is one type of linear transformation and it achieves two goals. By subtracting μ from every value of X_i, the numerator becomes 0. The normal curves are shifted so that each curve has a mean of 0 (Figure 6.3). Second, by dividing the numerator by the standard deviation, every normal curve has a unit standard deviation. Therefore, wide curves with big standard deviations and narrow curves with small standard deviations each assume a standard shape with a mean of 0 and a standard deviation of 1 (Figure 6.3).

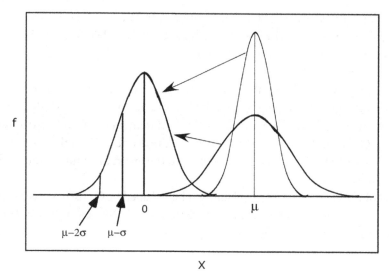

Figure 6.3 *z* Transform. The curve on the left has a mean of 0 and a standard deviation of 1 unit, and is what both the curves on the right would look like after the *z* Transformation.

Once the z transformation has been performed, the new normal curve will be that shown in Figure 6.1. The z transformation is based on population values for the mean and the standard deviation.

The Quincunx

A quincunx is a device resembling a pinball machine that was developed by Sir Francis Galton (1822–1911) to illustrate the theory of random errors (Figure 6.4).

Each pin deflects a falling ball either to the left or to the right. Despite the most careful construction of pins and balls, tiny imperfections or even air currents make each move at random to either side. Intuitively, it is very unlikely for any ball to move always to the left or always to the right, so that the bins at the ends have very few balls. Most balls tend to have roughly equal numbers of leftward or rightward deflections, accounting for the peaks in the central bins. The more pins, bins, and balls there are, the closer the distribution matches the normal Gaussian distribution.

Fascinating pictures of balls moving through the pins and into the bins can be seen at http://www.mathsisfun.com/data/quincunx.html and http://www.jcu.edu/math/isep/quincunx/quincunx.html.

Properties of the Normal Curve

The normal distribution curve has important mathematical properties. It is symmetrical about a mean (μ) of 0, and 68.26% of the measurements are within the limits of one standard deviation (σ) below to one standard deviation above the mean; this one standard

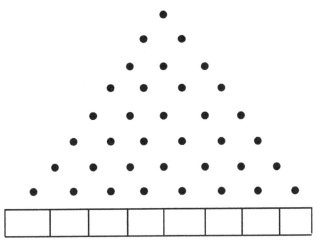

Figure 6.4 Quincunx consisting of regularly placed pins arranged vertically on a board. Steel balls much smaller than the space between the pins are dropped from the top, bounce off the pins, and end up in one of the bins at the bottom. If balls are dropped into bins, the following distributions might occur (Figure 6.5).

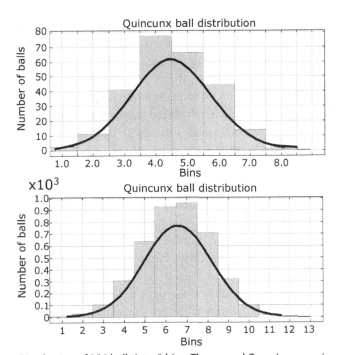

Figure 6.5 Upper: Distribution of 256 balls into 8 bins. The normal Gaussian curve is superimposed on the histogram. The fit is fair. Lower: Results after dropping 4096 balls into 12 bins. The histogram is more symmetrical. *(Constructed with applet from http://www.jcu.edu/math/isep/quincunx/quincunx. html.)*

deviation value is the point of inflection of the curve. The mean value is the most frequent measurement (the mode). 0.025 (or 2.5%) of the area under the curve is above a value of $X = mean + 1.96$ times the standard deviation; because the curve is symmetrical, there is an equal area below a value of $X = mean - 1.96$ times the standard deviation. These two areas added together give 0.05 (5%) of the area under the curve that is beyond the limits set by the mean ± 1.96 times the standard deviation. Figure 6.6 shows how the areas under the curve are often represented.

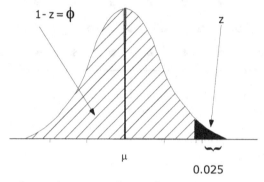

Figure 6.6 Components of normal curve. z is the area beyond some value on the horizontal X-axis.

Most texts and tables give the values of the total area under the curve beyond any given value of z (black area). The remaining area (cross-hatched area) to the left of the z demarcation is $1 - z$, often termed φ; this is the cumulative area from the left-hand end of the curve to the value of z. Occasionally some tables have different shaded areas, and the reader should check to see what the listed values refer to. Cumulative areas can be calculated at http://stattrek.com/online-calculator/normal.aspx and http://www.danielsoper.com/statcalc3/calc.aspx?id=2.

For a continuous distribution of this type, it makes little sense to ask about the probability of obtaining a given X value. The probability of an adult male human weighing 68.83997542001 kg is virtually 0. What does matter is the area under the curve between different values of X. As examples:

1. What proportion of the area under the curve lies between the mean μ and one standard deviation σ below the mean? From Figure 6.1, the area between these limits is 0.3413 or 34.13% of the total area.
2. What proportion of the area under the curve lies between the μ and 0.5 standard deviations below the mean? From tabulated areas under the curve, the area under the curve for $\mu - 0.5\sigma$ is 0.1914 (Figure 6.7(a)).
3. What proportion of the area under the curve lies between 0.5 and 1 standard deviations below the mean? From tabulated areas under the curve, the area under the curve for $\mu - 0.5\sigma$ is 0.1914, and for $\mu - \sigma$ is 0.3413. Therefore, the required area is $0.3413 - 0.1914 = 0.1499$ (Figure 6.7(b)).

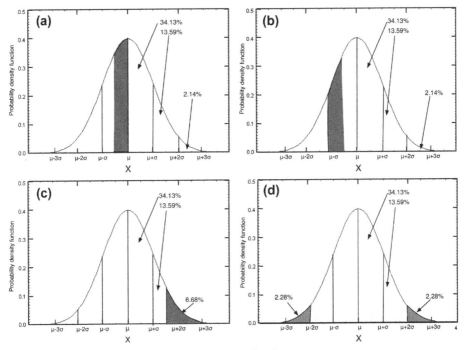

Figure 6.7 Areas under the curve.

4. What proportion of the area under the curve is >1.5 standard deviations above the mean? From tabulated areas under the curve, the area under the curve for $\mu + 1.5\sigma$ is 0.9332. The whole area under the curve is 1. Therefore the required area is $1 - 0.9332 = 0.0668$ (Figure 6.7(c)).

5. What proportion of the area under the curve is >2 standard deviations above and below the mean? From tabulated areas under the curve, the area under the curve for $\mu \pm 2\sigma$ is 0.0456 (Figure 6.7(d)).

6. 99.73% of the area under the curve lies between $\mu \pm 3\sigma$, 99.9937% between $\mu \pm 4\sigma$, and 99.999942% between $\mu \pm 5\sigma$.

Problem 6.1

Use the online calculator to determine the area under the normal curve between the limits of 0.75σ below the mean to 1.5σ above the mean.

All these areas can be calculated easily using http://davidmlane.com/hyperstat/z_table.html, http://easycalculation.com/statistics/normal-distribution.php, and http://psych.colorado.edu/~mcclella/java/normal/accurateNormal.html.

The normal curve can also be converted into a cumulative probability density curve with its characteristic S or sigmoid shape (Figure 6.8).

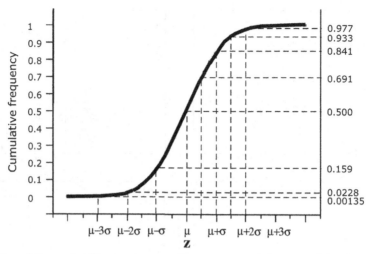

Figure 6.8 Cumulative probability density curve (frequency curve). Because of the changing slope of the curve, a change in the X-axis from μ to $\mu + 1\sigma$ changes the cumulative frequency from 0.500 to 0.691 for a difference of 0.191, whereas a one standard deviation change from $\mu + 2\sigma$ to $\mu + 3\sigma$ changes the cumulative frequency from 0.977 to 0.99865 (not shown) for a difference of 0.02165. These cumulative frequencies can be obtained easily online. The lower scale shows standard deviates (see below).

POPULATIONS AND SAMPLES

Initially, attention was paid to the sampling features of the mean of large samples; the sample standard deviation and the population standard deviation were assumed to be virtually identical. Gosset realized that some correction was required if inferences about small samples were to be made from the normal Gaussian curve. He introduced a value termed t, similar to z but with one important difference. Whereas for means

$$z = \frac{\overline{X_i} - \mu}{\sigma_{\overline{X}}},$$

where $\sigma_{\overline{X}} = \frac{\sigma}{\sqrt{N}}$ and $\sigma = \frac{\sum (X_i - \mu)^2}{N}$,

Gosset used an analogous expression

$$t = \frac{\overline{X_i} - \mu}{s_{\overline{X}}},$$

where $s_{\overline{X}} = \frac{s}{\sqrt{N}}$ and $s = \frac{\sum (X_i - \overline{X})^2}{N - 1}$.

There were two added features to his "Student's" t distribution. One was that $N - 1$ is a specific example of $N - k$, where k is the number of degrees of freedom, and second that the areas under the normal curve varied with the degrees of freedom. For large sample size, >200, the t and z distributions were identical, but for a sample of 11 with 10 degrees of freedom 95% of the area under the normal curve lies within the limits of $\mu \pm 2.228 s_{\overline{X}}$, not $\pm 1.96 \sigma_{\overline{X}}$ as for the z table.

DESCRIPTION OF THE DISTRIBUTION SHAPE

The mean μ gives the average size of the measurements, a measure of central tendency, and the square root of the variance gives the standard deviation σ, which is a measure of variability. Unfortunately, most real distributions are not exactly normal, and may even be very far removed from it. One common form of nonnormality is to have a few very large measurements, with the effect shown diagrammatically in Figure 6.9.

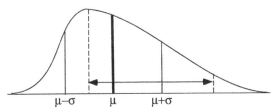

Figure 6.9 The dotted lines and double-headed arrow indicate the range within which two-thirds of the measurements lie.

The curve is no longer symmetrical, but is pulled to the right toward the larger measurements; it is *skewed* to the right. The mean is no longer near the most frequent measurement, but to the right of it. More importantly, the range from one standard deviation below to one standard deviation above the mean is not symmetrical and does not include a known proportion of the measurements. For some distributions with extreme skewing, the mean gives no useful information.

Many other types of nonnormality exist. One might guess that the distribution of serum electrolyte concentrations in healthy people approximates a normal distribution, but Elveback and her colleagues (Elveback et al., 1970; Elveback, 1972) showed that the distributions of several commonly obtained laboratory biochemical values are not normal in the Gaussian sense. Furthermore, they pointed out that to calculate mean and standard deviations from the data in the hope that the 2.5% with the highest values and the 2.5% with the lowest values could be declared abnormal (and therefore unhealthy) would lead to serious underdiagnosis of illness. In their studies, the distributions of commonly determined biochemical values were often leptokurtotic (excessively peaked), with more than 68% of the area between the limits of $\mu - \sigma$ and $\mu + \sigma$ and with excessively long tails (Figure 6.10). Therefore, the standard deviation of the leptokurtotic distribution is wider than that for a normal distribution, and this can have serious clinical consequences. For example, if the (leptokurtotic) distribution of serum calcium is

Figure 6.10 Normal, Leptokurtotic (for **Long-**tailed), and Platykurtotic (for **fl**at top) curves.

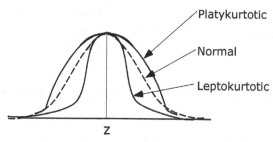

regarded as normal, the "normal" limits are too wide, and the upper critical normal value based on the calculated standard deviation would lead investigators to miss about 20% of patients with hyperparathyroidism. The problems of using the "normal range" to make clinical diagnoses has been discussed many times (Mainland, 1971; Murphy and Abbey, 1967). The International Federation of Clinical Chemistry recommends the term "reference range" rather than the poorly defined term "normal range" (Strike, 1981).

Other symmetrical curves are short-tailed and flat-topped (platykurtotic) so that fewer than 68% of the measurements are between the limits of $\mu - \sigma$ and $\mu + \sigma$ (Figure 6.10).

One approach to defining shape is by computing *moments*. The first moment about the mean is $\frac{\sum (X_i - \mu)}{N}$, that is, the average value of the deviations from the mean, and this is zero. The second moment about the mean is $\frac{\sum (X_i - \mu)^2}{N}$, the average of the squared deviations of X_i from the population mean, that is, the population variance. The third moment about the mean is $\frac{\sum (X_i - \mu)^3}{N}$, the average value of the sum of the cubed deviations from the mean; it is designated as m_3 or k_3. The fourth moment about the mean is $\frac{\sum (X_i - \mu)^4}{N}$, the average value of the sum of the deviations about the mean to the fourth power; it is designated as m_4 or k_4.

Skewness

With perfect symmetry, the third moment is zero, and if the distribution is nearly symmetrical the cubed numerator yields a small number because pluses and minuses almost cancel out. If the curve is skewed to the left, there will be more negative than positive numbers and k_3 will be negative. Conversely, skewing to the right yields a positive result. Because this expression has cubed units, it is customary to divide by the cube of the standard deviation to obtain a dimensionless measurement termed γ_1:

$$\gamma_1 = \frac{k_3}{\sigma^3}.$$

With sample data, the expression becomes:

$$g_1 = \frac{k_3}{s^3},$$ which is the above equation corrected for sample size.

Standard computer programs perform the calculations. A free online calculator can be found at http://www.wessa.net/skewkurt.wasp, and skewness can be calculated by the Skew function in Excel. The program gives the probability that $g_1 = 0$, or tables of g_1 can be consulted (see http://mvpprograms.com/help/mvpstats/distributions/SkewnessCriticalValues or http://www.engl.unt.edu/~leubank/researchmethods/appendicesa&b.html) to indicate if a positive or negative value of g_1 is large enough that the hypothesis that $g_1 = 0$ can be rejected.

Kurtosis

If the distribution is symmetrical, then kurtosis can be assessed with the fourth moment about the mean to calculate k_4 or m_4, and this can be made dimensionless and standardized to the standard deviation by

$$\gamma_2 = \frac{k_4}{\sigma^4}: \quad \text{the equivalent sample values are } g_2 = \frac{k_4}{s^4}.$$

γ_2 for a normal curve should be 3. It is customary to subtract 3 from the value of g_2; if $g_2 - 3$ is significantly below 0 then the curve is platykurtotic and if it is significantly above 0 then it is leptokurtotic. If either of these distorted normal curves is encountered, it is worth considering why they have occurred. A leptokurtotic curve might indicate the superimposition of two normal curves with the same mean but different standard deviations, and a platykurtotic curve might indicate the superimposition of two normal curves with similar standard deviations but different means (Zar, 2010). Platykurtosis often occurs when batches of data are collected at different times, with a slight shift in mean from one batch to the other. A free online calculator can be found at http://www.wessa.net/rwasp_skewness_kurtosis.wasp#output and http://www.calculatorsoup.com/calculators/statistics/descriptivestatistics.php. Kurtosis can also be calculated by the KURT function in Excel.

A rough assessment of kurtosis can be made with the ratio interquartile distance/1.35 (pseudostandard deviation or PSD). If the standard deviation $\ll$ PSD, the distribution is platykurtotic, and if the standard deviation $\gg$ PSD, the distribution is leptokurtotic (Hamilton, 1990).

Small sample sizes produce wide confidence limits.

Problem 6.2
Take the data from Table 4.15 and test them for skewness and kurtosis. Also calculate the PSD and decide if the curve is leptokurtotic or platykurtotic.

DETERMINING NORMALITY

Initially inspect the histogram, stem-and-leaf diagram, or box plots for asymmetry and outliers. Not only is the distribution seen clearly but any outliers are identified. Now that all of these graphics are incorporated into standard software programs, there is no excuse for not determining if a set of observations appears to be normal.

Skewing is easy to detect, but symmetrical distributions with straggling of the highest and lowest measurements are more difficult to judge by eye. The PSD described above is an easy way of assessing this. This is important to know because these straggling tail values can grossly distort the standard deviation and make comparisons between groups ineffi-cient. In addition, the mean ± 0.25 s should include about 40% of the measurements. If many more are included, this suggests that the upper part of the curve is narrower than it should be from a Gaussian distribution.

Some calculations yield a number that can be used to determine the likelihood that a given data set could represent a normal distribution. Shapiro and Wilk's test (Shapiro and Wilk, 1965), Lilliefors test (Lilliefors, 1967), and D'Agostino's test (D'Agostino and Pearson, 1973) are available in most statistical programs. Also see http://www.wessa. net/Ian.Holliday/rwasp_Shapiro-Wilks%20Test%20for%20Normality.wasp for the Shapiro—Wilk's test, http://www.wessa.net/rwasp_skewness_kurtosis.wasp#output for Agostino's test, and http://in-silico.net/statistics/lillieforstest, http://home.ubalt. edu/ntsbarsh/Business-stat/otherapplets/Normality.htm for the Lilliefors test. These tests are easy to do and interpret, but may not indicate where the distribution has departed from normality and thus may not indicate what to do about the problem.

A test for both skewness and kurtosis combined is the Jarque—Bera test (Jarque and Bera, 1980). The test value JB is calculated from:

$$JB = \frac{N}{6}\left(s^2 + \frac{(k-3)^2}{4}\right),$$

where s is the sample skewness and k is the sample kurtosis. The statistic JB has an asymptotic chi-square distribution with two degrees of freedom (Chapter 7), and tests the assumption that the data come from a normal distribution. It can be performed online at http://www.wessa.net/rwasp_skewness_kurtosis.wasp#output.

Graphic tests. Some tests are graphic: for example, the use of probability paper or normal quantile plots. In Figure 6.8, the typical sigmoid cumulative frequency curve is shown. If data points could be plotted on such a curve with an excellent fit, it is reason-able to conclude that the distribution from which those points came was normal. It is, however, difficult to assess S-shaped curves, and easier to assess straight lines. Fortunately the S-shaped curve can be made straight by plotting its points on probability paper (Figure 6.11).

There are other ways of plotting and assessing normal distributions. Normal quantile plots are standard on most computer programs. Figure 6.8 shows how for equal standard deviation increments the incremental change in the cumulative percentages became pro-gressively less as the distance from the mean increased. This was rectified in the

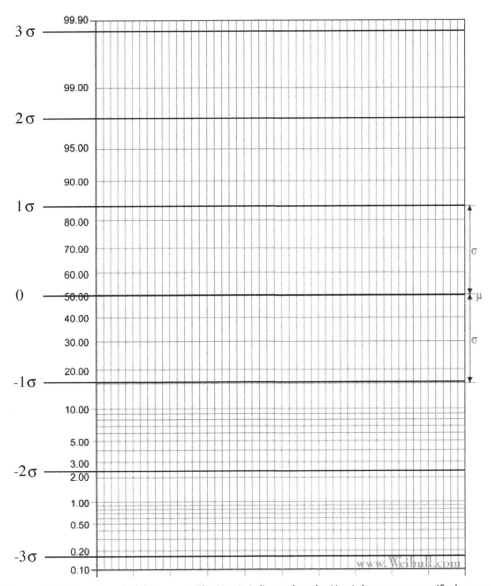

Figure 6.11 Normal probability paper. The X-axis is linear, but the Y-axis becomes magnified as one goes further away from the mean. The thick horizontal lines are placed 1, 2, and 3 standard deviations above and below the mean, as defined by the areas under the normal curve. Graphs for this and other distributions may be obtained free online from the ReliaSoft Corporation at http://www.weibull.com. (see Download Probability Plotting Papers).

probability paper that features in Figure 6.11 where the heavy horizontal lines demarcate standard deviation units rather than cumulative percentages. Thus, the vertical Y-axis is linear in standard deviation units, sometimes called standard normal deviates or normal equivalent deviates (NEDs). (The transformation of the S-shaped curve to the linear

NED scale is attributed to the pharmacologist J.H. Gaddum (1900–1965) (Eggert and Stick, 1984).) The cumulative percentages corresponding to various z values are shown in Table 6.1.

Table 6.1 Normal equivalent deviates (NEDs). The NED is the same as the area defined as $1 - z = \varphi$ in Figure 6.4

Cumulative percentage	Normal equivalent deviate
0.00135	−3
0.02775	−2
0.1589	−1
0.5	0
0.6915	0.5
0.8413	1
0.933	1.5
0.977	2
0.9986	3

With this information, plot the data on probability graph paper. The X-axis is the measurement of the variable, and on the Y-axis plot the observed cumulative percentages of the X variable. As an example, Table 6.2 gives data on the distribution of heights of eighteenth-century English soldiers in America (Komlos and Cinnirella, 2005).

Table 6.2 Distribution of heights. Discussion of columns in text below

Height (in)	Frequency	Cumulative frequency	% Cumulative frequency	NED
59	10	10	0.99	−2.330
60	14	24	2.15	−2.024
61	36	60	5.38	−1.609
62	50	110	9.87	−1.289
63	98	208	18.65	−0.891
64	172	380	34.08	−0.410
65	174	554	49.69	−0.008
66	184	738	66.19	0.418
67	119	857	76.86	0.734
68	127	984	88.25	1.188
69	60	1044	93.63	1.524
70	31	1075	96.41	1.800
71	22	1097	98.39	2.142
72	14	1111	99.64	2.687
73	4	1115	100.00	
Mean = 65.6 Sd = 2.54				

The mean of grouped data can be calculated using http://www.easycalculation.com/statistics/group-arithmetic-mean.php, and the mean and standard deviation from http://www.knowpapa.com/sd-freq.

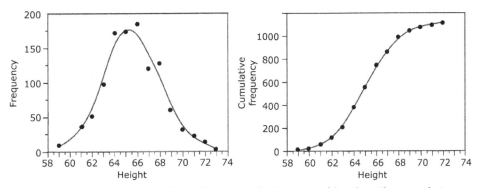

Figure 6.12 Frequency and cumulative frequency distributions of heights. The cumulative curve evens out the irregularities shown in the original distribution.

The resultant frequency and cumulative frequency distributions are shown in Figure 6.12.

One way of testing the normality of the distribution is to plot the cumulative percentage against the height on probability paper (Figure 6.13).

Another method that does not involve probability paper is to plot the NEDs on the Y-axis and the height on the X-axis. This involves calculating the cumulative percentage, transforming these values into NEDs (as shown in Table 6.1), from detailed tables, from Figure 6.6, or from online calculators http://stattrek.com/online-calculator/normal.aspx, http://sampson.byu.edu/courses/zscores.html or http://davidmlane.com/hyperstat/z_table.html (Figure 6.14). The calculators are more accurate but the results are similar.

UNGROUPED DATA

Table 6.3 shows the weight (in pounds) of 13 dogs. For ungrouped data, the individual frequencies are 1,1,1...1; the cumulative frequencies are 1,2,3...N; and the relative cumulative frequencies are $1/N$, $2/N...N/N$. Thus, because in Table 6.3 $N = 13$, the first relative cumulative frequency is $1/13 = 0.077$, the second is $2/13 = 0.154$, and so on.

Plotting the NED in column 4 against the actual values in column 2 gives Figure 6.15.

This is not as good a fit as shown in Figure 6.14, and some points are quite far from the theoretical line of normality. To determine if these data are consistent with a normal distribution, enter them into the programs http://stattrek.com/online-calculator/normal.aspx or http://www.wessa.net/rwasp_skewness_kurtosis.wasp#output. These show that skewness and kurtosis are not abnormal enough to allow rejection of the null hypothesis.

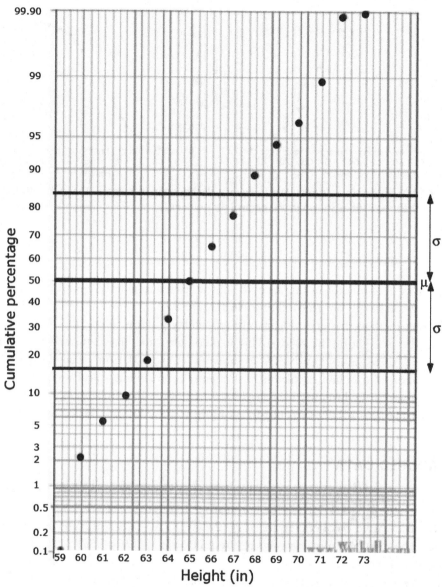

Figure 6.13 Probability paper showing cumulative heights. Apart from the ends, which are based on very small numbers, the distribution is reasonably linear. This suggests that the distribution is approximately normal, although it cannot be truly normal because it is truncated at each end.

The graphs in Figures 6.14 and 6.15 are *quantile* or Q–Q plots. To determine if these data are still compatible with a normal distribution, some programs, such as JMP, insert 95% confidence limits (Figure 6.16). Quantile plots can be implemented online by http://www.wessa.net/rwasp_harrell_davis.wasp#output, but without confidence

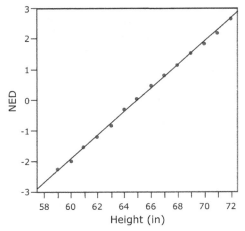

Figure 6.14 Using normal equivalent deviate (NED) to determine normality on ordinary graph paper. This is the equivalent of using probability paper.

Table 6.3 Dog data

Number	Weight (lbs)	Cumulative relative frequencies	NED
1	17.2	0.077	−1.426
2	20.8	0.154	−1.019
3	21.0	0.231	−0.736
4	21.2	0.308	−0.502
5	21.5	0.385	−0.292
6	24.2	0.462	−0.095
7	24.3	0.539	0.098
8	25.6	0.616	0.295
9	27.7	0.693	0.504
10	31.0	0.77	0.739
11	34.5	0.857	1.067
12	38.7	0.924	1.433
13	39.2	1.00	—
	$\sum X_i = 346.9$ $\overline{X} = 26.68$ $s = 7.12$		

limits. They can also be produced in Excel http://facweb.cs.depaul.edu/cmiller/it223/normQuant.html.

If the distribution had been perfectly normal, then all the points would have been on the line. These plots show exactly where the deviations from normality occur, and give a probability that can be used to decide if the distribution is sufficiently far from a normal distribution.

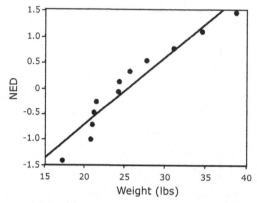

Figure 6.15 Dog data in normal equivalent deviate (NED) plot.

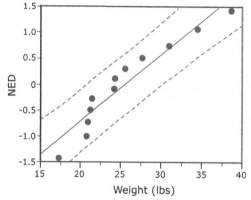

Figure 6.16 Normal quantile plot. The diagonal line indicates perfect normality. The vertical scale shows normal equivalent deviates (NEDs), and the horizontal scale shows the weight. The dashed curved lines show the 95% confidence limits.

Most computer programs produce similar figures. They can also be performed with Excel: see http://facweb.cs.depaul.edu/cmiller/it223/normQuant.html.

Problem 6.3
Draw a quantile plot of the data from Table 4.15.

HOW IMPORTANT IS NORMALITY?

The normal distribution curve plays a central part in statistical thinking and modeling. If the distribution is markedly abnormal, then even though a test statistic can be calculated, inferences drawn from it may be wrong. Furthermore, because statistics based on the normal distribution are very efficient, most people try to use normalizing transformations so that conventional statistics can be used. Alternatively, there are tests to use when distributions are markedly abnormal; these are called nonparametric tests.

How necessary is it to test normality and how much abnormality of the distribution can be tolerated? If a stem-and-leaf diagram, a box plot, or a histogram appear roughly normal and symmetrical by eye, then, as long as there are no extreme outliers, the distribution is normal enough, and more elaborate tests may not be needed. This attitude is supported by an article by Sall (with the appropriate title "Leptokurtophobia: irrational fear of non-normality") that appeared in the technical publication for JMP users, JMPer Cable (Sall, 2004). He pointed out that: "In large samples it is easy to detect non-normality, but it doesn't matter. In small samples, non-normality may matter, but you can't detect it." Sall concluded, however, that graphical testing, even if of limited use for detecting nonnormality, was of value looking for anomalies or a pattern that might be a clue to some hidden structure of the distribution.

REFERENCES

Cole, T.J., 2010. Babies, bottles, breasts: is the WHO growth standard relevant? Significance, Virtual Medical Issue 6−10.

D'Agostino Jr., R.B., Pearson, E.S., 1973. Tests of departure from normality. Biometrika 60, 613−622.

Eggert, P., Stick, C., 1984. The pattern of bilirubin response to phototherapy for neonatal hyperbilirubinemia. Pediatr. Res. 18, 682.

Elveback, L., 1972. A discussion of some estimation problems encountered in establishing "normal" values. In: Gabrieli, E.R. (Ed.), Clinically Oriented Documentation of Laboratory Data. Academic Press, New York.

Elveback, L.R., Guillier, C.L., Keating Jr., F.R., 1970. Health, normality, and the ghost of Gauss. J. Am. Med. Assoc. 211, 69−75.

Gridgeman, N.T., July 28, 1966. The normal curve. New Sci. 211−213.

Hamilton, L.C., 1990. Modern Data Analysis. A First Course in Applied Statistics. Brooks/Cole Publishing Co, Pacific Grove, CA.

Jarque, C.M., Bera, A.K., 1980. Efficient tests for normality, homoscedasticity and serial independence of regression residuals. Econ. Lett. 6, 3.

Komlos, J., Cinnirella, F., 2005. European Heights in the Early 18th Century (Online). Available: http://epub.ub.uni-muenchen.de/.

Lilliefors, H.W., 1967. On the Kolmogorov-Smirnov test for normality with mean and variance unknown. J. Am. Stat. Assoc. 64, 399−402.

Mainland, D., 1971. Remarks on clinical "norms". Clin. Chem. 17, 267−274.

Murphy, E.A., Abbey, H., 1967. The normal range—a common misuse. J. Chronic Dis. 20, 79−88.

Sall, J., 2004. Leptokurtophobia: Irrational Fear of Non-normality. JMPer Cable.

Shapiro, S.S., Wilk, M.B., 1965. An analysis of variance test for normality (complete samples). Biometrika 52, 591−611.

Strike, P.W., 1981. Medical Laboratory Statistics. John Wright and Sons, Ltd, Bristol.

Zar, J.H., 2010. Biostatistical Analysis. Prentice Hall, Upper Saddle River, NJ.

CHAPTER 7

Statistical Limits and the Central Limit Theorem

Contents

CENTRAL LIMIT THEOREM

In a 1966 publication, the mean height of 24,404 males in the US Army was reported as 68.4 in, with a standard deviation of 2.5 in (Newman and White, 1966). These figures are valuable for understanding biology and, more practically, for deciding what sizes to make uniforms! The question to ask is whether the sample mean of 68.4 in, is a good or a bad estimate of the theoretical population mean μ.

Imagine a theoretical normal population of heights of young adult males. In a sample S_1 of N subjects, the mean height might be 68.1 in. This is one estimate of the population mean, μ. A second sample S_2 of N subjects might have a mean value of 69.4 in. Which is the better estimate of μ? One way to answer this question would be to draw thousands of samples, each with N subjects, at random from the population. For each sample, calculate the mean and end up with thousands of mean heights taken from samples of size N. These means are themselves numbers, and the mean of all these means is the grand mean. With enough samples the grand mean will be very close to the population mean and can be termed μ with minimal inaccuracy. The standard deviation of these means can be calculated and will closely approximate σ, the population standard deviation of the mean. Because this standard deviation is not of individual measurements but of means, it is symbolized by a subscript $\sigma_{\overline{X}}$ and called the standard deviation of the mean. This is sometimes termed the standard error of the mean.

For a list of all websites referred to in this chapter, as clickable links, see the book companion website: www.booksite.elsevier.com/9780128023877.

Biostatistics for Medical and Biomedical Practitioners
http://dx.doi.org/10.1016/B978-0-12-802387-7.00007-X

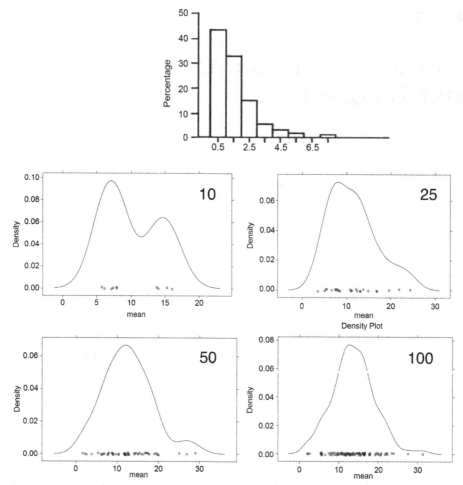

Figure 7.1 Upper panel shows a grossly abnormal distribution based on the upper panel of Figure 4.8. Below it are the distributions of means of repeated samples from this distribution, the numbers in the upper right-hand corners showing how many samples were taken. Despite the abnormal distribution, even 10 samples have a roughly normal distribution of means, and this distribution becomes more symmetrical as the sample size increases.

An important theorem in statistics is the central limit theorem. The theorem states that even if a distribution from which samples are drawn is not normal, the means of samples drawn at random from this population will be normally distributed (Figure 7.1).

Even for extreme distortions of the sample frequency curves, the sampling distribution of the mean is normal for sample sizes over 30, and for smaller sample sizes if the basic frequency distribution is closer to normal.

Therefore, the sample of very large numbers of means of heights should be normally distributed, and it is possible to draw a normal curve (of mean heights) (Figure 7.2).

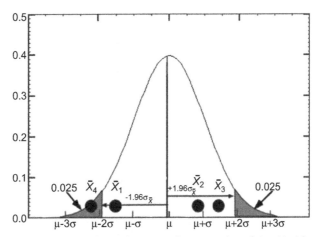

Figure 7.2 Normal Gaussian curve of sample means from samples of size N with population mean μ and standard deviation $\sigma_{\overline{X}}$. The two shaded area in the tails each include 2.5% of the area under the curve, that is, the area more than $1.96\sigma_{\overline{X}}$ above and below the mean. The unshaded area within the limits $\mu - 1.96\sigma_{\overline{X}}$ and $\mu + 1.96\sigma_{\overline{X}}$ (indicated by the two offset lines and arrow heads) includes 95% of the area under the curve.

In this example, the large black dots indicate the means of four samples, each of size N, drawn at random from this population. The population mean μ is approximated from the grand mean of the thousands of samples and $\sigma_{\overline{X}}$ from those thousands of means. Because this experiment is a thought experiment and we have actually not drawn these thousands of samples, we do not know what μ and $\sigma_{\overline{X}}$ are. We can, however, argue that 95% of these sample means (e.g., $\overline{X}_1$, $\overline{X}_2$, and $\overline{X}_3$) fall within the limits of $\mu \pm 1.96\sigma_{\overline{X}}$, and only 5% of them (e.g., $\overline{X}_4$) fall outside those limits. In other words, from the properties of the normal curve, the probability is 2.5% that a given mean is more than $1.96\sigma_{\overline{X}}$ above μ, 2.5% that it is more than $1.96\sigma_{\overline{X}}$ below μ, and 95% that it is between these limits.

Now if there is 5% probability that $\overline{Xi}$ is more than $\pm1.96\sigma_{\overline{X}}$ from μ, there is the same 5% probability that μ is $\pm1.96\sigma_{\overline{X}}$ from $\overline{Xi}$ (Figure 7.3(a)–(d)).

In samples 1 (Figure 7.3(a)), 2 (Figure 7.3(b)), or 3 (Figure 7.3(c)), the value of μ lies between the limits demarcated by the arrowheads. On the other hand, occasionally the limits set by $\overline{X} \pm 1.96\sigma_{\overline{X}}$ do not include μ (Figure 7.3(d)). However, this event should occur less than 2.5% of the time, or less than 5% of the time if the excessive deviation could be above or below the mean.

To recapitulate, if we draw thousands of samples of size N from a population with a mean of μ and a standard deviation of the mean of σ, then 95% of the means of those samples will be within $\mu \pm 1.96\sigma_{\overline{X}}$, so that there is a 95% probability that the unknown value of μ will be within those limits. Only 2.5% of the time will a sample mean be too small or too big for this prediction to be correct. Therefore a single sample of size N and

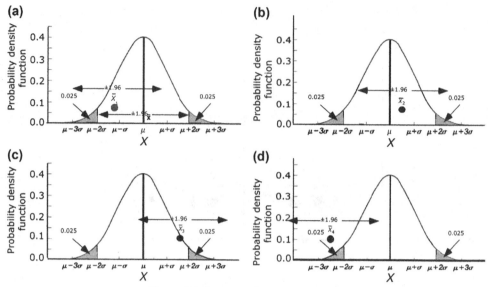

Figure 7.3 Reverse inference (see text).

its mean allow us to predict that the unknown value of μ would lie between $\overline{X}_1 \pm 1.96\sigma_{\overline{X}}$ 95% of the time. These limits are termed CL.

There is still one problem if we wish to avoid drawing thousands of samples. The CL described above are calculated using $\sigma_{\overline{X}}$, and this was obtained from the thousands of samples. Fortunately, there is an easy way of predicting $\sigma_{\overline{X}}$ from the single sample standard deviation:

$$\sigma_{\overline{X}} \approx \frac{s}{\sqrt{N}},$$

where s is the sample standard deviation and N is the sample size.

Therefore all that is needed is a single sample, calculate its mean and standard deviation, estimate the standard deviation of the mean as $\frac{s}{\sqrt{N}}$, and multiply this value by 1.96 to obtain the 95% CL about the mean.

Generalizations Based on a Single Sample

Our sample of measurements allows the determination of point estimates of central tendency and variation, but what use are these estimates? They are unlikely to be repeated in other samples drawn at random from the same population, but nevertheless are useful in making hypotheses about the parameters of the populations from which the samples were drawn. This is the beginning of scientific inference that often begins with determining confidence (or interval) estimates.

Setting CL

An interval estimate is a range that we believe will include the parameter being estimated with a given degree of confidence. The two ends of the range are called the CL for that parameter.

CL may be set for any given level of significance (Chapter 8). They are often specified as $(1 - \alpha)$ or $(100 - \alpha)\%$ where α is the significance level. Usually 0.95 (95%) limits are determined, corresponding to a significance level α of 0.05 (5%), but at times other CL are more useful.

The formula for CL may be written as

$$(1 - \alpha)\text{CL} = \overline{X} \pm z_{\alpha/2}\frac{s}{\sqrt{N}}$$

because $z_{\alpha/2}$ gives the area beneath one tail of the curve, and twice that value is α. In Figure 7.2, the lines demarcating the unshaded area show the CL.

Limits are not restricted to 95% confidence. In some data such as survival after cardiac surgery, 70% limits have been used, even though they are wide (Kirklin and Barratt-Boyes, 1993a,b). Alternatively, 99% CL are derived by multiplying $s_{\overline{X}}$ by 2.588. This allows more certainty about the limits within which μ lies, but the disadvantage is that the limits have become wider. Returning to the population mean for height, by using a big enough value for z we could even be 99.99999999999% sure that the limits are between $20''$ and $120''$, but those limits are so wide as to be useless.

For estimating results from small samples (<100), use an adjusted value of z that is called t. CL for the mean are then determined by multiplying the standard error by the appropriate value selected from the t table, and then subtracting that product from and adding it to the mean (Gardner and Altman, 1995). Thus if the mean of a series of 10 measurements is 57.5 and the standard deviation is 12.57, then the standard error of the mean is $\frac{12.57}{\sqrt{10}} = 3.98$. $t_{0.05}$ for 9 degrees of freedom is 2.262. Therefore, the 95% CL for the mean are $57.5 \pm 2.262 \times 3.98 = 57.5 \pm 9.00 = 48.5$ to 66.5. These limits are symmetrical about the observed mean. If the distribution is not normal, then the limits still tend to be symmetrical about the mean but will be wider because of the larger standard deviations. CL can be calculated online at http://easycalculation.com/statistics/confidence-limits-mean.php, http://ncalculators.com/statistics/confidence-interval-calculator.htm, and http://www.danielsoper.com/statcalc3/calc.aspix?id=96.

Problem 7.1

A data set has mean 93.2 and standard deviation of 13.7.
Set 95% CL for $N = 14$ and $N = 77$.

Confidence intervals with $N < 12$ are usually wide, and for larger N decrease rapidly (van Belle, 2002). In order to obtain narrow CL that allow efficient comparisons between two mean values, for example, we need a big value for N. What that value needs to be will be discussed in Chapter 11.

If there is concern about outliers and a trimmed mean $\overline{X_{trim}}$ is used, estimate the standard error of the trimmed mean as

$$s_{\overline{X_{trim}}} = \frac{1}{1 - 2\gamma} \frac{s_W}{\sqrt{N}}.$$

Here γ is the trimming fraction, usually $0.1N$ or $0.2N$, removed at each end of the distribution, and s_W is the Winsorized standard deviation (Wilcox, 1996) (Chapter 4). The CL are narrower for any given value of α because eliminating the outliers has reduced the standard error. The reasons for the outliers need careful examination (Chapter 9).

An assumption is that the sample standard deviation represents the population standard deviation, and this is one good reason for inspecting the distribution for abnormalities and unusually large outlying observations that might falsely inflate the estimate of the population standard deviation and the CL. What can we do to avoid this source of error other than inspecting the distribution carefully? One way is to increase the number of observations because this gives a more secure basis for assessing the standard deviation (Figure 7.4).

As sample size increases the standard deviation changes, sometimes exceeding and sometimes falling below the population standard deviation σ, but the swings about the mean value become smaller with increased N. On the other hand, as N increases the value of $s_{\overline{X}}$ becomes smaller because s is divided by greater values for $\sqrt{N}$. Because of this square root function, to halve the value of $s_{\overline{X}}$ for a given value of s we must increase

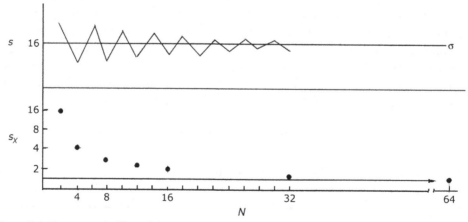

Figure 7.4 Upper panel: effect of increasing sample size on estimated population standard deviation. Lower panel: effect of increasing sample size on standard error of the mean.

sample size fourfold. To make $s_{\overline{X}}$ one-tenth as large we must increase sample size 100-fold. Although having a larger sample size gives a smaller value for $s_{\overline{X}}$ and decreases the confidence interval, the cost in time and money may not justify the increased size.

Finally, CL, as an indicator of the uncertainty of a test, provide only minimum estimates unless the distribution of errors is perfectly normal—an exceedingly unlikely event.

CL can be calculated for other statistics such as proportions, slopes, standard deviations, etc., and will be discussed in the appropriate chapters.

TOLERANCE LIMITS

Confidence intervals are determined for means by the formula $\overline{X} \pm t_{\alpha} s_{\overline{X}}$, and this formula is often incorrectly modified as $\overline{X} \pm t_{\alpha} s$ to set CL for individual data values. Such limits might be needed to evaluate when, for example, a single value for the concentration of a biological substance (glucose, calcium, etc.) is outside the usual limits and hence should be considered as possibly pathological. Unfortunately the standard formula was developed to examine the distribution of means around a population mean by making use of an estimate of the population standard deviation of the mean. When a single data point is to be evaluated from a sample, however, neither the population mean nor the population standard deviation is known (Figure 7.5).

What is needed is a tolerance interval, well known in industry. Tolerance limits define an interval that includes a designated proportion of the population (p) with a specified level of confidence (γ).

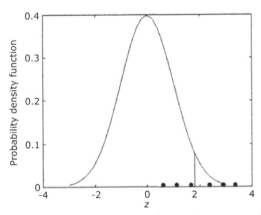

Figure 7.5 The Gaussian curve shows the distribution of means drawn at random from samples of the same size from a population; the horizontal scale is in standard units, with mean $= 0$ and standard deviation $= 1$. The short vertical line at 1.96z indicates the upper 2.5th percentile. As shown, the individual values that make up that mean are themselves scattered about the mean, and the upper 2.5th percentile for points has a z value >1.96. It is to allow for this added source of variability that tolerance limits were devised.

As described by Hahn and Meeker (1991), "Assume, for example, that measurements of the diameter of a machined part have been obtained on a random sample of 25 units from a machined process. A tolerance interval calculated from such data provides limits that one can claim, with a specified degree of confidence (e.g., $\gamma = 90\%$), contains the (measured) diameters of at least a specified proportion (e.g., p = 95%) of units from the sampled population. The two percentages in the preceding statement should not create any confusion when one recognizes that one (95% in the example) refers to the percentage of the population to be contained, and the other (90%) deals with the degree of confidence associated with the claim that the interval encloses (at least) 95% of the population."

Tolerance intervals can examine three types of questions: (Handbook)

1. What interval will contain p percent of the measurements? (Two-sided interval)
   This is calculated as $\overline{X} \pm k_2 s$, where k_2 is the two-sided tolerance factor.
2. What interval guarantees that p percent of measurements will not be below a lower limit? (One-sided interval)
   The lower limit X_L is calculated as $\overline{X} - k_1 s$, where k_1 is the one-sided tolerance factor.
3. What interval guarantees that p percent of measurements will not exceed an upper limit? (One-sided interval)
   The upper limit X_U is calculated as $\overline{X} + k_1 s$, where k_1 is the one-sided tolerance factor.

Some computer programs make these calculations, and one-sided limits can be determined online at http://statpages.org/tolintvl.html or by consulting a table of one-sided tolerance factors, for example, Table 6 in the book by Goldstein (1964), or Table A7 by Natrella (1963); the latter table is reproduced at http://water.usgs.gov/osw/bulletin17b/1963_Natrella.pdf.

Consider the weights of the first eight dogs from Table 6.4. They have mean weight 21.98 kg and standard deviation 2.66 kg. What are the lower tolerance weight limits for 99% of the population with a 95% probability of being correct? From the table, factor $k = 4.37$. Then the limit is $\overline{X} - ks$, that is $21.98 - 2.66 \times 4.37 = 10.36$. Therefore at least 99% of future observations will exceed 10.36 kg weight, and that statement will be correct 95% of the time. By the (incorrect) CL formula, the one tailed value would have been $21.98 - 2.66 \times 1.96 = 16.77$ kg, a value much too high. Transferring the concept to a serum electrolyte concentration, the lower limit set by CL would be too high for any single future measurement, and many patients would be regarded incorrectly as having an abnormally low concentration for serum electrolyte. The difference between tolerance and CL decreases as sample size decreases, but always persists.

REPORTING RESULTS

Most published reports give the point estimates for mean and standard deviation, and should also give the sample size. However, that is not sufficient. At the very least the CL (usually 95%) should be given, and many journals now insist on this because it gives the reader essential information. The presentation of CL is so important for all point estimates that everyone should read a simple book by Gardner and Altman entitled "Statistics with Confidence" (Gardner and Altman, 1995). CL should be provided not only because many journals require them, but because they provide added information (that investigators often ignore) about the data (Healy, 1992). Healy (1992) gives the example of a sample mean of 0.22 with a 95% confidence interval of 0.02–0.42. Because the confidence interval does not include zero it implies statistical significance at the 5% level (see later), but the lower limit is consistent with an effect that is too small to be of importance. Under these circumstances the investigator would be wise to put less emphasis on the significance of the test and more on the possible magnitude of the effect.

Graphic Representation

The question about what to include in a bar graph is not settled, and as pointed out in Chapter 4 the bar graph is an inefficient use of space. Usually in such a graph the mean is a bar with its height proportional to the mean, and a measure of variability is added as a vertical line (Figure 7.6, right panel). As shown in the figure, a box plot (left panel) presents far more useful data.

The box plot is more informative. Furthermore, the values for the mean and standard deviation are almost always present in the text and do not need to be shown graphically. The subject is discussed at length by Cumming et al. (2007).

Whether to give standard error or standard deviation is the most frequently asked question that I get. Some authors have commented on the confusion that this issue causes (Bunce et al., 1980; Gardner, 1975). In one sense the distinction is unimportant, because any two values of N, s, and $s_{\overline{X}}$ allow the remaining value to be calculated. When presenting data in the form of a bar graph (which is inferior to a box plot) there is a tendency to give the mean and standard error for two reasons. One is that it makes it easier to compare two or more means visually to determine if they are close together or far apart in terms of standard error, and this visual impression certainly reinforces any statistics that appear in the text. However, the visual impression is of value only if the numbers in the groups are similar. Furthermore, if N is large then the small value of the standard error tends to conceal what might be large variability (standard deviation) of the sample (Figure 7.7). Several issues about presenting data are discussed clearly in recent publications (Altman et al., 1983; Curran-Everett and Benos, 2004, 2007; Ludbrook, 2008; Morton, 2009). There is a tendency for journals to prefer the standard deviation (Bartko, 1985; Dawson-Saunders and Trapp, 1994). It is possible to present both numbers in the

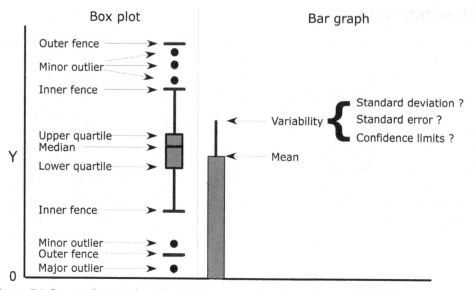

Figure 7.6 Bar graph on right with height representing the value on the Y-axis. A vertical line extending up from the top of the bar indicates variability, but there is little consistency about whether it represents standard deviation, standard error, or CL. Furthermore, the authors may not make this information available. Box plot (Velleman and Hoaglin, 1981) on left shows vastly more information for about the same space. (Other programs give slightly different box plots.)

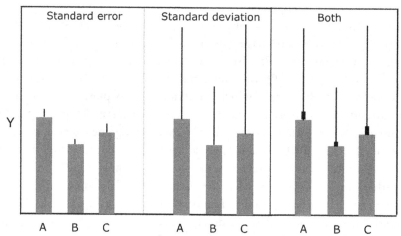

Figure 7.7 Comparison of bar graphs with standard error versus standard deviation.

same figure, for example, by making the standard error of the mean a thicker part of the line, or side by side, but this is seldom seen. If used, the two lines should be described (Figure 7.7).

The left-hand panel allows the reader to make judgments about differences of means among groups and is useful. The middle panel emphasizes the variability of the data and even suggests that groups A and C with their large standard deviations might have outliers. In addition, because the standard deviation and mean are about same size in bars A and C, it is almost certain that these represent distributions severely skewed to the right. The right-hand panel shows one way to include both numbers. There is no one right answer to the question about which deviation to show, but authors should make the basic data available to the reader (Brown, 1982). Variability is as much a feature of the data set as is the mean.

REFERENCES

Altman, D.G., Gore, S.M., Gardner, M.J., et al., 1983. Statistical guidelines for contributors to medical journals. BMJ 286, 1489–1493.

Bartko, J.J., 1985. Rationale for reporting standard deviations rather than standard errors of the mean. Am. J. Psychiatry 142, 1060.

Brown, G.W., 1982. Standard deviation, standard error. Which 'standard' should we use? Am. J. Dis. Child. 136, 937–941.

Bunce III, H., Hokanson, J.A., Weiss, G.B., 1980. Avoiding ambiguity when reporting variability in biomedical data. Am. J. Med. 69, 8–9.

Cumming, G., Fidler, F., Vaux, D.L., 2007. Error bars in experimental biology. J. Cell Biol. 177, 7–11.

Curran-Everett, D., Benos, D.J., 2004. Guidelines for reporting statistics in journals published by the American Physiological Society. Am. J. Physiol. Endocrinol. Metab. 287, E189–E191.

Curran-Everett, D., Benos, D.J., 2007. Guidelines for reporting statistics in journals published by the American Physiological Society: the sequel. Adv. Physiol. Educ. 31, 295–298.

Dawson-Saunders, B., Trapp, R.G., 1994. Basic & Clinical Biostatistics. Appleton & Lange.

Gardner, M.J., 1975. Understanding and presenting variation. Lancet 1, 230–231.

Gardner, M.J., Altman, D.G. (Eds.), 1995. Statistics with Confidence—Confidence Intervals and Statistical Guidelines. British Medical Journal. The Universities Press Ltd, Belfast.

Goldstein, A., 1964. Biostatistics, an Introductory Course. Macmillan Company.

Hahn, G.J., Meeker, W.Q., 1991. Statistical Intervals. A Guide for Practitioners. John Wiley and Sons, Inc.

Handbook, E.S. Tolerance Intervals for a Normal Distribution (Online). Available: http://itl.nist.gov/div898/handbook/prc/section2/prc263.htm.

Healy, M.J.R., 1992. Statistics from the inside. 3. Estimation. Arch. Dis. Child. 67, 149–150.

Kirklin, J.W., Barratt-Boyes, B.G., 1993a. Cardiac Surgery. Churchill Livingstone.

Kirklin, J.W., Barratt-Boyes, B.G., 1993b. The generation of knowledge from information, data, and analysis. In: Kirklin, J.W., Barratt-Boyes, B.G. (Eds.), Cardiac Surgery, second ed. Churchill Livingstone.

Ludbrook, J., 2008. The presentation of statistics in Clinical and Experimental Pharmacology and Physiology. Clin. Exp. Pharmacol. Physiol. 35, 1271–1274.

Morton, J.P., 2009. Reviewing scientific manuscripts: how much statistical knowledge should a reviewer really know? Adv. Physiol. Educ. 33, 7–9.

Natrella, M.G., 1963. Experimental Statistics. Dover Publications, Inc.

Newman, R.W., White, R.M., 1966. In: Damon, A., Stoudt, H.W., Mcfarland, R.A. (Eds.), The Human Body in Equipment Design. Harvard University Press.

van Belle, G., 2002. Statistical Rules of Thumb. Wiley Interscience.

Velleman, P.F., Hoaglin, D.C., 1981. Applications, Basics and Computing of Exploratory Data Analysis. Duxbury Press.

Wilcox, R.R., 1996. Statistics for the Social Sciences. Academic Press.

CHAPTER 8

Other Continuous Distributions

Contents

CONTINUOUS UNIFORM DISTRIBUTION

A uniform distribution, continuous or discrete, is one in which the random variable assumes all its values with equal probability. This distribution is used, for example, when determining if the incidence of a disease is constant month by month throughout the year.

If the continuous interval from which x is chosen extends from a to b, then the mean $\mu = \frac{a+b}{2}$, and the variance $\sigma^2 = \frac{(b-a)^2}{12}$ (Hogg and Tanis, 1977).

The probability of selecting a value of x in the range a to x is $\frac{x-a}{b-a}$.

The distribution can be used to assess waiting times. A physician sees one patient every 30 min from 8 am until 5 pm. What are the chances that a randomly arrived patient will have to wait less than 5 min? In each 30-min period the last 5-min meet the requirements, so that the probability is $5/30 = 0.167$. More formally, calculate $(30-25)/(30-0)$ to get the same answer.

EXPONENTIAL DISTRIBUTION

The times to failure, for example, of a heart valve or a transplanted kidney, or the survival time of a cancer patient often closely follow a curve defined as the exponential distribution, characterized by the quantity being studied growing or decaying at a rate proportional to its current value.

The continuous random variable X has an exponential distribution if its probability density function is given by

For a list of all websites referred to in this chapter, as clickable links, see the book companion website: www.booksite.elsevier.com/9780128023877.

Biostatistics for Medical and Biomedical Practitioners
http://dx.doi.org/10.1016/B978-0-12-802387-7.00008-1

$$f(X) = \frac{1}{\beta} e^{-\frac{x}{\beta}} \text{ when } x > 0 \text{ and } \beta > 0.$$

It can also be written as:

$$\int (x) = \lambda e^{-\lambda}.$$

Therefore, $\lambda = \frac{1}{\beta}$ and either formulation can be used. λ is sometimes termed the rate parameter, and β is termed the scale parameter.

The mean of this distribution is β, and the variance is β^2, or $\frac{1}{\lambda}$ and $\frac{1}{\lambda^2}$ respectively. Examples of exponential curves are given in Figure 8.1.

A negative rate constant estimates the time to failure, for example, of a heart valve, a transplanted kidney, or the whole person (death). It also estimates radioactive decay, where the amount of radioactivity emitted decays exponentially with time. In addition to playing a part in survival analysis (Chapter 35) it appears in Chapter 18 (Poisson distribution). Whereas the Poisson distribution deals with the number of random events that occur, the exponential distribution deals with the waiting time between those events.

As an example, patients arrive at a clinic randomly at an average rate of 20/h. Assume that this is a Poisson process in which the arrival times are independent of each other (Chapter 18). What is the probability that the first patient arrives more than 5 min after the clinic opens? An average of 20 patients per hour is equivalent to $\lambda = 1/3$ patients/ min. Because $\beta = 1/\lambda$, the function may be written as

$$f(X) = \beta e^{-\beta X} = \frac{1}{3} e^{-\left(\frac{1}{3}\right) X}. \text{ Therefore,}$$

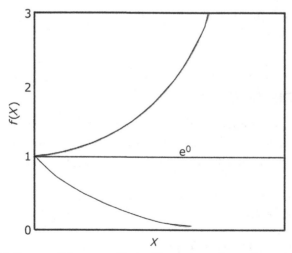

Figure 8.1 Exponential curves with positive, zero, and negative exponentials.

$$P(X > 5) = \int_5^\infty \frac{1}{3} e^{-\left(\frac{1}{3}\right)X} = e^{-\frac{5}{3}} = 0.189.$$

When the rate constant is positive, the exponential distribution characterizes growth processes such as the increase in bacteria or cancer cells with time.

LOGARITHMIC DISTRIBUTION

Many distributions are skewed to the right, making analysis awkward. One widely used solution is to use the logarithms of the observations, rather than the original observations themselves because these transformed values often resemble a normal distribution. This distribution is particularly useful in epidemiological studies in which values for variables such as smoking, calorie intake, exposure to an atmospheric pollutant, etc., cannot be negative (van Belle, 2002). A general discussion of logarithmic transformations is presented simply online by Motulsky (2009) (http://www.graphpad.com/faq/file/1487logaxes.pdf) who emphasized that an exponential decay curve could not be linearized by a logarithmic transformation unless it went to zero. He recommended using these transformations also for ratios (such as the odds ratio) and for growth curves.

There are difficulties when a confidence interval is determined for a lognormal distribution (Olsson, 2005; Zhou and Gao, 1997). Despite textbook recommendations, confidence limits of the mean of the normal distribution should not be determined by exponiating the confidence limits determined for the mean of the lognormal distribution. The limits so determined are the confidence limits for the median of the lognormal distribution. Cox suggested that the confidence limits for the mean of the normal distribution could be derived from (Zhou and Gao, 1997)

$$\overline{X} + \frac{s^2}{2} \pm z_{1-\alpha/2} \sqrt{\frac{s^2}{N} + \frac{s^4}{2(N-1)}}.$$

As an example, consider the lipoprotein a data in Figure 4.8. Table 8.1 shows that using the untransformed data, the 95% confidence limits are unrealistic in such a skewed

Table 8.1 Setting confidence limits for lognormal distributions

	Untransformed data	Log transformation; (exponiation)	Cox formula
Mean	1.51	0.8216	
s	1.3152	0.5138	
Upper 95% CL	4.0878	1.8286 → (6.2255)	1.4419
Lower 95% CL	−0.10678	−0.1854 → (0.8307)	0.4733

data set. After logarithmic transformation that provides a more symmetrical distribution, the lower 95% confidence limit is almost the same as the mean of the original distribution. When calculated from the modified Cox formula, the limits of 0.4733–1.4419 are more compatible with the raw data.

WEIBULL DISTRIBUTION

This distribution, developed by Waloddi Weibull (1887–1979), a Swedish engineer and mathematician (Weibull, 1951), is a versatile distribution that simulates many other functions. Its general formula is

$$f(x : \lambda k) = \left(\frac{x - \mu}{\lambda}\right)^{k-1} e^{\left(\frac{x-\mu}{\lambda}\right)^2} \text{ when } x \geq 0, \text{ and is zero if x} < 0.$$

This formula is not as complicated as it looks. k is a shape parameter, μ is a location parameter, and λ is a scale parameter. Changes in μ shift the curve to the left or the right, changes in λ alter the vertical and horizontal scales so that the total area under the curve is 1 unit, and changes in k change the shape of the curve. Figure 8.2 shows various shape parameters. The curves can fit many different distributions.

More complete but still relatively simple discussions are provided online at http://www.mathpages.com/HOME/kmath122/kmath122.htm, http://reliawiki.org/index.php/The_Weibull_Distribution, and by http://www.engineeredsoftware.com/nasa/weibull.htm.

This distribution is often used in time-to-failure analysis (Chapter 35). If the failure rate decreases over time, then $k < 1$. If $k = 1$, this becomes an exponential distribution. If the failure rate increases with time, then $k > 1$. When $k = 3.4$, this becomes the normal distribution.

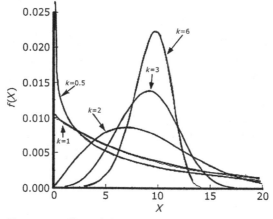

Figure 8.2 Effect of changing the shape parameter k.

CHI-SQUARE DISTRIBUTION

Draw at random a variable X_i from a normal distribution and transform it into a standard normal variate z_i by

$$z_i = \frac{X_i - \mu}{\sigma},$$

then if z_1, z_2,...z_n are independent standard normal deviates, the distribution of the random variable $\chi_n^2 = z_1{}^2 + z_2{}^2 + ...z_n{}^2$ is called the χ^2 distribution with n degrees of freedom.

The distribution of z^2 is called a χ^2 distribution with one degree of freedom, often written as χ_1^2. If there are two or more independent normal distributions of X, then $\chi_2^2 = z_1{}^2 + z_2{}^2$, termed χ^2 with two degrees of freedom, and in general $\chi_n^2 = z_1{}^2 + z_2{}^2 + ...z_n{}^2$ is termed χ^2 with n degrees of freedom.

This distribution has several properties:

1. If χ_n^2 and χ_m^2 are two independent χ^2 random variables, their sum $\chi_n^2 + \chi_m^2$ has a χ^2 distribution with $n + m$ degrees of freedom.
2. The mean value of χ^2 is v, the degrees of freedom, and its variance is $2v$.
3. The possible values of χ^2 run from 0 to infinity.
4. When v is greater than 30, $\sqrt{2\chi^2}$ is distributed approximately normally with unit standard deviation and mean $\sqrt{2v - 1}$.
5. If s^2 is the variance of a random sample of n measurements taken from a normal population with variance σ^2, then $\frac{(N-1)s^2}{\sigma^2}$ is distributed as $(N - 1)$ degrees of freedom, that is

$$\chi_{n-1}^2 = \frac{(n - 1)s^2}{\sigma^2}.$$

The distributions of χ^2 for different degrees of freedom is shown in Figure 8.3.

Because this distribution involves the square of z it is always positive. The probability is 0.05 that z is bigger than $+1.96$ or -1.96. If either of these events occurs, then z^2 exceeds 3.84. Thus the right tail of the curve is the same for negative and positive values of z.

The probabilities of any given value of χ^2 for given degrees of freedom can be obtained from standard tables or from online computer programs listed in Chapter 14.

This distribution can be used to determine the confidence limits for the variance. We construct the $100(1-\alpha)$ confidence limits for $\frac{(n-1)s^2}{\sigma^2}$ by selecting two values of χ^2 in the two tails of the distribution, $\chi_{\alpha/2}^2$ at the upper end and $\chi_{1-\alpha/2}^2$ at the lower end, with the value $\frac{(n-1)s^2}{\sigma^2}$ between them. These confidence limits can be calculated by the online program http://www.wessa.net/rwasp_hypothesisvariance4.wasp.

Another use of this distribution is to analyze categorical data, as discussed in detail in Chapter 14.

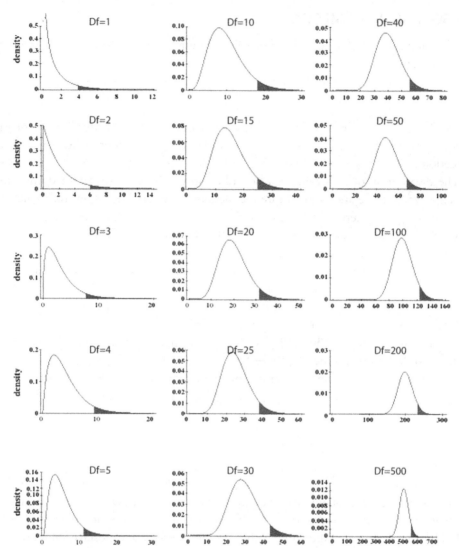

Figure 8.3 Chi-square for various degrees of freedom. The area under the curve representing 0.05 of the total area is shaded. The curves become more symmetrical as the degrees of freedom increase, and the peak of the curve is approximately at the corresponding degrees of freedom. If we draw at random one normal variate and square it, the probability of getting a value near the mean of zero is very high, and the probability of getting a large deviation from the mean is very low. Therefore, we get the curve as shown by the upper left for 1 degree of freedom. If we draw three normal variates at random and square them, the probability that they sum to a very small value near zero is lower, as shown by the curve for 3 degrees of freedom. By adding more squared normal variates, the sum tends to move further away from zero, as shown for increasing degrees of freedom.

VARIANCE RATIO (F) DISTRIBUTION

If we draw two random samples of size n_1 and n_2 from a normal distribution, and calculate their variances s_1^2 and s_2^2, these variances will not be identical. The distribution of the ratio of the two variances $\frac{s_1^2}{s_2^2}$ has been determined, and it is possible to determine the probability of the ratio exceeding any given value. The general form of the distribution is shown in Figure 8.4.

As generally used, this is a one-sided test, and we are usually interested only if the bigger variance exceeds the smaller variance by some critical ratio. Rarely we need to calculate values to the left of the distribution; for example, what is the value of F above which 95% of the distribution lies.

The distribution was discovered by R.A. Fisher in the 1920s. George Snedecor (1881−1974) named it the F distribution in Fisher's honor. The variance ratio is used extensively in analysis of variance and in regression statistics.

The distribution depends on the degrees of freedom υ_1 and υ_2 for the two variances. All statistical texts give tables of the critical values, and they can be found online at

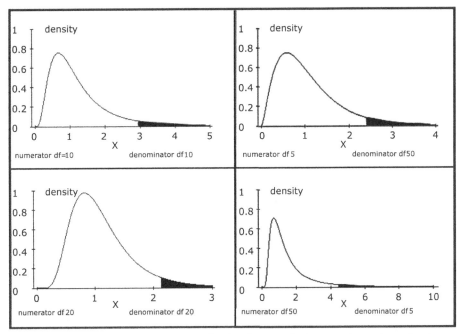

Figure 8.4 Typical F distributions. There is a family of curves. Each curve depends on the degrees of freedom in the numerator and the denominator, for example, 50 and 5, respectively. The shaded areas indicate the F value beyond which 0.05 of the curve occurs (one sided).

http://www.itl.nist.gov/div898/handbook/eda/section3/eda3673.htm, http://vassarstats. net/textbook/apx_d.html, and http://www.tutor-homework.com/statistics_tables/f-table-0.001.html. Online probabilities for given values of F and the degrees of freedom of the two components can be found at http://vassarstats.net/tabs.html, and http://www.statdistributions.com/f/.

REFERENCES

Hogg, R.V., Tanis, E.A., 1977. Probability & Statistical Inference. Macmillan Publishing Company, Inc, New York.

Motulsky, H.J., 2009. Statistical Principles: The Use and Abuse of Logarithmic Axes (Online). Available: http://helpdesk.graphpad.com/faq/viewfaq.cfm?faq=1487.

Olsson, U., 2005. Confidence intervals for the mean of a log-normal distribution. J. Stat. Educ. 13.

van Belle, G., 2002. Statistical Rules of Thumb. Wiley Interscience, New York.

Weibull, W., 1951. A statistical distribution function of wide applicability. J. Appl. Mech. Trans. Am. Soc. Mech. Eng. 18, 293–297.

Zhou, X.H., Gao, S., 1997. Confidence intervals for the log-normal mean. Stat. Med. 16, 783–790.

CHAPTER 9

Outliers and Extreme Values

Contents

OUTLIERS

In an example of the effect of raw and roasted peanuts on the growth of rats (Chapter 22), one rat in one pair of littermates showed an unusually small weight gain. This discrepant observation had the effect of reducing the difference in average weight gain on the two diets and making it impossible to reject the null hypothesis. Was it really an outlier and if so what should we do about it?

As defined by Grubbs (1969) "An outlying observation, or 'outlier,' is one that appears to deviate markedly from other members of the sample in which it occurs." There may be more than one outlier. First, eliminate errors of observation or recording. It is not uncommon to enter weight instead of height, or to misplace a decimal point. For the peanut example, a check of the weighing procedures may show that for this rat the scale had not been correctly calibrated, or checking the feeding logs may show that by mistake this rat missed one or more feedings. The rat might appear ill, and examination might disclose a lung infection. If errors of measurement or recording are detected, they are corrected if possible, and if not correctable (e.g., a scale that was incorrectly calibrated by some unknown and unrecoverable factor) the measurement is omitted with an explanation. If the rat missed a feed or was ill that also justifies removal, with an explanation. There are legitimate reasons for excluding data, but it is essential to describe why the data were removed.

If no apparent cause for the discrepancy is found, how discrepant is the measurement? One simple method is to make a box plot, looking for minor and major outliers, as defined by Tukey (1977) (Figure 4.20). By definition, a minor outlier is one that is

For a list of all websites referred to in this chapter, as clickable links, see the book companion website: www.booksite.elsevier.com/9780128023877.

Biostatistics for Medical and Biomedical Practitioners
http://dx.doi.org/10.1016/B978-0-12-802387-7.00009-3

141

more than 1.5 × interquartile distance above the 75th or below the 25th quartile, and this comes to a z value of 2.698 (one-sided). For a normal curve, only 0.35% of the area under the curve (about 1 in 285) is beyond this value. A major outlier is one that is 3 × interquartile distance above the 75th or below the 25th quartile, and this comes to a z value of 4.7215 (one-sided). For a normal curve, only 0.00012% of the area under the curve (about 1 in 833,333) is beyond this value.

Should the distribution be very skewed, there is a strong tendency for too many of the measurements to be declared outliers based on the Tukey limits as defined above. This bias can be reduced by using a skewness-adjusted box plot (Hubert and Vandervieren, 2008) that requires special programs for its use.

Grubb's Test

Other methods for making a decision depend on what we know of the variate that is being measured. *If there is reason to believe that the data should have been normally distributed,* there are tests to disclose outliers. A simple test is known as Grubbs' test or the extreme studentized deviate test (Grubbs, 1969). If we draw a sample of size N from a normal population, we can examine the difference between the mean and the extreme value of X, divided by the standard deviation:

$$T = \frac{\max|\overline{X} - X_i|}{s}$$

where $\max|\overline{X} - X_i|$ is the greatest deviation either above or below the mean. The standard deviation is calculated from all the data, including the suspected outlier. This ratio is called T. In a large number of random drawings it is possible to state that T exceeds a certain value 5% of the time, or 2.5% of the time, or 1% of the time, and so on. The relevant table is provided by Grubbs (1969) and appears also on the web at http://www.graphpad.com/quickcalcs/Grubbs1.cfm or www.sediment. uni-goettingen.de/staff/dunkl/software/pep-grubbs. Grubb's test allows only one outlier to be examined per sample. Sometimes, however, there may appear two or three outliers, and then a sequential test can be done. The greatest outlier is examined by Grubbs' test. If it is too extreme it is removed, and the next greatest outlier is examined, but assessed against a modified ratio (Rosner, 1977, 1995; Prescott, 1979) Alternatively, if there is suspicion about the two largest or the two smallest observations, Grubbs (1969) calculated the ratio $\frac{s_{12}^2}{s^2}$, where s^2 is the variance of the whole data set and s_{12}^2 is the variance of the data set after removing the two presumptive outliers. This ratio is then referred to a table of critical values (Grubbs, 1969) or at http://www.statistics4u.com/fundstat_eng/ee_grubbs_outliertest.html, or by using the free online programs at http://graphpad.com/quickcalcs/Grubbs1.cfm.

The difficulty with Grubb's test is that it is based on a presumed normal distribution.

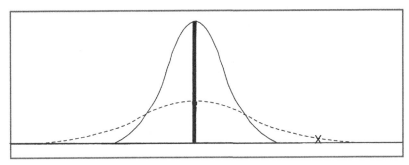

Figure 9.1 Contaminated distribution.

Slippage and Contamination

Even with a normal distribution, outliers may appear if there is contamination or slippage. In a study of the ability of people to identify the range of a distant object, the investigators were unaware that some people have no depth perception. Therefore, most people had errors that were normally distributed with a small deviation, and the others had errors with a much larger standard deviation (Figure 9.1).

The people without depth perception are represented by the dashed curve. A point from the upper (or lower) region of this curve (**X**) appears as an outlier in the main curve shown in solid lines.

Slippage implies that the data may come from a normal distribution in which the mean is larger than the control mean by some factor. For example, Karl Pearson recorded cranial capacities of 17 skulls found in an archeological site (Barnett and Lewis, 1984). Sixteen of these ranged from 1230 to 1540 ccs, but one was 1630 ccs (Figure 9.2).

The value at 1630 ccs is an outlier. If it is an outlier, what might have been the cause? Did it come from a diseased subject, or did the site from which the skulls were retrieved contain skulls from two different species (Figure 9.3)?

Here the second species with a larger cranial capacity is represented by the dashed curve. An individual from the upper part of this curve (**X**) appears as an outlier from the primary curve in solid lines. Slippage may also occur when a chemical or physical process becomes distorted.

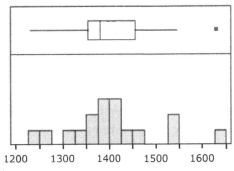

Figure 9.2 Cranial capacities.

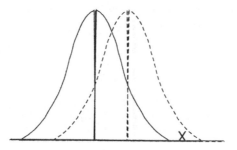

Figure 9.3 Slippage.

Robust Tests

Many tests are based on order statistics, one of the simplest being to use the median absolute deviation (MAD). The MAD (Chapter 3) is the median of the deviations from the median. In a normal distribution, there is a relationship among, MAD, standard deviation, and the interquartile distance (Wilcox, 1996).

$MAD \approx 0.6748\ \sigma$, so that $\sigma \approx 1.4826\ MAD$, and interquartile distance $\approx 2\ MAD$. From these relationships, X_i is unusually small if

$$\frac{0.6748(X_i - Median)}{MAD} < -1.28$$

and is unusually big if

$$\frac{0.6748(X_i - Median)}{MAD} > 1.28.$$

Dealing with Outliers

An outlier that is not due to an error requires careful consideration rather than exclusion based on a statistical test. Sometimes these outliers allow the investigator to develop new concepts. For example, in a study in which a low concentration of a gas is given to a group of people with normal lungs, all but one shows minimal changes in airway resistance but one subject had marked bronchoconstriction. Rather than discarding the data from this subject the investigator looks further, and finds that this subject has a medium-sized ventricular septal defect. This might lead to the hypothesis that children with congenital heart disease and a left-to-right shunt may have unusually reactive airways.

There are four ways of dealing with such an outlier. (1) Keep it in but use robust distribution-free methods of analysis; for example, using the median instead of the mean so that the size of the outlier has minimal effect. (2) Transform the data, for example, by logarithm or square root, to remove outliers. (3) Retain the outlier, and use conventional parametric analysis, accepting the loss of power that this will produce. (4) Omit the outlier, but report what you have done. Kruskal, an eminent statistician, wrote: "As to practice, I suggest that it is of great importance to preach the doctrine that apparent outliers should always be reported, even when one feels that their causes are known or when one rejects them for whatever good rule or reason. The immediate pressures of practical statistical analysis are almost uniformly in the direction of suppressing announcements of observations that do not fit the pattern; we must maintain a strong seawall against these pressures" (Barnett and Lewis, 1984). After all, if the observations do not fit the expected pattern, perhaps it is the expected pattern that is wrong.

EXTREME VALUES

Sometimes we wish to know how large or how small an extreme value may be. An engineer might want to know, when designing a bridge, what the highest water level might be, a level perhaps reached only once in a 100 years, or what the highest possible wind force could be. A hospital administrator might want to know the maximal number of hospital beds required in a severe influenza epidemic. Alternatively, the minimum breaking strain of a metal bar or a surgical suture is needed. It was this last problem as applied to cotton threads that was the starting point for Tippett's investigations of this subject. Subsequently, Fisher and particularly Gumbel (1891−1966) contributed to the field.

Consider the extreme high value. Some type of distribution needs to be assumed, based on prior knowledge. One common distribution for this purpose is the cumulative distribution function.

$F(y) = e^{-e^{-y}}$. In this equation, $F(y)$ is the probability of getting a value of y or less. If y = 3, then $F(y)$ is 0.9514, the probability of getting 3 or less.

This distribution is one of a family of distributions referred to as the exponential type; these include the exponential, chi-square, logistic, Weibull, and many others (Gumbel, 1958; Gumbel and Lieblein, 1954) (Chapter 8). To do the analysis, the **maximum** value in each of several members of a set is noted, and several sets are inspected; the sets may be rainfall per year, red cell diameter per sample of blood, number of patients with severe influenza per year, etc. These maximal values are ranked from smallest to largest, assigned ranks 1 to n, and then transformed into cumulative frequencies $P_i = i/(n + 1)$, where i is the rank of the ith observation starting from the smallest. The data are plotted on special extreme-value probability paper. Figure 9.4 shows an example using the largest size of a red blood cell from 14 blood samples selected from the data of Chen and Fung (1973).

Similar methods can be used to determine extreme minima. These are required in fatigue studies; for example, what is the lowest number of stress cycles will a prosthetic valve or an orthopedic prosthesis tolerate before breaking? (Freudenthal and Gumbel, 1954, 1953).

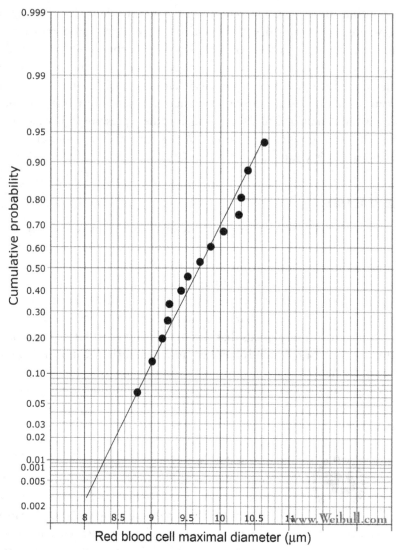

Figure 9.4 Extreme value of red cell diameters, measured in several samples each with 100 red blood cells. Ninety percent of samples have maximal red cell diameters <10.6 μm. Graph paper from http://www.reliasoft.com/pubs/paper_normal.pdf.

Graph papers for lognormal plots can be obtained online at http://www.reliasoft.com/pubs/paper_lognormal.pdf, http://www.printablepaper.net/, http://www.humboldt.edu/geology/for_download/graphpaper/4x3_cycle_log_bw.pdf, and http://www.printfreegraphpaper.com/. It is possible for the curves to be alinear and based on other distributions (Freudenthal and Gumbel, 1954), and then other functions and graph papers are needed. The appendix shows how these plots can be hand-generated.

APPENDIX

Professional statistics programs will produce extreme value diagrams, but they are easy to do by hand. Set out a table (below), based on the red blood cell data of Chen and Fung (1973).

Rank	Largest diameter (μm)	Cumulative probability $i/(1 + N)$
1	8.8	0.0667
2	9	0.1333
3	9.15	0.2
4	9.24	0.2667
5	9.28	0.3333
6	9.45	0.4
7	9.52	0.4667
8	9.7	0.5333
9	9.85	0.6
10	10.05	0.6667
11	10.23	0.7333
12	10.3	0.8
13	10.4	0.8667
14	10.65	0.9333

Then construct Figures 9.5 as recommended by Santner (1973): Draw two parallel horizontal lines as shown below.

1. Label the lower one "Reduced variate" and mark it off in a linear scale from −2 to 6. This reduced variate is in standard form, with location parameter μ = 0, and scale parameter β = 1, much like the z transform. In this form, on the reduced variate scale

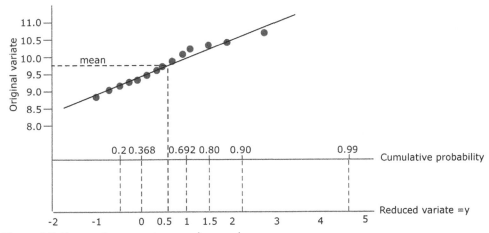

Figure 9.5 How to draw an extreme value graph.

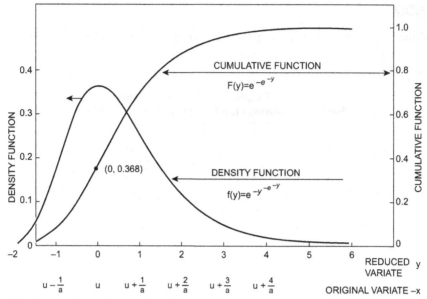

Figure 9.6 Figure 1 from Santner (1973). *(Reproduced with permission from the US Environmental Protection Agency.)*

the mode is 0, the mean is 0.577, and the standard deviation of y is 1.28255. Original values can be recalculated (Santner, 1973).

2. Using the formula $F(y) = e^{-e^{-y}}$ or Figure 1 in Santner (Figure 9.6), add cumulative probability units to the upper line. The vertical dashed lines show corresponding values.

3. Add a suitable original scale to the vertical axis (arithmetic or logarithmic as appropriate), and then plot the original values against the cumulative probabilities.

REFERENCES

Barnett, V., Lewis, T., 1984. Outliers in Statistical Data. John Wiley & Sons, New York.
Chen, P.C., Fung, Y.C., 1973. Extreme-value statistics of human red blood cells. Microvasc. Res. 6, 32–43.
Freudenthal, A.M., Gumbel, E.J., 1953. On the statistical interpretation of fatigue tests. Proc. R. Soc. A 216, 309–332.
Freudenthal, A.M., Gumbel, E.J., 1954. Minimum life in fatigue. J. Am. Stat. Assoc. 49, 575–597.
Grubbs, F.E., 1969. Procedures for identifying outlying observations in samples. Technometrics 11, 1–21.
Gumbel, E.J., 1958. Statistics of Extremes. Dover Publications, Inc., Mineola, NY.
Gumbel, F.J., Lieblein, J., 1954. Some applications of extreme value methods. Am. Stat. 8, 14–17.
Hubert, M., Vandervieren, E., 2008. An adjusted boxplot for skewed distributions. Comput. Stat. Data Anal. 52, 5186–5201.
Prescott, P., 1979. Critical values for a sequential test for many outliers. Appl. Stat. 28, 36–39.
Rosner, B., 1977. Percentage points for the RST many outliers. Technometrics 19, 307–312.
Rosner, B., 1995. Fundamentals of Biostatistics. Duxbury Press, New York.

Santner, J.F., 1973. An Introduction to Gumbel, or Extreme-Value Probability Paper (Online). U.S. Environmental Protection Agency, Cincinnati, OH 45268. http://nepis.epa.gov/Exe/ZyNET.exe/900N0900.TXT?ZyActionD=ZyDocument&Client=EPA&Index=Prior+to+1976&Docs=&Query=&Time=&EndTime=&SearchMethod=1&TocRestrict=n&Toc=&TocEntry=&QField=&QFieldYear=&QFieldMonth=&QFieldDay=&IntQFieldOp=0&ExtQFieldOp=0&XmlQuery=&File=D%3A%5Czyfiles%5CIndex%20Data%5C70thru75%5CTxt%5C00000006%5C900N0900.txt&User=ANONYMOUS&Password=anonymous&SortMethod=h%7C-&MaximumDocuments=1&FuzzyDegree=0&ImageQuality=r75g8/r75g8/x150y150g16/i425&Display=p%7Cf&DefSeekPage=x&SearchBack=ZyActionL&Back=ZyActionS&BackDesc=Results%20page&MaximumPages=1&ZyEntry=1&SeekPage=x&ZyPURL.

Tukey, J.W., 1977. Exploratory Data Analysis. Addison-Wesley Publishing Co, Menlo Park, CA.

Wilcox, R.R., 1996. Statistics for the Social Sciences. Academic Press, San Diego.

PART 3

Hypothesis Testing

CHAPTER 10

Hypothesis Testing: The Null Hypothesis, Significance, and Type I Error

Contents

HYPOTHESES

Statistical inference is often based on a test of significance, "a procedure by which one determines the degree to which collected data are consistent with a specific hypothesis…" (Matthews and Farewell, 1996). Hypotheses may be specific, for example, that the slope relating two variables is 1, the line of identity. More often the hypothesis is that two (or more) sample statistics could have been drawn from the same population. The principles to be discussed are illustrated by referring to sample and population means, but apply equally to all other types of statistics. This is the null hypothesis or H_0, and if it is accepted then we believe that the two samples could have come from the same population.

If we choose to reject the null hypothesis, then there is an alternative hypothesis, H_A, that has three forms:

1. $\overline{X_1} \neq \overline{X_2}$; $\overline{X_1}$; and $\overline{X_2}$ come from different populations and $\overline{X_1}$ is bigger or smaller than $\overline{X_2}$.
2. $\overline{X_1} < \overline{X_2}$; $\overline{X_1}$; and $\overline{X_2}$ come from different populations and $\overline{X_1}$ is smaller than $\overline{X_2}$.
3. $\overline{X_1} > \overline{X_2}$; $\overline{X_1}$; and $\overline{X_2}$ come from different populations and $\overline{X_1}$ is bigger than $\overline{X_2}$.

SIGNIFICANCE

How do we make the decision to accept or reject the null hypothesis? Fisher recommended defining the probability that a particular difference between two means allowed us to reject the null hypothesis of no difference. A decision of this sort has many implications, so that to make it as certain as possible we try to minimize the chances of rejecting the null hypothesis (of no difference) when it is actually correct. This is known as a Type I error,

For a list of all websites referred to in this chapter, as clickable links, see the book companion website: www.booksite.elsevier.com/9780128023877.

Biostatistics for Medical and Biomedical Practitioners
http://dx.doi.org/10.1016/B978-0-12-802387-7.00010-X

symbolized by α. The value of α is assigned a probability (p or P) that is commonly termed "significance."

Fisher's proposal was sensible, but the pendulum has swung the other way, and investigators draw conclusions based on an inadequate understanding of what Fisher really intended. As proposed by Fisher, the statistical test is only one of the factors allowing us to decide whether or not to reject the null hypothesis. The magnitude of the difference and the plausibility of the hypothesis are other important factors. Fisher thus introduced a degree of subjectivity into the assessment, something quite the opposite of what happens when we slavishly accept a given level of significance. Fisher wrote: "If p is between 0.1 and 0.9 there is no reason to suspect the hypothesis tested. If it is below 0.02 it is strongly indicated that the hypothesis fails to account for the whole of the facts. We shall not often be led astray if we draw a conventional line at 0.05 and consider that higher values of χ^2 indicate a real discrepancy" (Fisher, 1956). He was here referring to the null hypothesis. That he was not rigid in his approach is shown by his statement that "the state of opinion derived from a test of significance is provisional, and capable, not only of confirmation, but of revision" and "A test of significance… is intended to aid the process of learning by observational experience" (Fisher, 1956). In another publication, cited by Curran-Everett (2009), Fisher wrote: "we prefer it, draw the line at one in fifty (the 2 per cent. point), or one in a hundred (the 1 per cent. point). Personally, the writer prefers to set a low standard of significance at the 5 per cent. point, and ignore entirely all results which fail to reach this level. A scientific fact should be regarded as experimentally established only if a properly designed experiment rarely fails to give this level of significance."

Nothing can put this point better than the remarks of John Tukey (1991): "The worst, i.e., most dangerous feature of 'accepting the null hypothesis' is the giving up of explicit uncertainty: the attempt to paint with only the black of perfect equality and the white of demonstrated direction of inequality. Mathematics can sometimes be put in such black-and-white terms, but our knowledge or belief about the external world never can.

The black of 'accept the null hypothesis' is far too black. It treats 'between −101 and +1,' 'between −101 and +101,' and 'between −1 and +1' all alike, when their practical meanings are often very, very different.

The white of demonstrated direction of inequality is too white. On its face, it treats 'between +1 and +101,' 'between+1 and +3,' and 'between +99 and +101' as if they were the same when their practical meaning is quite different."

He continued: "Long ago, Fisher (1926, foot of page 504) recognized that truly solid knowledge did not come from analyzing a single experiment—even when that gave a confident direction with a very, very small error rate, like one in a million—but rather that solid knowledge came from a demonstrated ability to repeat experiments, each of which showed confident direction at a reasonable error rate, like 5%. This is unhappy for the investigator who would like to settle things once and for all, but consistent with the best accounts we have of scientific method, which emphasize repetition, preferably under varied circumstances."

An example of this caveat was reported by Crease (2010) in discussing the search for dark matter by astrophysicists. Physicists collect over time the outputs from a detector displayed in different energy levels (bins). If one particular bin shows an increased number of hits compared to what was expected at that energy level, it may provide evidence for a new particle. In one such experiment, the DAMA/LIBRA experiment at the Gran Sasso National Laboratory in Italy, the excess of energy in a particular bin had a confidence level of 8.2σ. This indicates a very low probability of falsely rejecting the null hypothesis, considering that 5σ has a probability of 3.0018676e-7. Nevertheless, subsequent experiments failed to confirm this finding.

As a corollary to this, we cannot ignore prior probabilities when assessing the results of a study. Millard (Borenstein et al., 2009) provided an example by citing a report from The Guardian newspaper at http://www.guardian.co.uk/football/2010/jul/12/paul-psychic-octopus-wins-world-cup about the ability of an octopus named Paul who in eight successive years correctly predicted the winner of the World Cup (soccer). Although the probability of this occurring by chance alone was $1/256 = 0.0039$, to draw the conclusion that the octopus was able to predict the results of a soccer match defies credibility, no matter what the P value was.

Ioannidis (2005) published a provocative article entitled "Why most published research findings are false." He pointed out that when the prior probability of a relationship is low (and this is true for many relationships) a value of $P < 0.05$ for the Type I error α would almost certainly lead to an exaggerated tendency to reject the null hypothesis. From his analysis he set out some important corollaries, including the following:

1. The smaller the size of the studies conducted in a scientific field, the less likely the research findings are to be true.
2. The smaller the effect sizes in a scientific field, the less likely the research findings are to be true.
3. The greater the financial and other interests and prejudices in a scientific field, the less likely the research findings are to be true. Although this is an ethical and not a statistical matter, the bias is so pervasive (Chapter 2) that we should be cautious in rejecting the null hypothesis based on a borderline value of 0.05 for the Type I error.

Schuemie et al. (2014) introduced an empirical calibration to correct the error, and estimated that up to 54% of tests deemed significant at the 0.05 level were actually not in favor of rejecting the null hypothesis. The exact proportion of erroneous statistical conclusions is disputed (see the Symposium in the journal "Biostatistics," volume 15, issue 1, 2014), but it is almost certainly much greater than 5%. This bias has recently been emphasized (Colqhoun, 2014) who showed that the Type I error of 5% now in vogue was more of the order of 36%, and that to keep it below 5% one should use a 3 sigma deviation from the mean, not 2 sigma as is now used.

Sterne and Davey Smith (2001) agreed that the smaller the value of P, the less the chance of a Type I error, but they (along with many others), regarded 0.05 as unsafe per se, and preferred to see a value of $P < 0.001$ for safety. Figure 10.1 summarizes their view.

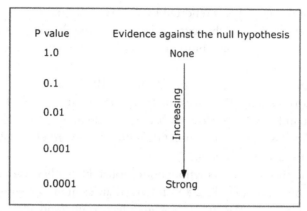

Figure 10.1 Degree of evidence against null hypothesis. *(Based on Sterne and Davey Smith (2001).)*

It is commonplace to see in the Methods section of a scientific publication the phrase: "Statistical significance was set at $P < 0.05$." All that this means is that the reader is given the user's definition of the term "statistical significance" and little of substance is provided. It would be more useful to abandon the term "statistical significance" and provide the reader with important information such as the exact P value *and* the confidence limits of the mean or other relevant parameter.

The value of $\alpha = 0.05$ is arbitrary, and values of 0.01 or 0.10 may be used. Much of the time, however, we wish to evaluate how much uncertainty there is in rejecting the null hypothesis, and it is preferable to give the exact P value, whether it be 0.036 or 0.12, and the confidence limits associated with it, and do not even need to mention the term "significant" (Colquhoun, 1971). In fact, quotations from statisticians indicate the unpopularity of the current usage of the term "statistical significance":

...it is better to regard the level of significance as a measure of the strength of the evidence against the null hypothesis rather than showing whether the data are significant or not at a certain level.

Sterne and Davey Smith (2001)

...the function of significance tests is to prevent you from making a fool of yourself, and not to make unpublishable results publishable.

Colquhoun (1971)

Statistical "significance" by itself is not a rational basis for action.

Deming (1943)

In biologic experimental work, for instance, a.... common abuse is to use a statistical test to try to "prove" a hypothesis...... The scandal is that the "significant" results are published as though they had meaning.

Feller (1969)

Because of these and other caveats, it is better to treat p values as nothing more than useful exploratory tools or measures of surprise. In any search for new physics, a small p value should only be seen as a first step in the interpretation of the data, to be followed by a serious investigation of an alternative hypothesis. Only by showing that the latter provides a better explanation of the observations than the null hypothesis can one make a convincing case for discovery.

Demortier (2008)

P values of 0.036, 0.047, or 0.063 are all important pieces of information, and an arbitrary designation of significance may conceal information. As the sports commentator Vin Scully remarked: "Statistics are used much like a drunk uses a lamppost: for support, not illumination."

A final point to consider was raised by Binder (1963), who wrote "It is surely apparent that anyone who wants to obtain a significant difference enough can obtain one—if his only consideration is obtaining that significant difference." (Significance can always be attained by a large enough sample size—see Chapter 11.)

The apparent importance of 0.05 and 0.01 was in part due to the lack of computing facilities in the 1930s. Statistical tables were difficult and expensive to produce, so that initially only the 0.05 and 0.01 values were provided for certain tests (Barnard, 1992).

In practice, the 0.05 value of P is used in at least two ways. It may be used as a critical value for making a decision by deductive inference to accept or reject the null hypothesis. If an investigator is testing 500 chemical agents for their ability to reduce bacterial growth or enzyme activity, there is no doubt about the population mean value that is the control value of growth. What the investigator seeks are those agents worth pursuing in more detail. Therefore in a large batch of experiments, the 0.05 cutoff allows the investigator to concentrate on the more promising agents, knowing that less than 5% of the time the null hypothesis will be rejected falsely (Type I error). Furthermore, although the null hypothesis might not be true, the difference is unlikely to be important. In this usage there are multiple samples, and no inverse logic is used to determine a population mean. However, in most experiments investigators use P as support for a hypothesis, and the exact value of P does not have the same critical importance.

In summary, those who understand statistical methods and philosophy attach only minor importance to the calculated P values, whereas those who merely make the calculations and do not think about them overestimate their importance. Recently the American Psychological Association endorsed this approach, stating: "Estimation based on effect sizes, confidence intervals, and meta-analysis usually provides a more informative analysis of empirical results than does statistical significance testing, which has long been the conventional choice in psychology" (Cumming et al., 2011).

This cautious approach to deciding about statistical significance has even been endorsed by the US Supreme Court (Ziliak, 2011). A pharmaceutical company was sued for failing to warn investors about adverse effects that were not statistically significant. The Supreme Court found on behalf of the plaintiffs. At one point in the judgment Justice Sotomayor wrote:

"… argument rests on the premise that statistical significance is the only reliable evidence of causation. This premise is flawed," and again "medical professionals and researchers do not limit the data they consider to the results of randomized clinical trials or to statistically significant evidence…." The FDA similarly does not limit the evidence it considers for purposes of assessing causation and taking regulatory action to statistically significant data. In assessing the safety risk posed by a product, the FDA considers factors such as "strength of the association," "temporal relationship of product use and the event," "consistency of findings across available data sources," "evidence of a dose-response for the effect," "biologic plausibility," "seriousness of the event relative to the disease being treated," "potential to mitigate the risk in the population," "feasibility of further study using observational or controlled clinical study designs," and "degree of benefit the product provides, including availability of other therapies." …[The FDA] "does not apply any single metric for determining when additional inquiry or action is necessary."

More than a P value is required in assessing a hypothesis.

REFERENCES

Barnard, G.A., 1992. Review of statistical inference and analysis: selected correspondence of R. A. Fisher by J T Bennett. Stat. Sci. 7, 5—12.

Binder, A., 1963. Further considerations on testing the null hypothesis and the strategy and tactics of investigating theoretical models. Psychol. Rev. 70, 107—115.

Borenstein, M., Hedges, L.V., Higgins, J.P.T., et al., 2009. Introduction to Meta-analysis. John Wiley & Sons, Chichester, England.

Colquhoun, D., 1971. Lectures on Biostatistics. Clarendon Press, Oxford.

Colqhoun, D., 2014. An investigation of the false discovery rate and the misinterpetation of P values. R. Soc. Open. Sci. 1, 140216. http://dx.doi.org/10.1098/rsos.140216.

Crease, R.P., 2010. Discovery With Statistics [Online]. Available: http://physicsworld.com/cws/article/indepth/43309.

Cumming, G., Fidler, F., Kalinowski, P., et al., 2011. The statistical recommendations of the American Psychological Association Publication Manual: effect sizes, confidence intervals, and meta-analysis. Aust. J. Psychol. 12 Oct ed.

Curran-Everett, D., 2009. Explorations in statistics: hypothesis tests and P values. Adv. Physiol. Educ. 33, 81—86.

Deming, W.E., 1943. Statistical Adjustment of Data. John Wiley & Sons, Inc, New York.

Demortier, L., 2008. P values and nuisance parameters. In: Prosper, H.B., Lyons, L., De Roeck, A. (Eds.), PHYSTAT LHC Workshop on Statistical Issues for LHC Physics, 2007. CERN, Geneva.

Feller, W., 1969. Are life scientists overawed by statistics? Sci. Res. 4, 24—29.

Fisher, R.A., 1956. Statistical Methods and Scientific Inference. Oliver and Boyd, Edinburgh.

Ioannidis, J.P., 2005. Why most published research findings are false. PLoS Med. 2, e124.

Matthews, D.E., Farewell, V.T., 1996. Using and Understanding Medical Statistics. Karger, Basel.

Schuemie, M.J., Ryan, P.B., Dumouchel, W., et al., 2014. Interpreting observational studies: why empirical calibration is needed to correct p-values. Stat. Med. 33, 209—218.

Sterne, J.A., Davey Smith, G., 2001. Sifting the evidence-what's wrong with significance tests? BMJ 322, 226—231.

Tukey, J.W., 1991. The philosophy of multiple comparisons. Stat. Sci. 6, 1.

Ziliak, S.T., 2011. Matrixx v. Siracusano and Student v. Fisher. Statistical significance on trial. Significance 8, 131—134.

CHAPTER 11

Hypothesis Testing: Sample Size, Effect Size, Power, and Type II Errors

Contents

BASIC CONCEPTS

Statistical Power

If the null hypothesis is rejected when it is true, we have committed a Type I error, with a probability symbolized by α. On the other hand, accepting the null hypothesis of no difference between the two means if they really are from different populations produces a Type II error with a probability symbolized by β.

Consider two populations of means, each population having different grand means, but the normal curves characterizing the distributions of those means overlap (Figure 11.1).

If H_0 is true (i.e., that the two means come from the same population), then a single sample mean falling to the right of the heavy vertical line is unlikely and can lead to rejection of the null hypothesis; the probability of falsely rejecting the null hypothesis is the Type I error, symbolized by α. If, however, H_A is true, as shown in the lower part of the diagram, then more than 50% of the time the single sample mean will fall to the left of the heavy vertical line and the null hypothesis would not be rejected. This is the Type II error. The chance of making a Type II error (the probability of accepting the null hypothesis if it is false) is symbolized by β. If the chances of making a Type II error are 0.67, then the chances of not making a Type II error are $1 - 0.67 = 0.33$; there is a 33% probability of making the correct assumption that there are two different groups.

For a list of all websites referred to in this chapter, as clickable links, see the book companion website: www.booksite.elsevier.com/9780128023877.

Biostatistics for Medical and Biomedical Practitioners
http://dx.doi.org/10.1016/B978-0-12-802387-7.00011-1

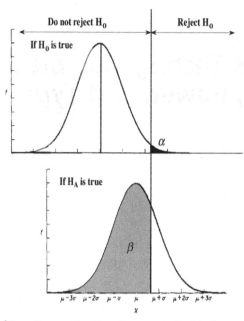

Figure 11.1 Illustration of Type II error. The Type I error α is the black area in the upper panel and is constant and determined by the investigator. The Type II error β is grey-shaded in the lower panel, and varies with the value of H_A.

This value, $1 - \beta$, is known as the power of the test, that is, its ability to correctly reject the null hypothesis. The power is lowest when the means are close together and highest when they are farthest apart (Figure 11.2).

In this diagram A is a reference curve showing the distribution of means of samples of size N from a population. B is a similar curve derived from means of samples also of size N from a different population. The black triangle indicates the upper tail that includes 0.025 of the A distribution. A decision to accept or reject the null hypothesis that the mean of B differs from the mean of A depends on whether a *single sample mean* from B falls to the right (reject null hypothesis and state that there are probably two different distributions) or left (do not reject null hypothesis that the sample comes from the A distribution) of the shaded area.

In the upper panel, the two distribution means are close together, and there is about a 90% chance of accepting the null hypothesis as shown by the grey-shaded marking of curve B. Because the null hypothesis is actually wrong, we have committed a Type II error with a probability of about 0.9. In the middle panel, with the two distribution means farther apart, about two-thirds of the B samples fall to the left of the decision line, so that the chances of making a Type II error are about 0.67. In the bottom panel, with the distribution means far apart, there is only a 0.025 chance that the sample from B will be considered as coming from the A distribution, that is, the Type II error is about 0.025.

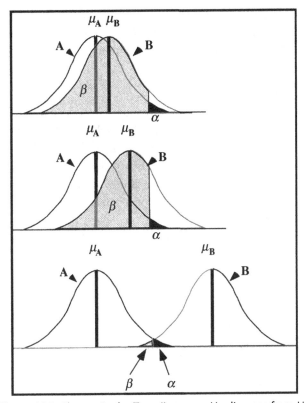

Figure 11.2 Change in the Type II error as H_A diverges from H_0.

Effect Size

As shown in Figure 11.2, the power of the test is closely related to the difference between the means, also known as the effect size. The difference might be between the two sample means, or one sample mean and a population mean. The effect size may be classified as:

1. Absolute effect size, sometimes symbolized as Δ. If in treating a group of patients with hypertension the pressure falls by an average of 10 mm Hg, then $\Delta = 10$ mm Hg. What we do with the information depends on how important that effect size is. It is unlikely that a pharmaceutical company would spend millions of dollars to produce a new antihypertensive drug with an effect size of 3 mm Hg, but they might do so for an effect size of 15 mm Hg.

2. Relative effect size, usually symbolized as δ, is the actual effect size relative to the standard deviation. Therefore, $\delta = \frac{\Delta}{\sigma}$, where σ is a general estimate of variability that we approximate by the sample values. (Not all texts use these symbols as defined above, and sometimes δ represents the absolute difference.) Relative effect size is used in determining how many measurements or subjects will be needed for an adequate study (see below).

There are several slightly different formulas for calculating the relative effect size that takes into account the variability of the two (or more) groups that are to be compared. Cohen's d and Hedges' g are the two most often used (Durlak, 2009).

Calculation of Power

We can calculate the power for any values of μ and $\overline{X}$ if we know N and an estimate of σ derived from the sample standard deviation s. Consider the heights of adult European males in the eighteenth century (Komlos and Cinnirella, 2005) with a mean of $66''$ and a standard deviation of $4.47''$ (curve C in Figure 11.3). We draw at random a group of 30 subjects today and wish to determine if their mean height is consistent with our previous population sample; this distribution of means is curve E shown in Figure 11.3.

The shaded area to the right of the vertical line X_c at $1.96 s_{\overline{X}}$ represents $\alpha/2$, or 0.025 of the area under curve C, and represents the α error. Reject the null hypothesis with $\alpha = 0.05$ if

$$z - \frac{\overline{X} - \mu}{s_{\overline{X}}} \geq 1.96.$$

This can be rearranged to give

$$\overline{X} - \mu > z_{\alpha/2}\, s_{\overline{X}}.$$

Rearrangement and substitution give

$$\overline{X} \geq 1.96 \times \frac{4.47}{\sqrt{30}} + 66 \quad \text{or} \quad \overline{X} \geq 67.60.$$

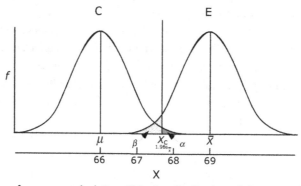

Figure 11.3 Diagram for power calculation. C is the distribution of the control population means around a "population" mean $\mu = 66$, E is the distribution of our sample means around a single observed sample mean $\overline{X} = 69$. The shaded area to the right of X_c for the C distribution (H$_0$) is the significance level α, the grey-shaded area to the left of X_c is the Type II or β error, and the total area to the right of X_c for the E distribution (H$_A$) is the power $1 - \beta$.

Therefore any mean value for height in the series of 30 subjects greater than a critical value of $67.60''$ leads to rejection of the null hypothesis, and we conclude that heights of adult males today are probably greater than $66''$.

Now consider what happens if H_A is true. The grey-shaded area to the left of the critical line X_c is the β error, and this is given by $1 -$ area under curve E to the right of X_c. We can calculate this error if we know how many standard error units $\overline{X}$ is from μ.

Consider the true mean difference $\overline{X} - \mu$:

$$\delta = \frac{\overline{X} - \mu}{\frac{s}{\sqrt{N}}} = \frac{\overline{X} - 66}{\frac{4.47}{\sqrt{30}}} = \frac{\overline{X} - 66}{0.8161}.$$

Therefore if $\overline{X}$ is 69, the above equation becomes

$$\delta = \frac{69 - 66}{0.8161} = 3.676.$$

In other words, if H_A is true, a mean value of $69''$ is 3.676 standard errors from the "population" mean of $66''$. But X_c is 1.96 standard errors from $66''$, so the area between X_c and $69''$ is represented by $z = 3.676 - 1.96 = 1.716$. This is z_b, which represents how many standard error units X_c is below $\overline{X}$. This area referred to $z = 1.716$ is 0.0431. Therefore if H_A, the sample mean of $69''$, is true, there is 0.0431 chance of rejecting the alternative hypothesis. The power is $1 - \beta = 0.9568$.

More generally,

$$z_\beta = \delta - z_\alpha.$$

Simplify the calculation by using the following relationship:

$$z_\beta = \delta - z_\alpha = \frac{\overline{X} - \mu}{\frac{s}{\sqrt{N}}} - \frac{X_c - \mu}{\frac{s}{\sqrt{N}}} = \frac{\overline{X} - X_c}{\frac{s}{\sqrt{N}}}$$

Thus, $z_\beta = \frac{69 - 67.6}{0.8161} = 1.7155$, as shown above (with slight difference due to rounding off).

This discussion implies using a two-tailed test for z, so that $z = 1.96$ includes 0.025 of the area under curve C at each end. To use a one-tailed test with 0.05 of the area under curve C at one end, use $z = 1.645$ to calculate the β error. (If the sample size is <100, use the t table instead of the z table, but as long as $N > 10$ the error is under 0.01 (Zar, 2010).) It is not worth worrying about this small error in view of the fact that we are guessing the standard deviation.

If we compare two independent samples, then the standardized deviation δ is

$$\frac{\overline{X_1} - \overline{X_2}}{\sqrt{\frac{2\sigma^2}{N}}},$$

and proceed as before.

How can we reduce the Type II error? For a given biological system the difference between the mean of the two populations is determined by the system and not subject to manipulation, except perhaps by selecting subgroups and increasing homogeneity. What we can do is to increase the sample size, with the effect shown in Figure 11.4.

There remains the question of how much to increase the sample size so that the power of the test is high. In theory we would like a power of 0.9, but in practice often settle for 0.8. Whether we can achieve this increased sample size depends on the availability of samples, and the cost and manpower needed to obtain them. In principle, solve the equation $t_{0.05} = \frac{\overline{X_1} - \overline{X_2}}{\frac{s_{\overline{X_1} - \overline{X_2}}}{\sqrt{N}}}$ (or whatever other value we want for α) for N by assigning the critical value of t, the difference between the means (the desired effect size), and the standard deviation. From our knowledge of previous studies in a particular field or a pilot study we guess the standard deviation of the population. This can be wrong, as a result of misleading sample size calculations. It is therefore best to take any sample size calculations as only approximations and wise to plan for a larger sample size (Schulz and Grimes, 2005).

With an estimated standard deviation decide what difference between the means would be important, and calculate the relative effect size $\delta = \frac{\overline{X_1} - \overline{X_2}}{s}$. Use the population standard deviation, not the standard deviation of the mean.

Then use tables in which the number of subjects is listed for given values of δ, α, and $1 - \beta$ (Beyer, 1966; Cohen, 1988; Kraemer, 1988). Some publications give

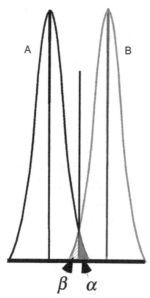

Figure 11.4 Effect of markedly increasing the sample size. For a mean difference similar to that in the middle panel of Figure 11.3, the Type II error has been reduced from 0.67 to 0.025.

nomograms to determine these numbers (Gore and Altman, 1982). An excellent discussion with examples is given by DiMaggio (DiMaggio, 2012). Alternatively, there are computer programs to make the calculation. An extensive interactive freeware program is termed G*Power at http://www.psycho.uni-duesseldorf.de/abteilungen/aap/gpower3/download-and-register (Faul et al., 2007; G*Power) and is very useful for calculating power for all types of statistical tests. Power calculations in the protocol are required by most grant agencies to show that the proposed study is feasible in terms of subjects, time, and money. Another extensive program (Macintosh and Windows) is available at http://biostat.mc.vanderbilt.edu/wiki/Main/PowerSampleSize. Two programs that cover a wide range of statistical tests are http://www.sample-size.net and http://www.powerandsamplesize.com. Other simpler programs online are http://www.biomath.info/power/index.htm, <http://www.statisticalsolutions.net/pss_calc.php>.

Lehr (1992) pointed out that for $\alpha = 0.05$, and power $(1 - \beta) = 0.80$, sample size can be closely approximated by a simple relationship

$$n = \frac{ks^2}{\delta^2},$$

where $k = 8$ for a paired t-test and 16 for an unpaired t-test (see below) and δ is the difference to be detected (effect size). This is very close to the exact number from the more complex calculation, and seeing that we have to guess the value of s, a simple formula seems preferable. For other values of α and β there is a simple table (Table 11.1).

Table 11.1 Values of k for the Lehr equation

Power $1 - \beta$	α (Two samples)			α (One sample)
	0.01	0.05	0.10	0.05
0.80	23.5	16	12.5	8
0.90	30	21	17.5	11
0.95	36	26	22	13
0.975		31		16

Problem 11.1
Determine the sample sizes needed for determining a mean change in the myocardial blood flow from 1 to 1.3 ml/g min (paired samples) if the standard deviation is 0.4 with $\alpha = 0.05$ and power of 0.8, 0.85, or 0.9.

Problem 11.2
Repeat the calculations if the standard deviation is 0.64 ml/g min.

The Type I error of falsely rejecting the null hypothesis, as previously stated, has nothing to do with the importance of any difference, but is more an issue of consistency of data and the comfort that we feel in deciding to reject the null hypothesis. The degree of certainty is under our control, and we can make the requirement as stringent as we please. On the other hand, the Type II error is more insidious. If we do not have enough power and decide to accept the null hypothesis we may neglect a difference that might be important. If an intervention doubles flow to an ischemic region of the myocardium but because of lack of power of the test we cannot reasonably reject the null hypothesis of no effect, we might be induced to ignore a very useful intervention. That is why if we cannot reject the null hypothesis it is better to regard the effect of the intervention as unproven rather than nonexistent. In fact, Williams et al. (1997) found that failure to achieve a high enough power was the most common statistical error made in publications in the *American Journal of Physiology*, often because investigators were unaware of the need to assess the power of their negative results. Similar failures to achieve adequate power have been reported in many other fields and journals (Burback et al., 1999; Dimick et al., 2001; Freedman et al., 2001; Moher et al., 1994; Weaver et al., 2004; Yusuf et al., 1985). This subject is so important that readers should also go to excellent explanatory writings by Berkowitz that can be downloaded from <www.columbia.edu/~mvp19/RMC/M6/M6.doc>.

A major study drawing attention to this problem in Medicine was by Freiman et al. (1978) who examined 71 randomized trials that compared the effects of two drugs or treatments and concluded that there was no statistically significant difference between their effects (Figure 11.5).

They showed that in many of those studies the responses were quite large, but the sample sizes were too small to show a 25% difference between the two treatments, let alone a 50% difference between them. In some instances this led the investigators to discontinue studying the new treatment and to conclude that it was of no benefit. This is undesirable; a 25% improved cure rate in any disease would be very welcome.

It is possible to make the Type I error as small as you like, for example, reducing it from 0.05 to 0.01 (or even smaller) so that the risk of falsely rejecting the null hypothesis becomes very small indeed. However, the cost of making the Type I error smaller is making the Type II error bigger (Figure 11.6).

If for curve C the Type I error is set at 0.05, with 0.025 in each tail (solid-shaded area), then the Type II error is shown by the grey-shaded area for curve E. If the Type I error is made 0.01, with 0.005 in each tail of curve C, then the Type II error has increased to include the horizontally shaded area under curve E.

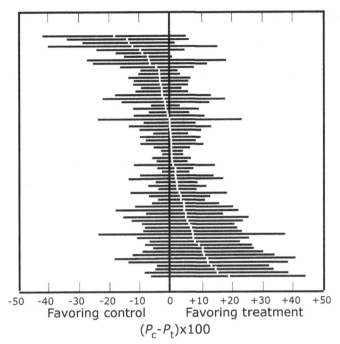

Figure 11.5 Trials comparing two therapeutic agents. Modified from Freiman et al. by arranging mean differences in order. Each horizontal line represents one clinical trial. The white central dot is the mean and the black bars demarcate 90% confidence limits. The thick vertical black line indicates no difference. Because the confidence limits include zero difference, P is greater than 0.05 in all these tests. Almost all the mean differences (effect size) are <15%.

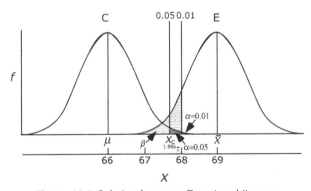

Figure 11.6 Relation between Type I and II errors.

Post hoc Power Analysis

Power analysis may be used in several ways. It is best used in planning experiments and is now required by most grant agencies. The investigator decides on the effect size desired, a value for the Type I error α (usually 0.05), and a value for the power that is $1 - \beta$, the Type II error and is usually set at 0.8—0.9. Then the number to be used is determined from tables or programs. These numbers are provisional, depending on preliminary observations of means and standard deviations. Julious and Owen (2006) observed that if a variance obtained in a previous study was based on small sample sizes and used as if it were the population variance, its use in the standard formulas could underestimate the future sample size needed to achieve a given power. They provide tables of corrections, but in general it is safe to increase the predicted sample size by about 20—30%. If some patients or animals are expected to leave the study prematurely, even bigger numbers will be needed. Sometimes, however, there are no previous studies to provide data, and a pilot study might need to be done. A sample size of 12 in each group may be adequate (Julious, 2005; van Belle, 2002).

How should we think about results in which the null hypothesis could not be rejected, with $\alpha > 0.05$, but with a sample size too small to provide adequate power? Many statistical programs allow post hoc calculations of power, but this may not be the best way to assess the data (Kraemer, 1988; Sterne et al., 2001; Williams et al., 1997). In fact, by definition a P value of >0.05 indicates that the power was too low to reject the null hypothesis for that effect size. Investigators have argued that a "nonsignificant" result indicates either too small a standardized difference or too small a sample *size*, and results might or might not be important. In place of the post hoc power analysis, Walters (2009) suggested using confidence intervals to help distinguish statistical significance from clinical importance (Figure 11.7).

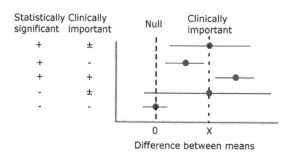

Figure 11.7 Distinction between statistical significance and importance, showing a useful way of evaluating a "nonsignificant" result by plotting means and confidence limits. + yes; − no; ± possible.

Based on figure published by Walters (2009). Any one of these rows presents information more useful than merely stating that the power was low.

ADVANCED AND ALTERNATIVE CONCEPTS

Hypothesis Testing and Maximum Likelihood; The Bayes Factor

Fisher considered only the null hypothesis, but if the null hypothesis is rejected an alternative hypothesis must be considered (Neyman and Pearson, 1928). The philosophical differences between these two approaches are discussed by Goodman (Goodman, 1993; Goodman and Royall, 1988; Goodman, 1999) who emphasized that Fisher was not using the P value to indicate the area beyond a critical value in which future results from that population would fall. He was interested in that single measurement. Now it is true that the single sample on which we base our decision to accept or reject the null hypothesis is either from the control population or else from another population. What the rest of the area under the curve from that point out to infinity has no real meaning to us. Whether the mean of another sample from the population being examined will be close to or far from the mean of the first sample is unknown. The best that we can do is to make a statement of belief that the sample does or does not come from the control population. On the other hand, we can be more comfortable if we can compare our belief that the sample comes from the control population with our belief that it comes from another specified population.

To illustrate this point, Goodman discusses the subject of mathematical likelihood. Consider Figure 11.8 that features the upper two panels of Figure 11.2.

The Bayes factor, also known as the likelihood ratio, is the ratio:

$$\frac{\text{Probability of data (null hypothesis)}}{\text{Probability of data (alternative hypothesis)}}$$

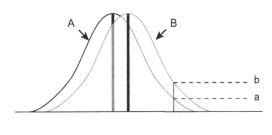

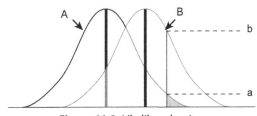

Figure 11.8 Likelihood ratios.

In the upper panel, with the two means close together, the probability of "a" is about 50% the probability of "b." The exact probability is used, not the area beyond the critical value. In the lower panel, "a" is about 16% of "b." Curve B has a better likelihood of being correct in the lower panel, even though in terms of a Type I error the null hypothesis would not be rejected. The calculations of likelihood are presented in Goodman's article.

REFERENCES

Beyer, W.H., 1966. Handbook of Tables for Probability and Statistics. The Chemical Rubber Company, Cleveland, OH.

Burback, D., Molnar, F.J., St John, P., et al., 1999. Key methodological features of randomized controlled trials of Alzheimer's disease therapy. Minimal clinically important difference, sample size and trial duration. Dement. Geriatr. Cogn. Dis. 10, 534–540.

Cohen, J., 1988. Statistical Power Analysis for Behavioral Sciences. Lawrence Erlbaum Associates, Hillsdale, NJ.

DiMaggio, C., 2012. http://www.columbia.edu/~cjd11/charles_dimaggio/DIRE/styled-4/code-12.

Dimick, J.B., Diener-West, M., Lipsett, P.A., 2001. Negative results of randomized clinical trials published in the surgical literature: equivalency or error? Arch. Surg. 136, 796–800.

Durlak, J.A., 2009. How to select, calculate, and interpret effect sizes. J. Pediatr. Psychol. 34, 917–928.

Faul, F., Erdfelder, E., Lang, A.G., et al., 2007. G*Power 3: a flexible statistical power analysis program for the social, behavioral, and biomedical sciences. Behav. Res. Methods 39, 175–191.

Freedman, K.B., Back, S., Bernstein, J., 2001. Sample size and statistical power of randomised, controlled trials in orthopaedics. J. Bone Joint Surg. Br. 83, 397–402.

Freiman, J.A., Chalmers, T.C., Smith Jr., H., et al., 1978. The importance of beta, the type II error and sample size in the design and interpretation of the randomized control trial. N. Engl. J. Med. 299, 690–694.

G*Power. Available: http://www.psycho.uni-duesseldorf.de/abteilungen/aap/gpower3/download-and-register.

Goodman, S.N., 1993. P values, hypothesis tests, and likelihood: implications for epidemiology of a neglected historical debate. Am. J. Epidemiol. 137, 485–496. discussion 497–501.

Goodman, S.N., 1999. Toward evidence-based medical statistics. 1: the P value fallacy. Ann. Intern. Med. 130, 995–1004.

Goodman, S.N., Royall, R., 1988. Evidence and scientific research. Am. J. Public Health 78, 1568–1574.

Gore, S.M., Altman, D.G., 1982. Statistics in Practice. Devonshire, Torquay, UK.

Julious, S.A., 2005. Sample size of 12 per group rule of thumb for a pilot study. Pharm. Stat. 4, 287–291.

Julious, S.A., Owen, R.J., 2006. Sample size calculations for clinical studies allowing for uncertainty about the variance. Pharm. Stat. 5, 29–37.

Komlos, J., Cinnirella, F., 2005. European Heights in the Early 18th Century (Online). Available: http://epub.ub.uni-muenchen.de/572/1/european_heights_in_the_Early_18th_Century.

Kraemer, H.C., 1988. Sample size: when is enough enough? Am. J. Med. Sci. 296, 360–363.

Lehr, R., 1992. Sixteen s-squared over d-squared: a relation for crude sample size estimates. Stat. Med. 11, 1099–1102.

Moher, D., Dulberg, C.S., Wells, G.A., 1994. Statistical power, sample size, and their reporting in randomized controlled trials. JAMA 272, 122–124.

Neyman, J., Pearson, E., 1928. On the use and interpretation of certain test criteria for purposes of statistical inference. Biometrika 20, 175–240.

Schulz, K.F., Grimes, D.A., 2005. Sample size calculations in randomised trials: mandatory and mystical. Lancet 365, 1348–1353.

Sterne, J.A., Davey Smith, G., 2001. Sifting the evidence-what's wrong with significance tests? BMJ 322, 226–231.

van Belle, G., 2002. Statistical Rules of Thumb. Wiley Interscience, New York.

Walters, S.J., 2009. Consultants' forum: should post hoc sample size calculations be done? Pharm. Stat. 8, 163–169.

Weaver, C.S., Leonardi-Bee, J., Bath-Hextall, F.J., et al., 2004. Sample size calculations in acute stroke trials: a systematic review of their reporting, characteristics, and relationship with outcome. Stroke 35, 1216–1224.

Williams, J.L., Hathaway, C.A., Kloster, K.L., et al., 1997. Low power, type II errors, and other statistical problems in recent cardiovascular research. Am. J. Physiol. 273 (Heart and Circulation Physiology 42), H487–H493.

Yusuf, S., Collins, R., Peto, R., et al., 1985. Intravenous and intracoronary fibrinolytic therapy in acute myocardial infarction: overview of results on mortality, reinfarction and side-effects from 33 randomized controlled trials. Eur. Heart J. 6, 556–585.

Zar, J.H., 2010. Biostatistical Analysis. Prentice Hall, Upper Saddle River, NJ.

## PART 4

Discrete and Categorical Distributions

CHAPTER 12

Permutations and Combinations

Contents

PERMUTATIONS

Consider the problem of selecting k objects from a set of n objects and arranging them in order; we can select all the objects in the population ($k = n$) or a subset of them. Such an arrangement is a permutation of n objects, taken k at a time. For example, a license plate with seven characters (numbers, letters) is a permutation of length 7 out of 36 objects (0, 1,…9, A, B,…Z). The order of the objects is important. License plate 2NNP386 is not the same as license plate 2PNN836, even though they use the same characters. The number of possible permutations depends on whether the same selection can appear more than once ("with replacement" into the selection pool), or is excluded from future selection ("without replacement" or withdrawn from the selection pool).

For the license plate, both letters and numbers can be selected with repetition. The number of possible permutations of n objects, taken k at a time, is n^k.

Proof: The first position can be filled in n ways. The second position can be filled in n ways, and because these choices are independent, the first two positions can be filled in $n \times n = n^2$ ways. Similarly, the first three positions can be filled in n^3 ways, and so on. Therefore, the number of possible license plate permutations is $36^7 = 78,364,164,096$.

If the objects are chosen without repetition, then the number of permutations is given by $\frac{n!}{(n-k)!}$.

Proof: The first position can be chosen in n ways, leaving $n - 1$ objects. The second position can therefore be filled in $(n - 1)$ ways, so that the first two positions can be filled in $n(n - 1)$ ways. The third position can be filled in $(n - 2)$ ways, so that the first three positions can be filled in $n(n - 1)(n - 2)$ ways. Therefore, the first k positions can be filled in $n(n - 1)(n - 2)…(n - k + 1)$ ways. This can be rewritten as

For a list of all websites referred to in this chapter, as clickable links, see the book companion website: www.booksite.elsevier.com/9780128023877.

Biostatistics for Medical and Biomedical Practitioners
http://dx.doi.org/10.1016/B978-0-12-802387-7.00012-3

$$[n(n-1)(n-2)...(n-k+1)] \times \frac{[(n-k)(n-k-1)...1]}{[(n-k)(n-k-1)...1]}$$

$$= \frac{[n(n-1)(n-2)...(n-k+1)] \times [(n-k)(n-k-1)...1]}{[(n-k)(n-k-1)...1]}$$

$$= \frac{n!}{(n-k)!}$$

$[(n! = n(n-1)(n-2)(n-3)...(1).$ Therefore, $5! = 5 \times 4 \times 3 \times 2 \times 1 = 120).]$

If all the objects are chosen, then $k = n$, and the formula reduces to $n!$ because by definition $0! = 1$.

COMBINATIONS

Sometimes the order of the arrangements has no meaning, and we are interested only in how many of each type of object we have. Such an unordered selection is called a combination of n objects taken k at a time.

The number of combinations of k items chosen from a total of n items is less than the number of permutations. Because any k items can be arranged in $k!$ ways, dividing the number of permutations of n objects taken k at a time by the number of permutations of k objects, which is $k!$, gives $\frac{n!}{(n-k)!}$ divided by $k! = \frac{n!}{k!(n-k)!}$. This is denoted by $\binom{n}{k}$ or $_nC_k$.

These problems and many variations on them are described well by Ash (1993) and Ross (1984).

Note that $\binom{n}{k} = \binom{n}{n-k}$, because both sides of the equation can be written $\frac{n!}{k!(n-k)!}$.

Thus, if we choose a committee of 4 people out of 12 applicants, we can do this in

$$\frac{12!}{4!(12-4)!} = \frac{12 \times 11 \times 10 \times 9 \times 8 \times 7 \times 6 \times 5 \times 4 \times 3 \times 2 \times 1}{(4 \times 3 \times 2 \times 1)(8 \times 7 \times 6 \times 5 \times 4 \times 3 \times 2 \times 1)}$$

$$= \frac{12 \times 11 \times 10 \times 9}{4 \times 3 \times 2 \times 1} = 495$$

ways. Therefore, there are also 495 ways in which the other eight applicants can be not chosen. These calculations can be done online at http://stattrek.com/online-calculator/combinations-permutations.aspx, http://www.mathsisfun.com/combinatorics/combinations-permutations-calculator.html, http://www.calctool.org/CALC/math/probability/combinations, http://www.statisticshowto.com/calculators/permutation-calculator-and-combination-calculator/, and http://www.calculatorsoup.com/calculators/discretemathematics/combinations.php.

In some permutation problems, there may be sets of identical objects, for example, A,A,A,B,B,C. To know how many permutations are there, calculate

$$\frac{N!}{n_1!n_2!...n_k!},$$

where N is the total and n_1, n_2,...n_k are the numbers of identical objects n_i in each set over k sets.

Therefore for the alphabetic problem above the number of permutations is

$$\frac{6!}{3!2!1!} = 60.$$

Example. How many permutations can be made from the word Tennessee? In this example, $n_1 = 1$, $n_2 = 4$, $n_3 = 2$, and $n_4 = 2$, and $N = 9$, so that the number of permutations is

$$\frac{9!}{1!4!2!2!} = 7560.$$

To see the effect of this calculation, consider two five member sets: a,e,i,o,u and b,e,e,b,e. The first of these, with no duplications, has $5! = 120$ permutations. The second has fewer permutations because of the duplications, and there are $5!/(2!3!) = 10$ permutations.

Examples

1. The Dean wishes to select a committee of 5 from a senior faculty of 30 members. In how many ways can this be done?

   Answer:

   Because the order of selection is not important, we need the combinations. The answer is $\frac{30!}{5!25!} = 142,506$.

2. Out of 30 senior faculty, 10 are women. The Dean wants to select 3 women and 2 men. How many combinations are there?

   3 women can be selected in $\frac{10!}{3!7!} = 120$ ways.

   2 men can be selected in $\frac{20!}{2!18!} = 190$ ways.

   These are independent combinations, so that the final set of 5 people can be selected in $120 \times 190 = 22,800$ ways.

3. Of the 10 women, 6 are clinicians and 4 are from basic sciences. Of the 20 men, 15 are clinicians and 5 from basic sciences. How many combinations of 2 female clinicians, 1 female basic scientist, 1 male clinician, and 1 male basic scientist are there?

   This is equivalent to selecting 2 female clinicians out of 6, 1 female basic scientist out of 4, 1 male clinician out of 15, and 1 male basic scientist out of 5. Therefore the numbers of

---

(Continued)

Examples—cont'd

combinations are respectively: $\frac{6!}{2!4!} = 15$, $\frac{4!}{1!3!} = 4$, $\frac{15!}{1!14!} = 15$, and $\frac{5!}{1!4!} = 5$. As these are independent, the total number of combinations is $15 \times 4 \times 15 \times 5 = 4500$.

4. A poker hand consists of any 5 cards from a deck of 52 cards. What are the chances of having the ace of spades?

The number of combinations of 5 cards is $\frac{52!}{5!47!} = 2,598,960$.

The number of combinations of any 4 cards that do not include the ace of spades are $\frac{51!}{4!47!} = 249900$. Therefore, the number of 5 card hands that include the ace of spades is determined from $\frac{249,900}{2,598,960} = 0.096$, or $\sim 1/10.4$.

This can be calculated more simply as five chances of drawing an ace of spades out of 52 cards $= \frac{5}{52} = 0.096$.

Problem 12.1

What are the chances of a flush (all the 5 cards of the same suit)?

Problem 12.2

What are the chances of having a straight, that is, a numerical sequence, no matter what the suits are?

Problem 12.3

What are the chances of getting a straight flush, i.e., a numerical sequence of the same suit?

REFERENCES

Ash, C., 1993. The Probability Tutoring Book. An Intuitive Course for Engineers and Scientists, p. 470.
Ross, S., 1984. A First Course in Probability. Macmillan Publishing Company.

CHAPTER 13

Hypergeometric Distribution

Contents

INTRODUCTION

If we select a sample of 5 marbles from a jar containing 15 red and 10 green marbles, then the probability that the first marble is red is $15/25 = 0.600$. If that marble is put back in the jar, the jar is shaken, and another marble is picked, the probability that the next marble will also be red is still 0.600. On the other hand, if the marble is not replaced, then the jar will contain 14 red and 10 green marbles. The chances that the next marble picked will be red are now $14/24 = 0.5833$. An experiment in which sampling is done without replacement and in which the population size is not large cannot be a Bernoulli trial, because the probability of success alters after each member of the sample is chosen. To answer the question "What is the probability of getting 2 red and 3 green marbles from the above population of marbles?", use the hypergeometric distribution.

GENERAL FORMULA

The formula envisages a total population of N objects, with X having characteristic A (success) and $N–X$ not having it. Choose a sample of n objects from the total population, and ask what is the probability that r objects have A. That is, what is $P(X = r,n)$?

$$P(X = r) = \frac{\binom{X}{r}\binom{N-X}{n-r}}{\binom{N}{n}} = \frac{\left(\frac{X!}{r!(X-r)!}\right)\left(\frac{(N-X)!}{(n-r)!(N-X-n+r)!}\right)}{\frac{N!}{n!(N-n)!}}.$$

This is the probability function.

For a list of all websites referred to in this chapter, as clickable links, see the book companion website: www.booksite.elsevier.com/9780128023877.

Biostatistics for Medical and Biomedical Practitioners
http://dx.doi.org/10.1016/B978-0-12-802387-7.00013-5

Thus in our example above, $N = 25$, $X = 15$, $n = 5$, $k = 2$. Therefore,

$$P(X = 2,\ n = 5) = \frac{\left(\frac{15!}{2!(15-2)!}\right)\left(\frac{(25-15)!}{(5-2)!(25-15-5+2)!}\right)}{\frac{25!}{5!(25-5)!}} = \frac{\left(\frac{15!}{2!13!}\right)\left(\frac{10!}{3!7!}\right)}{\frac{25!}{5!20!}} = 0.2372.$$

The mean value is

$$mean = \frac{nX}{N} = \frac{5 \times 15}{25} = 3$$

and

$$\text{Variance} = \frac{nX(N-X)}{N^2}\left(1 - \frac{n-1}{N-1}\right) = \frac{5x25(25-15)}{25^2}\left(1 - \frac{5-1}{25-1}\right) = 1.67$$

The calculation can be done online at http://stattrek.com/online-calculator/ hypergeometric.aspx, http://www.adsciengineering.com/hpdcalc/, or http://easy calculation.com/statistics/hypergeometric-distribution.php.

Problem 13.1

A chest physician selects at random 6 patients out of a group of 16 patients, 5 of whom are hyperreactors to inhaled particles. What is the probability that the sample contains (1) 2 hyperreactors?, (2) 5 hyperreactors?

(Because of the risk of arithmetic errors, always do this type of calculation by using an online calculator. Some of these calculators supply added information, such as cumulative probabilities.)

FISHER'S EXACT TEST

Fisher's exact test is based on the hypergeometric distribution. Consider sampling a population of size N that has c_1 objects with A and c_2 with not-A. Draw a sample of r_1 objects and find a with A. Then

	A	not-A	Total
In sample	a	b	r_1
Not in sample	c	d	r_2
	c_1	c_2	N

There are $\binom{N}{r_1}$ possible samples. Of these, $\binom{c_1}{a}$ is the number of ways of choosing A in a sample of size c_1, $\binom{c_2}{b}$ is the number of ways of choosing not-A in a sample of size $N - c_1 = c_2$; and because these are independent, there are $\binom{c_1}{a}\binom{c_2}{b}$ ways of choosing a

As and b not-As. Therefore, the probability of choosing a As $= \dfrac{\binom{c_1}{a}\binom{c_2}{b}}{\binom{N}{r_1}} =$

$\dfrac{\frac{c_1!}{a!c!}\times\frac{c_2!}{b!d!}}{\frac{N!}{r_1!r_2!}} = \dfrac{c_1!c_2!r_1!r_2!}{N!a!b!c!d!}$; the last form is the way in which Fisher's exact test formula is usually given. Doing this calculation for all combinations more extreme than the one presented produces the probability given in Fisher's exact test.

Example 13.1

A medical clinic has 30 patients, 20 women and 10 men. A random sample of 5 patients is drawn. What is the probability that there will be 2 men?

A sample of 5 patients out of 30 can be chosen in $\binom{30}{5}$ ways $= 142{,}506$ ways.

A sample of 2 men and 3 women can be drawn in $\binom{10}{2} \times \binom{20}{3}$ ways $= 51{,}300$ ways. Therefore,

$$P(2\ \text{men},\ 3\ \text{women}) = \dfrac{\binom{10}{2} \times \binom{20}{3}}{\binom{30}{5}} = 51{,}300/142{,}506 = 0.359985.$$

Alternatively,

	Women	Men	Total
In sample	3	2	5
Not in sample	17	8	25
	20	10	30

The probability in Fisher's exact test is thus $\frac{20!10!5!25!}{3!2!17!8!30!} = 0.359985$.

This test can be done online at http://research.microsoft.com/en-us/um/redmond/projects/mscompbio/FisherExactTest/, http://www.danielsoper.com/statcalc3/calc.aspx?id=29, http://www.langsrud.com/fisher.htm, or http://www.quantitativeskills.com/sisa/statistics/fisher.php?n11=3&n12=2&n21=17&n22=8. Note that the probability of 0.359985 is the probability of that particular distribution given the marginal totals. Often we need to know the probability of that distribution and more extreme disparities (Chapter 15), and http://research.microsoft.com/en-us/um/redmond/projects/mscompbio/FisherExactTest/ and http://www.quantitativeskills.com/sisa/statistics/fisher.php?n11=3&n12=2&n21=17&n22=8 give these accumulated probabilities as well.

MULTIPLE GROUPS

More than two groups can be involved (Hogg and Tanis, 1977). If there are $n_1, n_2, n_3 \ldots n_k$ objects in each class, and $n_1 + n_2 + n_3 \ldots + n_k = n$, then

$$P(X_1 = x_1, \; X_2 = x_2 \ldots X_n = x_n) = \frac{\binom{n_1}{x_1}\binom{n_2}{x_2} \cdots \binom{n_k}{x_k}}{\binom{n}{r}},$$

where $x_1 + x_2 + x_3 \ldots + x_k = r$.

REFERENCE

Hogg, R.V., Tanis, E.A., 1977. Probability & Statistical Inference. Macmillan Publishing Company, Inc., New York.

CHAPTER 14

Categorical and Cross-Classified Data: Goodness of Fit and Association

Contents

BASIC CONCEPTS

Introduction

Members of a population may be classified into different categories: for examples, male or female; or improved, the same, or worse after one or more treatments. The frequency with which members of the sample representing the population of interest occur in each category can be determined, so that each category shows a count (Table 14.1).

These categories are *mutually exclusive*, so that no one patient can be in two different categories at the same time, and they are also *exhaustive*, that is, there are enough categories to account for all the members of that particular population. This is not

For a list of all websites referred to in this chapter, as clickable links, see the book companion website: www.booksite.elsevier.com/9780128023877.

Biostatistics for Medical and Biomedical Practitioners
http://dx.doi.org/10.1016/B978-0-12-802387-7.00014-7

Table 14.1 Table of categories

	Improved	Unchanged	Worse	Total
Treatment A	17	7	2	26

essential, but if the categories are not exhaustive, interpretation may be difficult. If an investigation of the effects of a treatment used only the categories improved and the same, it would be difficult to make sensible judgments without knowing how many became worse. The categories represent *nominal* or *qualitative* variables, also termed *attributes*, and do not represent measurements or even a particular order of the variables.

Goodness of Fit

Often we wish to compare a distribution of counts in different categories with some theoretical distribution. For example, in a classical genetics experiment (Mendel, 1965) tall plants are crossed with short plants to provide an F1 generation, and these are crossed with others of the F1 generation to provide a second (F2) generation. Counts of 120 plants of the F2 generation are listed in Table 14.2a.

Table 14.2a Hypothetical Mendelian experiment

	Tall	Short	Total
Observed counts	94	26	120

In classical Mendelian genetics with the phenotype determined by dominant and recessive alleles, there should be a 3:1 ratio in which only one-quarter of the F2 generation have two recessive genes and are short, whereas three-quarters of them have at least one dominant gene and are tall. Is the result of F2 crosses in our series of 120 plants consistent with the hypothesis that we are dealing with classical Mendelian inheritance? The observed ratio of Tall:Short is 3.62:1 which differs from 3:1, but if the 3:1 ratio is true in the population, the relatively small sample might by chance have a ratio as discrepant as 3.62:1.

To analyze this, adopt the null hypothesis that the sample is drawn from a population in which the Tall:Short ratio is 3:1. If this is true, then a sample of 120 F2 crosses is expected to provide $0.75 \times 120 = 90$ tall plants and $0.25 \times 120 = 30$ short plants (Table 14.2b).

Table 14.2b Chi-square analysis of Mendelian experiment

	Tall	Short	Total
Observed (O)	94	26	120
Expected (E)	90	30	120
Deviation (O − E)	+4	−4	0
$(O - E)^2$	16	16	
χ^2	0.178	0.533	$\chi^2_T = 0.711$

The expected frequencies (symbolized by f_e or E) appear below their respective observed frequencies (symbolized by f_o or O), and the deviations $(O - E)$ appear in the line below the expected frequencies. Whether a given deviation is small or big depends not on its absolute size but on how big the deviation is relative to the numbers used in the experiment. Thus a deviation of 10 is large and perhaps important with 30 counts but small and probably unimportant with 1000 counts. To evaluate the relative size of the deviation, it is squared and then divided by the expected value in that column; the ratio $\frac{(O-E)^2}{E}$ is termed χ^2, also sometimes written as chi-square. The values of χ^2 for each column are added up to give a total $\chi^2_T = 0.711$. This is a measure of the overall discrepancies between O and E for each cell, and the larger the discrepancy the larger will be the value of χ^2_T.

Does this value of 0.711 helps to support or refute the null hypothesis? One way of deciding would be to draw a large number of samples of 120 plants from a population with a 3:1 ratio of Tall:Short plants, calculate χ^2 for each sample, and determine how often any given value of χ^2_T occurred. Large values of χ^2_T would occur infrequently, and we could estimate the probability of getting a value as big as or bigger than any given χ^2_T. If the probability of getting $\chi^2_T = 0.711$ is low, we would tend to reject the null hypothesis, but if the probability is high, then we would not be able to reject the null hypothesis. Fortunately, we do not have to do these experiments because of the similarity of the distribution of chi-square to the χ^2 distribution described in Chapter 8. (There is some possibility for confusion in the use of symbols here. Most but not all texts distinguish between these two distributions.) A brief explanation of the equivalence is given by Altman (1992, p. 246).

For the example above, the $\chi^2_T = 0.711$ is referred to a table of the χ^2 distribution, and with 1 df, P = 0.399, so that if the null hypothesis is true, then about 40% of the time, samples of 120 plants drawn from this population could have ratios as deviant from 3:1 as 3.62:1 or even more. Such an estimate would not allow us to be comfortable in rejecting the null hypothesis; we conclude that there is an acceptable fit between the observed and expected results.

Continuity Correction

Because the χ^2 distribution is continuous and if we examine only two groups, in a large series of experiments in which the null hypothesis is known to be true, the values obtained cause us to reject the null hypothesis more than the expected number of times for any critical value of χ^2_T (type I error). To reduce the error, Yates' correction for continuity is often advised, especially if the actual numbers are small (Yates, 1934). (Yates (1902−1994) was Fisher's assistant at Rothamsted and became head of the unit when Fisher moved to University College London.) To make this correction, the absolute value of the deviation (written as $|O - E|$) is made smaller by 0.5: +4 becomes +3.5, and −4 becomes −3.5. The result is to make χ_T^2 smaller than it would have been without the correction (χ_T^2 becomes 0.544 in Table 14.2b), and the excessive number of type I errors is abolished. Yates' correction for continuity is made also with 2 × 2 tables, but *should not be used* for larger tables. The correction is used only when there is one degree of freedom (see below).

The need for such a correction is disputed (Adler, 1951; Conover, 1974; Maxwell, 1976; Rhoades and Overall, 1982; Upton, 1982). Yates (1984) analyzed the defects in alternative approaches. Some of the issues are discussed clearly by Ludbrook (Ludbrook and Dudley, 1994) who compared these various corrections. For the same data set he obtained two-sided values for P ranging from 0.0281 to 0.0673. Yates' correction certainly increases the risk of accepting the null hypothesis falsely (type II error). If, however, the decision about statistical significance or not depends on whether or not Yates' or some other correction is used, it is better to consider the results of the test as borderline or, better still, to use another test such as Fisher's exact test (Camilli, 1990; Yates, 1984) (see below).

The chi-square test is not restricted to two categories. Continuing with the genetic example, with two pairs of dominant−recessive alleles—one for Tall versus Short, one for Green versus Yellow—the expected ratios for the F2 plants are 9 tall green, 3 tall yellow, 3 short green, and 1 short yellow, or 9:3:3:1. Assume that an experiment gives the results shown in Table 14.2c.

Table 14.2c Extended Mendelian experiment

	Tall green	Tall yellow	Short green	Short yellow	Total
Observed (O)	94	22	33	11	160
Expected (E)	90	30	30	10	160
Deviation ($O - E$)	4	−8	3	1	
$(O - E)^2$	16	64	9	1	
χ^2	0.178	2.133	0.300	0.100	$\chi_T^2 = 2.711$

The calculations show a value of χ_T^2 of 2.711 with 3 df, and from the χ^2 table P = 0.438, so that we would not on this basis reject the null hypothesis.

In general, we are interested in large values of chi-square, because it is these that answer the question about whether or not to reject the null hypothesis, and so pay attention to the area on the right-hand side of the chi-square curve where values above certain critical values are found. On the other hand, even if the null hypothesis is true, there should be a certain degree of variation between the observed and experimental data, and if the two sets of data are too much alike, we might be suspicious about why that occurred. Fisher once reviewed a series of experiments reported by Mendel, and after combining their individual chi-squares obtained a total chi-square of 42 with 84 df (Fisher, 1936). The area under the chi-square curve on the left-hand side gives the probability of getting this value, and it is about 0.00004. Therefore either a very unusual event had occurred, or else someone had manipulated the data to make it agree so closely with theory. There is evidence that this was done by a gardener who knew what answers the Abbott Mendel wanted to get.

Degrees of Freedom

The concept of degrees of freedom may be understood by examining the observed data in Table 14.2a. If the marginal total of 120 plants is fixed, then by choosing any number N_T (not negative and <120) for the counts in Tall, the counts in Short must be $120 - N_T$. Therefore, we are free to pick only one of the two numbers and so have lost one degree of freedom. With more observed categories, for example, four categories (tall green, tall yellow, short green, short yellow), then we could choose any numbers for the counts in any three of these categories, but the counts in the fourth category must be such that all four counts add up to 160 (Table 14.2c). Once again we have lost one degree of freedom, and we look up the value of chi-square in the table for $4 - 1 = 3$ df.

2 × 2 Contingency Tables

Both the examples above compared one observed and one theoretical distribution. Frequently, however, we wish to compare two or more observed distributions. Table 14.3a shows the binary outcomes of two forms of treatment for a disease set out in a 2 × 2 table, also known as a fourfold table; this is the most common contingency table.

Table 14.3a Typical 2 × 2 table

	Alive	Dead	Total
Treatment A	60	40	100
Treatment B	30	20	50
Total	90	60	150

Table 14.3b shows some symbols commonly used to indicate different components of the table. a, b, c, d are the counts for each *cell*, defined as the intersection of a row category and a column category. In larger contingency tables, the cells may be indicated by a_1, $a_2,...a_m$; $b_1, b_2,...b_m$; $n_1, n_2,...n_m$, or may be indicated by the row and column that characterize that cell. Thus r_2c_3 indicates the cell in the second row and the third column, and r_ic_j indicates the cell in the ith row and the jth column. By adopting the convention of

Table 14.3b Notation for 2 × 2 table

	Alive	Dead	Total
Treatment A	$a = n_{11}$	$b = n_{12}$	$R_1 = n_1.$
Treatment B	$c = n_{21}$	$d = n_{22}$	$R_2 = n_2.$
Total	$C_1 = n._1$	$C_2 = n._2$	$N = n..$

Table 14.3c 2 × 2 table as proportions

	Alive	Dead	Total
Treatment A	0.40	0.27	0.67
Treatment B	0.20	0.13	0.33
Total	0.60	0.40	1.00

citing rows before columns the symbols can be shortened to n_{ij} or f_{ij}, where i indicates the ith row and j indicates the jth column. Therefore the cell counts in 2 × 2 table may be defined as n_{11}, n_{12}, n_{21}, and n_{22}, where the first number in the subscript indicates the row and the second number indicates the column. The totals of each row or column, known as marginal totals, are referred to as R_1 and R_2 (for the first and second rows) and C_1 and C_2 (for the first and second columns), or may be referred to as $n_1.$ and $n_2.$, where the dot indicates summation of all the columns in that row, and as $n._1$ and $n._2$, where the dot indicates summation of all the rows in that numbered column. The grand total of all the cell counts is the same as the sum of the two marginal row totals or the two marginal column totals, and is symbolized by N or $n....$ In larger $m \times n$ contingency tables, the marginal totals in the rows and columns are designated as R_1, $R_2,...R_i...R_m$ and C_1, $C_2,...C_j...C_n$, respectively, or else as $n_1.$, $n_2.,...n_i.,...n_m.$ and $n._1$, $n._2,...n._j,...n._n$, respectively.

Table 14.3c shows each of the counts as a proportion of the total; thus the 60 patients alive after treatment A represent $60/150 = 0.40$ of the total number of 150 patients. The proportion of survivors after treatment A ($60/100 = 0.6$) is the same as the proportion of survivors after treatment B ($30/50 = 0.6$), so that the two different treatments did not affect the survival rate. Survival was *independent* of the type of treatment used; other words used to express the same idea are that survival was *not associated* with the type of treatment or was *not contingent* on the type of treatment. Table 14.4a shows a different set of results obtained by treating this disease with two different treatments.

Table 14.4a

	Alive	Dead	Total
Treatment A	60	40	100
Treatment B	70	30	100
Total	130	70	200

In Table 14.4b, the probabilities p (in parentheses) have subscripts that indicate what they refer to: p_{11} indicates the probability in row 1 and column 1 (the upper left-hand cell), whereas p_{21} indicates the probability in the second row, first column (the lower left-hand cell). The probability $p_1.$ indicates the probability of the marginal total in row 1; the dot indicates that all the columns in row 1 are summed.

Table 14.4b

B	Alive	Dead	Total
Treatment A	0.30 (=p_{11})	0.20 (=p_{12})	0.50 (=$p_{1.}$)
Treatment B	0.35 (=p_{21})	0.15 (=p_{22})	0.50 (=$p_{2.}$)
	0.65 (=$p_{.1}$)	0.35 (=$p_{.2}$)	1.00 (=$p_{..}$)

A higher proportion of patients survived after treatment B than after treatment A, 0.35 versus 0.30, respectively, but is there an association between the type of treatment and the outcome, or are the observed differences due to chance variation in relatively small samples from a population in which a larger study would show no association between treatment and outcome? These tables allow us to evaluate association or contingency, and are known as *contingency tables*, defined as *tables that show the association between variables where the variables have been classified into mutually exclusive categories and the cell entries are frequencies.* There are at least two requirements to be fulfilled for the analysis to be valid. There should be no systematic change in the proportion of survivors in each group in different periods throughout the study, and the outcome for any one patient should not affect the outcome for any other patient.

To answer the question, begin by adopting the null hypothesis (H_0) that the two groups *do* come from the same population, and that any differences in the observed proportions in the two samples are due to chance variation. Then calculate how likely those differences are to occur if the null hypothesis is true; if the probability of such differences is very low, then it might be better to reject the null hypothesis. Most computer programs carry out all the necessary calculations, but this is a test that can be done readily by hand, with the merit of showing how the contributions to the total chi-square are derived (Table 14.5a).

Table 14.5a Layout for chi-square analysis

	Category 1		Category 2		Total
	O_{11}	E_{11}	O_{12}	E_{12}	$O_{11} + O_{12}$
					(=$E_{11} + E_{12}$)
Treatment 1	$(O-E)_{11}$	$(O-E)^2_{11}$	$(O-E)_{12}$	$(O-E)^2_{12}$	
		χ^2_{11}		χ^2_{12}	
	O_{21}	E_{21}	O_{22}	E_{22}	$O_{21} + O_{22}$
					(=$E_{21} + E_{22}$)
Treatment 2	$(O-E)_{21}$	$(O-E)^2_{21}$	$(O-E)_{22}$	$(O-E)^2_{22}$	
		χ^2_{21}		χ^2_{22}	
Total	$O_{11} + O_{21}$		$O_{12} + O_{22}$		$O_{11} + O_{21}$
					$+ O_{12} + O_{22}$

$$\chi_T^2 = \sum_{i=1}^{m} \sum_{j=1}^{n} \frac{(O_{ij} - E_{ij})^2}{E_{ij}} = \chi_{11}^2 + \chi_{12}^2 + \chi_{21}^2 + \chi_{22}^2$$

Put the observed count (O) in the upper left-hand corner of each cell, the expected count (E) in the upper right-hand corner of each cell, the deviation ($O - E$) below each observed count, the squared deviation below the expected count, and then divide the squared deviation by the expected count (which is just above it) to give the value of χ^2 for that cell. The values of χ^2 for all the four cells are added up to give χ_T^2, and this total value is looked up in the tables of the distribution of χ^2 for the appropriate degrees of freedom. The first step is to calculate the expected counts in each cell. Given the null hypothesis, the subtotals in the two columns represent better estimates of the proportion surviving or dying in the population of patients with that disease (Table 14.5b).

Table 14.5b Basic analysis

	Alive		Dead		Total
Treatment A	**60**	65	**40**	35	100
	−5	25	5	25	
	0.385		0.714		
Treatment B	**70**	65	**30**	35	100
	5	25	−5	25	
	0.385		0.714		
Total	130		70		200

Observed numbers in bold type, chi-square in italics.
$\chi_T^2 = 2.198$, 1 df, P = 0.1382.

(These computations can also be performed on freeware designed for larger tables see below.) If out of a total of 200 patients 130 survive, then in a sample of 100 patients $130 \times 100/200$ are expected to survive. More generally, the expected value in any cell is (row subtotal × column subtotal)/N, and this applies to any sized chi-squared table. Another way of obtaining the same result is to point out that the proportion surviving in the pooled results is $130/200 = 0.65$. Then this proportion multiplied by the marginal total in a sample (100) gives an expected value of $100 \times 0.65 = 65$. This value is the expected count in the upper left-hand cell. In a similar fashion, the expected counts in the other three cells can be calculated. Once these expected values are obtained, it is easy to obtain the deviations, the squared deviations, and the χ^2 values for each cell, as well as the χ_T^2.

Probability for any chi-square total and degrees of freedom may be found online at http://www.fourmilab.ch/rpkp/experiments/analysis/chiCalc.html, http://www.stat.tamu.edu/~west/applets/chisqdemo.html, http://vassarstats.net/tabs.html#csq, and http://stattrek.com/online-calculator/chi-square.aspx. The chi-square computation itself may be performed online for 2 × 2 tables at http://www.statstodo.com.

Problem 14.1

The table below shows data for maternal age and the babies' birth weight. Are these independent?

	Birth weight (g)	
Maternal age	**<2,500**	**>2,500**
<25 years	64	216
>25 years	47	273

Note: (1) once the expected counts in one cell have been obtained, the expected counts in the other three cells may be obtained by subtracting the expected counts from the marginal totals; (2) in a 2 × 2 table, the absolute deviations are the same in all four cells; and (3) the sum of the deviations in any row or column is zero.

The degrees of freedom can be calculated using the argument described above for the first goodness-of-fit test. If the four marginal totals are given, then the count in any one of the four cells could be any number (provided it was not negative and was less than the total counts in the whole study). Once that count was chosen, however, then the other three counts are forced by the marginal totals.

A more general way of calculating degrees of freedom is (number of rows − 1)(number of columns − 1).

Therefore, in Table 14.5a the degrees of freedom are $(2 - 1)(2 - 1) = 1$.

The value for total chi-square in Table 14.5a is 2.198 that, with one degree of freedom, does not allow us to reject the null hypothesis with confidence. What would happen if we increased the sample size? Assume that we examine another 100 patients in each treatment group and that the proportions alive and dead do not change (Table 14.5c).

Table 14.5c Change in sample size

	Alive		Dead		Total
Treatment A	**120**	130	**80**	70	200
	−10	100	10	100	
	0.769		1.429		
Treatment B	**140**	130	**60**	70	200
	10	100	−10	100	
	0.769		1.429		
Total	260		140		400

Observed numbers in bold type.
$\chi_T^2 = 4.3960$, 1 df, P = 0.036.

Comparing Tables 14.5a and 14.5c, all the observed and expected numbers, the deviation between observed and expected numbers, the marginal totals, and the total number of patients have been doubled, so that the proportion surviving in each treatment group is the same for both sample sizes; for simplicity, Yates' correction has been omitted. However, because the deviations are squared, the χ^2 contributions for each cell and thus the χ^2_T have doubled (apart from small rounding-off errors), so that the null hypothesis can be rejected at the 0.05 level for the larger sample size even though it could not be rejected for the smaller sample size. This is reasonable. If a difference between two treatments is consistent as samples get bigger, then we feel more comfortable about rejecting the null hypothesis that there is no difference between the two treatments. For this reason, chi-square tests must always be done with absolute numbers and not with percentages or numbers per unit. On the other hand, expressing the individual proportions as percentages allows the investigator to assess important differences, even if they are not used in subsequent calculations.

It is possible to estimate the sample size needed to have a desired probability of rejecting the null hypothesis for any given difference; the way to do this is given below.

Practical Issues

1. Because in general the expected values will not be whole numbers, calculate them and the chi-square to three decimal places to minimize rounding-off errors.
2. For 2 × 2 tables, many but not all statisticians use Yates' correction for continuity; that is, decrease the absolute size of the deviation by 0.5. Table 14.5a should therefore be as follows:

	Alive		Dead		Total
Treatment A	**60** −4.5 *0.312*	65 20.25	**40** 4.5 *0.579*	35 20.25	100
Treatment B	**70** 4.5 *0.312*	65 20.25	**30** −4.5 *0.579*	35 20.25	100
Total		130		70	200

Observed numbers in bold type.
$\chi^2_T = 1.78$, 1 df, $P = 0.182$.

This correction has made the total chi-square smaller, so that the null hypothesis is even less likely to be rejected.

3. None of the expected frequencies should be too small. As a rule of thumb, Cochran suggested that 80% of the cells should have expected frequencies >5 and that none should be below 1 (Cochran, 1954). A very small expected value could lead to a big squared deviation that, divided by the small expected value, gives a very large contribution to the χ^2_T. This tends to inflate the χ^2_T and we should hesitate to accept a conclusion based on a single

---

Practical Issues—cont'd

   large value of χ^2. In addition, a very small expected value makes the theoretical basis for using the χ^2 table suspect. It would be better to use Fisher's exact test (see below). If the expected value is <5, we can use the chi-square technique, but should be cautious about interpreting the results. If more than 20% of the cells (in larger contingency tables) have expected values <5, either combine adjacent rows or columns to increase the size of the expected numbers (if that makes sense) or do not use the chi-square test. These criteria are frequently used, but not all statisticians agree with them.

4. Problems about whether to use Yates' correction or about too small an expected value can be dealt with by using Fisher's exact test. Computer programs can calculate the probability by this test for any sample size, so that this test may be preferred for any 2×2 table.

5. Some authorities (Daniel, 1995) distinguish between tests of independence and tests of homogeneity. For the first of these, a sample is drawn from a population, and then the members of the sample are classified into each of the categories; the entries into each cell are determined only after the sample has been drawn, and the totals in the rows and columns are therefore not under control of the investigator. This test answers the question of whether the two criteria of classification are independent. For the second type of test, independent samples are drawn from two or more populations, so that one set of marginal totals can be fixed in advance, whereas the other set of marginal totals is a function of the classification criteria. This type of test answers the question about whether the two or more sets of samples are homogeneous in relation to the criteria of classification. Although conceptually these two types of tests are different, their mathematical analyses are identical.

Odds Ratio

The chi-square test gives the probability of rejecting the null hypothesis falsely. If this probability is low, then we may elect to conclude that the differences between the two groups are not likely to have occurred by chance. What the test does not indicate is the magnitude of the difference between the proportions (effect size) in the two treatment groups. To find out the magnitude of the difference between the proportions in the two treatment groups consider the proportions themselves in each group (Fleiss, 1981). Return to the data in Tables 14.4a and 14.4b. Define the odds (risk) of dying with treatment A as Ω_A:

$$\Omega_A = \frac{\Pi(\text{Dead}|A)}{\Pi(\text{Alive}|A)}.$$

In other words, the risk of dying with treatment A is the ratio of two conditional probabilities, the probability (Π) of dying with treatment A and the probability of not dying with treatment A. Ω_A is the odds that death will occur if treatment A is present.

$$\Pi(\text{Dead}|A) \text{ may be estimated by } \frac{p_{12}}{p_{1\cdot}},$$

$$\text{and } \Pi(\text{Alive}|A) \text{ may be estimated by } \frac{p_{11}}{p_{1\cdot}}.$$

Therefore, Ω_A may be estimated by

$$O_A = \frac{p_{12}/p_{1\cdot}}{p_{11}/p_{1\cdot}} = \frac{p_{12}}{p_{11}}.$$

Thus from Table 14.4b, $O_A = \frac{0.20}{0.30} = 0.667$.
In a similar fashion, define Ω_B, the risk of dying with treatment B, as:

$$\Omega_B = \frac{\Pi(\text{Dead}|B)}{\Pi(\text{Alive}|B)}.$$

This ratio can be estimated by

$$O_B = \frac{p_{22}/p_{2\cdot}}{p_{21}/p_{2\cdot}} = \frac{p_{22}}{p_{21}}$$

$$= \frac{0.15}{0.35} = 0.429.$$

These two ratios (Ω_A, Ω_B) can be compared in several ways, but most often one is divided by the other to give ω, the *odds ratio*. This ratio $\omega = \frac{\Omega_A}{\Omega_B}$ can be estimated as

$$o = \frac{O_A}{O_B} = \frac{p_{12}/p_{11}}{p_{22}/p_{21}} = \frac{p_{12} \times p_{21}}{p_{11} \times p_{22}} = \frac{0.20 \times 0.35}{0.30 \times 0.15} = 1.56,$$

where o is the sample odds ratio.

This may also be symbolized by $\widehat{OR}$.

This ratio can be interpreted as the risk of dying with treatment A is 1.56 times the risk of dying with treatment B.

Because the proportions given in Table 14.4b are the same as the individual cell values given in Table 14.4a divided by the total number of patients, this ratio can be determined simply by using the original cell counts a, b, c, d. Thus

$$o = \frac{b \times c}{a \times d}$$

$$= \frac{40 \times 70}{60 \times 30} = 1.56.$$

In this form the ratio is also termed the cross-product ratio, because to obtain it we multiply the counts in two cells on one diagonal and divide that product by the product of the counts in the two cells on the other diagonal (see Table 14.5d). In Table 14.5d, the

Table 14.5d

	Alive	Dead	Total
Treatment A	60	40	100
Treatment B	70	30	100
Total	130	70	200

thick line indicates which product goes in the numerator; in this instance, emphasizing the risk of dying on treatment A. To focus on the "risk" of surviving on treatment A, then the other product would go in the numerator.

Thus to focus on survival,

$$o = \frac{a \times d}{b \times c} = \frac{60 \times 30}{40 \times 70} = 0.64.$$

This answer is the reciprocal of the one obtained above. For either form of calculation, the chances of dying are about two-thirds for treatment B.

Odds versus risk ratios and their confidence limits are discussed in detail in Chapter 20. Odds ratios can be calculated online at http://statpages.org/ctab2x2.html, http://www.hutchon.net/ConfidOR.htm, and http://vassarstats.net/odds2x2.html.

Problem 14.2

What was the odds ratio for the data in Problem 14.1?

Cautionary Tales

Selecting Samples

We should not be so involved with the mechanics of doing these tests that we forget to think about the data and what they mean. A good example can be found in an article published in the *New England Journal of Medicine* in 1965 (Binder et al., 1965). Investigators in the departments of Internal Medicine and Radiology at the Yale University School of Medicine noted a lack of association between achalasia of the esophagus and hiatus hernia, and to see if this impression was correct they reviewed the records of all patients with a diagnosis of achalasia of the esophagus in the previous 11 years. Forty-three of these patients were found. The X-ray films of a control group of 43 patients of similar age and sex distribution, who were scheduled for a radiological examination of the upper

(Continued)

Selecting Samples—cont'd

Table 14.6a Achalasia data

	Hernia	No hernia	Total
Achalasia	1	42	43
No achalasia	9	34	43
Total	10	76	86

gastrointestinal tract in May 1964, were reviewed by a radiologist with no knowledge of the patients' clinical history. The results are set out in a fourfold table, Table 14.6a.

The total chi-square for this example is 5.54 with 1 df, so that P = 0.0093. The cross-product ratio to evaluate the association between achalasia and hernia is $\frac{1 \times 34}{9 \times 42} = 0.0899$. These results show that the null hypothesis of no difference in the incidence of hiatus hernia whether there is or is not achalasia of the esophagus can be rejected, and that the chance of someone with achalasia of the esophagus also having a hiatus hernia is only 9% of that of someone without achalasia. The investigators concluded that "Hiatus hernia is found very much less frequently in patients with achalasia than in the normal hospital population." In the discussion, they speculated about the mechanisms of these two lesions and found it reasonable that they should not occur together, inasmuch as achalasia represents undue tightness of the esophageal sphincter whereas hiatus hernia is associated with undue laxness of the esophageal sphincter.

In a letter to the journal a few weeks later, a note of warning was introduced (Muench, 1965). Dr Muench (from Harvard!) pointed out that patients having a barium examination of their upper gastrointestinal tract probably did so because they had some upper gastrointestinal tract symptoms, and could not be taken as representative of the whole hospital population. He hypothesized that if the investigators had done a barium examination of the upper gastrointestinal tract of every hospitalized patient, they might have found a large number with neither achalasia nor hernia, and the resultant fourfold table might resemble Table 14.6b.

Table 14.6b Hypothetical extension of achalasia data

	Hernia	No hernia	Total
Achalasia	1	42	43
No achalasia	9	340	349
Total	10	382	392

The rationale for increasing the number only in the lower right-hand cell is that patients with symptoms that lead to a radiological examination of the upper gastrointestinal tract will already have been included in the study, and the others are unlikely to have either of the two diseases in question. It is true that asymptomatic disease might be revealed by the X-ray examination, but in general most people do not have either of these relatively uncommon diseases. The choice of the actual number of 340 was arbitrary, but

Selecting Samples—cont'd

it does correspond to what one might find in a medium-sized hospital. From this new table of data, χ^2_T at 0.0099 is not different from zero, and the cross-product ratio is $\frac{1 \times 340}{9 \times 42} = 0.8995$. There does not seem to be an association between achalasia and hiatus hernia when one takes account of the whole hospital population.

Dr Muench went one step farther. He considered what might have happened if the whole population of a small town, both those in and out of hospital, had been given a radiological examination of the upper gastrointestinal tract. Once again, he used the reasonable assumption that most of the people outside hospital would have neither disease, and postulated a table such as Table 14.6c.

Table 14.6c Further hypothetical extension of achalasia data

	Hernia	No hernia	Total
Achalasia	1	42	43
No achalasia	9	3,400	3,409
Total	10	3,442	3,452

Now χ^2_T is still small, partly because of the huge number who have neither disease, but the cross-product ratio is $\frac{1 \times 3400}{9 \times 42} = 8.9947$, indicating a tendency for achalasia to be associated with hiatus hernia in the whole population!

This is an instructive example. People who have any given investigation are not representative of all patients in a hospital, and patients in hospital are not representative of all people in a population. The number of people who have neither of two diseases is almost certainly very large, even if not well known, and attempts made to define associations without including them may well lead to incorrect conclusions.

Spurious Associations (Berkson's Fallacy)

Berkson (1946) studied the apparent association between diabetes and cholecystitis that had been found in an investigation at the Mayo Clinic, and concluded that the association could be spurious if the occurrence of two disorders in the same person increases the probability that they will be admitted to a hospital or clinic, and if the proportions of these patients are not the same in the hospital and the general population. He pointed out that 2×2 tables differed if based on experimental or clinical data. The experiment starts with equally matched subjects that are divided into two groups (experimental and control), the experiment is performed, and the results (effect or no effect) are obtained. In the clinical setting the groups A and not-A have already been determined without knowing from which populations they were drawn from.

Berkson began with four assumptions:

1. In the whole population, cholecystitis, diabetes mellitus, and refractive errors are unrelated.
2. It is possible to have more than one of these diseases.

(Continued)

Selecting Samples—cont'd

3. The chances of a disease causing hospital admission (or death) vary from disease to disease.

4. Having more than one disease increases the chances of hospital admission.

Tables 14.7a and 14.7b give estimates of three diseases in a large population area. (The presentation is based on descriptions by Berkson (1946) and Mainland (1953).)

Table 14.7a Population prevalences

	A	Not-A	Total		A	Not-A	Total
B	3,000	97,000	100,000	B	3,000	97,000	100,000
Not-B	297,000	9,603,000	9,900,000	X	59,400	930,600	990,000
Total	300,000	9,700,000	10,000,000	Total	62,400	1,027,600	1,090,000

| | A in control group—3% | | | A in B group—3% | |
| | A in B group—3% | | | A in X group—3% | |

X in 20% of any group.
Fractional admission rate: A—0.15, B—0.10, X—0.20.

Table 14.7b Estimated hospital populations

Group	Population number	Fractional admission rate	Hospital population
A	237,600	0.15	35,640
B	77,600	0.10	7,760
X	930,600	0.2	186,120
AB	2,400		564
AX	59,400		19,008
BX	19,400		5,432
ABX	600		233

How were these calculated? X occurred in 20% of the subjects; for example, of 297,000 with A but not B there were 59,400 with X, and we are told this is the same for all groups. Therefore, people with only A in the general population come to 297,000 − 59,400 = 237,600. Similar calculation applies to B and X. To calculate the number with AB, we take all with A and B (3000) and subtract the 20% who also have X, leaving 2400 with only A and B. Similarly calculate AX and BX. Finally calculate the number with all three diseases as 3000 with A and B, of whom 20% also have X to get 600.

For the three sets with single diseases, multiply the numbers of patients by the fractional admission rate to see how many are admitted. For those with A and B, first apply the fractional admission rate for A. Thus of 2400 with A and B, 2400 × 0.15 = 360 are admitted because they have A. This leaves 2040 who also have B, and with a fractional admission rate of 0.10 another 2040 × 0.10 = 204 are admitted because they have B. Therefore a total of 360 + 204 = 564 are admitted with both A and B. Similar

Selecting Samples—cont'd

calculations apply to AX and BX, and ABX. Now we collect up the admissions for the three diseases. For example, A and B occur together in $564 + 233 = 797$ patients (Table 14.8).

Table 14.8 Hospital admission with A or B

	A	Not A	Total
B	797	13,192	13,989

A with B—$797/13,989 = 5.7\%$

These data appear to show some relationship between A and B, yet we know from the population data they are unrelated. The concentration in the hospital population is due to the selective and differential admission rates.

If instead of admission rates we think about rates of admission to an autopsy room, a clinic, or physician's office, then it is likely that different diseases have different probabilities of being included in an investigation of an association between different diseases. Unless these associations are studied in populations in which this selection bias does not occur, little faith can be placed in the results. Some examples of this error were found in about 25% of studies surveyed by Roberts et al. (1978).

Simpson's Paradox

In 1951, Simpson described an apparent paradox, in that successes of individual groups seem reversed when the groups are combined (Simpson, 1951). He showed that it was possible for two subgroups each to have $A_1 > B_1$ and $A_2 > B_2$, yet on pooling them $A_{1+2} < B_{1+2}$. This paradox was the basis for a suit for gender discrimination against the University of California in Berkeley. The plaintiffs alleged that the University discriminated against admitting women to graduate studies (Bickel et al., 1975). A simplified set of data based on that publication illustrates the problem (Table 14.9).

Table 14.9 University selection data

	Total applications	Admit	Deny	% admitted
Department A				
Men	400	200	200	50
Women	200	100	100	50
Department B				
Men	150	50	100	33
Women	450	150	300	33
Totals				
Men	550	250	300	45
Women	650	250	400	38

(Continued)

Selecting Samples—cont'd

In each department the admission rate for men and women is the same. When the two departments are combined, however, the fact that more women apply for the department with the lower admission rate explains the apparent gender discrimination. Other versions of this example are described by Williams (1978).

Similar examples are scattered throughout the literature. In 1934, Cohen and Nagel examined deaths from tuberculosis in New York City and Richmond, VA for white and nonwhite residents (Cohen and Nagel, 1934) (Table 14.10).

Table 14.10 An early example of Simpson's paradox

	Total population		Deaths		Deaths/100,000	
Race	NYC	Richmond	NYC	Richmond	NYC	Richmond
White	4,675,174	80,895	8,365	131	179	162
Nonwhite	91,709	46,733	513	155	560	332
Total	4,766,883	127,628	8,878	286	186	226

For both whites and nonwhites, the death rate per 100,000 population was higher in New York than Richmond, but for the total population the rates were higher in Richmond than New York: 226 versus 187. The cause of this paradox lies in the greater risk of tuberculosis in nonwhites who made up a bigger percentage of the population in Richmond than they did in New York City.

Charig et al. compared the effects of A—open surgery versus B—percutaneous lithotomy for kidney stones (Charig et al., 1986; Julious and Mullee, 1994). They found that the success rate for treatment A was 273/350 (78%) and for treatment B was 289/350 (83%). Therefore treatment B was slightly more effective. When, however, the data were separated in the results for large and small kidney stones, the results were as shown in Table 14.11.

Table 14.11 Renal calculi

	Treatment A		Treatment B	
Small stones	81/87 (93%)	a	234/270 (87%)	b
Large stones	192/263 (73%)	c	55/80 (69%)	d
Both	273/350 (78%)		289/350 (83%)	

Here, each individual group (stone size) showed that treatment A was better, yet combining them showed the reverse. What happened is that doctors preferred to offer the better treatment (open surgery) to patients with the larger stones, and offered treatment B to more patients with smaller stones. As a result, the total outcome for treatment B depends mainly on the larger number of patients with small stones (who on the whole do well) in cell b as compared with the number for treatment A (who do less well) in cell c.

This phenomenon of a lurking confounder is common and must be sought. Other examples are the paradox that low birth weight babies of smoking mothers have a lower

Selecting Samples—cont'd

perinatal mortality than those from nonsmoking mothers, despite the fact that exposure to smoking during pregnancy is known to be harmful (Hernandez–Diaz et al., 2006; Wilcox, 2006), drawing incorrect conclusions from a study on treatment of meningococcal disease (Perera, 2006), in evaluating trends for the Scholastic Aptitude Test (SAT) (Bracey), and a study of medical aid society enrollment in South Africa (Morrell, 1999).

Larger Contingency Tables

Contingency tables need not be restricted to a 2 × 2 format. For example, patients with migraine were treated with a new agent, sumatriptan, during attacks (Treatment of migraine attacks with sumatriptan, 1991). As part of the study, investigators evaluated the effect of placebo and three different regimens of sumatriptan on recurrence of the headache within 24 h. The results are set out in Table 14.12a.

Table 14.12a Extended contingency table

	P/P		6 mgS/P		6 mgS/6 mgS		8 mgS/P		Total
No recurrence	**85**	74.576	**194**	199.119	**190**	195.390	**103**	102.915	572
	14.424	108.660	−5.119	26.204	−5.390	29.052	0.085	0.007	
		1.457		*0.132*		*0.149*		*0.000*	
Recurrence	**15**	25.424	**73**	67.881	**72**	66.610	**35**	35.085	195
	−14.424	108.660	5.119	26.204	5.390	29.052	−0.085	0.007	
		4.274		*0.386*		*0.436*		*0.000*	
Total	100		267		262		138		767

Observed numbers in bold type.
$\chi_T^2 = 6.833$, 3 df, P = 0.0774.
P/P = placebo on two occasions; 6 mgS/P = 6 mg sumatriptan plus placebo; 6 mgS/6 mgS = 6 mg sumatriptan on both occasions; 8 mgS/P = 8 mg sumatriptan and placebo.

The sum of deviations in any row or any column equals zero, but unlike the 2 × 2 table, the deviations in different rows need not be the same. Yates' correction is not made for any table larger than a 2 × 2 table.

This is a 2 × 4 table (2 rows, 4 columns). Therefore the degrees of freedom are $(2 − 1)(4 − 1) = 3$. The value for χ_T^2 indicates that if the null hypothesis is true, then 7.74% of the time one might get results with the differences shown here by random variation, so that we might not feel safe in concluding that there was an association between the treatment regimen and the duration of freedom from headache; nevertheless, the possibility of an effective treatment should be pursued, perhaps with greater numbers of patients.

These larger chi-square tables can be analyzed online at http://home.ubalt.edu/ntsbarsh/Business-stat/otherapplets/Catego.htm, http://in-silico.net/statistics/chi2test/upload, http://www.quantpsy.org/chisq/chisq.htm, http://easycalculation.com/statistics/goodness-of-fit.php, and http://vassarstats.net/index.html.

Problem 14.3

Assume that the data on maternal age and birth weight are:

Maternal age (year)	Birth weight (g)		
	<2500	2,500–3,000	>3,000
<20	21	14	30
20–25	43	56	116
>25	47	56	217

Is there any association?

In 2 × 3 or larger tables, it is unsafe to do the calculation if the expected value in any cell is under 1. If this happened, it is best to try to combine adjacent cells. Combination of cells can also be done if the total chi-square is not significant but the deviations in adjacent cells go in the same direction. Then it might be appropriate to combine cells to try to obtain a greater deviation, providing that pooling the data from these cells is meaningful. Consider the data in Table 14.12b in which the proportions with recurrent headaches on placebo alone are compared with the other three groups, all of which received at least 6 mg of sumatriptan, and had more than expected or the same number of recurrent headaches.

Table 14.12b Pooling cells

Headaches	P/P		Rest		Total
No recurrences	**85** 10.424 9.924	74.576 98.486	**487** −10.424 −9.924	497.424 98.486	572
		1.321		*0.198*	
Recurrences	**15** −10.424 −9.924	25.424 98.486	**180** 10.424 9.924	169.576 98.486	195
		3.874		*0.581*	
Total	100		667		767

$\chi_T^2 = 5.974$, 1 df, P = 0.0145.

We have gained ability to reject the null hypothesis.

Caution is needed when making such combinations. If we imagine a study with 20 columns and 6 rows, we could end up making dozens of combinations of cells for the analysis, but how should we interpret a significant value of chi-square for any one of them? Just as for multiple t-tests (Chapter 24) we might achieve statistical significance at the 0.05 level when in reality the null hypothesis is true. It is best to make as few comparisons as possible, to combine cells only if combination makes physiological or clinical sense, and preferably to use significant results after the combination as a reason to repeat the experiment to test that particular hypothesis.

Fisher's Exact Test

When the total number of counts in a fourfold table <30, or if $N < 50$ and the smallest expected value is <5, the chi-square test may be inaccurate, and is better replaced by Fisher's exact test (also called the Fisher–Irwin test). If there is no association between the row and column classifications, the exact probability of obtaining any set of cell counts given the marginal totals can be calculated as:

$$P = \frac{R_1!R_2!C_1!C_2!}{a!b!c!d!N!}$$

where the symbol ! indicates the factorial of the number referred to. This is based on the hypergeometric function (Chapter 13).

Table 14.13 shows data reported by Basile et al. (1991) about the activity of benzodiazepine receptors in patients who died from fulminant liver failure and a control group who died from cardiovascular causes.

Table 14.13 Data for Fisher's test

	Diazepam equivalents (ng/g tissue)		
	Under 100	Over 100	Total
Liver disease	2	9	11
Control	5	3	8
Total	7	12	19

The proportion with low activity in the control group is $5/8 = 0.625$, and the proportion with low activity in those with liver disease is $2/11 = 0.182$. Are these proportions different enough to allow us to reject the null hypothesis?

If the marginal totals are fixed, there are eight different combinations of cell counts possible (Figure 14.1).

From the formula above, the probabilities of getting each of these combinations of cell counts are given in Table 14.14.

0	11	11
7	1	8
7	12	19

4	7	11
3	5	8
7	12	19

1	10	11
6	2	8
7	12	19

5	6	11
2	6	8
7	12	19

2	9	11
5	3	8
7	12	19

6	5	11
1	7	8
7	12	19

3	8	11
4	4	8
7	12	19

7	4	11
0	8	8
7	12	19

Figure 14.1 All possible combinations with fixed marginal totals.

Table 14.14 Probabilities of each combination

$P(a = 0)$	0.000158768
$P(a = 1)$	0.006112566
$P(a = 2)$	0.061125665
$P(a = 3)$	0.229221243
$P(a = 4)$	0.366753989
$P(a = 5)$	0.256727792
$P(a = 6)$	0.073350798
$P(a = 7)$	0.006549178
	0.999999999

These results are plotted in Figure 14.2, which plots the probabilities on the vertical axis against the value of a shown above, that is, the chances of getting any given number with low receptor activity values in the group with liver disease.

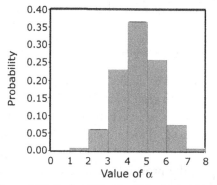

Figure 14.2 Probabilities for Fisher's exact test.

As expected from an exhaustive set of mutually exclusive events, the sum of the probabilities equals 1. From Table 14.14, the probability of getting α equal to 2 if the null hypothesis is true is 0.0611, not strong evidence against the null hypothesis. However, we must also consider the probability of $\alpha = 1$ or 0, which would be more extreme departures from the hypothesis of equal proportions. These probabilities are 0.0061 and 0.00015, and the three probabilities together sum to 0.0674, equivalent to one tail of the distribution, namely the probability of getting 2 or less with low values in those with liver disease. From this study, then, we have no compelling reason to reject the null hypothesis. (Consider the possibility that there is a difference, and do more tests.) As described here, the test is a one-sided test, which is the more usual requirement. Should a two-sided test be wanted, then according to many statisticians the probability as calculated above should be doubled if the sample sizes in the two groups are similar (Armitage et al., 2002; Everitt, 1992). However, because the distribution is not symmetrical (see Figure 14.2), others recommend calculating both tails separately (Zar, 2010). This is the procedure adopted by major software programs such as SAS and SPSS. An interactive freeware Internet program for doing this and many other aspects of the chi-square test may be found at http://statpages.org/ctab2x2.html, http://www.graphpad.com/quickcalcs/contingency1.cfm, http://research.microsoft.com/en-us/um/redmond/projects/mscompbio/FisherExactTest/default.aspx, http://www.quantpsy.org/fisher/fisher.htm, http://www.danielsoper.com/statcalc3/calc.aspx?id=29, or http://vassarstats.net/.

Calculating by hand, even with a calculator that gives factorials, is tedious and fraught with errors. Use programs such as those listed above.

Problem 14.4

Examine the data relating gender (M, F) to drinking dietary soft drinks:

	Dietary soda	Nondietary soda
Male	3	9
Female	7	4

Because of the small numbers, perform Fisher's test.

Fisher's exact test (like most tests) has relatively low power when N is small (Everitt, 1992). Thus a significant difference with the test may be reason to reject the null hypothesis, but with small total numbers failure to reach a low level of α may merely reflect a low power of the test; Table 14.14 is a good example of this low power.

It is possible with the aid of a computer program to do Fisher's exact test for tables larger than 2×2, for example, by using the interactive freeware found online at http://vassarstats.net/.

Determining Power and Sample Size

To assess the degree of effect, that is, the size of the difference, between observed and expected distributions that are independent of sample size, several indexes have been suggested. An important one is w (Cohen, 1988), defined as:

$$w = \sqrt{\sum_{i=1}^{m} \frac{\left(pO_{ij} - pE_{ij}\right)^2}{pE_{ij}}}$$

where m is the number of cells.

Here pO_{ij} and pE_{ij} are the observed and expected proportions in any cell, and the fraction is summed for all cells in the table. The expected proportions for any cell are obtained by multiplying the marginal proportions for the row and column which that cell shares. For example, consider Table 14.15, which shows in the upper left-hand corner of each cell the observed proportions $\left(pO_{ij}\right)$ of migrainous patients with and without recurrent headaches after treatment with various combinations of placebo and sumatriptan, taken from the raw data in Table 14.12a.

Table 14.15 Sumatriptan data as proportions

	P/P		6 mgS/P		6 mgS/6 mgS		8 mgS/P		Total
No	0.1108	0.0972	0.2529	0.2596	0.2477	0.2547	0.1343	0.1342	0.7457
recurrence	0.0136	0.000185	−0.0067	0.000045	−0.007	0.000049	0.0001	0.000	
		0.00190		0.000173		0.000192		0.000	
Recurrence	0.0196	0.0331	0.0952	0.0885	0.0939	0.0868	0.0456	0.0457	0.2543
	−0.0135	0.000182	0.0067	0.000045	0.0071	0.00005	0.0001	0.000	
		0.00550		0.000507		0.000581		0.000	
Total	0.1304		0.3481		0.3416		0.1799		1.0000

P/P = placebo on two occasions; 6 mgS/P = 6 mg sumatriptan plus placebo; 6 mgS/6 mgS = 6 mg sumatriptan on both occasions; 8 mgS/P = 8 mg sumatriptan and placebo.

The expected proportions $\left(pE_{ij}\right)$ are set out in the upper right-hand corners of each cell. The expected proportion $\left(pE_{ij}\right)$ of those with no recurrence who had only placebo (p/p) is calculated as (marginal proportion with p/p × marginal proportion with no recurrences) = $0.1304 \times 0.7457 = 0.0972$. This is quicker than calculating the expected numbers and then turning them into proportions. Then to calculate w, sum the values of fractions such as $\frac{(0.1108-0.0972)^2}{0.0972}$ for each cell, and take the square root of the sum. This value of w indicates the amount of departure from no association between no recurrences and placebo treatment. If observed and expected values are the same, then $w = 0$. The more w exceeds zero, the less likely is it that the null hypothesis is true.

Another way of calculating w is to note that

$$\frac{\left(p_{O_{ij}} - p_{E_{ij}}\right)^2}{p_{E_{ij}}} = \frac{\left(O_{ij}/N - E_{ij}/N\right)^2}{E_{ij}/N} = \chi^2/N.$$

Therefore, if the values of χ^2 for each cell have already been calculated,

$$w = \sqrt{\frac{\chi_T^2}{N}};$$

this involves little extra calculating.

The maximum value of w for perfect association is $\sqrt{k-1}$, where k is the smaller of the number of rows or column. The index is higher with better association, but its maximum values change as the number of cells changes.

The index w is used in the tables provided by Cohen to evaluate the power of a given chi-square test. To use these tables, a value for α, the type I error, is selected, and the table is selected for the degrees of freedom involved in the test, the total number of counts, N, and the calculated value of w. For example, in the study shown in Table 14.20, $w = \sqrt{0.0019 + 0.000173 + 0.000192 + 0.0055 + 0.000507 + 0.000581} = 0.094$. This is almost the same as $\sqrt{\frac{6.834}{767}} = 0.095$, taken from Table 14.12a. With this value, 3 df, and $\alpha = 0.05$, the table gives the power as 0.63. Therefore the type II error (β) is $1 - 0.63 = 0.37$. Clearly, the test had low power and the number of subjects was too small to be sure that the degree of difference observed was not due to chance. If we multiply the value of $\frac{(p_{O_i} - p_{E_i})^2}{p_{E_i}}$ in each cell by N, the product is the value of χ^2 for that cell.

Power calculations are available in many computer programs and online programs such as http://statpages.org/ctab2x2.html and http://www.biomath.info/power/index.htm for 2×2 tables. There is an extensive freeware program called G*Power, at http://www.psycho.uni-duesseldorf.de/abteilungen/aap/gpower3/download-and-register. Details of its use have been published and should be consulted (Koopmans, 1987). An easy graphically determined power is available at http://homepage.stat.uiowa.edu/~rlenth/Power/index.html. Also see http://www.real-statistics.com/chi-square-and-f-distributions/power-chi-square-tests/.

Problem 14.5

Confirm the power calculation for Table 14.12a by using http://homepage.stat.uiowa.edu/~rlenth/Power/index.html and use it to determine the number needed for a power of 0.8.

Any 2×2 table can be analyzed by a chi-square test or as proportions, and sample sizes for proportions can be obtained from several online sources (Chapter 16).

To determine sample size required to give a particular power, consider the same example in which we want to determine what sample size would give a power of 0.8. Look up in a companion set of tables for $\alpha = 0.05$, degrees of freedom $= 3$, and $w = 0.094$ how many total counts (=patients) are needed for a power of 0.8. Approximately 1090 patients would be needed to achieve the desired level of significance, that is, another 323 patients would be needed. Of course, if we gathered another 323 patient results, the chi-square test would not reach significance unless the additional patients behaved in the same way as those already studied. If the new patients did not show as big differences as the old patients did, then the total chi-square would not be significant, and we would probably conclude that any differences related to the drug dosages were small indeed. Implicit assumptions are that the added patients are similar to those already studied and the different groups are incremented in rough proportion to their present numbers. If any cells have expected numbers below 5, the total sample size needed may be very large.

ADVANCED CONCEPTS

Cochran—Mantel—Haenszel Test and Confounders

In Simpson's paradox, the paradoxical conclusions were usually due to ignoring a third factor, for example, the relative number of applications per department in the Berkeley study, or the size of the kidney stones. These sometimes disregarded third factors may be confounders, in which all the relationship between X and Y is due to their individual relationship with the third factor S, or may be modifiers, in which the strength of the association between X and Y depends on the level of the S factor. To deal with this problem, the Cochran—Mantel—Haenszel (C-M-H) test is used. If there are three nominal variables, for example, two 2×2 contingency tables for testing independence and a third nominal variable that indicates repeats, we need to know if it is appropriate to merge the different repeats and obtain a larger and more representative sample. For example, let us compare two species of snail counted above and below the tide line to determine if there is any relationship between species and site. This is a simple 2×2 table for nominal variables. If we do this in two different months, can we combine the two data sets? There is actually a third nominal variable, the lurking confounder of time, much like the confounder of the size of the kidney stones cited earlier.

To test the independence between cause and effect at two different levels of the possible confounder, there is a method based on the hypergeometric distribution known as the C-M-H (or sometimes just as the Mantel—Haenszel) test. The null hypothesis is that the deviation $O - E = 0$; because in a 2×2 table the deviations are of the same magnitude in each cell, calculate only the deviation in any one cell. As shown above, the expected value can be determined as $O_{ij} - \frac{R_i O_j}{N}$. Thus for the upper left cell, the deviation is $O_{11} - \frac{R_1 C_1}{N}$. Do this calculation for each stratum, subtract 0.5 for Yates' continuity correction, and then square the deviations. (This calculation is equivalent to summing all the observed numbers O_{ij} and subtracting the sum of all the expected numbers.) Pool these squared deviations for each stratum, and obtain a weighted mean by dividing the sum of the squared deviations by the sum of their respective variances, calculated as $Variance = \frac{R_1 C_1 R_2 C_2}{N^2(N-1)}$ for each stratum. The final formula becomes

$$\chi^2_{MH} = \frac{\left\{\left|\sum\left(O_{ij} - \frac{R_i C_j}{N}\right) - 0.5\right|\right\}^2}{\sum\left(\frac{R_1 R_2 C_1 C_2}{N^2(N-1)}\right)}, \text{ sometimes written as}$$

$$\chi^2_{MH} = \frac{\left\{\left|\sum\left(a - \frac{(a+b)(a+c)}{N}\right) - 0.5\right|\right\}^2}{\frac{\sum(a+b)(a+c)(b+d)(c+d)}{N^2(N-1)}}.$$

This value is distributed like χ^2 with 1 df.

The combined odds ratio is:

$$OR_{MH} = \frac{\sum\left(\frac{ad}{N}\right)}{\sum\left(\frac{bc}{N}\right)}.$$

As an example, investigators wished to determine the association between thiazide diuretics and hip fractures (LaCroix et al., 1990). They studied subjects in East Boston, Iowa, and New Haven, and data for incidence rates of hip fracture are shown in Table 14.16.

Although all the odds ratios are >1, none of the chi-squares are close to $P = 0.05$. Is it reasonable to combine the data from the groups and obtain a combined odds ratio? (Although the data are not shown here, in East Boston the incidence rates in men and women were almost the same.)

Table 14.16 Hip fracture data

Age	Number East Boston			Number Iowa			Number New Haven		
	Men	Women	Total	Men	Women	Total	Men	Women	Total
65–74	11	17	28	7	17	24	8	15	23
≥75	15	42	57	9	49	58	12	40	52
Total	26	59	85	16	66	82	20	55	75
Chi-square	1.48, $P = 0.33$			2.04, $P = 0.16$			1.11, $P = 0.29$		
Odds ratio	1.812			2.24			1.78		

In these tables, there seems to be an association between the age and gender. The combined odds ratio is $OR_{MH} = \frac{\frac{11 \times 42}{85} + \frac{7 \times 49}{82} + \frac{8 \times 40}{75}}{\frac{15 \times 17}{85} + \frac{9 \times 17}{82} + \frac{8 \times 40}{75}} = \frac{13.88}{7.27} = 1.91$. This is the weighted average of the three odds ratios. The Cochran–Mantel–Haenszel test (Mantel, 1963; Mantel and Haenszel, 1959) is then

$$\sum O_{11} = 11 + 7 + 8 = 26$$

$$\sum E_{11} = \frac{26 \times 28}{85} + \frac{16 \times 24}{82} + \frac{20 \times 23}{75} = 19.38.$$

$$v_{EB} = \frac{26 \times 59 \times 57 \times 28}{85^2 \times 84} = 4.03, \quad v_I = \frac{16 \times 66 \times 58 \times 24}{82^2 \times 81} = 2.70.$$

$$v_{NH} = \frac{20 \times 55 \times 23 \times 52}{75^2 \times 74} = 3.16.$$

Therefore
$\chi^2_{MH} = \frac{(|26-19.38|-0.5)^2}{4.03+2.70+3.16} = 3.79$. With 1 df, this indicates that $P = 0.0581$ so that there are significant age differences.

We can use more groups. An example of the Berkeley admissions data alluded to above uses some data (Internet Project, Simpson's Paradox). The number of applicants admitted and rejected by four different departments was sorted by gender (Table 14.17).

Table 14.17 Berkeley admission data by department and gender

	A		B		C		D	
	M	F	M	F	M	F	M	F
Admitted	512	89	353	17	138	131	53	94
Rejected	313	19	207	8	279	244	138	299
Total	825	108	560	25	417	375	191	393

For the data as a whole, ignoring the departments, refer to Table 14.18.

The χ^2 total is 211.90, $P < 0.00001$, and the odds ratio is 1.94, suggesting that males are admitted disproportionately more than females. As mentioned above, this was the basis for a complaint to the US Government about discrimination against women in the

Table 14.18 Admission data pooled across departments

		Stratum		
		M	F	Total
Status	Admitted	1,056	331	1,387
	Rejected	937	570	1,507
	Total	1,993	901	2,894

admissions policy of the Graduate Division. If we examine each of the four departments separately, we notice that the four χ^2 total values are respectively 17.25, 0.25, 0.30, and 1.001, with respective odds ratios of 0.35, 0.80, 0.92, and 1.22.

The Mantel–Haenszel test gives

$$\chi^2_{MH} = \frac{\left\{\left|\left(512 - \frac{601 \times 825}{933}\right) + \left(353 - \frac{370 \times 560}{585}\right) + \left(138 - \frac{269 \times 417}{792}\right) + \left(53 - \frac{147 \times 191}{584}\right)\right| - 0.5\right\}^2}{\left(\frac{601 \times 332 \times 825 \times 108}{933^2 \times 932}\right) + \left(\frac{370 \times 215 \times 560 \times 25}{585^2 \times 584}\right) + \left(\frac{269 \times 523 \times 417 \times 375}{792^2 \times 791}\right) + \left(\frac{147 \times 437 \times 191 \times 393}{584^2 \times 583}\right)}$$

$$= \frac{-19.43 - 1.19 - 3.63 + 4.92}{21.91 + 5.57 + 44.34 + 24.25} = \frac{\{|-19.33| - 0.5\}^2}{96.07} = \frac{354.57}{96.07} = 3.69$$

This, with 1 df, does not quite reach the 0.05 significance level. Does this substantiate the complaint? No, it does not, because the odds ratio for the whole data set is

$$o_{MH} = \frac{\frac{512 \times 19}{933} + \frac{353 \times 8}{585} + \frac{138 \times 244}{792} + \frac{53 \times 299}{584}}{\frac{89 \times 313}{933} + \frac{17 \times 207}{585} + \frac{131 \times 279}{792} + \frac{94 \times 138}{584}} = \frac{84.90}{104.23} = 0.81.$$ In other words, there was a

tendency for fewer males to be admitted!

Pooling Data

How can we best combine data from several small 2×2 tables, each with a trend that does not reach statistical significance? First examine the tables to determine if the direction of the trend is similar in all the samples. If the different samples show trends in opposite directions, there is not much sense in combining them. Once we decide to combine them, we have a choice of several methods. The simplest would be to combine all the original data from each table to produce a larger single 2×2 table. The next simplest might be to combine the χ^2 values from each of the k tables and refer the total chi-square to the chi-square table with k degrees of freedom, because the sum of k chi-squares is distributed like chi-square with k degrees of freedom. The first method could produce misleading results if the proportions in the different groups differ markedly from each other (Armitage et al., 2002). The second method may lack power. Statistical consultation is required.

Testing for Trends in Proportions (Cochran–Armitage Test)

A $2 \times k$ table may have the k groups arranged in some natural order, for examples, time, age groups, or degrees of severity of an illness. A chi-square test examines the null hypothesis that the proportions of the variables in the two rows are the same. However, there might be a significant trend in the proportions from group 1 to group k. To test this, use an analogy to the testing of linearity with ANOVA (Chapter 25), by comparing the total variability of a variate with the amount of variability due to linear regression; if the difference between these is small, there is good evidence for a linear relationship. To do this for the chi-square test, assign a quantitative variable x_i to the k groups. This variable might be ascending integers from 1 to k if, for example, the groups were arranged in decades by age; they might be estimated magnitudes, for example, estimated thyroid weights for different groups of enlarged thyroid glands; or they might merely indicate an order of magnitude, such as -1 for normal tonsils, 0 for moderately enlarged tonsils, and 1 for very enlarged tonsils (Armitage et al., 2002).

For example, Table 14.19 shows the proportion of deaths from coronary heart disease in workers exposed to increasing concentrations of carbon disulfide (Hernberg

Table 14.19 Social class and ischemic deaths

Heart disease (xⱼ)	Concentration score				Total
	0	**1**	**2**	**3**	
Yes (n_{1i})	3	5	6	5	19 $(R_1 = n_i.)$
No	340	157	18	552	667 (R_2)
Total $(n_1.)$	343 (C_1)	162 (C_2)	124 (C_3)	57 (C_4)	686 (N)
Proportion %	0.87	3.09	4.83	8.77	

et al., 1973).

Does the proportion of coronary heart disease tend to increase with carbon disulfide concentration? Inspection shows that the proportions do increase, but is the change significant? Start by calculating the standard chi-square with 3 df; it is 14.23, and $P = 0.0026$. Then compute a component of chi-square (χ^2_{lin}) that is due to a linear trend. If this is similar to the standard chi-square, then there is probably a trend. This is calculated as

$$\frac{N\left[N\sum n_{1i}x_i - n_{i\cdot}\sum n_{\cdot i}x_i\right]^2}{n_{i\cdot}(N - n_{i\cdot})\left[N\sum n_{\cdot i}x_1^2 - \left(\sum n_{\cdot i}x_i\right)^2\right]}$$

$$= \frac{N\left[N\sum n_{1i}x_i - R_1\sum C_ix_i\right]^2}{R_1 R_2\left[N\sum C_1x_1^2 - \left(\sum C_ix_i\right)^2\right]} \text{ (alternative symbols)}$$

Thus from Table 14.19

$$\chi^2_{\text{lin}} = \frac{686[686(0 \times 3 + 1 \times 5 + 2 \times 6 + 3 \times 5) - 19(0 \times 343 + 1 \times 162 + 2 \times 124 + 3 \times 57)]^2}{19 \times 667\left[686(0^2 \times 343 + 1^2 \times 162 + 2^2 \times 124 + 3^2 \times 57) - (0 \times 343 + 1 \times 162 + 2 \times 124 + 3 \times 57)^2\right]}$$

$$= 13.84$$

Therefore the difference between the two, which tests departure from a linear trend, is

$$\chi^2_T - \chi^2_{\text{lin}} = 14.23 - 13.84 = 0.39 \text{ with 2 df, and } > 0.99.$$ Therefore, reject the null hypothesis of departure from linear trend and conclude that most of the total chi-square is

due to the linear trend in the direction of increasing coronary heart disease as the concentration of carbon disulfide increases. The selection of n_{1i} or n_{2i} is arbitrary; one could replace n_{1i} and $n_{.i}$ by n_{2i} and $n_{.2}$ in the formula above. Furthermore, the scores assigned are also arbitrary. If the calculation of the linear chi-square is repeated replacing n_{1i} and $n_{.i}$ by n_{2i} and $n_{.2}$, and assigning scores of -1, 0, 1, and 2, exactly the same result will be obtained.

Trends can be assessed for tables larger than $2 \times k$; see Armitage et al. (2002).

Problems with $R \times C$ Tables

The cross–product ratio cannot be calculated for chi-square tables larger than 2×2, and in large tables it is possible for a few cells to contribute most of the total chi-square. Even if the total chi-square is big enough to be significant, it would be useful to determine which of the individual χ^2 appears to be significant on its own. To do this, use the fact that, if the null hypothesis is true,

$$z = \frac{(O - E)}{\sqrt{E}},$$

has an approximately standard normal distribution (as long as E is not too small) (Koopmans, 1987) that can be read from the z table at http://davidmlane.com/hyperstat/z_table.html, or http://www.fourmilab.ch/rpkp/experiments/analysis/zCalc.html. Thus if z calculated in this way is 2.08, 0.0188 of the area under the standard probability curve is above $z = 2.08$ (one tail). If the null hypothesis is true, the deviation that produced this value of χ^2 is unlikely to have arisen by chance, and we should pay attention to that particular cell in our assessment. The ratio z can be positive or negative. If positive, it indicates a greater than expected frequency, and if negative, a lesser than expected frequency. The square of this z is the same as χ^2. The z statistic, calculated in this way, is what is used when the alternative hypothesis is one-sided. Thus if

$$H_0 : p_1 = p_2 \text{ and } H_A : p_1 < p_2 \text{ or } p_1 > p_2,$$

calculate the square root of chi-square and refer to the z table for the level of α to determine if the null hypothesis can be rejected.

Another approach to the multiplicity problem when chi-squared testing with multiple rows and columns is to calculate adjusted standardized residuals as

$$\text{Adjusted residual } (z_{ij}) = \frac{\text{Observed} - \text{Expected}}{\sqrt{\text{Expected} \times \text{Row total proportion} \times \text{Column total proportion}}}.$$

These can be computed from $z_{ij} = \dfrac{O_{ij} - \frac{R_i C_j}{N}}{\sqrt{\frac{R_i C_j}{N}\left(1 - \frac{R_i}{N}\right)\left(1 - \frac{C_j}{N}\right)}}.$

Essentially this formula relates the magnitude of the difference to its standard deviation that is a function of sample size. If the variables in the contingency table are independent, then the terms z_{ij} are approximately normally distributed with mean zero and standard deviation of 1. Therefore any adjusted residuals over 1.96 should occur less than 5% of the time if the null hypothesis is true, allowing us to decide where there are significant departures from the null hypothesis of equal proportions in each group.

With many cells, correction for multiplicity can be made by multiplying each P value by $(r-1)(c-1)$ to produce the equivalent of a Bonferroni type adjustment (Chapter 24). Only if the adjusted P value is below 5% should the null hypothesis be rejected at the 5% level.

Multidimensional Tables

The typical $r \times c$ contingency table that assesses independence or association between two categories is computationally simple and relatively easy to interpret. In more complex tables, however, interactions among several categories are common. Their analyses are more complex but can be done with current computer programs. However, their interpretation involves investigating possible interactions among the categories, an issue absent from $r \times c$ tables. With a multidimensional table we may consider doing multiple $r \times c$ tables that cover all the possibilities. This procedure is inefficient. It provides many different $r \times c$ tables for consideration, with the caveat that the more tests that are done, the more false positive results there will be. More importantly, the possibility of interaction cannot readily be evaluated.

Only the three-dimensional table will be discussed here (Everitt, 1992). Figure 14.3 shows how a $2 \times 2 \times 2$ table is constructed.

The left panel shows eight cells specified by rows (r), columns (c), and layers (l). The right-hand panel shows that the cells can be designated in standard format. The observed number in the cell in the first row, first column, and first layer is O_{111}; in the second row, second column, and first layer is O_{221}; and in the second row, second column, and second layer is O_{222}, and so on. (There may be more than two categories in each row, column, or layer; for example, Rubik's cube is a $4 \times 4 \times 4$ matrix.) To represent

Figure 14.3 Diagram of 2 x 2 x 2 lay-out.

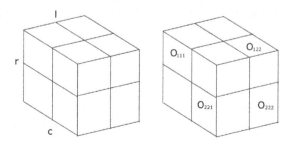

this three-dimensional structure in two dimensions either a tree-like table or else an extended two-way table with subgroups can be constructed.

Table 14.20 shows data from a study examining the mortality rates of two cardiac surgeons operating on children with congenital heart disease. Because different forms of congenital heart disease have different operative risks, the patients are classified by a RACHS scale, in which grades 1–3 are relatively simple lesions with a low expected operative mortality, and grades 4–6 are more complex lesions with a higher expected operative mortality.

Table 14.20 Three-way table: surgical results

| | Survival | | | | |
| | Dead | | Alive | | |
	RACHS 1–3	RACHS 4–6	RACHS 1–3	RACHS 4–6	Total
Surgeon 1	14	10	397	44	465
Surgeon 2	4	2	342	49	397
Total	18	12	739	93	862

The table is regarded as having three categories, arranged in rows (r), columns (c), and layers (l). The observed number in any cell can be represented by O_{ijk}, for $i = \cdot 1,2\ldots r$; $j = 1,2\ldots c$; and $k = 1,2\ldots l$. Single variable marginal totals can be obtained by summing all the values for the other two categories:

Thus, for example,

$O_{1\cdot\cdot}$ = number of patients operated on by Surgeon 1 = $(14 + 10) + (397 + 44) = 465$

$O_{\cdot 1\cdot}$ = number of deaths = $(14 + 4) + (10 + 2) = 30$

$O_{\cdot\cdot 1}$ = number of children with RACHS $1 - 3 = (14 + 4) + (397 + 342) = 739$

Two-variable marginal totals can be obtained by summing the O_{ijk} over any single subscript:

For example, the number of children who died with Surgeon 1, summed over all RACHS grades, is $n_{11*} = (14 + 10) = 24$.

In a three-way table of this type, any of the categories might be dependent or independent. In this table, for example, the outcomes (survival) depend on the severity of the lesions, and possibly depend on the surgeon; it is this last possibility that was being assessed.

Similar to 2×2 tables, calculate the expected frequencies in any cell as

$$E_{ijk} = \frac{n_{i\cdot\cdot} \cdot n_{\cdot j\cdot} \cdot n_{\cdot\cdot k}}{N^2}.$$

Then calculate the total chi-square as:

$$\chi_T^2 = \sum_{\substack{r \\ i=1}} \sum_{\substack{c \\ j=1}} \sum_{k=1}^{l} \frac{\left(O_{ijk} - E_{ijk}\right)^2}{E_{ijk}}.$$

Using the table, the degrees of freedom are $rcl - r - c - 1 + 2 = 2 \times 2 \times 2 - 2 - 2 - 2 + 2 = 4$.

E_{111} is $\frac{465 \times 30 \times 757}{862^2} = 14.212$; the other expected frequencies can be calculated in similar fashion. The value of the total chi-square is 52.34 with 4 df, $P < 0.0001$, so that we would reject the null hypothesis of independence among the three categories.

If we do not reject the null hypothesis, there is no reason to proceed further. If we do accept it, then examine interactions. If two of the variables are associated while the third is completely independent, we would test hypotheses of *partial independence*. Alternatively, we could ask if two of the variables are *conditionally independent*, that is, if they are independent within each level of the third variable, but apparently dependent when the third variable is included because both of them depend on the third variable.

The hypotheses of partial independence are:

$H_0^{(1)}: p_{ijk} = p_{i \cdot \cdot} p_{\cdot jk}$ (row classification independent of column and layer classification);
$H_0^{(2)}: p_{ijk} = p_{\cdot j \cdot} p_{i \cdot k}$ (column classification independent of row and layer classification);
$H_0^{(3)}: p_{ijk} = p_{\cdot \cdot k} p_{ij \cdot}$ (layer classification independent of row and column classification).

Although direct computation of these subgroups is not complicated, it is easier to use log-linear models. These are presented fairly simply by Everitt (1992) and by Fienberg (1977). Some useful examples are described by Fisher and van Belle (1993), in Chapter 7.

As an example, consider again the data on surgical mortality (Table 14.21). These were analyzed by the interactive freeware program http://statpages.org/#CrossTabs. They can also be analyzed in the Frequency section of http://vassarstats.net/.

Table 14.21 Mortality rate by surgeon (p-proportion)

Surgeon 1					Surgeon 2				
	Dead	Alive		p		Dead	Alive		p
Simple	14	397	411	0.034	Simple	4	342	346	0.012
Complex	10	44	54	0.23	Complex	2	49	51	0.041
	24	441	465			6	391	397	

$$G^2 = 0.3, \quad PP = NS \qquad G^2 = 9.2, \quad PP < 0.005 \qquad G^2 = 15.62, \quad P < 0.001$$
$$\chi^2 = 0.305, \quad PP = 0.581 \qquad \chi^2 = 8.493, \quad PP = 0.004 \qquad \chi^2 = 22.486, \quad PP < 0.0001$$

There are differences between the mortality rates for the two surgeons, but how do we evaluate these? When the complete table is analyzed by log-linear analysis,

Table 14.22 Partial independence

Surgeon vs RACHS				Surgeon vs Survival				RACHS vs Survival			
	Simple	Complex			Dead	Alive			Dead	Alive	
Surgeon 1	411	54	465	Surgeon 1	24	441	465	Simple	18	739	757
Surgeon 2	346	51	397	Surgeon 2	6	391	397	Complex	12	93	105
	757	105	862		30	832	862		30	832	862

$G^2 = 26.33$ with 4 df, $P < 0.00$. (G^2 is distributed like chi-square.) Therefore reject the null hypothesis of independence, and then find out where the associations are. To do this, test for partial independence in which two of the variables are examined for association and the third is completely independent (Table 14.22). Do this by ignoring the third component in each analysis.

Each of these tables has 1 df. In the first panel, for example, the association between the surgeon and severity is examined, independent of survival. We conclude that the choice of surgeon and severity of disease are not related (first panel, perfectly reasonable), and also conclude that survival and severity are associated (third panel, also reasonable). In the middle panel, however, the significant difference in mortality rates is important and is what we wanted to examine, but does not allow for differences in severity of disease. Because these log–linear analyses are additive, determine if the difference between surgical mortalities explains all the overall difference shown for Table 14.21. In this table $G^2 = 26.33$ with 4 df. If we concentrate on the data in the center panel of Table 14.22, after subtracting $G^2 = 9.2$ with 1 df, we are left with $G^2 = 17.13$ with 3 df, and now $P < 0.001$. In other words, disease severity does play a role in the surgical mortalities. If from the overall results in Table 14.22 we subtract the G^2 results from both the panels that involve disease severity, we get $G^2 = 26.33 - 0.3 - 15.62 = 10.41$ with degrees of freedom $4 - 1 - 1 = 2$, and $P = 0.0055$. Therefore, even after allowing for disease severity there is a significant difference between the mortality rates for the two surgeons.

REFERENCES

Adler, F., 1951. Yates' correction and the statisticians. J. Am. Stat. Assoc. 46, 490–501.

Altman, D.G., 1992. Practical Statistics for Medical Research. Chapman & Hall, London, p. 611.

Armitage, P., Berry, G., Matthews, J.N.S., 2002. Statistical Methods in Medical Research. Blackwell, Oxford.

Basile, A.S., Hughes, R.D., Harrison, P.M., Murata, Y., Pannell, L., Jones, E.A., Williams, R., Skolnick, P., 1991. Elevated brain concentrations of 1,4-diazopines in fulminant hepatic failure. N. Engl. J. Med. 325, 473–478.

Berkson, J., 1946. Limitations of the fourfold table analysis to hospital data. Biom. Bull. 2, 47–53.

Bickel, P.J., Hammel, E.A., O'Connell, J.W., 1975. Sex bias in graduate admissions: data from Berkeley. Science 187, 398–404.

Binder, H.J., Clemett, A.R., Thayer, W.R., Spiro, H.M., 1965. Rarity of hiatus hernia in achalasia. N. Engl. J. Med. 272, 680–681.

Bracey, G. Those Misleading SAT and NAEP Trends: Simpson's Paradox at Work. http://www.huffingtonpost.com/gerald-bracey/on-knowing-when-youre-bei_b_39647.html.

Camilli, G., 1990. The test of homogeneity for 2×2 contingency tables: a review of and some personal opinions on the controversy. Psychol. Bull. 108, 135–145.

Charig, C.R., Webb, D.R., Payne, S.R., Wickham, J.E., 1986. Comparison of treatment of renal calculi by open surgery, percutaneous nephrolithotomy, and extracorporeal shockwave lithotripsy. Br. Med. J. (Clin. Res. Ed.) 292, 879–882.

Cochran, W.G., 1954. Some methods for strengthening the common c^2 tests. Biometrics 10, 417–451.

Cohen, M., Nagel, E., 1934. An Introduction to Logic and Scientific Method. Harcourt Brace and Co, New York.

Cohen, J., 1988. Statistical Power Analysis for Behavioral Sciences. Lawrence Erlbaum Associates, Hillsdale, NJ, p. 567.

Conover, W.J., 1974. Some reasons for not using the Yates continuity correction on 2×2 contingency tables. J. Am. Stat. Assoc. 69, 374–376.

Daniel, W.W., 1995. Biostatistics. A Foundation for Analysis in the Health Sciences. John Wiley & Sons, Inc., New York, p. 780.

Everitt, B.S., 1992. The Analysis of Contingency Tables. Chapman & Hall, London, p. 164.

Fienberg, S.E., 1977. The Analysis of Cross-Classified Categorical Data. The MIT Press, Cambridge, p. 151.

Fisher, L.D., van Belle, G., 1993. Biostatistics. A Methodology for the Health Sciences. John Wiley and Sons, New York, p. 991.

Fisher, R.A., 1936. Has Mendel's work been rediscovered? Ann. Sci. 1, 115–137.

Fleiss, J.L., 1981. Statistical Methods for Rates and Proportions. John Wiley & Sons, New York, p. 321.

Hernandez-Diaz, S., Schisterman, E.F., Hernan, M.A., 2006. The birth weight "paradox" uncovered? Am. J. Epidemiol. 164, 1115–1120.

Hernberg, S., Nurminen, M., Tolonen, M., 1973. Excess mortality from coronary heart disease in viscose rayon workers exposed to carbon disulfide. Scand. J. Work Environ. Health 10, 93–99.

Internet Project, Simpson's Paradox http://wps.aw.com/wps/media/objects/15/15719/projects/ch2_simpson/index.html#top.

Julious, S.A., Mullee, M.A., 1994. Confounding and Simpson's paradox. BMJ (Clin. Res. Ed.) 309, 1480–1481.

Koopmans, L.H., 1987. Introduction to Contemporary Statistical Methods. Duxbury Press, Boston, p. 683.

LaCroix, A.Z., Wienpahl, J., White, L.R., Wallace, R.B., Scherr, P.A., George, L.K., Cornoni-Huntley, J., Ostfeld, A.M., 1990. Thiazide diuretic agents and the incidence of hip fracture. N. Engl. J. Med. 322, 286–290.

Ludbrook, J., Dudley, H., 1994. Issues in biomedical statistics: analysing 2×2 tables of frequencies. Aust. N. Z. J. Surg. 64, 780–787.

Mainland, D., 1953. The risk of fallacious conclusions from autopsy data on the incidence of diseases with applications to heart disease. Am. Heart J. 45, 644–654.

Mantel, N., Haenszel, W., 1959. Statistical aspects of analysis of data from retrospective studies of disease. J. Natl. Cancer Inst. 22, 719–748.

Mantel, N., 1963. Chi-square tests with one degree of freedom: extensions of the Mantel–Haenszel procedure. J. Am. Stat. Assoc. 58, 690–700.

Maxwell, E.A., 1976. Analysis of contingency tables and further reasons for not using Yates; correction in 2×2 tables. Can. J. Stat. Sect. C Appl. 4, 277–290.

Mendel, G., 1965. Experiments in Plant Hybridisation. Oliver and Boyd, Edinburgh.

Morrell, C.H., 1999. Simpson's paradox: an example from a longitudinal study in South Africa. J. Stat. Educ. 7, 3.

Muench, H., 1965. Hiatus hernia in achalasia. N. Engl. J. Med. 272, 1134.

Perera, R., 2006. Statistics and death from meningococcal disease in children. BMJ (Clin. Res. Ed.) 332, 1297–1298.

Rhoades, H.M., Overall, J.E., 1982. A sample size correction for Pearson chi-square in 2 × 2 contingency tables. Psychol. Bull. 91, 418–423.

Roberts, R.S., Spitzer, W.O., Delmore, T., Sackett, D.L., 1978. An empirical demonstration of Berkson's bias. J. Chronic Dis. 31, 119–128.

Simpson, E.H., 1951. The interpretation of interaction in contingency tables. J. R. Stat. Soc. Ser. B 13, 238–241.

Group TSSIS, 1991. Treatment of migraine attacks with sumatriptan. N. Engl. J. Med. 325, 316–321.

Upton, G.J.G., 1982. A comparison of alternative tests for the 2 × 2 comparative trial. J. R. Stat. Soc. A 145, 86–105.

Wilcox, A.J., 2006. Invited commentary: the perils of birth weight—a lesson from directed acyclic graphs. Am. J. Epidemiol. 164, 1121–1123 discussion 1124–25.

Williams, B., 1978. A Sampler on Sampling. John Wiley & Sons, New York.

Yates, F., 1934. Contingency tables involving small numbers and the χ^2 test. J. R. Stat. Soc. A Suppl. 1, 217–235.

Yates, F., 1984. Tests of significance for 2 × 2 contingency tables. J. R. Stat. Soc. A 147, 426–463.

Zar, J.H., 2010. Biostatistical Analysis. Prentice Hall, Upper Saddle River, NJ, p. 044.

CHAPTER 15

Categorical and Cross-Classified Data: McNemar's Test, Kolmogorov—Smirnov Tests, Concordance

Contents

PAIRED SAMPLES: MCNEMAR'S TEST

The chi-squared tests in Chapter 12 are unpaired tests. It is, however, sometimes appropriate to pair data (McNemar, 1947). Catalona et al. (1975) compared the reactivity to DNCB and PHA in each of 28 patients with genitourinary tract malignances; that is reactivity to both agents, one on each arm, was tested in each patient. The data are shown in Table 15.1.

Table 15.1 Paired data set

		DNCB		
		Reactive	Nonreactive	Total
PHA	Reactive	13	3	16
	Nonreactive	4	8	12
	Total	17	11	28

For a list of all websites referred to in this chapter, as clickable links, see the book companion website: www.booksite.elsevier.com/9780128023877.

Biostatistics for Medical and Biomedical Practitioners
http://dx.doi.org/10.1016/B978-0-12-802387-7.00015-9
221

This 2 × 2 table resembles a typical 2 × 2 chi-square table, but it is not because the results are pairs of results; the units are pairs, not individuals. The table shows that 13 patients reacted to both agents, three patients reacted to PHA but not to DNCB, four patients reacted to DNCB but not to PHA, and eight patients did not react to either agent. By chi-square analysis, χ^2_T is 6.39 and $P = 0.0115$; the odds ratio is 8.667. No clear interpretation of the chi-square and the odds ratio can be obtained. The odds ratio implies that the proportion of reactors to DNCB is higher in those who are also reactors to PHA, and the chi-square value indicates that we can reject the null hypothesis that this proportion is similar in those who do and who do not react to PHA. However, that was not the scientific question being investigated, which was whether there was a difference in the reactivity of the patients to the two agents, and the chi-square test does not help to evaluate this question. To make this judgment, use McNemar's test. The proportion of PHA reactive patients who also react to DNCB is $\frac{a}{a+b}$, $\left(= \frac{13}{13+3} \right)$, and the proportion of DNCB reactive patients who react to PHA is $\frac{a}{a+c}$, $\left(= \frac{13}{13+4} \right)$. The only way that these two proportions can differ is if b (3) and c (4) are unequal, so it is these two cells that we focus on; those who react to both agents, or who react to neither, do not help to evaluate differences between reactivity to these agents. Therefore, focus attention on the two sets of discordant results; three patients who react to PHA but not to DNCB, and four patients who react to DNCB but not to PHA. There is no real difference between these, and if formal testing were needed one could use a 2 × 1 chi-square or the binomial theorem. Although hardly necessary, these calculations can be done online at http://www.graphpad.com/quickcalcs/McNemar1.cfm and http://vassarstats.net/.

To see an example of a significant difference by McNemar's test, consider the data presented in Table 15.2, based on a study done of the response of preterm infants with a patent ductus arteriosus to indomethacin, a drug purported to lead to closure of the ductus arteriosus. Because the chance of there being a persistent ductus arteriosus depends on the degree of prematurity, infants were paired based on their weight at birth, and one member of the pair chosen at random was given indomethacin whereas the other member of the pair was given a placebo.

Because this is a paired test, compare the 27 pairs of patients whose ductuses closed with indomethacin but not with placebo with the 13 pairs of patients whose ductuses

Table 15.2 Paired patent ductus arteriosus study

Indomethacin	Placebo	
	Closed	Open
Closed	65	27
Open	13	40

closed with placebo but not with indomethacin. The null hypothesis of no difference in responsiveness to the two agents gives us an expected number of $\frac{13+27}{2} = 20$, so that $\chi^2_T = \frac{(|27-20|-0.5)^2}{20} + \frac{(|13-20|-0.5)^2}{20} = 4.22$ which, with one degree of freedom, gives $P = 0.04$. It is thus reasonable to reject the null hypothesis, and to believe that indomethacin is more likely than the placebo to cause closure of the ductus arteriosus. If we had analyzed this table with the chi-square test, then $\chi^2_T = 26.954$, and $0.0001 > P$, but we would have difficulty in drawing conclusions from the analysis.

(Excluding the Yates' adjustment for discontinuity, this calculation is the same as $\frac{(27-13)^2}{27+13}$, or more generally $\frac{(b-c)^2}{b+c}$, where b and c are the two discordant frequencies (McNemar, 1947).) As a rule of thumb, there should be at least 10 discordant pairs for accurate computation of χ^2_T.

It is of interest to analyze these data as an unpaired chi-squared test. To extract the correct numbers, remember that the count in each cell indicates the response of two infants. Therefore, the number of ductuses that closed with indomethacin is 92—the 65 members of the pairs in which both members closed with indomethacin and placebo and the 27 members of the pairs closed with indomethacin but not with placebo. The remaining numbers can be worked out similarly, and the results (with Yates' correction) are given in Table 15.3.

Table 15.3 Unpaired patent ductus arteriosus study

	Closed		Open		Total
Indomethacin	**92**	85	**53**	60	145
	7		−7		
	6.5	42.25	−6.5	42.25	
		0.50		*0.70*	
Placebo	**78**	85	**67**	60	145
	7		−7		
	−6.5	42.25	6.5	42.25	
		0.50		*0.70*	
Total	170		120		290

$\chi^2_T = 2.40$, 1 d.f., and $P = 0.12$; that is, we cannot reject the null hypothesis. This example shows that a paired test is more sensitive than an unpaired test.

If the number of discordant observations is very small relative to the number of concordant observations, then McNemar's test is still valid but the difference between the groups, although significant, becomes trivial when related to the sample size. Assume, for example, the results shown in Table 15.4.

Table 15.4 Hypothetical paired study

	Group A	
Group B	**Success**	**Failure**
Success	4000	27
Failure	13	3000

McNemar's test gives the same conclusion as for the data in Table 15.2, namely a significant difference between groups A and B. Nevertheless, common sense tells us that either there is a success in both groups or a failure in both groups, and that very seldom will there be discordance. Once again, the distinction between statistical significance and importance needs to be considered. Furthermore, although the concordant cells a and d play no part in the McNemar test per se, they are a factor in estimating the variance of the difference between $\widehat{p_1} = \frac{a+c}{N}$ and $\widehat{p_2} = \frac{a+b}{N}$ (Selvin, 1995)

$$\text{Variance } \widehat{p_1} - \widehat{p_2} = \frac{(a+d)(b+c) + 4bc}{N^2}.$$

Thus if a and d are very large, so are the variance and the resulting confidence limits.

Bowker's Test

A similar paired test with three or more categories, the Bowker test (Bowker, 1948), can also be done. Consider three categories of improved, unchanged, and worse, with the two treatments given to paired patients (Table 15.5).

Table 15.5 Paired test with three categories

		Treatment A			
		Improved	**Unchanged**	**Worse**	**Total**
Treatment B	Improved	50	18	35	103
	Unchanged	7	20	9	36
	Worse	8	12	30	50
	Total	65	50	74	189

To perform Bowker's test, do three separate McNemar tests: Improved versus Unchanged, Improved versus Worse, and Unchanged versus Worse. Each of these gives a value for χ^2, calculated as $\frac{(b-c)^2}{b+c}$. These are summed to give the total Bowker χ^2. This is then evaluated by a chi-square distribution with degrees of freedom $\nu = \binom{k}{2}$, where k is the number of categories (that can be more than 3). For the example above, the chi-squares for each of the individual McNemar tests are $\frac{(18-7)^2}{18+7} = 4.84, \frac{(35-8)^2}{35+8} = 16.95$, and $\frac{(9-8)^2}{9+8} = 0.059$.

Thus the total chi-square is 21.85 with 3 d.f., and $P = 0.00007$ (the 0.05 value is 7.81). Therefore the universal null hypothesis H_0: $p_{12} = p_{21}$, $p_{13} = p_{31}$, and $p_{23} = p_{32}$

can be rejected. The investigator then inspects the individual paired tests to decide which of the alternative hypotheses to consider.

TESTING ORDERED CATEGORICAL DATA: KOLMOGOROV–SMIRNOV TESTS

If the categories to which the data are assigned are ordered, the chi-square test may not be the best test to use. Kolmogorov–Smirnov (K-S) tests were developed to compare ordered distributions. Kolmogorov type tests are designed to compare an observed sample distribution and a specified theoretical distribution, and are termed K-S one-sample tests. Smirnov type tests are designed to compare two (or occasionally more) observed distributions, and are termed K-S two-sample tests. These tests do not depend on parameters of the distributions, but assume that the distribution of the underlying variable is continuous. They are therefore applicable to ordinal but not nominal data.

In principle, these tests obtain the cumulative frequencies for each of the distributions, observed or theoretical, plot the cumulative frequencies for each distribution on the vertical (Y) axis against the ordered groups on the horizontal (X) axis, convert the cumulative absolute frequencies to cumulative relative frequencies (i.e., as fractions of the total number), and then examine the vertical differences between the cumulative frequencies for the two distributions at each ordered group (Figure 15.1, based on Table 15.6 below).

If the distributions are consistent with having come from the same population, then the vertical differences are unlikely to be large. The sampling distributions of the maximal differences, if the null hypothesis is true, have been determined. Therefore, if the maximal vertical difference exceeds the $1 - \alpha$ quantile, the null hypothesis can be rejected at the level α.

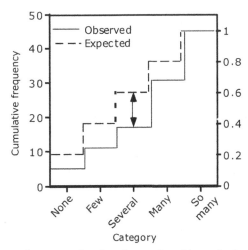

Figure 15.1 The cumulative frequency for the observed and hypothesized distributions is plotted against the ordered frequencies for the number of ectopic beats (see below). The left-hand vertical scale is in absolute cumulative numbers, the right-hand vertical scale is the relative cumulative frequency. The vertical double arrow indicates the maximal vertical difference.

K–S One-Sample Test

After surviving a myocardial infarction, patients may be studied for 24 h to determine how many ventricular ectopic beats per hour they have, as a means to assess their risk of sudden death. The average hourly number of these ectopic beats is assessed as none, few (1–10), several (11–30), many (31–300), and so many ($\geq$300). If the numbers in each group are 5, 6, 6, 14, and 14, for a total of 45, is there any evidence that the numbers in each group are or are not randomly distributed? The null hypothesis H_0 is that the numbers should be the same in each group, namely, 9 in each group (Figure 15.1 above).

We could treat this as a one by five contingency table, and ask if there was any relationship between the frequency category and the number in it by performing a chi-square test (Table 15.6).

Table 15.6 One-sample test

	None	Few	Several	Many	So many	Total
Observed	5	6	6	14	14	45
Expected	9	9	9	9	9	45
Difference	−4	−3	−3	5	5	
Difference^2	16	9	9	25	25	
χ^2	1.778	1.000	1.000	2.778	2.778	9.334

$\chi^2_T = 9.334$, 4 d.f., $P = 0.0533$.

This does not quite reach the 5% level of significance. In this example, it would not matter if we interchanged the positions of any of the columns. In the chi-square test, the categories are merely names. However, we know that the categories are ordered, and should ask if we can make use of this information to create a more sensitive test.

One approach is to use the one-sample K–S test. To do this, H_0 is the same null hypothesis that the observed distribution does not differ significantly from some expected distribution of interest. Then the observed and expected numbers are cumulated (Table 15.7), and their absolute deviations are calculated. A variation used here is to make all the cumulative numbers fractions of the total.

Table 15.7 Layout for the Kolmogorov–Smirnov test

	None	Few	Several	Many	So many	Total
Observed	5	6	6	14	14	45
Cumulative observed (Co)	5	11	17	31	45	
Relative Co	**5/45 = 0.111**	**11/45 = 0.244**	**17/45 = 0.378**	**31/45 = 0.689**	**1**	
Expected	9	9	9	9	9	45
Cumulative expected (Ce)	9	18	27	36	45	
Relative Ce	**9/45 = 0.200**	**18/45 = 0.400**	**27/45 = 0.600**	**36/45 = 0.800**	**1**	
Relative |Difference|	**0.089**	**0.156**	**0.222**	**0.111**	**0**	

If the null hypothesis is true, then none of the relative differences should be very big. The sampling distribution of these differences has been worked out, and tables give the critical values of the maximal fractional difference for different total numbers. The largest relative difference is 0.222, and the 0.05 critical value for $N = 45$ is 0.1984, so that $P < 0.05$ that the null hypothesis is true, that is, we can reject the null hypothesis at the 0.05 level. An online program is available at http://home.ubalt.edu/ntsbarsh/Business-stat/otherapplets/ks.htm (which needs at least six categories of data), http://www.physics.csbsju.edu/stats/KS-test.n.plot_form.html (which needs at least 10 data categories), http://www.wessa.net/rwasp_Reddy-Moores%20K-S%20Test.wasp#charts, and http://vassarstats.net/ksm.html. We would obtain a different maximal fractional difference if we change the order of the columns (Table 15.8).

Table 15.8 Revised Kolmogorov–Smirnov test to change the order of data

	None	Many	Few	Several	Very many	Total
Observed	5	14	6	6	14	45
Cumulative observed (Co)	5	19	25	31	45	
Relative Co	**0.111**	**0.422**	**0.556**	**0.689**		
Expected	9	9	9	9	9	45
Cumulative expected (Ce)	9	36	18	27	45	
Relative Ce	**0.200**	**0.800**	**0.400**	**0.600**		
Relative |difference|	**0.089**	**0.378**	**0.156**	**0.089**	**0**	

In this instance, the deviation from the null hypothesis is even greater; the critical value for 0.01 is 0.237, so that $P < 0.01$.

As in most hypothesis tests, there are three possibilities if H_0 is rejected. The usual two-sided test is H_0: Observed distribution = Expected distribution.

H_A: Observed distribution $\neq$ Expected distribution.

However, one-sided tests are also possible. There are two of these:

a. H_0: Observed distribution = Expected distribution

H_A: Observed distribution > Expected distribution,

and

b. H_0: Observed distribution = Expected distribution

H_A: Observed distribution < Expected distribution.

For (a), calculate the greatest vertical difference by which the observed distribution exceeds the expected distribution; for (b), calculate the greatest vertical difference by which the observed distribution falls below the expected distribution. The test is done in the same way, but Table 15.8 is examined under one-sided values for α.

Critical values for the one-sample K-S test may be found at http://www.york.ac.uk/depts/maths/tables/kolmogorovsmirnov.ps, for N up to 40. For larger values of N an approximate formula is given (e.g., $1.22/\sqrt{N}$ for one sided $\alpha = 0.05$), but a more accurate estimate comes from $\sqrt{\frac{-\ln(\alpha/2)}{2N}} - \frac{0.16693}{N}$ (Zar, 2010). For $N = 45$ the first formula yields $\frac{1.22}{\sqrt{45}} = 0.1819$, and the more accurate formula yields $\sqrt{\frac{-\ln 0.025}{2 \times 45}} - \frac{0.16693}{45} = 0.1987$.

Problem 15.1

Test the following distribution for difference from a uniform distribution: 4, 11, 19, 31, 42, 50, 63, 68.

K–S Two-Sample Test

This can be used to compare two (or more) distributions, to find out if they could have been drawn from a single population or from two populations with the same distributions. Unlike some other tests, which test differences between the means or the medians, these tests are sensitive to differences in shapes of the distributions as well.

The assumptions behind the test are that the samples are random samples, that the two samples are mutually independent, that the measurement scale is at least ordinal, and for exact results, the random variables should be continuous. If the variables are discrete, the test remains valid but becomes conservative.

Set up the two cumulative frequency distributions, just as in Table 15.8. Because the total numbers (m, n) in each group can be different, the relative cumulative frequency distributions must be calculated. The maximal vertical difference between these distributions is obtained, multiplied by mn, and the result compared with the quantile values in the appropriate table. Such tables can be found at http://www.scribd.com/doc/53565230/103/Table-I-Kolmogorov-Smirnov-Two-Sample-Statistic, and http://home.ubalt.edu/ntsbarsh/Business-stat/otherapplets/ks.htm. Alternatively the maximal difference is significant at $\alpha = 0.05$ (two-tailed) if it exceeds $1.36\sqrt{\frac{N_1+N_2}{N_1 N_2}}$, where N_1 and N_2 are the respective sample sizes (Campbell, 1989; Siegel and Castellan, 1988). As an example, consider a study of the occurrence of nausea after two different chemotherapeutic agents (Table 15.9).

Table 15.9 Comparison of the degree of nausea after two chemotherapeutic agents

Group		None	Vague	Slight	Mild	Moderate	Severe	Very severe
A	Observed O_A	9	18	15	10	11	10	9
A	Cumulative O_A	9	27	42	52	63	73	82
A	Relative O_A	0.1098	0.3297	0.5122	0.6341	0.7683	0.8902	1
B	Observed O_B	5	10	12	13	13	10	10
B	Cumulative O_B	5	15	27	40	53	63	73
B	Relative O_B	0.0685	0.2055	0.3699	0.5479	0.7260	0.8630	1
	Relative D	0.0413	0.1242	0.1423	0.0862	0.0423	0.0272	

The largest difference is 0.1423. The critical value for $\alpha = 0.05$ is $1.36\sqrt{\frac{N_1+N_2}{N_1 N_2}} = 1.36\sqrt{\frac{82+73}{82\times73}} = 0.2188$. Because this exceeds the maximal difference, reject the hypothesis that the two distributions are significantly different. This is the same conclusion as obtained from the online program at http://home.ubalt.edu/ntsbarsh/Business-stat/otherapplets/ks.htm. For $\alpha = 0.025$ or 0.01 the above formula is used with factors 1.48 and 1.63, respectively, in place of 1.36.

Problem 15.2

Use the K-S test to determine if the following two distributions are comparable

8	17	31	47	52	73	89	98
4	6	19	36	44	68	93	99

CONCORDANCE (AGREEMENT) BETWEEN OBSERVERS

Two Categories

At times, we want to know how close the agreement (concordance) is between two sets of data; for example, if two radiologists examine the films of an upper gastrointestinal barium study, how often will they agree or disagree about the presence of an ulcer? If two ophthalmologists examine patients for papilledema, how often will they agree or disagree? The results of such studies can be set out in 2×2 tables, but neither chi-square nor McNemar's tests are appropriate to answer the question. Consider the data set out in Table 15.10.

Table 15.10 Interobserver agreement

	Radiologist A		
Radiologist B	**Ulcer**	**No ulcer**	**Total**
Ulcer	20	4	24
No ulcer	9	85	94
Total	29	89	118

Here both radiologists diagnose ulcers in 20 patients, and agree that there are no ulcers in 85 patients. However, radiologist A diagnoses ulcers in 9 patients whom radiologist B regards as having no ulcer, whereas radiologist B diagnoses ulcers in 4 patients whom radiologist A considers as being normal. How can we specify the degree of agreement of these two radiologists? The percentage of agreement is

$$\left(\frac{a+d}{N}\right) \times 100;$$

and, for example, in Table 15.10 is $\left(\frac{20+85}{118}\right) \times 100 = 89.0\%$. However, this index does not take account of the degree of agreement expected by chance. We can calculate the expected values in each cell if the null hypothesis is true as we did for the chi-square test: the expected value for a is $\frac{29 \times 24}{118} = 5.90$, and the expected value for d is $\frac{89 \times 94}{118} = 70.9$. Now calculate the percentage of agreement using the expected numbers to get $\left(\frac{5.90+70.9}{118}\right) \times 100 = 65.1\%$. How much better than chance agreement did they do? One way of assessing this is to use the κ (kappa) statistic (Cohen, 1960).

$$\kappa = \frac{p_o - p_e}{1 - p_e},$$

where p_o is the observed proportion of agreements, and p_e is the chance expected proportion of agreements. The agreement expected by chance is obtained by adding the chance-expected agreements in cells a and d—in which both observers agree or disagree with the diagnosis—and dividing by the total number of observations. The expected value in cell a is $\frac{R_1 \times C_1}{N}$, and in cell d is $\frac{R_2 \times C_2}{N}$. Therefore, the proportion of expected agreements is

$$\frac{\frac{R_1 \times C_1}{N} + \frac{R_2 \times C_2}{N}}{N} = \frac{R_1 \times C_1 + R_2 \times C_2}{N^2}$$

If the observed and chance-expected agreements are the same, the numerator and thus κ will be zero. If the observed agreement is perfect and the chance agreement is zero, then the numerator and denominator will be 1, and so will κ. If the observed agreement is less than the chance-expected agreement, then κ will be negative.

In the example given in Table 15.10, $\kappa = \frac{0.89-0.65}{1-0.65} = 0.69$. This result can be evaluated in two ways. One is by computing the standard error of κ when the null hypothesis is true, that is, when $\kappa = 0$, from the formula developed by Fleiss, Cohen and Everitt (Fleiss, 1981) and implemented at http://graphpad.com/quickcalcs/Kappa2.cfm, The standard error by this formula is 0.081, so that $z = 0.69/0.081 = 8,52$, $P < 0001$. This indicates that the null hypothesis is unlikely and that the two observers have systematic differences in the way they interpret the X-ray films. The other way to evaluate κ

is to assess qualitatively the degree of agreement as $<0 =$ poor; $0-0.20 =$ slight; $0.21-0.40 =$ fair; $0.41-0.60 =$ moderate; $0.61-0.80 =$ substantial; $0.81-1.00 =$ almost perfect (Landis and Koch, 1977).

More than Two Categories

There may be more than two categories to be evaluated. For example, two physicians may be evaluating four grades of pneumonia: $+$, $++$, $+++$, or $++++$, based on considering fever, white blood cell count, cognitive state, physical findings in the lungs, and chest X-ray findings (Table 15.11).

Table 15.11 Interrater agreement. Agreement shown in bold enlarged type

		Physician A				
		+	++	+++	++++	Total
Physician B	+	**72**	18	7	1	98
	++	22	**53**	6	1	82
	+++	9	7	**24**	4	44
	++++	3	10	7	**6**	26
	Total	106	88	44	12	250

It is often easier to work after these numbers have been turned into proportions of the total (Table 15.12a). Then both N and N^2 are 1, and can be omitted from the equation.

Table 15.12a Observed interrater agreement as proportions. Agreement shown in bold enlarged type

		Radiologist A				
		+	++	+++	++++	Total
Radiologist B	+	**0.288**	0.072	0.028	0.004	0.392
	++	0.088	**0.212**	0.024	0.004	0.328
	+++	0.036	0.028	**0.096**	0.016	0.176
	++++	0.012	0.040	0.028	**0.024**	0.104
	Total	0.424	0.352	0.176	0.048	1.000

From these data calculate the expected proportions as usual as R_iC_j (Table 15.12b).

Table 15.12b Expected proportions. The expected proportion in any cell is the product of the corresponding marginal row and column proportions. Thus, $0.166 = 0.424 \times 0.392$

		Radiologist A				
		+	++	+++	++++	Total
Radiologist B	+	**0.166**	0.138	0.069	0.019	0.392
	++	0.139	**0.115**	0.058	0.016	0.328
	+++	0.075	0.062	**0.031**	0.008	0.176
	++++	0.044	0.037	0.018	**0.005**	0.104
	Total	0.424	0.352	0.176	0.048	1.000

Then the observed agreement from Table 15.12a (bold figures) is $0.288 + 0.212 + 0.096 + 0.024 = 0.62$. The expected agreement, also in bold figures (Table 15.12b), is $R_1C_1 + R_2C_2 + R_3C_3 + R_4C_4 = (0.424 \times 0.392) + (0.352 \times 0.328) + (0.176 \times 0.176) + (0.048 \times 0.104) = 0.32$.

Then

$$\kappa = \frac{0.62 - 0.32}{1 - 0.32} = 0.44.$$

There are interactive online calculators that include the option of comparing the concordance among more than two observers: http://graphpad.com/quickcalcs/Kappa2.cfm, http://www.singlecaseresearch.org/calculators/pabak-os.

Weighted Kappa

If the categories are nominal, this form of kappa set out above has to be used. Sometimes, however, the categories form an ordered array, just as in the example above. Then diagnosing + instead of ++ is not as serious an error as diagnosing + instead of +++ or ++++. To deal with this, each observed value is weighted in one of the two ways (Cohen, 1968). If each category is regarded as one step different from the adjacent one, use unit weights. If the error is proportionately more serious as the disagreement becomes more marked, then a quadratic weight is given. The effect of weighting is to minimize small discrepancies. If there are k ordered categories, then categories may differ by $1, 2 \ldots k - 1$ distances, with $k - 1$ being the maximum discrepancy. Then for linear weights, use

$$\text{weight} = 1 - \frac{|\text{distance}|}{\text{maximal possible distance}},$$

and for quadratic weights, use

$$\text{weight} = 1 - \frac{|\text{distance}|^2}{\text{maximal possible distance}^2}.$$

Linear and quadratic weights for the pneumonia data shown above are given in Tables 15.13a and 15.13b.

Table 15.13a Linear weights for $k = 4$

		Physician A			
		+	++	+++	++++
Physician B	+	1	$1 - 1/3 = 0.67$	$1 - 2/3 = 0.33$	0
	++	0.67	1	0.67	0.33
	+++	0.33	0.67	1	0.67
	++++	0	0.33	0.67	1

Table 15.13b Quadratic weights for $k = 4$

		Physician A			
		+	++	+++	++++
Physician B	+	1	$1 - (1/3)^2 = 0.89$	$1 - 4/9 = 0.56$	0
	++	0.89	1	0.89	0.56
	+++	0.56	0.89	1	0.89
	++++	0	0.56	0.89	1

Multiply each of the data cells by the corresponding weight, both for the observed data and for the expected data. Then add the probabilities for all the k^2 cells in the observed set to give p_o, and do the same for all the cells in the expected data table to give p_e. For the data in Table 15.12a, quadratic weighting gives the results in Tables 15.14a and 15.14b.

Table 15.14a Weighted observed probabilities

		Physician A			
		+	++	+++	++++
Physician B	+	**0.288**	0.064	0.016	0
	++	0.078	**0.212**	0.021	0.002
	+++	0.020	0.025	**0.096**	0.014
	++++	0	0.020	0.025	**0.024**

Table 15.14b Weighted expected probabilities

		Physician A			
		+	++	+++	++++
Physician B	+	**0.166**	0.122	0.032	0
	++	0.124	**0.115**	0.052	0.009
	+++	0.042	0.055	**0.031**	0.007
	++++	0	0.021	0.016	**0.005**

Then $p_o = 0.905$. Also $p_e = 0.797$. The quadratic weighted kappa is

$$\kappa = \frac{0.905 - 0.797}{1 - 0.797} = 0.53.$$

With linear weighting, kappa $= 0.48$.

Both of these weighted kappa estimates are a little higher than the unweighted kappa. Because hand calculations are tedious and prone to arithmetic error, it is better to use an online program that provides values for unweighted and both weighted kappa statistics, as well as standard errors and confidence intervals: http://faculty.vassar.edu/lowry/kappa.html.

There are advantages of using the quadratic weighting that turns out to be the equivalent of the intraclass correlation (Norman and Streiner, 1994).

Problem 15.3

Two subjects A and B are given a series of stimuli and asked to assess the degree of discomfort as 1 (least uncomfortable), 2, 3, and 4 (most uncomfortable). The following matrix shows their ratings. Calculate kappa (weighted and unweighted).

		Subject A			
	Degree	1	2	3	4
Subject B	1	16	3	1	1
	2	3	17	2	2
	3	4	6	14	3
	4	1	1	5	16

Uebersax (2008) has described clearly some of the issues involved in the rating comparisons. We need to know why they are being done, and how we interpret any differences that are found. If, for example, different radiologists disagree about the presence or absence of cancer on a mammogram, is this because they are using different criteria? And if so, can these criteria be clarified? As Uebersax wrote, "…the aim is more to understand the factors that cause raters to disagree, with an ultimate goal of improving their consistency and accuracy. For this, one should separately assess whether raters have the same definition of the basic trait (that different raters weight various image features similarly) and that they have similar widths for the various rating levels." The suggestion by Feinstein and Cicchetti of reporting p_{pos} and p_{neg} (see below) as well makes it easier to determine where agreements and disagreements occur.

Cautionary Tales

Do not accept the kappa statistic unreservedly. Like all omnibus statistics that uses a single number to summarize a batch of data, there are unseen dangers lurking, even with as simple a procedure as kappa.

Kraemer (1977) and Viera and Garrett (2005) pointed out that if a finding was rare (low prevalence), kappa might be very low despite what appears to be good agreement. As an example, the latter authors cited a study by Metlay et al. (1997) of pneumonia in which tactile fremitus was diagnosed with 85% agreement but with kappa only 0.01, and provided an explanation based on the rarity of the finding. Feinstein and Cicchetti (Cicchetti and Feinstein, 1990; Feinstein and Cicchetti, 1990) studied other paradoxes associated with kappa, and found that the same high percentage of agreement between two observers could produce either a high or a low value of kappa, depending on the distribution of the marginal subtotals (Tables 15.15a and 15.15b).

Table 15.15a Two rater agreement tables with similar percentage agreement but different kappa values

Observer B	Observer A Yes	No	Total
Yes	87	7	94
No	6	4	10
Total	93	11	104

Table 15.15b

Observer B	Observer A Yes	No	Total
Yes	72	12	84
No	2	24	26
Total	74	36	110

Tables based on examples provided by Feinstein and Cicchetti (1990).

In both sets of data there is substantial agreement between the two observers, with the observed agreement p_o being 0.88 in panel a and 0.87 in panel b. Nevertheless, the kappa values for each are very different, being 0.31 for panel a and 0.69 for panel b.

Subsequently, Cicchetti and Feinstein (1990) recommended that in addition to kappa the investigator should report the value of p_{pos} and p_{neg}. To calculate p_{pos}

$$P_{pos} = \frac{a}{\frac{R_+ + C_+}{2}} = \frac{2a}{R_+ + C_+}.$$

In this formula, use the format for the usual 2×2 table, where a is the number of positive agreements between the two observers, and R_+ and C_+ are the respective row and column subtotals associated with a. Thus, for observers a and b

$$p_{pos} = \frac{2 \times 87}{93 + 94} = 0.93 \text{ for observer a, and } p_{pos} = \frac{2 \times 72}{74 + 84} = 0.91 \text{ for observer b.}$$

To calculate p_{neg}

$$p_{neg} = \frac{d}{\frac{R_- + C_-}{2}} = \frac{2d}{R_- + C_-}.$$

Here d is the number of negative agreements between the two observers, and R_- and C_- are the associated row and column subtotals. Kappa is the weighted sum of the two proportions. Thus, for observers a and b

$$p_{neg} = \frac{2 \times 4}{11 + 10} = 0.38 \text{ for observer a and } p_{neg} = \frac{2 \times 24}{36 + 26} = 0.77 \text{ for observer b.}$$

These precautions have been emphasized by others (Byrt et al., 1993; Flight and Julious, 2014). The kappa statistic is affected by bias, the frequency at which raters choose a particular category, because this unbalances the table. The bias index (BI) is $BI = \frac{b-c}{N}$, and larger values of BI yield a larger kappa. It is also affected by the prevalence index (PI), defined as $PI = \frac{a-d}{N}$; the higher the PI the more unbalanced the table the lower the value for kappa. Both of these can be dealt with in a single formula (PABAK)

$$PABAK = \frac{\frac{(a+d)}{2N} - 0.5}{1 - 0.5} = 2p_o - 1.$$

If BI and PI are small, kappa and *PABAK* are similar. If they are large, the two measures differ, and caution is needed in interpreting the data.

INTRACLASS CORRELATION

Although there are variations of the kappa statistic for more than two raters, they are used less often than the intraclass correlation (Chapter 25).

For further discussion of concordance, see Fleiss (1981), Kramer and Feinstein (1981), and Randolph at http://www.eric.ed.gov/PDFS/ED490661.pdf. Because all of these measures of concordance—chi-square and odds ratio, kappa, Cramer's φ, and many others not mentioned here all use the same few cell numbers deployed in different ways, they are closely related to each other.

REFERENCES

Bowker, A.H., 1948. A test for symmetry in contingency tables. J. Am. Stat. Assoc. 43, 572—574.

Byrt, T., Bishop, J., Carlin, J.B., 1993. Bias, prevalence and kappa. J. Clin. Epidemiol. 46, 423—429.

Campbell, R.C., 1989. Statistics for Biologists. Cambridge University Press, London.

Catalona, W.J., Tarpley, J.L., Potvin, C., et al., 1975. Correlations among cutaneous reactivity to DNCB, PHA-induced lymphocyte blastogenesis and peripheral blood E rosettes. Clin. Exp. Immunol. 19, 327—333.

Cicchetti, D.V., Feinstein, A.R., 1990. High agreement but low kappa: II. Resolving the paradoxes. J. Clin. Epidemiol. 43, 551—558.

Cohen, J., 1960. A coefficient of agreement for nominal scales. Educ. Psychol. Meas. 20, 37—46.

Cohen, J., 1968. Weighted kappa: nominal scale agreement with provision for scaled disagreement or partial credit. Psychol. Bull. 70, 213—220.

Feinstein, A.R., Cicchetti, D.V., 1990. High agreement but low kappa: I. The problems of two paradoxes. J. Clin. Epidemiol. 43, 543—549.

Fleiss, J.L., 1981. Statistical Methods for Rates and Proportions. John Wiley & Sons.

Flight, L., Julious, S.A., 2014. The disagreeable behaviour of the kappa statistic. Pharm. Stat. 14, 74—78.

Kraemer, H.C., 1977. Ramifications of a population model for κ as a coefficient of reliability. Psychometrika 44, 461—472.

Kramer, M.S., Feinstein, A.R., 1981. Clinical biostatistics. LIV. The biostatistics of concordance. Clin. Pharmacol. Ther. 29, 111—123.

Landis, J.R., Koch, G.G., 1977. The measurement of observer agreement for categorical data. Biometrics 33, 159—174.

McNemar, Q., 1947. Note on the sampling error of the difference between correlated proportions or percentages. Psychometrika 12, 153—157.

Metlay, J.P., Kapoor, W.N., Fine, M.J., 1997. Does this patient have community-acquired pneumonia? Diagnosing pneumonia by history and physical examination. JAMA 278, 1440—1445.

Norman, G.R., Streiner, D.L., 1994. Biostatistics. The Bare Essentials. Mosby.

Selvin, S., 1995. Practical Biostatistical Methods. Wadsworth Publishing Company.

Siegel, S., Castellan, Jr., N.J., 1988. Nonparametric Statistics for the Behavioral Sciences. McGraw-Hill, New York.

Uebersax, J., 2008. Statistical Methods for Rater Agreement (Online). Available: http://john-uebersax.com/stat/agree.htm.

Viera, A.J., Garrett, J.M., 2005. Understanding interobserver agreement: the kappa statistic. Fam. Med. 37, 360—363.

Zar, J.H., 2010. Biostatistical Analysis. Prentice Hall.

CHAPTER 16

Binomial and Multinomial Distributions

Contents

BASIC CONCEPTS

Introduction

Observations that fall into one of two mutually exclusive categories are dichotomous or binary. Any population with only two categories is a binomial population; newborn infants are male or female or the outcome of a treatment is cure or failure. We can ask certain questions about binomial populations. For example, what is the likelihood that in a family of five children there will be three girls? What is the probability that 5 patients out of 50 will die from meningitis? How likely is it that 7 out of 20 people with a certain type of seizure will develop paralysis?

The allocation to each category must be unambiguous. The number of items (counts) in one group (for example, r successes), gives information about the proportion of the total number (n) attributed to one of the groups. It is usual to define the proportion of the number of one of the groups to the total (r/n) as π for a theoretical population, and as p

For a list of all websites referred to in this chapter, as clickable links, see the book companion website: www.booksite.elsevier.com/9780128023877.

Biostatistics for Medical and Biomedical Practitioners
http://dx.doi.org/10.1016/B978-0-12-802387-7.00016-0

for a sample from that population. Therefore, $\pi = \frac{\text{number of newborn girls}}{\text{total number of newborns}}$ in an infinitely large number of births, but the same proportion is p if related to a smaller number of births in a particular hospital at a given period. Because this is a dichotomous variable in which the total probability must add to 1, if the probability of one of the two categories is π, then the probability of the other category must be $1 - \pi$. In a sample, the probability of one category is p, and the other is $1 - p$, also called q. By convention, the probability of one category is a success and of the other category is a failure, without equating the terms "success" and "failure" with the merit or desirability of the outcome. An examination of the dichotomous outcomes of a study is often termed a Bernoulli trial if:

1. The number of trials is defined.
2. In each trial, the event of interest either occurs ("success") or does not occur ("failure").
3. The trials are independent, that is, the outcome of one trial does not affect the outcome of the next trial.
4. The probability of success does not change throughout the trial.

Example 16.1

The proportion π for male births is approximately 0.5. (Actually, about 51.2% of newborns are males in the US.) If a family has five children, how often would there be three girls? no girls? four boys? To approach this problem, consider what happens by flipping a fair coin many times, and recording whether it comes down heads (H) or tails (T). This is a good analogy, because for heads in coin tossing π is exactly 0.5. Table 16.1 gives the possible results for the first few tosses.

Table 16.1 Binomial table.

Number of tosses	Possible combinations				
1		1H	1T		
2	1HH	2HT	1TT		
3	1HHH	3HHT	3HTT	1TTT	
4	1HHHH	4HHHT	6HHTT	4HTTT	1TTTT
5	1HHHHH	5HHHHT	10HHHTT	10HHTTT	5HTTTT	1TTTTT

H = head; T = tail. The numbers (coefficients) indicate how many possible combinations are there for each set.

Example 16.1—cont'd

Turning this figure through 90° gives a tree diagram (Figure 16.1).

Toss #

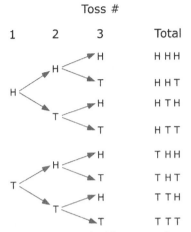

Figure 16.1 Binomial table as tree diagram.

Consider the numbers of possible combinations of heads and tails for any given number of tosses.

First toss: a head (H) or a tail (T)

Second toss: HH, HT, TH, or TT. The difference between the two middle combinations is the order in which the outcomes occur. If order is immaterial, the outcomes are HH, 2HT, TT.

Third toss: HHH (three heads) once, HHT, HTH, THH (two heads and one tail), HTT, THT, TTH (one head and two tails), or TTT (three tails) once.

Fourth toss: Four heads (HHHH) once; three heads and one tail, and there are four ways of doing this (HHHT, HHTH, HTHH, THHH); two heads and two tails, and there are six ways of doing this (HHTT, HTHT, HTTH, TTHH, TTTH, THHT); one head and three tails, with four possible combinations; and four tails (TTTT) once.

Fifth toss: HHHHH, with only one such combination possible; four heads and one tail, with five possible combinations; three heads and two tails, with 10 possible combinations (work this out for practice); two heads and three tails, also with 10 possible combinations; one head and four tails, with five possible combinations; and five tails, with only one such combination.

Isolating the numbers of possible combinations (the coefficients) in the above diagram gives Table 16.2.

Each line begins and ends with a 1, because there can be only one combination with all heads and one with all tails. In each line, except the first, the number of combinations is the sum of the two nearest combinations in the preceding line. Thus, 5 for 5 tosses is the sum of 1 and 4 which are above it in line 4, 10 is the sum of the 4 and the 6 above it in line 4, and

(Continued)

Example 16.1—cont'd

Table 16.2 Bernoulli coefficients

Number of tosses			Numbers of combinations					
1				1		1		
2			1		2		1	
3		1		3		3		1
4	1		4		6		4	1
5	1	5		10		10		5

so on. In each line, the pattern of coefficients is symmetrical because the coefficient for, say, $5 - 1$ heads $= 4$ heads is 5, and this is the same as the coefficient for $5 - 4$ heads $= 1$ head. More generally, in n trials, the coefficient for k successes is the same as for $n - k$ successes. This pattern is termed Pascal's triangle, described in a letter to Fermat in 1654, but this pattern was known in China in the twelfth century.

These numbers of combinations, also termed coefficients, are one of the two items needed to work out the probabilities. The other is the probability of getting any particular combination. The second item is easy to calculate. With the assumption that the results of one toss do not influence any of the other results, then to get any combination with two tosses multiply the probabilities of each result. Thus, the probability of getting one head is 0.5. The probability of getting two heads is $0.5 \times 0.5 = 0.5^2 = 0.25$. The probability of getting three heads is $0.5 \times 0.5 \times 0.5 = 0.5^3 = 0.125$. The probability of getting two heads and a tail is $0.5^2 \times 0.5 = 0.5^3 = 0.125$, and so on for other numbers of tosses and combinations. Now all we need to do is to multiply the probability of getting any particular combination by the number of times that combination occurs, that is, by the coefficient.

For example, for four tosses, we get the following probabilities:

P(Four heads) $= 0.5 \times 0.5 \times 0.5 \times 0.5 = 0.5^4 = 0.0625$.

P(Three heads and one tail) $=$ P(three heads) $\times$ P(one tail) $\times$ number of combinations $= 0.5^3 \times 0.5 \times 4 = 0.25$ because there are four ways of having three heads and one tail: HHHT, HHTH, HTHH, THHH.

P(Two heads and two tails) $= 0.5^2 \times 0.5^2 \times 6 = 0.375$, because there are six possible combinations: HHTT, HTHT, HTTH, TTHH, TTTH, THHT.

P (One head and three tails) $= 0.5^1 \times 0.5^3 \times 4 = 0.25$.

P (Four tails) $= 0.5^4 = 0.0625$.

Adding up all these probabilities gives $0.0625 + 0.25 + 0.375 + 0.25 + 0.0625 = 1.0000$.

Example 16.2

Perform similar calculations when π is not 0.5. Take a six-sided die, call the number 1 a success, and any of the numbers 2–6 a failure. Then the probability of getting a success is 1/6, and the probability of getting a failure is 5/6.

For one toss of the die, the probability of one success = 1/6, and the probability of one failure = 5/6.

For two tosses, the probability of two successes is $1/6 \times 1/6 = (1/6)^2 = 1/36$. The probability of one success and one failure is $1/6 \times 5/6 \times 2 = (1/6)^1 \times (5/6)^1 \times 2 = 10/36$. The probability of two failures is $5/6 \times 5/6 = (5/6)^2 = 25/36$.

For three tosses, the probability of one success is $1/6 \times 1/6 \times 1/6 = (1/6)^3 = 1/216$. The probability of two successes and one failure is $1/6 \times 1/6 \times 5/6 \times 3 = (1/6)^2 \times (5/6)^1 \times 3 = 15/216$. The probability of one success and two failures is $1/6 \times 5/6 \times 5/6 \times 3 = (1/6)^1 \times (5/6)^2 \times 3 = 75/216$. The probability of three failures is $5/6 \times 5/6 \times 5/6 = (5/6)^3 = 125/216$. The sum of these probabilities is $(1 + 15 + 75 + 125)/216 = 1$, as expected.

Bernoulli Formula

With greater numbers of tosses, the calculations of the probabilities (especially the coefficients) become increasingly tedious. Fortunately, Jakob Bernoulli (1654–1705), belonging to one of a large, famous, and disputatious family of Swiss physicists and mathematicians, showed that these expressions were the expansion of the algebraic expression $(\pi + [1 - \pi])^n$, where n represents the number of observations. For there to be X successes (with probability π of each success), there must therefore be $n - X$ failures. The probability for any value of r and n is: $_nC_r\pi^r[1 - \pi]^{n-r}$, where $_nC_r$ (also written $\binom{n}{r}$) represents the number of possible combinations of r successes and $n - r$ failures (i.e., the binomial coefficient). This is the probability function.

From the combinatorial theory (Chapter 12) $_nC_r$ is: $\frac{n!}{r!(n-r)!}$.

Thus in our example, the probability would be $\frac{n!}{r!(n-r)!}\pi^r[1 - \pi]^{n-r}$. This formula has two components. The first, the binomial coefficient, $\frac{n!}{r!(n-r)!}$, gives the number of possible arrangements of r successes and $n - r$ failures as set out in part in Table 16.2. The second factor involving π is the probability for any of the different ways of getting r successes and $n - r$ failures.

Therefore the probability of getting four successes out of six tosses is

$$\frac{6!}{4!(6-4)!}(1/6)^4(5/6)^{6-4} = \frac{720}{24 \times 2} \times \frac{1}{1296} \times \frac{25}{36} = 0.008038.$$

The probability of getting one success out of six tosses is

$$\frac{6!}{1!(6-1)!}(1/6)^1(5/6)^{6-1} = \frac{720}{120} \times \frac{1}{6} \times \frac{3125}{7776} = 0.401878.$$

To determine the probability of getting 7 successes out of 12 total trials in which $p = 0.37$, this would be calculated from

$$_{12}C_7(0.37)^7(1-0.37)^{12-7} = \frac{12!}{7!(12-7)!}(0.37)^7(1-0.37)^{12-7}$$

$$= 792 \times 0.0009493 \times 0.09924 = 0.07461.$$

What is the probability that 5 patients out of 50 with meningitis will die? To answer this question, we need information about the average proportion of these patients who die. Assume that the probability is $p = 0.1$. Then the probability that we want is

$$_{50}C_5(0.1)^5(1-0.1)^{50-5} = \frac{50!}{5!(50-5)!}(0.1)^5(1-0.1)^{50-5}$$

$$= 2118760 \times 0.000010 \times 0.008727964 = 0.1849.$$

Free online binomial calculators are available at http://www.stat.tamu.edu/~west/applets/binomialdemo.html, http://stattrek.com/online-calculator/binomial.aspx, and http://vassarstats.net/binomialX.html.

Problem 16.1

In an influenza epidemic the mortality rate is 0.7%. What is the probability of death in 3 out of the next 50 patients?

Binomial Basics

The mean of a binomial distribution is $n\pi$ and its variance is $n\pi(1-\pi)$. Because both π and $1-\pi$ are less than one, their product is even smaller, so that the variance of a binomial distribution is less than the mean. If the mean and variance are calculated as proportions of 1, rather than as numbers based on the sample size, then divide the mean by n and the variance by n^2 to give π and $\frac{n\pi(1-\pi)}{n^2} = \frac{\pi(1-\pi)}{n}$, respectively.

Even if π and $1-\pi$ are unknown, there is an upper bound for the variance. The product of π and $1-\pi$ is 0.25 when both have the value 0.5, and this product value is greater than any other product of π and $1-\pi$. For example, the product of 0.4 and 0.6 is 0.24, the product of 0.2 and 0.8 is 0.16, and so on. Therefore the variance is greatest when π is 0.5, but cannot exceed $0.25/n$.

The Normal Approximation

The binomial distribution is approximately normal when $n > 10$ if $\pi = 0.5$, but requires larger values of n when π is not 0.5. The normal approximation can be used if $n\pi$ and $n(1-\pi) > 9$ (Hamilton, 1990).

Figure 16.2 shows the distribution for different values of n when $p = 0.1, 0.3,$ or 0.5.

Fitting a Binomial Distribution to a Set of Trial Results

In a typical Mendelian recessive gene, for example, for Tay-Sachs disease, the probability of a child having Tay-Sachs disease if both parents carry the recessive gene is 0.25. One hundred such families with five children are examined, and the children with Tay-Sachs disease are identified (Table 16.3). Does the observed distribution fit a binomial distribution?

Calculate the expected probabilities of having 0, 1, 2, 3, 4, or 5 children with the disease.

$$P(r = 0) = 1 \times 0.25^0 \times 0.75^5 = 0.237305$$

$$P(r = 1) = 5 \times 0.25^1 \times 0.75^4 = 0.395508$$

$$P(r = 2) = \frac{5!}{2!3!} \times 0.25^2 \times 0.75^3 = 0.263672$$

$$P(r = 3) = \frac{5!}{2!3!} \times 0.25^3 \times 0.75^2 = 0.087891$$

$$P(r = 4) = 5 \times 0.25^4 \times 0.75^1 = 0.014648$$

$$P(r = 5) = 1 \times 0.25^5 \times 0.75^0 = 0.0009766.$$

These add up to 1.0000006, the difference from one being due to rounding off errors. Now compare observed and expected numbers by a chi-square test, as in Table 16.3 (Chapter 14).

The observed and expected values are similar. The total chi-square is 6.18 with 4 degrees of freedom, so that $P = 0.1861$. There is therefore no convincing evidence against the null hypothesis that these samples are drawn from a population in which the mean probability of the occurrence of the disease is 0.25.

Cumulative Binomial Probabilities

Some problems call for an estimate of more than one probability. For example, if for a Mendelian recessive characteristic the risk of a child with the recessive disease is 0.25, how likely is that there will be families of five children with two or more diseased children? This could be calculated by working out the probabilities of having 0 or 1 affected child, adding these together and then subtracting that total from 1. If the sample sizes

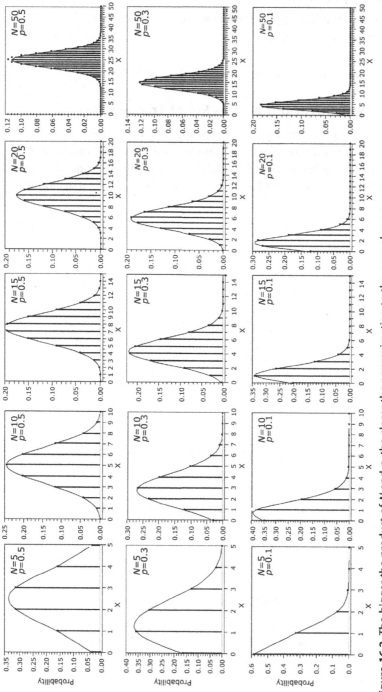

Figure 16.2 The bigger the product of N and p, the closer the approximation to the normal curve.

Table 16.3 The expected values show the theoretical distribution for the recessive population

Number of involved children (r)	Observed f	Expected f	χ^2
0	26	23.73	0.22
1	37	39.55	0.16
2	22	26.37	0.72
3	11	8.79	0.56
4	4	1.46	4.42
5	0	0.10	0.10
Total	100		6.18

were larger, however, this could be very time-consuming. For example, in samples of 100 people, what is the probability that there will be more than 20 with the type B blood group that occurs in about 14% of the population? Fortunately, there are tables in which cumulative probabilities have been calculated and listed for varying values of π (Hahn and Meeker, 1991; Kennedy and Neville, 1986; McGhee, 1985). The calculations can be done easily on the free interactive Web sites http://onlinestatbook.com/analysis_lab/binomial_dist.html, http://stattrek.com/online-calculator/binomial.aspx, http://www.stat.tamu.edu/~west/applets/binomialdemo.html, or http://www.danielsoper.com/statcalc3/calc.aspx?id=71.

Example 16.3

Using the blood group data above, $n = 100$, $p = 0.14$. From the calculator, $p > 20 = 0.0356$.

Confidence Limits

Continuity Correction

A binomial series consists of the probabilities of discrete events—three children, seven teeth, etc. Because these events are discrete they are represented by integers. When this probability set is examined as if it were a continuous distribution, an error appears as shown in Figure 16.3.

For the sample illustrated above, with $n = 20$ and $p = 0.3$, the probability of $P \geq 10$, that is, the probability of getting 10 or more, can be calculated from the binomial theorem. This probability is 0.0480 (using the online calculator referred to above). But with the normal approximation and the formula:

$$z = \frac{X_i - p}{\sqrt{Npq}} \quad \text{(see below)}$$

$$z = \frac{10 - 20 \times 0.3}{\sqrt{20 \times 0.3 \times 0.7}} = \frac{4}{2.0494} = 1.95, \quad P = 0.02559.$$

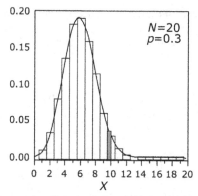

Figure 16.3 Diagram of continuity correction.

As shown in Figure 16.3, this value must be incorrect. The value 10 really extends from 9.5 to 10.5, so that calculating the probability from the continuous curve using only 10 and above ignores the shaded area in the figure. To allow for this, subtract 0.5 from 10 and then

$$z = \frac{9.5 - 20 \times 0.3}{\sqrt{20 \times 0.3 \times 0.7}} = \frac{3.5}{2.0494} = 1.71, \ \ P = 0.0463.$$

This is much closer to the true probability. When N is large, the correction is less important.

Calculating confidence limits depends upon whether the distribution can be considered approximately normal or not. Using the continuity correction, for a one-tailed test, $z = \frac{(r - np) - 0.5}{\sqrt{npq}}$. (Do not correct if $r - np \leq 0.5$.) For two-tailed tests, delete the fractional part of $r - np$ if it lies between 0 and 0.5, and replace it by 0.5 if the fractional part lies between 0.5 and 1.0. Therefore, 7.3 becomes 7; 8.73 becomes 8.5; 5.0 becomes 4.5; 3.5 becomes 3.0. Confidence limits can be calculated online from http://statpages.org/confint.html, http://www.danielsoper.com/statcalc3/calc.aspx?id=85, http://www.graphpad.com/quickcalcs/ConfInterval2.cfm, and http://www.biyee.net/data-solution/resources/binomial-confidence-interval-calculator.aspx.

For example, if $N = 20$ and $p = 0.3$, what are the confidence limits for p? From the calculator, the 95% confidence limits for p are 0.1189–0.5428, a very wide range because of the small sample size.

In larger samples, the binomial estimate of p is approximately normally distributed about population proportion π with standard deviation $\sqrt{\frac{\pi(1-\pi)}{n}}$. For the true but unknown standard deviation substitute the sample estimate $\sqrt{\frac{pq}{n}}$.

Hence, the probability is approximately 0.95 that π lies between the limits: $\pi - 1.96\sqrt{\frac{pq}{n}}$ and $\pi + 1.96\sqrt{\frac{pq}{n}}$. With the correction for continuity, use $p \pm \left(1.96\sqrt{\frac{pq}{n}} + \frac{1}{2n} \right)$.

Example 16.4

If the proportion of people with group *B* blood in a sample of 100 people is 0.14, what are the 95% confidence limits for that proportion?

$p = 0.14$, $q = 0.86$, $n = 100$. The 95% confidence limits are

$$p \pm \left(1.96\sqrt{\frac{pq}{n}} + \frac{1}{2n} \right) = 0.14 \pm \left[1.96\sqrt{0.14 \times 0.86/100} + 1/200 \right]$$

$$= 0.14 \pm [1.96 \times 0.034699 + 0.005] = 0.14 \pm 0.073$$

$$= 0.067 - 0.213.$$

(The exact interval is 0.0612–0.2072, so that the approximation is close).

Other slightly more complex formulas can be used, with Wilson's method being highly accurate (see below) (Curran-Everett and Benos, 2004).

Problem 16.2

A study (Jousilahti et al., 1998) showed that serum cholesterol in men in 1992 had the following distribution:

<5.0 mmol/l-6%; 5–6.4 mmol/l-37%; 6.5–7.9 mmol/l-41%; >8.0 mmol/l-16%.

Set 95% confidence limits for those with serum cholesterol 5.0–6.4 mmol/l in a sample of 200 men.

Comparing Two Binomial Distributions

This can be done with the chi-square or the *z*-test, although tests based on other features of the binomial distribution are possible (Snedecor and Cochran, 1989). Tables or graphs for performing these comparisons can be found in Armitage (1975), Gardner and Altman (1995), and Goldstein (1964).

Estimating Sample Size

If two binomial distributions are not significantly different, this may be because they are very similar (that is, that the null hypothesis is true) or else that the null hypothesis may not be true but the numbers in each sample are too small to allow us to reach that conclusion with confidence. To determine a sample size that is big enough to give us confidence in detecting a difference that exists, calculate the approximate numbers that should be used.

A simple way is to use the normal approximation with the formula:

$$N = [p(1-p)]\left[\frac{z_{1-\alpha/2}}{d}\right]^2,$$

p is the average of the two proportions p_1 and p_2, and d is their difference $p_1 - p_2$.

If $p = 0.4$ and the difference $d = 0.04$, then $N = [0.4(1-0.4)]\left[\frac{1.96}{0.04}\right]^2 = 576$.

Alternatively, to determine the sample size, use the free online program http://www.stat.ubc.ca/~rollin/stats/ssize/b2.html or http://www.cct.cuhk.edu.hk/stat/proportion/Casagrande.htm.

Comparing Probabilities

We may be interested in comparing the ratio of two of the probabilities p_i/p_j (Neter et al., 1978). A $1 - \alpha$ confidence interval can be created from

$$\log_e L = \log(p_i/p_j) - z(1-\alpha/2)\left(\sqrt{\frac{1}{n_1} + \frac{1}{n_2}}\right) \text{ and }$$

$$\log_e U = \log(p_i/p_j) + z(1-\alpha/2)\left(\sqrt{\frac{1}{n_1} + \frac{1}{n_2}}\right).$$

In the above example, consider the ratio of two blood types, A and B; $pA/pB = 0.43/0.12 = 3.58$. If this ratio is based on the observation of 100 individuals, 43 with A and 12 with B, what is the 95% confidence interval for this ratio?

Then $\log L = \log(43/12) - 1.96\sqrt{1/43 + 1/12}$, and $\log U = \log(43/12) + 1.96\sqrt{1/43 + 1/12}$

Then $\log L = 1.2763 - 1.96 \times 0.6399 = 0.2764$, and $\log U = 0.8322$. Therefore, the lower and the upper limits are the antilogarithms of these values, and these are 1.8897–6.7952. These limits would be different for different sample sizes.

ADVANCED OR ALTERNATIVE CONCEPTS

Exact Confidence Limits

Wilson's method for determining confidence limits (Newcombe, 1998) seems to be the most accurate method available. It involves solving the two formulas for the lower (L) and upper (U) confidence limits of a binomial proportion, and includes the continuity correction:

$$L = \frac{2np + z^2 - 1 - z\sqrt{\{z^2 - 2 - 1/n + 4p(nq+1)\}}}{2(n+z^2)}$$

$$U = \frac{2np + z^2 + 1 + z\sqrt{\{z^2 + 2 - 1/n + 4p(nq+1)\}}}{2(n+z^2)}.$$

For 95% confidence limits, $z = 1.96$, and the equations reduce to

$$L = \frac{2np + 2.84 - 1.96\sqrt{\{1.84 - 1/n + 4p(nq + 1)\}}}{2(n + 3.84)}$$

$$U = \frac{2np + 4.84 + 1.96\sqrt{\{5.84 - 1/n + 4p(nq + 1)\}}}{2(n + 3.84)}.$$

For the example used above, the confidence limits are 0.0829–0.2278, for an interval of 0.145. If p is very low and the lower limit is <0, it is set at zero. If p is very high and the upper limit is >1, it is set at 1.

The continuity correction is not needed for larger sample sizes, and a simpler formula can then be used:

$$\frac{2np + z^2 \pm z\sqrt{z^2 + 4npq}}{2(n + z^2)}.$$

With the same proportions as used previously, the 95% confidence limits are from 0.0852 to 0.2213, quite close to the more exact formulation. This method seems to be more accurate than other proposed methods. It can be performed online at http://vassarstats.net/.

Problem 16.3

Calculate 95% confidence limits as in Problem 16.3, using Wilson's method.

Multinomial Distribution

This is an extension of the binomial distribution to more than two groups. If there are more than two mutually exclusive categories, X_1 is the number of trials producing type 1 outcomes, X_2 is the number of trials producing type 2 outcomes,...X_k is the number of trials producing type k outcomes, then the event $(X_1 = x_1, X_2 = x_2,...X_k = x_k)$ follows a multinomial distribution if there are n independent trials, each trial results in one of k mutually exclusive outcomes, the probability of a type i outcome is p_i, and this probability does not change from trial to trial. Then the distribution of the event $(X_1 = x_1, X_2 = x_2,...X_k = x_k)$ is given by

$$P(X_1 = x_1......X_k = x_k) = \frac{n!}{x_1!x_2!...x_k!}p_1^{x_1}p_2^{x_2}...p_k^{x_k}.$$

where $\sum_{i=1}^{k} p_i = 1$, and $x_1, x_2,...x_k$ are nonnegative integers satisfying $\sum_{i=1}^{k} x_1 = n$.

The mean of each X_1 is given by $\mu_i = np_i$ and its variance is given by $\sigma_i^2 = np_i(1 - p_i)$.

Consider the four main blood group phenotypes. The probabilities of A, B, AB, and O are respectively 0.43, 0.12, 0.05, and 0.40. In a study of 17 randomly selected subjects, what is the probability of choosing 5 As, 2 Bs, 1 AB, and 9 Os at random?

By the formula,

$$P(A = 5; B = 2; AB = 1; O = 9) = \frac{17!}{5!2!1!9!} 0.43^5 0.12^2 0.05^1 0.40^9 = 0.01133.$$

This calculation can be done online at http://stattrek.com/online-calculator/multinomial.aspx.

In repeated random samples of size 17, the mean number of persons with type A is $17 \times 0.43 = 7.3$, with variance $17 \times 0.43 \times 0.57 = 4.1667$ and standard deviation about 2.04.

Explanations of the formula with examples are given by Ash (1993), Hogg and Tanis (1977), Murphy (1979), and Ross (1984).

Problem 16.4

Using the serum cholesterol data above, in repeated random samples of 75 subjects, what is the probability of choosing, in the order of ascending concentrations, 3, 26, 43, and 9, respectively.

APPENDIX

1. Calculation of sample size for unequal numbers.

Let sample sizes be n_1 and n_2, and let $k = n_1/n_2$. Then modified sample size $N' = N(1 + k)^2/4k$. That is, calculate N for the total sample size, assuming equal sample sizes. Then compute N'. Then the two sample sizes are $N'/(1 + k)$ and $kN'(1 + k)$.

REFERENCES

Armitage, P., 1975. Sequential Medical Trials, p 194.
Ash, C., 1993. The Probability Tutoring Book. An Intuitive Course for Engineers and Scientists, p 470.
Curran-Everett, D., Benos, D.J., 2004. Guidelines for reporting statistics in journals published by the American Physiological Society. Am. J. Physiol. Endocrinol. Metab. 287, E189–E191.
Gardner, M.J., Altman, D.G., 1995. Statistics with confidence—confidence intervals and statistical guidelines. Br. Med. J. Universities Press, Belfast.
Goldstein, A., 1964. Biostatistics, An Introductory Course. Macmillan Company.
Hahn, G.J., Meeker, W.Q., 1991. Statistical Intervals. A Guide for Practitioners. John Wiley and Sons, Inc.
Hamilton, L.C., 1990. Modern Data Analysis. A First Course in Applied Statistics. Brooks/Cole Publishing Co.
Hogg, R.V., Tanis, E.A., 1977. Probability & Statistical Inference. Macmillan Publishing Company, Inc.
Jousilahti, P., Vartiainen, E., Pekkanen, J., et al., 1998. Serum cholesterol distribution and coronary heart disease risk: observations and predictions among middle-aged population in eastern Finland. Circulation 97, 1087–1094.
Kennedy, J.B., Neville, A.M., 1986. Basic Statistical Methods for Engineers and Scientists. Harper and Row.
McGhee, J.W., 1985. Introductory Statistics. West Publishing Company.
Murphy, E.A., 1979. Probability in Medicine. Johns Hopkins University Press.
Neter, J., Wasserman, W., Whitmore, G.A., 1978. Applied Statistics. Allyn and Bacon, Inc.
Newcombe, R.G., 1998. Interval estimation for the difference between independent proportions: comparison of eleven methods. Stat. Med. 17, 873–890.
Ross, S., 1984. A First Course in Probability. Macmillan Publishing Company.
Snedecor, G.W., Cochran, W.G., 1989. Statistical Methods. Iowa State University Press.

CHAPTER 17

Proportions

Contents

INTRODUCTION

Previous chapters dealing with categories used the proportions within each group. It may be easier to work with proportions rather than the absolute numbers.

A proportion is the relationship of a part to the whole and can be given as a fraction of 1 or as a percentage. A ratio is the relationship of one part to another part. Thus if out of 100 patients with a myocardial infarction 30 of them die, the proportion who die is $30/100 = 0.3$ or 30%, whereas the ratio of those who die to that who survive is $30/70 = 0.43$ or 43%.

PROPORTIONS AND BINOMIAL THEOREM

If there are 37 deaths in 192 people with a certain disease, the number who survive is $192 - 37 = 155$. The proportion of deaths (p) is determined by number with the attribute/total number $= 37/192 = 0.1927$. The proportion that survives is $155/192 = 0.8073$. This is the value $1 - p$, also symbolized by q (Chapter 16). In repeated samples from this population, the value of p would vary; the sample value p is a point estimate of the population value π. From the binomial theorem, the distribution of p is approximately normal as long as np and $nq > 9$. The standard deviation σ of such a binomial is as follows:

$$\sigma = \sqrt{p(1-p)} = \sqrt{pq}$$

For a list of all websites referred to in this chapter, as clickable links, see the book companion website: www.booksite.elsevier.com/9780128023877.

Biostatistics for Medical and Biomedical Practitioners
http://dx.doi.org/10.1016/B978-0-12-802387-7.00017-2

The standard error (se_p) of the sample proportion p that estimates the population proportion π is equivalent to the standard error of a mean value, and is estimated by dividing the standard deviation by $\sqrt{n}$. Therefore, $\sigma_p = \sqrt{\frac{pq}{n}}$. Therefore in the above example

$$\sigma_p = \sqrt{\frac{0.1927 \times 0.8073}{192}} = 0.02846.$$

Therefore, the 95% confidence limits of π are $p \pm 1.96 \times 0.02846 = 0.1369$ to 0.2485.

As the formula for the standard error of a proportion comes from the approximation of the discrete binomial distribution to the normal distribution, we need a continuity correction. Test the null hypothesis by

$$z = \frac{|p - \pi| - \dfrac{1}{2n}}{se_p}.$$

The effect of the correction is to make the difference slightly smaller, and for large sample sizes the correction is unimportant.

If the sample size n is large relative to the population size N, use the finite population correction

$$\sigma_p = \sqrt{\frac{N - n}{N - 1}} \sqrt{\frac{pq}{n}}$$

If n is 5% of N, the correction factor is 0.98 and can be ignored. If n is 10% or 20% of N, then the correction factor is about 0.95 and 0.90, respectively, and cannot be ignored. If the effect is ignored, the calculated standard deviation will be too large and give poor estimates for determining Type I and II errors.

CONFIDENCE LIMITS

The observed proportion is a point estimate. To determine its confidence limits, use the Wald method, with the 95% limits determined from $p \pm z_{\alpha/2}\sqrt{\frac{pq}{N}}$. This method yields inaccurate results if N is small or p is close to 0 or 1. A simple way to obtain more accurate limits is to use the Agresti–Coull adjustment (Agresti and Coull, 1998; Agretsi and Caffo, 2000) by adding two successes and two failures to the observed counts. Thus, $p_a = \frac{X+2}{N+4}$, and the adjusted value of $p(p_a)$ is substituted for the value of p in the Wald formula above.

Thus, if $p = \frac{37}{192} = 0.1927$, then the Wald limits are $0.1927 \pm 1.96\sqrt{\frac{0.1927 \times 0.8703}{192}}$ $= 0.1927 \pm 0.0558 = 0.1369$ to 0.2485. With the adjustment, the adjusted value of

p is $p = \frac{37+2}{192+4} = 0.1990$, and the adjusted Wald limits are 0.1990 ± 1.96 $\sqrt{\frac{0.1990 \times 0.8010}{192}} = 0.1990 \pm 0.0565 = 0.1425$ to 0.2555.

Confidence limits may be obtained online from http://www.causascientia.org/math_stat/ProportionCI.html (a Bayesian calculator), http://www.graphpad.com/quickcalcs/ConfInterval2.cfm, and http://www.mccallum-layton.co.uk/stats/ConfidenceIntervalCalcProportions.aspx. The first two are exact.

Problem 17.1

19 out of 113 (16.8%) men have a serum cholesterol of <5.0 mmol/l. What are the 95% and 99% confidence limits for this proportion?

One particular use of confidence limits is to determine the upper 95% limit for a proportion if zero events occur. If a surgeon operates on 10 patients without a death, what is the upper 95% limit of deaths? It can be determined easily by the rule of 3 (Hanley and Lippman-Hand, 1983; van Belle, 2002). The upper 95% limit for the proportion is determined by $3/N$. Thus, the upper 95% mortality proportion for the surgical procedure is 3/10 or 0.3 (or 30%). If there were no deaths in 50 operations the upper 95% limit would be $3/50 = 0.06$ or 6%.

The corollary to this is to determine how many surgical operations must be observed in order to find at least one death if we know the average mortality. Thus, if the mortality of a procedure is 1%, there is a 95% chance of observing 1 death in $3/0.01 = 300$ operations. This calculation does not allow for differences in surgical skills.

SAMPLE AND POPULATION PROPORTIONS

To compare any observed value of p with the population value π, use the normal distribution curve.

$$z = \frac{\pi - p}{\sigma_p}$$

Thus, to determine if the sample value of $p = 0.1927$ could have come from a population in which $\pi = 0.3$, calculate

$$z = \frac{0.3 - 0.1927}{0.02846} = 3.770.$$

Therefore, $p = 0.000008$, and we would reject the null hypothesis. We could have drawn the same conclusion by looking at the 95% confidence limits, except that this calculation tells us how strong our rejection is.

SAMPLE SIZE

To compare two proportions, we need to know how many subjects we will need to minimize Type I and II errors. The Type I error (the risk of declaring two proportions different when in fact they come from the same population) is set by us and is typically 0.05 or 0.01. The Type II error is made if we declare that two proportions are not significantly different when in fact they really do come from different populations. This is discussed in detail in Chapter 11, but one way to minimize this error is to increase the sample size N.

The basic formulas are discussed by Fleiss (1981) and Bland (1995). They are relatively complex and approximate, can be written in several ways, and are best replaced by free online calculation at http://statpages.org/proppowr.html, http://www.stat.ubc.ca/~rollin/stats/ssize/b2.html, or http://www.cct.cuhk.edu.hk/stat/proportion/Casagrande.htm.

A simplified approximation was devised by Lehr (1992) who used the equation

$$n = \frac{16pq}{(p_1 - p_2)^2},$$

where p is the average of p_1 and p_2, and q is $1 -$ average p. This gives the number in each group for a power of 0.8 (Type II error $\beta = 0.2$) and a Type I error $\alpha = 0.05$ (two-tailed). If a power of 0.9 is wanted, the constant is changed from 16 to 21. According to Lehr, this estimate is slightly low for Fisher's exact test and slightly high for a 2×2 chi-square test. As with all sample size calculations, these are estimates, not precise numbers.

As an example, consider how many subjects (equal-sized groups) are needed to show a difference between a remission rate of 0.7 for one treatment and 0.6 for another. We wish to set $\alpha = 0.05$ and $\beta = 0.2$, that is, power $= 0.8$. By Lehr's formula, $n = \frac{16 \times 0.65 \times 0.35}{(0.7 - 0.6)^2} = 364$ as the number required in each group. The more formal calculation online gives 356 in each group or 376 if the continuity correction is used. For a power of 0.9, Lehr's formula gives 478 in each group, and the online calculation gives 476, or 496 with the continuity correction. The major advantage of using an online calculator is that it allows for unequal group sizes.

In estimating the numbers needed, we need to have some idea of the effect size that we want. Take 0.50 as the null hypothesis, that is, there is no difference between the two groups. Then either select an effect size based on previous work, or else try to decide what minimum effect size to detect. For example, suppose the null hypothesis is that the probability of survival of a disease under standard treatment is 0.50, we would probably not be interested in a treatment that changed the proportion to only 0.49. Cohen (1988) classified effect size of the difference from 0.50 as small (<0.05, i.e., 0.45−0.55), medium (0.15, i.e., 0.35−0.65), and large (0.25, i.e., 0.25−0.75).

He pointed out that large differences were rare. For example, in presidential elections in the US there has never been a division as extreme as 65:35, and even a division of 55:45 would be regarded as a landslide victory. Cohen gives tables, and online calculators are available. As always, it takes a huge number of measurements or counts to detect a small difference.

Problem 17.2

In two different populations of men serum cholesterol concentrations below 5.0 mmol/l occur in 6% and 9% respectively. What sample size is needed to show that this difference is significant with $\alpha = 0.05$ and $\beta = 0.2$. (Assume equal-sized groups.)

COMPARING PROPORTIONS

To compare two proportions, for example, the survival of patients with a given disease who have two different treatments, let the proportion surviving in group 1 be p_1 and that in group 2 be p_2. If these two proportions are similar, we conclude that treatment did not affect survival. If they are quite different, then we can ask if the null hypothesis is true. To do this, calculate the standard error of the difference as

$$S_{p_1 - p_2} = \sqrt{\left(\frac{p_1 q_1}{n_1}\right)\left(\frac{p_2 q_2}{n_2}\right)}$$

Then relate the difference $p_1 - p_2$ to the standard error of the difference;

$$z = \frac{p_1 - p_2}{\sqrt{\left(\frac{p_1 q_1}{n_1}\right)\left(\frac{p_2 q_2}{n_2}\right)}}$$

For example, if treatment 1 gives a survival proportion of $37/192 = 0.1927$ and treatment 2 gives a survival of $17/168 = 0.1012$, could that difference have occurred by chance? Calculate z as

$$z = \frac{0.1927 - 0.1012}{\sqrt{\left(\frac{0.1927 \times 0.8073}{192}\right)\left(\frac{0.1012 \times 0.8988}{168}\right)}} = \frac{0.0915}{\sqrt{0.0008102 + 0.0005414}} = 2.4888$$

Therefore, P $= 0.0128$ (two-sided) and we can reasonably reject the null hypothesis and believe that treatment 2 might be better.

The 95% confidence limits for the difference are $0.0915 \pm 1.96 \times 0.03676 = 0.05474$ to 0.1291. Because this does not include zero, it confirms the results of the z test.

The continuity correction can be done by using

$$z = \frac{|p_1 - p_2| - \frac{1}{2}\left(\frac{1}{n_1} + \frac{1}{n_2}\right)}{se_{(p_1 - p_2)}}$$

Sample sizes for adequate power are provided by Cohen (1988) and an online calculator is available at select-statistics. co.u/sample-size-calculator-two-proportions, http://www.fon.hum.uva.nl/Service/Statistics/Binomial_proportions.html, http://in-silico.net/statistics/ztest/two-proportion, or http://www.measuringusability.com/ab-calc.php or http://www.sample-size.net.

POOLING SAMPLES

If there are several small samples from a population, with X_1 successes in N_1 trials, X_2 successes in N_2 trials, up to X_k successes in N_k trials, then an average proportion of successes can be calculated as

$$\bar{p} = \frac{X_1 + X_2 + \dots X_k}{N_1 + N_2 + \dots N_k}.$$

REFERENCES

Agresti, A., Coull, B.A., 1998. Approximate is better than "exact" for interval estimation of binomial proportions. Am. Stat. 52, 119–126.

Agretsi, A., Caffo, B., 2000. Simple and effective confidence intervals for proportions and differences of proportions result from adding two Successes and two failures. Am. Stat. 54, 280–288.

Bland, M., 1995. An Introduction to Medical Statistics. Oxford University Press.

Cohen, J., 1988. Statistical Power Analysis for Behavioral Sciences. Lawrence Erlbaum Associates.

Fleiss, J.L., 1981. Statistical methods for rates and proportions, John Wiley & Sons.

Hanley, J.A., Lippman-hand, A., 1983. If nothing goes wrong, is everything alright? J. Am. Med. Assoc. 249, 1743–1745.

Lehr, R., 1992. Sixteen s-squared over d-squared: a relation for crude sample size estimates. Stat. Med. 11, 1099–1102.

van Belle, G., 2002. Statistical Rules of Thumb. Wiley Interscience.

CHAPTER 18

The Poisson Distribution

Contents

INTRODUCTION

The results of a study may be counts of the numbers of discrete events that occur per unit of measurement: the unit may be time, space, or mass.

1. Examples with unit time are:
   a. number of disintegrations per minute of a radioactive isotope,
   b. number of telephone calls per hour to a given number,
   c. number of births per day in a busy Metropolitan Hospital,
   d. (a famous historical example) annual number of people kicked to death by mules in different Austrian cavalry corps.
2. Examples with unit space are:
   a. number of flaws per cm length of silk suture material,
   b. number of red cells per hemocytometer field,

For a list of all websites referred to in this chapter, as clickable links, see the book companion website: www.booksite.elsevier.com/9780128023877.

Biostatistics for Medical and Biomedical Practitioners
http://dx.doi.org/10.1016/B978-0-12-802387-7.00018-4

    c. number of mutant bacteria per 100 µl of a bacterial suspension,

    d. number of diseased white-footed mice (carriers of the agent that causes Lyme disease) per acre of woodland.

3. An example with unit mass is the number of seeds of poisonous plants per 100 g of grass seeds.

We expect variation from one unit to the next and also expect some average number of births, bacteria, or poisonous seeds. What form of distribution does this type of variation take?

The mathematical distribution of rare events that occurs randomly in time or space is called after a French mathematician, Siméon-Denis Poisson (1781−1840). The term *random* implies that any one section of space or time interval has the same probability as any other of experiencing or not experiencing an event. For the counts to fit a Poisson distribution, they must obey the following assumptions:

1. The probability that a single event occurs in a very small time interval or region is proportional to the length of that interval or size of that region. Assume that there is a constant λ, such that the probability of observing one event in a small time interval Δt is $\lambda \Delta t$, and the probability of observing no events is $1 - \lambda \Delta t$; the probability of observing more than one event is essentially zero, being the probability of a rare event raised to some power.

2. The probability of observing an event in a small time interval or region does not change over the whole period of observation. The process shows stationarity.

3. An event that occurs in one time interval or region is independent of events occurring in other time intervals or regions. An event does not influence or is not influenced by any other events.

If the events meet these assumptions, then the probability of k events occurring in a time period t for a Poisson variable with parameter λ is:

$$P(X = k) = \frac{e^{-\lambda}\lambda^k}{k!},$$

where $k = 0,1,2,3...$, and e is the base of the natural (or Napierian) logarithms, and is approximately 2.71828. The parameter λ represents the expected number of events per unit time, whereas the parameter λ represents the expected number of events over the time period t. These are parameters that reflect a population value, hence the Greek symbols. Sample values should be given other symbols, but some authorities still use the Greek symbols and rely on the reader to differentiate between population and sample values; others use m, μ, or $\overline{X}$ instead of λ.

The Poisson distribution is asymmetrical, especially for low values of the Poisson parameter λ (Figure 18.1). As the value for the Poisson variate (or mean count) increases, the distribution becomes more symmetrical and approaches the normal distribution.

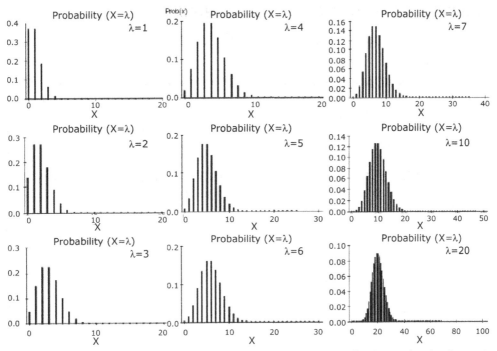

Figure 18.1 Poisson distribution for $\lambda = 1, 2, 3, 4, 5, 6, 7, 10$, and 20. After $\lambda = 5$, the distribution is fairly normal.

RELATIONSHIP TO THE BINOMIAL DISTRIBUTION

The Poisson distribution approximates the binomial distribution closely when n is very large and p is very small. It is the limiting form of the binomial distribution when $n \rightarrow \infty$, $p \rightarrow 0$, and $np = \mu$ are constant and <5. In the binomial distribution, the mean is given by np, and the standard deviation by $\sqrt{npq}$. If n is large and p is very small, as in the Poisson approximation to the binomial, then the mean is still np, but the standard deviation is now $\sim\sqrt{np}$, because q is almost 1. Therefore, the limiting value of the standard deviation, as the binomial distribution approaches the Poisson distribution, is the square root of the mean. This mathematical distribution can be applied to a binomial distribution in which the probability of an event, p, is very small and n is large, and also to a rare, random event in which we know the number of events that occur but do not know the number that do not occur. We know how many people in the cavalry corps were kicked to death by mules, but there is no way of knowing how many were not kicked to death by mules. We can count how many telephone calls were made to a particular number, but cannot know how many were not made. We know how many people were struck by lightening, but not how many were not struck. For the binomial example, we could calculate the probabilities of 0, 1, 2, etc., events from the binomial distribution, but when p is very small and n is very big, the Poisson calculation is simpler.

GOODNESS OF FIT TO A POISSON DISTRIBUTION

Example 18.1

Here is an example of how to calculate the Poisson distribution. It shows the process, although in practice we use a computer program. Free online programs are available: http://stattrek.com/online-calculator/poisson.aspx, http://easycalculation.com/statistics/poisson-distribution.php, and http://vassarstats.net/poissonfit.html, this last being the most convenient.

The data recorded by von Bortkiewicz (1898) on the chances of a Prussian cavalryman being kicked to death by a mule were taken from 14 cavalry corps over 20 years, for a total of 200 readings (Table 18.1). This is an important example historically, because it was the first time that the Poisson distribution function had been used in practice, and it introduced the Poisson distribution to a wide audience.

Table 18.1 Deaths from mule kicks in the cavalry corps

Number of deaths per corps per year (x)	Frequency (f)	fx (observed)
0	109	0
1	65	65
2	22	44
3	3	9
4	1	4
5	0	0
6	0	0
Sum	200	122

There is variation from corps to corps. In 109 corps there were no such deaths, but in 1 corps in 1 year there were 4 deaths. Was this a random event, could there have been inadequate training in that corps of how to handle mules, or was there one particularly vicious mule in that corps?

First, calculate the average number of deaths per corps per year. There were 122 deaths to be averaged over 200 corps-years, for a mean of 0.61 per corps-year. This is the value of $\overline{X}$, an estimate of λ in the Poisson equation.

The equation tells us that no deaths $[P(X = 0)]$ will be given by

$$P(X = 0) = \frac{e^{-0.61}0.61^0}{0!} = 0.543351 \quad (\text{because } 0.61^0 \text{ and } 0! \text{ both equal } 1).$$

By applying the formula, the remaining probabilities can be calculated.

$$P(X = 1) = \frac{e^{-0.61}0.61^1}{1!} = 0.331444$$

$$P(X = 2) = \frac{e^{-0.61}0.61^2}{2!} = 0.101090$$

Example 18.1—cont'd

$$P(X = 3) = \frac{e^{-0.61}0.61^{\mathbf{3}}}{\mathbf{3!}} = 0.020555$$

$$P(X = 4) = \frac{e^{-0.61}0.61^{\mathbf{4}}}{\mathbf{4!}} = 0.003135$$

$$P(X = 5) = \frac{e^{-0.61}0.61^{\mathbf{5}}}{\mathbf{5!}} = 0.000382$$

$$P(X = 6) = \frac{e^{-0.61}0.61^{\mathbf{6}}}{\mathbf{6!}} = 0.000039.$$

The figures in bold type show differences from the formula in the immediately preceding line.

The sum of these six probabilities is 0.999996. The remainder is the probability of getting more than 6 deaths, and is very small.

If the data are truly random, then they will fit a Poisson process with the mean value of 0.61. Taking each calculated probability and multiplying it by 200, the total number of observations, gives the fourth column in Table 18.2, a column-labeled expected frequency. Note how closely the observed and expected frequencies agree. To determine objectively how good the fit is, do a χ^2 test (Chapter 14). The total χ^2 is very small, and indicates a good fit between observed and expected frequencies. The probability of falsely rejecting the null hypothesis (Type I error, or α) can be determined from the χ^2 tables, with $k - 2$ degrees of freedom, where k is the highest number of events observed. (Two degrees of freedom are lost. One is the usual loss because of the mean, and the other because the mean is used to calculate all the other terms.) In this example, the risk of falsely rejecting the null hypothesis is low.

If the data do not indicate randomness, with excess numbers in some bins and too few in others, they may fit a distribution called a contagious distribution (other terms are clumped, aggregated, overdispersed, or clustered), that has application to epidemics. Detecting and modeling such data will be presented in Chapter 19.

Table 18.2 Analysis of mule data

Number of deaths per corps per year (x)	Observed frequency (f)	fx	Expected frequency $= np$	χ^2
0	109	0	108.67	0.0010
1	65	65	66.29	0.0251
2	22	44	20.22	0.1567
3	3	9	4.11	0.2998
4	1	4	0.63	0.2173
5	0	0	0.08	0.0078
Sum	200	122	200.01	0.7077

Problem 18.1

In 1910, Rutherford and Geiger (1910) described the radioactive decay counts of polonium and discovered alpha particles. Their observations are provided in the Table 18.3.

Does this fit a Poisson distribution?

Table 18.3 Alpha particle experiment

Particles/unit	Number of units
0	57
1	203
2	383
3	525
4	532
5	408
6	273
7	139
8	45
9	27
10	10
11	4
12	0
13	1
14	1
Total	2608

Example 18.2

The numbers of bacteria counted in 10 agar plates are shown below (Observed). Because these are counts they should fit a Poisson distribution, and failure to do so reflects on the method of preparing the samples.

The mean of these counts is 534.4. This is the expected number to be obtained, and calculating the chi-square value for each observed number gives (Table 18.4).

Table 18.4 Bacterial counts

Observed (O)	Expected (E)	O − E	x^2
545	534.4	10.6	0.21
531	534.4	−3.4	0.02
530	534.4	−4.4	0.04
525	534.4	−9.4	0.17
533	534.4	−1.4	0.00
529	534.4	−5.4	0.05
529	534.4	−5.4	0.05
535	534.4	0.6	0.00
543	534.4	8.6	0.14
544	534.4	9.6	0.17
Total			0.85

A total chi-square of 0.85 with 9 degrees of freedom shows that $P > 0.999$, so that there is no reason to reject the null hypothesis that these counts could have come from a Poisson distribution.

THE RATIO OF THE VARIANCE TO THE MEAN OF A POISSON DISTRIBUTION

If X_1, X_2, X_3...X_n come from a Poisson distribution with mean λ, then $\frac{\sum (X_i - \lambda)^2}{\lambda}$ is approximately distributed as χ_n^2.

If the value of λ is not known but calculated from the data, then the ratio is distributed like χ^2 with $n - 1$ degrees of freedom (Dixon and Massey, 1983; Selvin, 1991).

The variance of a Poisson variable is the same as the mean (see Appendix below). Therefore, if the data fit a Poisson distribution, the ratio of variance to mean should be 1. But the variance is also obtained from $\sum \frac{(X_i - \lambda)^2}{n-1}$. Therefore,

$$\chi^2 = \frac{\sum (X_i - \lambda)^2}{\lambda} = \frac{\sum (X_i - \lambda)^2 (n - 1)}{\lambda (n - 1)} = \frac{s^2 (n - 1)}{\lambda}.$$

If the agreement is perfect, then the ratio of variance to mean will be exactly 1, and chi-square will equal $n - 1$. If the agreement is not perfect, then the value of chi-square can be referred to a table of chi-square values to assess the probability that the distribution is compatible with a Poisson distribution. If $n > 31$, $\sqrt{2\chi^2}$ is distributed normally about $\sqrt{2\upsilon - 1}$ with unit variance, or alternatively, the variable $d = \sqrt{2\chi^2} - \sqrt{2\upsilon - 1}$ is a normal variable with zero mean and unit variance. (υ is the number of degrees of freedom.) Then if the absolute value of $d < 1.96$, the hypothesis that the distribution is consistent with a Poisson distribution cannot be rejected.

Example 18.3

The standard deviation of the deaths in the mule example was 0.611. The ratio of the variance to the mean is 0.611/0.61 = 1.0016, very close to the exact ratio of 1. Alternatively, refer to the chi-squared table with $n = 199$. Now 1.0016 × 199 = 199.318, and this is close to the 50% value of chi-square.

Example 18.4

In 80 samples of shrimps taken from a river, the mean was 5.3125 and the variance was 13.53 (Elliott, 1983).

$$\chi^2 = \frac{s^2 (n - 1)}{\lambda} = \frac{13.534 \times 79}{5.3125} = 201.2585.$$

(Continued)

Example 18.4—cont'd

The normal variable d is

$$d = \sqrt{2\chi^2} - \sqrt{2\upsilon - 1} = \sqrt{402.5170} - \sqrt{157} = +7.532.$$

Because d is $\gg 1.96$, reject the null hypothesis that the distribution is compatible with a Poisson distribution at the 0.01 level. The high and positive value for d, with the variance much greater than the mean, suggests that this is a contagious distribution. This example is better analyzed as a negative binomial distribution (Chapter 19).

Problem 18.2

Use the polonium data to test the fit to a Poisson distribution by the method of Example 18.4.

Example 18.5

Examine the problem of the successive bacterial counts shown in Table 18.4 by using the ratio of the variance to the mean: $\chi^2 = \frac{s^2(n-1)}{\lambda} = \frac{458.4 \times 9}{534.4} = 7.72$. For chi-square with 9 degrees of freedom, P-0.56, so that there is no reason to reject the null hypothesis (see online calculators http://www.fourmilab.ch/rpkp/experiments/analysis/chiCalc.html, or http://www.stat.tamu.edu/~west/applets/chisqdemo.html, or http://www.danielsoper.com/statcalc3/calc.aspx?id=).

SETTING CONFIDENCE LIMITS

The variance of a Poisson variable is the same as the mean. Therefore, it is possible to set confidence limits about the mean number of counts.

Normal Approximation

If $\overline{X}$ is >100, an approximate $100(1 - \alpha)$ confidence interval for λ is,

$$\overline{X} \pm z_{1-\alpha/2}\sqrt{\overline{X}}.$$

Example 18.6

Consider counting a dilute suspension of red blood cells under a microscope. The suspension is pipetted onto a hemocytometer slide and then covered with a coverslip so that the thickness of the suspension is constant. In the first square, 400 red blood cells are counted. What are the 95% confidence limits of the number of red blood cells per square?

Example 18.6—cont'd

Because these are counts, and because 400 is a very tiny portion of the millions of red blood cells present, the counts should fit a Poisson distribution. Therefore, the standard deviation of the counts is $\sqrt{400} = 20$ and 95% confidence limits for the counts per square are $400 \pm (20 \times z_{0.05}) = 400 \pm (20 \times 1.96) = 400 \pm 39.2 = 360.8 - 439.2$. Thus, the population counts per square range from 361 to 439 with a probability of 95%. However, most red cell counts are reported per mm^3, so we need to correct for the actual volume examined. The volume that is examined is the area of counting chamber examined multiplied by the depth of the fluid under the coverslip. Assume that this is 10^{-4} mm^3. Then had the cells been counted over 1 mm^3, the total number would have been 400×10^4, and the corresponding 95% confidence limits would therefore be $360.8 \times 10^4 - 439.2 \times 10^4$, or $3.61 - 4.39$ million per mm^3. It is essential to use the actual observed counts to set the confidence limits. If we had taken the calculated number of cells per mm^3, namely 4 million, then the standard deviation would have been 2000, and the confidence limits would have been calculated as $4 \times 10^6 \pm 1.96 \times 2000 = 4 \times 10^6 \pm 3920 = 3.996 - 4.004$ million per mm^3. These limits are too narrow. The precision depends on the actual number counted. Had the number counted been 4 million, then the narrower confidence limits would have been appropriate. These calculations can be done online at http://www.danielsoper.com/statcalc3/calc.aspx?id=86 and http://statpages.org/confint.html.

Problem 18.3

If the mean number of polonium counts was 425, what are the 95% confidence limits for this mean?

Exact Method

If $\overline{X} < 100$, the approximation ceases to be accurate, and must be replaced. Exact confidence limits can be calculated by using the mathematical link between the Poisson and chi-squared distributions (Armitage et al., 2002). These limits are

$$\lambda_L = 0.5\chi^2_{2\lambda,1-\alpha/2} \quad \text{and} \quad \lambda_U = 0.5\chi^2_{(2\lambda+2),\alpha/2}.$$

For 95% confidence limits, $\alpha = 0.5$, and $\alpha/2 = 0.025$. For 99% limits, $\alpha = 0.01$ and $\alpha/2 = 0.005$.

Problem 18.4

What are the 95% confidence limits for a mean count of 4?

Example 18.7

10 deaths are observed from AIDS in 1 week in an urban hospital. What are the exact 95% confidence limits for the number of deaths per 4 weeks?

The 95% confidence limits for 10 counts are

$$\lambda_L = 0.5_{\chi^2_{20,0.975}} \text{ and } \lambda_U = 0.5_{\chi^2_{22,0.025}}.$$

These limits are thus 4.80 and 18.39 deaths per week, or 19.18–73.56 deaths per 4 weeks. These can be determined online at http://statpages.org/confint.html or http://www. danielsoper.com/statcalc3/calc.aspx?id=86.

With the normal approximation, the limits would have been $10 \pm 1.96\sqrt{10} = 10 \pm 6.20 = 3.80$ to 16.20 per week. These limits, even if incorrect, are not very far from the true limits.

Example 18.8

A physician observes two deaths from a rare form of cancer in 1 year. If deaths from this form of cancer are random, what are the 95% confidence limits of annual deaths? The normal approximation gives $2 \pm 1.96\sqrt{2} = 2 \pm 2.77$, or -0.23 to 4.77 per year. The exact method and the calculators at http://statpages.org/confint.html or http://www.danielsoper.com/statcalc3/calc. aspx?id=86 give limits of

$$\lambda_L = 0.5_{\chi^2_{4,0.975}} \text{ and}$$
$$\lambda_U = 0.5_{\chi^2_{6,0.025}}, \quad ; \text{ these are 0.24 to 7.22 per year.}$$

If one-sided upper and lower $(100 - \alpha)$ limits are wanted, replace $\alpha/2$ by α in the respective equations. Therefore, the upper 95% limit becomes $\lambda_U = 0.5_{\chi^2_{(2\lambda+2),\alpha}}$ and the lower 95% limit becomes $\lambda_L = 0.5_{\chi^2_{2\lambda,1-\alpha}}$. In the cancer example, the one-sided upper 95% confidence limit would be

$$\lambda_U = 0.5_{\chi^2_{(6),0.05}} = 6.30.$$

THE SQUARE ROOT TRANSFORMATION

It is desirable to have the variances of different groups homogeneous when testing for differences between the means, because if the group variances differ markedly, then comparisons between groups become less efficient (Chapter 25). This could be a problem for Poisson distributions because as their means increase, so do their variances. Therefore, it may be useful to use a transformation that keeps the variances stable. Such a transformation is the square root transformation. If a random variable X has a

Poisson distribution with mean λ, then the reexpression $\sqrt{X}$ or $\sqrt{X+0.5}$ if some counts have zero values has a more normal distribution with a mean that is a function of λ and a variance of about $\frac{1}{4}$, as long as λ is >30 (Bartlett, 1936; Bishop et al., 1975; Zar, 2010). The mean and variance are no longer interdependent after the transformation. Freeman and Tukey (1950) suggested that for small values of $\lambda < 3$ it is better to use $\sqrt{X_i} + \sqrt{X_i + 1}$. This transformation is also used if there are many zero values in a data set that has <15 counts. In addition to stabilizing the variance, the distribution becomes closer to a normal distribution.

CUMULATIVE POISSON PROBABILITIES

Often we want the combined probabilities of counts over certain ranges, rather than the absolute probability of each count. For this, we make use of the cumulative Poisson distribution.

Example 18.9

A nursing supervisor has to determine the duty roster for a busy delivery service. If too few nurses are assigned, then patients will not receive good care. If too many are assigned, then several nurses will not have anything to do, and the costs of medical care will be unnecessarily increased. If there were some way to know how many deliveries were likely to occur, then the supervisor could arrange for a certain number of nurses to be on duty and for a certain number to be at home but available in an emergency.

Assume that over a long time in which deliveries have been recorded there are an average of 16 deliveries per 8-h shift. The delivery rate per shift is likely to be a Poisson variate, so it is possible to calculate the probability of any given number of deliveries per shift. The calculations below are provided to illustrate the process of cumulating probabilities.

It is easy to calculate the probabilities of 0, 1, 2, etc., events.

$P(X = 0) = e^{-16} = 0.000000113$

$P(X = 1) = 0.000000113 \times 16 = 0.000001801$

$P(X = 2) = 0.000001801 \times 16/2 = 0.0000144.$

....

These results are displayed in Figure 18.2 left panel.

The most likely numbers of deliveries per shift are 15 and 16. However, 16 would not be a safe upper number to pick, because higher numbers of deliveries per shift are fairly frequent.

Now calculate a cumulative probability from these data.

$P(X = 0) = 0.000000113$

$P(X \le 1) = P(X = 0) + P(X = 1) = 0.000000113 + 0.000001801 = 0.000001914$

$P(X \le 2) = P(X \le 1) + P(X = 2) = 0.000001914 + 0.0000144 = 0.000016314.$

....

(Continued)

Example 18.9—cont'd

The results appear in Figure 18.2 right panel.

The supervisor can be sure that about 95% of the time, there will not be more than 22–23 deliveries per shift. Therefore, with this knowledge and the experience of knowing what happens if there are too few or too many nurses on duty per shift, the supervisor can decide how many nurses to allocate per shift.

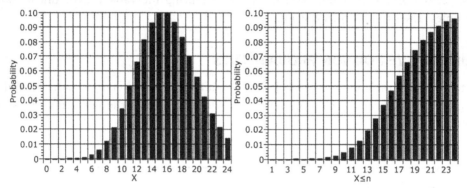

Figure 18.2 Probabilities of $P(X = n)$ in left panel and $P(X \leq n)$ in right panel for a Poisson with mean number of events being 16.

These calculations are very tedious, and it is best to use tables of the cumulative Poisson distribution or an online program such as http://stattrek.com/Tables/poisson.aspx, http://easycalculation.com/statistics/poisson-distribution.php, http://www.solvemymath.com/online_math_calculator/statistics/discrete_distributions/poisson/cdf_poisson.php, or http://www.danielsoper.com/statcalc3/calc.aspx?id=86. In these, the mean number of events (e.g., 16) and some higher number (e.g., 21) are entered, and the cumulative probability up to that number is calculated. The second number is reentered until the desired probability is achieved.

The same process can be used to set the probability for a range of values. For example, in Example 18.9, what proportion of the counts lies between 9 and 15? From the calculator the cumulative probability up to 9 deliveries per shift is 0.0433, and up to 15 per shift is 0.4667. Therefore, the probability of being between these limits is $0.4667 - 0.0433 = 0.4234$.

Tables for selected values of λ up to 5 are available online at http://sites.stat.psu.edu/~mga/401/tables/poisson.pdf and http://mat.iitm.ac.in/home/vetri/public_html/statistics/poisson.pdf.

Problem 18.5

Assume that an emergency room gets an average of 3 patients per hour. What is the 95% probability of seeing 6 patients in the next hour? What is the probability of seeing 32 patients in the next 8 h?

DIFFERENCES BETWEEN MEANS OF POISSON DISTRIBUTIONS

Comparing the mean counts in two Poisson distributions depends in part on the size of the means and the size of the samples from which they come, and on whether the counts are based on the same or different units.

Comparison of Counts Based on Same Units

Assume that the counts in the two groups are both >10, and that each is based on the same unit of time or space. Then the normal approximation to the Poisson distribution can be used. Let the counts in the two groups be λ_1 and λ_2. Then,

$$z = \frac{\text{Difference between the counts}}{\text{Square root of the variance of the difference between the counts}} = \frac{\lambda_1 - \lambda_2}{\sqrt{\lambda_1 + \lambda_2}}.$$

If the sum of the mean counts in the two groups is >5 but under 20, then use the formula with the continuity correction:

$$\frac{\lambda_1 - \lambda_2 - 1}{\sqrt{\lambda_1 + \lambda_2}}.$$

Example 18.10

If there are 33 counts in the first group, and 26 counts in the second group, $z = \frac{33-26}{\sqrt{33+26}} = 0.91$, and the null hypothesis of no difference would be accepted with P = 0.36 (two sided).

These differences can be tested online at http://www.quantitativeskills.com/sisa/statistics/t-thlp.htm.

An alternative normal approximation is based on the square root transformation (Anscombe, 1948).

$$z = \left| \sqrt{2\lambda_1 + \frac{3}{4}} - \sqrt{2\lambda_2 + \frac{3}{4}} \right|.$$

Example 18.11

Thus $z = \left| \sqrt{2 \times 33 + \frac{3}{4}} - \sqrt{2 \times 26 + \frac{3}{4}} \right| = 0.9071$. This is similar to the previous result.

Some texts give tables for evaluating differences between the means of two Poisson distributions.

Comparison of Counts Not Based on Same Units

Often the two counts being compared are not based on the same unit rate or space. For example, we may want to compare the number of abnormal cells in an organ after two methods of treatment, but the number of cells (n, m) in the microscopic fields differs in the two groups. Then we must obtain a proportion that bases the count in each group on a common unit. Let the resulting two rates be μ_1 and μ_2 where $\mu_1 = \lambda_1/n$ and $\mu_2 = \lambda_2/m$. First, calculate a pooled weighted average to estimate the common rate, assuming that the null hypothesis is true. This is

$$\lambda_p = \frac{\lambda_1 n + \lambda_2 m}{n + m} = \frac{\mu_1 + \mu_2}{n + m},$$

where λ_p is the pooled rate. Then the standard error of the difference between the two rates is

$$\sqrt{\frac{\lambda_p}{n} + \frac{\lambda_p}{m}}.$$

The test of the significance of the difference between the two count rates is thus

$$z = \frac{\lambda_1 - \lambda_2}{\sqrt{\frac{\lambda_p}{n} + \frac{\lambda_p}{m}}}.$$

This can also be written as,

$$z = \frac{\lambda_1 - (\lambda_1 + \lambda_2)\left(\frac{n_1}{n_1 + n_2}\right)}{\sqrt{(\lambda_1 + \lambda_2)\left(\frac{n_1}{n_1 + n_2}\right)\left(1 - \frac{n_1}{n_1 + n_2}\right)}},$$

where λ_1 and λ_2 are the two sets of counts, and n_1 and n_2 are the respective sample sizes.

Example 18.12

Let there be 11 abnormal cells out of 1800 cells in treatment 1, and 27 abnormal cells out of 1450 cells in treatment 2. Then the two rates per 1000 cells are $11/1.8 = 6.11$ and $27/1.45 = 18.62$, for a difference between rates of 12.51. The standard error of the difference between these two rates is based on the pooled average rate of $(11 + 27)/(1.8 + 1.45) = 11.69$. The standard error of the difference is thus

$$\sqrt{\frac{11.69}{1.8} + \frac{11.69}{1.45}} = 3.82.$$

Therefore, $z = \frac{12.51}{3.82} = 3.27$, and the null hypothesis can be rejected with $P < 0.0018$ (two sided).

Example 18.12—cont'd

By the second method, this gives

$$z = \frac{11 - (11 + 27)\left(\dfrac{1800}{1800 + 1450}\right)}{\sqrt{(11 + 27)\left(\dfrac{1800}{1800 + 1450}\right)\left(1 - \dfrac{1800}{1800 + 1450}\right)}} = \frac{-10.0462}{3.0643} = 3.2785.$$

This formula saves having to calculate pooled rates.

Another useful method for small mean counts is to calculate the pooled value of λ, as above, and then to calculate z_1 for the smaller value of λ, and z_2 for the larger value of λ, from

$$z_1 = 2\left(\sqrt{\mu_1 + 1} - \sqrt{\lambda_p \times n}\right) \text{ and } z_2 = 2\left(\sqrt{\mu_2} - \sqrt{\lambda_p \times m}\right).$$

Calculate the sum of z_1^2 and z_2^2. This is referred to the chi-square table with one degree of freedom.

This method can be extended to k groups. The first formula, i.e., that for z_1, is used for all samples where the value of λ is less than λ_p, and the formula for z_2 is used when λ is greater than λ_p. Then testing is done with the formula

$$\chi^2 = \sum_{i=1}^{k} z_i^2 \text{ for } k - 1 \text{ degrees of freedom.}$$

Example 18.13

For the data in Example 18.12, we have

$$z_1 = 2\left(\sqrt{11 + 1} - \sqrt{11.69 \times 1.8}\right) \text{ and } z_2 = 2\left(\sqrt{27} - \sqrt{11.69 \times 1.45}\right).$$

Therefore $z_1 = -2.2461$ and $z_2 = 2.1581$, and the sum of their squares is 9.7024. From the table for one degree of freedom, $P = 0.0018$, the same as shown above.

If μ_1 and μ_2 are large, but n and m are small, then use the square root transformation. With this transformation, the variance is approximately 0.25. Therefore, the variance of the difference between $\sqrt{\mu_1}$ and $\sqrt{\mu_2} = (\sqrt{\mu_1} + \sqrt{\mu_2}) \approx 0.5$. Under the null hypothesis, the difference d between the means of the square roots has mean zero and variance $\frac{0.25}{n} + \frac{0.25}{m}$. Therefore,

$$z = \frac{d}{0.5\sqrt{\dfrac{1}{n} + \dfrac{1}{m}}}.$$

Example 18.14

In 11 soil samples from one area there are an average of 34 pathogenic bacteria, and from another area 15 soil samples give an average of 69 pathogenic bacteria. Are these significantly different?

$$d = \sqrt{69} - \sqrt{34} = 2.476.$$

$$z = \frac{2.476}{0.5\sqrt{1/11 + 1/15}} = 12.47, \text{ with } P < 0.001.$$

Comparing the Ratio of Two Poisson Variates

To compare the ratio of two Poisson variates, use a method recommended by Armitage et al. (2002).

Example 18.15

Let $X_1 = 13$, and $X_2 = 4$. Then $\widehat{F} = \frac{13}{4+1} = 2.60$. Entering the F table with degrees of freedom $2(4 + 1) = 10$, and $2 \times 13 = 26$, we find that $F = 2.59$ with $\alpha(2) = 0.05$. Therefore, we can reject the two-sided null hypothesis that the two mean values are equal at the 0.05 level of probability.

Using this for the values in Example 5.16 of 33 and 26, we have

$$\widehat{F} = \frac{33}{(26 + 1)} = 1.22.$$

For degrees of freedom 54 and 66, we have $\alpha(2) \approx 0.50$, and once again the null hypothesis cannot be rejected.

This is based on the test for comparing proportions in paired samples. If X_1 and X_2 are counts following Poisson distributions with means μ_1 and μ_2, respectively, X_1 can be taken as the proportion of the total frequency $X_1 + X_2$. Then X_1 follows a binomial distribution with parameters $X_1 + X_2$, equivalent to n, and $\mu_1/(\mu_1 + \mu_2)$, equivalent to r in the binomial equation. μ_1/μ_2, the desired ratio, is thus equivalent to $\pi/(1 - \pi)$. Tables give the 95% confidence limits for π, and calculating $\pi/(1 - \pi)$ gives the 95% confidence limits for μ_1/μ_2.

Example 18.16

The number of bacteria growing on two culture plates is 13 and 31. Then the 95% confidence limits for the ratio 13/31 are calculated by taking the proportion of bacteria in the first plate as $13/44 = 0.2955$, and from http://statpages.org/confint.html the confidence limits for π are 0.1676 and 0.4520. For each of these values we then calculate the 95% confidence limits of $\pi/(1 - \pi)$ as $0.1676/(1 - 0.1676) = 0.2013$, and $0.4520/(1 - 0.4520) = 0.8248$.

To compare the ratio of two rates derived from Poisson variables, use a similar approach, but multiply the final values for the upper and lower limits by the ratio of the two measurement units.

Example 18.17

Assume that the two culture plates above had different areas. The 13 bacteria in plate one were based on an area of 6.3 cm^2, whereas the 31 bacteria in plate two were based on an area of 10.9 cm^2; the number of bacteria per cm^2 would then be $13/6.3 = 2.0635$ and $31/10.9 = 2.8440$, and their ratio would be 0.7256. Then the lower limit of the ratio per cm^2 would be $0.2013 \times (10.9/6.3) = 0.3483$, and the upper limit would be $0.8248 \times (10.9/6.3) = 1.427$ (see Daly et al., 1991).

DETERMINING THE REQUIRED SAMPLE SIZE

There are at least three different ways of determining sample sizes, power, and differences between Poisson means, depending on the underlying assumptions. They give similar results for sample sizes >100, but differ for smaller numbers.

If two Poisson distributions have means λ_1 and λ_2, a simple formula to determine the required number of observations to give a difference with $\alpha = 0.05$ is (see van Belle http://vanbelle.org/chapters/webchapter2.pdf)

$$N = \frac{4}{\left(\sqrt{\lambda_1} - \sqrt{\lambda_2}\right)^2}.$$

Thus, if the means are 30 and 40, the number of events per group needed will be $N = \frac{4}{(\sqrt{30} - \sqrt{40})^2} = 5.57$, or a total of about 12. If the two means are closer together, such as 7 and 11, the number needed per group is $N = \frac{4}{(\sqrt{7} - \sqrt{11})^2} = 8.89$, or a total of about 18.

Slightly different sample sizes are given by http://www.quantitativeskills.com/sisa/statistics/t-test.php?mean1=33&mean2=26&N1=000&N2=000&SD1=00.00&SD2=00.00&CI=95&Submit1=Calculate. For the above example, this calculator gives 11 in each group.

Sometimes we are interested in calculating sample size for detecting a difference between two Poisson counts when there is a background count rate. Examples might be analyzing two Poisson radiation counts against a background of radiation, or evaluating the significance of two sedatives in producing phocomelia (as with thalidomide) when there is already a low incidence of phocomelia in the absence of drugs. Let the background rate be λ^*, and the two experimental rates be λ_1 and λ_2. Then,

$$N = \frac{4}{\left(\sqrt{\lambda^* + \lambda_1} - \sqrt{\lambda^* + \lambda_2}\right)^2}.$$

Taking the example of rates of 7 and 11 used above, but add a background of 3, then we have,

$$N = \frac{4}{\left(\sqrt{3+7} - \sqrt{3+11}\right)^2} = 11.9 \text{ for a total of about 24.}$$

We may need to determine how large a sample size is needed to determine λ so that the upper or lower confidence bounds do not differ from the sample estimate by more than a specified percentage. These bounds can be determined easily from graphs published by Hahn and Meeker (1991).

Example 18.18

A problem concerns the accuracy of the microsphere method of measuring regional blood flow. Microspheres are tiny (usually 15 μm in diameter) spheres that when well mixed with blood in the heart are distributed to all the organs and regions within organs in proportion to the flows to those regions and organs. The microspheres are trapped in the organs. At the end of the experiment, the organs are removed, cut up into appropriate pieces, and the microspheres are counted by virtue of radioactivity or contained dye. The question asked is how many microspheres need there be in, say, the left atrial wall for flow to be measured within 10% of the true flow with a probability of 95%. The concept here is that if flows showed stationarity (i.e., did not change from measurement to measurement) and we were to repeat the microsphere injection several times, there would be different numbers of microspheres trapped each time, simply because there would be slight changes in the mixing and distribution of the microspheres with each injection. What critical number of microspheres is needed?

Let the critical average number of microspheres be X. If we require the 95% confidence limits of X to be within 10% of the true flow that would be given by the average number of microspheres for all the injections, then the 95% confidence limits will be $\pm 0.1X$. Because the distribution of the microspheres is a Poisson variate, the 95% confidence limits are given by $1.96\sqrt{X}$. These two numbers are equal. Therefore,

$0.1X = 1.96\sqrt{X}$. Square to remove the square root, so that

$0.01X^2 = 3.84X$. Multiply by 100 to remove the decimal point, so that

$X^2 = 384X$, and $X = 384$.

Therefore if there are 384 microspheres per piece of tissue to be measured, the requirements will be satisfied. (There are, of course, other technical points to be covered before the method can be accurate: see Heymann et al. (1977).)

This same method could be used for other degrees of precision, for example 5%, or for other confidence limits, for example, 99%, by substituting the appropriate figures in the above equations.

Hahn and Meeker also give a simple computational formula for determining sample size:

$$n = \lambda^* \left[\frac{z_{(1-\alpha/2)}}{d}\right]^2,$$

where λ^* is the desired mean rate, and d is the $100(1 - \alpha)$ confidence interval of length $\pm d$, usually given as a percentage of λ^*. This approximation works well if $n > 10$.

Example 18.19

We wish to determine how many water samples of fixed volume to count to determine if the mean number of pathogenic *Escherichia coli* bacteria is 3, with 95% confidence limits of 20% of the mean value, that is $3 \times 0.2 = 0.6$. Then,

$$n = 3\left(\frac{1.96}{0.6}\right)^2 = 32.$$

Waiting Times

One common extension of Poisson statistics is calculating the probability of the time between events. For example, what is the time between the arrival of individual patients at an emergency room, or between the arrival of nerve impulses (interspike interval)? If the process is a Poisson process, then the waiting times can be fitted to a negative exponential distribution (Brown and Rothery, 1993):

$$f(t) = \lambda e^{-kt}.$$

This distribution has mean $= 1/\lambda$ and variance $1/\lambda^2$.

As an example, consider a bacterial species that in a specific culture medium has an exponentially distributed lifetime with a mean of 100 h. What proportion of them will die before 40 h?

From their mean lifetime, $\lambda = 1/100$. The probability of dying before 40 h is,

$$1 - e^{-40/100} = 0.33, \quad \text{or} \quad 33\%.$$

These types of statistics are also used when calculating how rapidly participants in a clinical trial will appear at each cooperating center (Jones, 2010).

APPENDIX

The formula for the variance of a Poisson distribution follows naturally from the equivalent formula for the binomial distribution. In the latter, the mean is $N\pi$ and the variance is $N\pi(1 - \pi)$. As π becomes smaller, the expression $(1 - \pi)$ approaches 1. Therefore the variance becomes $N\pi$.

REFERENCES

Anscombe, F.J., 1948. The transformation of Poisson, binomial, and negative-binomial data. Biometrika 36, 246–254.

Armitage, P., Berry, G., Matthews, J.N.S., 2002. Statistical Methods in Medical Research. Blackwell.

Bartlett, M.S., 1936. The square root transformation in analysis of variance. J. R. Stat. Soc. Suppl. 3, 68–78.

Bishop, Y.M.M., Fienberg, S.E., Holland, P.W., 1975. Discrete Multivariate Analysis: Theory and Practice. The MIT Press.

Brown, D., Rothery, P., 1993. Models in Biology: Mathematics, Statistics and Computing. John Wiley & Sons, Inc.

Daly, L.E., Bourke, G.J., McGilvray, J., 1991. Interpretation and Uses of Medical Statistics. Blackwell Scientific Publications.

Dixon, W.J., Massey Jr., F.J., 1983. Introduction to Statistical Analysis. McGraw-Hill Book Publishers.

Elliott, J.M., 1983. Some Methods for the Statistical Analysis of Samples of Benthic Invertebrates. Freshwater Biological Association, Ambleside, Cumbria.

Freeman, M.F., Tukey, J.W., 1950. Transformations related to the angular and the square root. Ann. Math. Stat. 21, 607–611.

Hahn, G.J., Meeker, W.Q., 1991. Statistical Intervals. A Guide for Practitioners. John Wiley and Sons, Inc.

Heymann, M.A., Payne, B.D., Hoffman, J.I.E., et al., 1977. Blood flow measurements with radionuclide-labelled particles. Prog. Cardiovasc. Dis. 20, 55–79.

Jones, B., 2010. The waiting game: how long is long enough? Significance 2, 40–41.

Rutherford, E., Geiger, H., 1910. The probability variations in the distribution of alpha particles. Phil. Mag. 20, 698–704.

Selvin, S., 1991. Statistical Analysis of Epidemiologic Data. Oxford University Press.

von Bortkiewicz, L., 1898. Das gesetz der kleinen Zahlen (The Law of Small Numbers) (B.G. Taubner).

Zar, J.H., 2010. Biostatistical Analysis. Prentice Hall.

CHAPTER 19

Negative Binomial Distribution

Contents

INTRODUCTION

This distribution is used to solve two different problems. The first resembles a Bernoulli trial, in which the number of successes in the first n trials has a binomial distribution $(p + q)^n$ with parameters n and p. If we ask instead, what random variable r will give the number of trials at which the kth success is achieved, then we use the negative binomial distribution, because it is derived from the expansion of $(q - p)^{-k}$, where $p = \mu/k$ and μ is the mean number of events.

The parameters of this distribution are the arithmetic mean μ (a measure of location), and k (a measure of dispersion), which is not necessarily an integer. If k is an integer, the distribution is known as the Pascal distribution. The negative binomial distribution is appropriate when

The experiment consists of x repeated trials.

Each trial can result in just two possible outcomes. One of these outcomes is success and the other is failure.

The probability of success, denoted by p, is the same on every trial.

The trials are independent; that is, the outcome of one trial does not affect the outcome on other trials.

The experiment continues until r successes are observed, with r specified in advance.

PROBABILITY OF r SUCCESSES

Suppose that independent trials, each with probability p of being a success, are done until there are r successes. If X is the number of trials required, then;

$$P(X = n) = \binom{n-1}{r-1} p^r (1-p)^{n-r}, \text{ where } n = r, r+1, \ldots$$

For a list of all websites referred to in this chapter, as clickable links, see the book companion website: www.booksite.elsevier.com/9780128023877.

Biostatistics for Medical and Biomedical Practitioners
http://dx.doi.org/10.1016/B978-0-12-802387-7.00019-6

In order for the rth success to occur in the nth trial, there must be $r - 1$ successes in the first $n - 1$ trials, and the nth trial must be a success. The probability of $r - 1$ successes in the first $n - 1$ trials is $\binom{n-1}{r-1} p^{r-1}(1-p)^{n-r}$ by the binomial theorem, and the probability of the second event is p. Multiplying these two together gives $\binom{n-1}{r-1} p^{r}(1-p)^{n-r}$ the required probability (Ross, 1984).

Example 19.1 Probability of successes

What is the probability of getting 3 heads in 8 tosses of a coin? $p = 0.5$, $X = n$ (number of heads) $= 3$, $r =$ number of tosses. The formula provides the results in Table 19.1.
  Therefore, the probability of getting the third head in the eighth toss is 0.08203125.

Table 19.1

$r =$ number of tosses for $X = 3$	Probability $X = 3$
3	0.125
4	0.1875
5	0.1875
6	0.15625
7	0.1171825
8	0.08203125
9	0.0546875
10	0.003525625
	etc

Example 19.2

Let P(head $= p = 0.5$). Then to get 17 heads in 30 tosses, we have,

P(16 heads in 29 tosses and heads on 30th toss)

$$= \binom{29}{16} p^{16}(1-p)^{13} p = \binom{29}{16} p^{17}(1-p)^{13} = \frac{29!}{16!13!} 0.5^{17} 0.5^{13} = 0.0632.$$

A free online calculator at http://stattrek.com/Tables/NegBinomial.aspx solves similar problems easily.

Example 19.3

How might we apply this to a medical problem? An oncologist wants to recruit 6 patients with breast cancer to test a new therapeutic agent to prepare for a large randomized trial. Assume that the probability of a patient agreeing to the trial is $p = 0.25$. What is the probability that $N = 16$ patients will have to be interviewed to obtain 6 (=r) consents?

$$p = \binom{N-1}{r-1} p^r (1-p)^{N-r} = \frac{15!}{5!10!} 0.25^6 0.75^{10} = 0.0413.$$

This probability may be of little use, and a more important question is what is the average number of interviews to obtain 6 consents. The mean μ of a negative binomial distribution is $r/p = 6/0.25 = 24$.

Problem 19.1

What is the probability that the oncologist will obtain 8 consents in 30 interviews?

OVERDISPERSED DISTRIBUTION

The negative binomial distribution has a more important use for a contagious or over-dispersed distribution, one with clumps of objects rather than a random distribution. In such a distribution, the variance is much greater than the mean, whereas in a Poisson distribution the variance is approximately equal to the mean, and in a binomial distribution the variance is less than the mean. Unlike the Poisson, the probability of any time or space being occupied by an event is not constant, and the occurrence of an event may affect the occurrence of other events.

An early example of this distribution was provided by Greenwood and Yule (1920), who examined the number of accidents in 414 machinists followed for 3 months (Table 19.2).

If the accidents are independent events, then a Poisson distribution would be suitable. As shown, however, the Poisson distribution has a deficit of those with no accidents and an excess of those with one or more accidents. When a negative binomial distribution is fitted, however, the observed and expected numbers match, suggesting that some machinists are accident-prone. The negative binomial is preferred to the Poisson distribution when events are more likely to recur in one group than another (Glynn and Buring, 1996).

The mean of a negative binomial is kq/p, and the variance is kq/p^2. The variance is also given as $\mu + \frac{\mu^2}{k}$.

Table 19.2 Accidents and machinists

Observed		Expected	
Number of accidents	Number of machinists	Poisson	Negative binomial
0	296	256	299
1	74	122	69
2	26	30	26
3	8	5	11
4	4	1	5
5	4	0	2
6	1	0	1
7	0	0	1
8	1	0	0
Total	414		

The expression $1/k$ is a measure of the excess variance due to possible clumping. As $1/k$ approaches zero, the distribution converges to the Poisson. As $1/k$ approaches infinity, the distribution approaches the logarithmic.

USES OF THE NEGATIVE BINOMIAL

It is used extensively to model temporal and geographic variations in parasitic infections of plants, animals, and humans, in all of which zero infestation is frequent but a few have excessive numbers of infestations; for example, the variations in schistosomal infection in different regions of East Africa (Clements et al., 2006), the burden of parasitic infections in host wildlife (Shaw et al., 1998), the counts of *Wucheria bancrofti* (the cause of filariasis) in human blood (Alexander et al., 2000), the prevalence of *Plasmodium falciparum* infestation of mosquitos (Billingsley et al., 1994), and the pattern of childhood susceptibility to malaria (Mwangi et al., 2008). It has been used to model accident statistics in many fields—occupational health, automobile accidents (Ramirez et al., 2009), or falls in the home (Iinattiniemi et al., 2009). Some have used this distribution to model the sizes of family practices in Canada (Anderson et al., 1986), the rate of consultations in a practice Iinattiniemi et al., 2009; (Kilpatrick, 1977), or the number of episodes of psychiatric illness (Smeeton, 1986). The distribution model has even been extended to evaluating founder germ cell numbers (Zheng et al., 2005) and vasopressin mRNA distribution in the supraoptic nucleus (McCabe et al., 1990).

There are several methods for determining k and so being able to test for the fit to a negative binomial distribution. Consultation with a statistician is recommended.

Many negative binomial distributions are monotonic with a huge peak for those with no episodes. This is not a requirement for the negative binomial that could resemble a skewed Gaussian curve (Mwangi et al., 2008; Torgerson et al., 2003).

Example 19.4

Table 19.3 shows data from a survey of the number of episodes of psychiatric illness in a general practice (21).

The Poisson distribution fits poorly, but the negative binomial shows a good fit, with $k = -0.23$.

Table 19.3 Psychiatric episodes

Number of episodes ($X = r$)	Observed number (f)	Expected Poisson	Expected negative binomial
0	45,067	36,945	45,061
1	7917	17,634	7959
2	3256	4208	3209
3	1550	670	1537
4	762	80	794
5	434	7.6	428
6	243		237
7	127		134
8	77	1.6	77
9	50		45
10	26		26
11	15		15
12	10		9
13	5		5
≥14	7		8
$\overline{X} = 0.4757$	$N = 59,737$ $s = 1.3112$		

Fitting the distribution is not the end of the exercise. Once the value of k is determined, the investigator can then consider why that form of contagious distribution had occurred and postulate mechanisms that might lead to better understanding. One way of thinking about the meaning of k is that it indicates variation among individuals in their intrinsic level of contact that is responsible for departure from randomness.

Other comparable distributions are the zero-inflated Poisson and the zero-inflated negative binomial distributions referred to in Chapter 34.

REFERENCES

Alexander, N., Moyeed, R., Stander, J., 2000. Spatial modelling of individual-level parasite counts using the negative binomial distribution. Biostatistics 1, 453–463.

Anderson, J.E., Willan, A.R., Gancher, W.A., 1986. The negative binomial model and the denominator problem in a rural family practice. Fam. Pract. 3, 174–183.

Billingsley, P.F., Medley, G.F., Charlwood, D., et al., 1994. Relationship between prevalence and intensity of *Plasmodium falciparum* infection in natural populations of *Anopheles* mosquitoes. Am. J. Trop. Med. Hyg. 51, 260–270.

Clements, A.C., Moyeed, R., Brooker, S., 2006. Bayesian geostatistical prediction of the intensity of infection with *Schistosoma mansoni* in East Africa. Parasitology 133, 711–719.

Glynn, R.J., Buring, J.E., 1996. Ways of measuring rates of recurrent events. BMJ (Clin. Res. Ed.) 312, 364–367.

Greenwood, M., Yule, G.U., 1920. An inquiry into the nature of frequency distributions of multiple happenings, with particular reference to the occurrence of multiple attacks of disease or repeated accidents. J. R. Stat. Soc. 83, 255–279.

Iinattiniemi, S., Jokelainen, J., Luukinen, H., 2009. Falls risk among a very old home-dwelling population. Scand. J. Prim. Health Care 27, 25–30.

Kilpatrick Jr., S.J., 1977. Consultation frequencies in general practice. Health Serv. Res. 12, 284–298.

McCabe, J.T., Kawata, M., Sano, Y., et al., 1990. Quantitative in situ hybridization to measure single-cell changes in vasopressin and oxytocin mRNA levels after osmotic stimulation. Cell. Mol. Neurobiol. 10, 59–71.

Mwangi, T.W., Fegan, G., Williams, T.N., et al., 2008. Evidence for over-dispersion in the distribution of clinical malaria episodes in children. PLoS One 3, e2196.

Ramirez, B.A., Izquierdo, F.A., Fernandez, C.G., et al., 2009. The influence of heavy goods vehicle traffic on accidents on different types of Spanish interurban roads. Accid. Anal. Prev. 41, 15–24.

Ross, S., 1984. A First Course in Probability. Macmillan Publishing Company.

Shaw, D.J., Grenfell, B.T., Dobson, A.P., 1998. Patterns of macroparasite aggregation in wildlife host populations. Parasitology 117 (Pt 6), 597–610.

Smeeton, N.C., 1986. Distribution of episodes of mental illness in general practice: results from the Second National Morbidity Survey. J. Epidemiol. Community Health 40, 130–133.

Torgerson, P.R., Shaikenov, B.S., Rysmukhambetova, A.T., et al., 2003. Modelling the transmission dynamics of *Echinococcus granulosus* in dogs in rural Kazakhstan. Parasitology 126, 417–424.

Zheng, C.J., Luebeck, E.G., Byers, B., et al., 2005. On the number of founding germ cells in humans. Theor. Biol. Med. Model 2, 32.

## PART 5

Probability in Epidemiology and Medical Diagnosis

CHAPTER 20

Some Epidemiological Considerations: Odds Ratio, Relative Risk, and Attributable Risk

Contents

BASIC CONCEPTS

Introduction

The odds ratio (OR) in Chapter 14 gave a point estimate of how much a proportion of successes in one group differs from the proportion of successes in another group. By definition, "odds" is the probability of an event occurring, divided by the probability that an event does not occur. The OR is the odds of an outcome occurring in one group, divided by the odds of an outcome occurring in another group. A comparable ratio is the relative risk (RR) ratio, and the following discussion describes the relationships and uses of each of these ratios.

Care is needed to use the correct estimates of disease incidence, because there are many deceptively similar ratios in use. Three common estimates are (1) the incidence rate (or density) which is the number of new incidences of the disease per unit time,

For a list of all websites referred to in this chapter, as clickable links, see the book companion website: www.booksite.elsevier.com/9780128023877.

Biostatistics for Medical and Biomedical Practitioners
http://dx.doi.org/10.1016/B978-0-12-802387-7.00020-2

(2) the cumulative incidence which is the proportion of study subjects who develop the outcome of interest at any time during the follow-up period, and (3) the incidence odds, the ratio of the number of subjects experiencing the outcome to those not experiencing the outcome (Pearce, 1993). The latter two are not rates and are discussed below. The data must be collected over the same time period. Detailed evaluations of these different estimates are described by Kleinbaum et al. (1982).

Cohort Study

Consider a population study that follows a large population from time t_0 to time t_n, noting who has a putative risk factor (cause or exposure) at onset and at the end of the period noting how many have response (disease) in those with and without risk factor. This is a prospective cohort study. The data might have been collected previously and we are examining the records, but as long as one moves forward from time t_0 to time t_n it is still a prospective study. People who have the disease at the outset are excluded. Then calculate the RR as

$$RR = \frac{\text{Incidence of disease in exposed group}(p_e)}{\text{Incidence of disease in unexposed group}(p_u)}.$$

More generally, RR is defined as "the ratio of the probability of an outcome in one group to the probability of the outcome in another group."

Most often, the data are represented by a 2×2 table (Table 20.1). Methods for dealing with more complex tables are discussed in epidemiology texts.

Table 20.1 represents a typical data table relating an input (exposure) to an output (disease). In discussing how to make various calculations (see below) I will use the format of Table 20.2 (left side) rather than the format of (right side) that appears in some texts.

One way to avoid errors due to use of the wrong symbols is to specify the conditional probability in each cell. Thus, the probability of disease (D+) given exposure (E+) is

Table 20.1 Factors and definitions

	Disease				
	Yes	No	Total	Odds of disease	Probability of disease
Exposure	a	b	R_1	a/b	$a/(a+b) = a/R_1 = p_e$
No exposure	c	d	R_2	c/d	$c/(c+d) = c/R_2 = p_u$
Total	C_1	C_2	N		$C_1/N = p_t$
Odds of exposure	a/c	b/d			

p_e is the probability of disease in the exposed population; p_u is the probability of disease in the unexposed population; p_t is the probability of disease in the whole population whether exposed or not. Another incidence is the probability of exposure in the whole population, R_1/N, denoted by p_{ex}.

Table 20.2 Left side—format used in this chapter; right side—alternative format used in some texts. Total number N is $a + b + c + d$, and this and cells a and d are unaffected by the different arrangements

	Disease	No disease	Disease	No disease
Exposure	a	b	a	c
No exposure	c	d	b	d

written as $P(D+|E+)$, the probability of no disease in exposed subjects is $P(D-|E+)$. These are unambiguous. $P(D+|E+) = a/N$, $P(D-|E+) = b/N$ (in Table 20.2, left side), and so on. Because N is common to all these proportions, we can work with either absolute numbers or proportions.

As an example, 122,612 normotensive people and 18,310 with systolic hypertension were followed to determine the incidence of cardiovascular (CV) deaths in each group (Table 20.3) (Kelly et al., 2008).

Table 20.3 Data on blood pressure and strokes

	CV death	No CV death	Total	Incidence
Hypertension	2,134	16,176	18,310	0.116548
Normotension	3,882	118,730	122,612	0.0316608
Total	6,016	134,906	140,922	0.0426903

The incidence rate of CV deaths in hypertensives (p_e) [$P(D+|E+)$] is $2134/18,310 = 0.116548$, and in normotensives (p_u) [$P(D+|E-)$] is $3882/122,612 = 0.0316608$. The RR is therefore

$$0.116548/0.0316608 = 3.6811.$$

This study gives an estimate of the incidence of new CV deaths in each group over the time period. Because the data are set out as a 2×2 contingency table, the OR is

$$\frac{2134 \times 118730}{16176 \times 3882} = \frac{253369820}{62795232} = 4.0349.$$

The OR and the RR are similar.

For the whole population the risk p_t is $6016/140,922 = 0.0426903$.

The online calculator at http://www.medcalc.org/calc/relative_risk.php gives the RR and confidence limits, and http://statpages.org/ctab2x2.html gives the OR as well.

Cross-sectional Study

An alternative to a cohort study is a cross-sectional study. This is done at one time on a series of subjects who are not followed; the studies can be divided into two groups. In one, patients are matched for risk factor, and response is determined in each group.

In the other, patients are matched for response, and the risk factor is calculated for each group. The latter is known as a case–control study and is retrospective. The choice of which type of study to do is often practical. If the response of interest is rare, for example, a congenital disease with an incidence of about 1/10,000 live births, then it takes a huge number of people to be followed prospectively in a cohort study to obtain enough responses to evaluate. It is less costly and time-consuming to select 500 patients with the disease and 500 without the disease, and then look back to determine which group differed in antecedent factors. Because the subjects are selected (based on factor or response) and not chosen at random, no population incidence rate can be determined. For this reason, we cannot calculate RR, but must use the OR. An example is shown in Table 20.4 in a cross-sectional study relating exposure to second-hand smoke to ischemic strokes (He et al., 2008).

Table 20.4 Relation of stroke to second-hand smoke exposure

	Stroke	No stroke	Total	Incidence
Exposure	83	394	477	0.174004
No exposure	89	643	732	0.121585
	172	1,037	1,209	0.142266

The incidence rate of stroke in those exposed to cigarette smoke [P(D+|E+)] is $83/477 = 0.174,004$, and in those not exposed [P(D+|E−)] is $89/732 = 0.121,585$. Because the data are set out as a 2×2 contingency table, the OR is

$$\frac{83 \times 643}{394 \times 89} = \frac{53369}{35066} = 1.5220.$$

Odds and risk ratios can be calculated online from http://vassarstats.net/odds2x2.html or http://statpages.org/ctab2x2.html. Be careful entering data into each cell.

The "RR" from the table is $0.174004/0.121585 = 1.4311$. This is not a true RR because each group is selected, and may or may not approximate the true RR, depending on the relative rarity of the response in the population (p_t). The difference is shown in the artificial example in Table 20.5(a)–(d).

RR and OR are similar only if the population prevalence p_t is very low because then the data in the "total" and "no stroke" columns are similar. The RR is $\frac{\frac{a}{a+b}}{\frac{c}{c+d}}$. If a and c are very small relative to b and d, this ratio approximates $\frac{\frac{a}{b}}{\frac{c}{d}}$ which is another way of writing the OR. Therefore, although it is RR that we want, the OR is a reasonable estimate of RR if the response (disease) is relatively rare. It is only in the study of Table 20.5(d) that we can even approximate a true population prevalence.

Table 20.5 Comparison of odds ratio and relative risk

	S	No S	T	S	No S	T	S	No S	T	S	No S	T
Smoker	63	50	113	63	542	605	63	1259	1322	63	12,593	12,656
Nonsmoker	33	50	83	33	539	572	33	1260	1293	33	12,732	12,765
Total	96	100	196	96	1,081	1,177	96	2519	2615	96	25,325	25,421

        Table 20.5(a)   Table 20.5(b)   Table 20.5(c)   Table 20.5(d)

S-stroke; No S- no stroke; T-total

	Group			
	a	b	c	d
OR	1.91	1.90	1.91	1.93
"RR"	1.40	1.80	1.87	1.926
p_t	0.49	0.08	0.037	0.0038

Table 20.5(e) Analysis of tables 20.5 (a)–(d)

OR-odds ratio; "RR"-approximate relative risk; p_t-population prevalence (total stroke/population)

Problem 20.1

A study of the relationship between prehypertension and the presence or absence of diabetes mellitus produced the following data (Shrier and Steele, 2006) (Prehypertension was defined as systolic pressure 120–139 mm Hg or diastolic pressure 80–89 mm Hg.):

	No prehypertension	Prehypertension	Total
Diabetes	445	652	1,097
No diabetes	794	738	1,532
Total	1,239	1,390	2,629

Calculate the OR and "RR." Is this a true RR?

Confidence Limits

Both the OR and the RR are point estimates, and we should determine their confidence limits. For the odds, the population value is usually written as Ωi, and the ratio of two odds Ωi and Ωj as ω. The corresponding sample values are $O i$ and $O j$, and their ratio is o or $\widehat{OR}$.

Because the ORs do not follow a normal distribution, Woolf used the logarithm to base e of the OR (Woolf, 1955; Gardner and Altman, 1995)

$$\text{Standard error } \log_e \widehat{OR} = \sqrt{\frac{1}{a} + \frac{1}{b} + \frac{1}{c} + \frac{1}{d}}.$$

For Table 20.3, the standard error of $\log_e \widehat{OR}$ is $\sqrt{\frac{1}{2134} + \frac{1}{3882} + \frac{1}{16176} + \frac{1}{118730}} = 0.01811$. To determine the 95% confidence interval, calculate the lower (L) and upper (U) limits in logarithmic units as:

$$L = \log_e \widehat{OR} - \left[N_{1-\alpha/2} \times \text{SE} \log_e \widehat{OR} \right], \text{ and}$$
$$U = \log_e \widehat{OR} + \left[N_{1-\alpha/2} \times \text{SE} \log_e \widehat{OR} \right].$$

The only difference between these expressions is the sign between the first and second parts of the right-hand side of the equations.

$$L = \log_e 4.035 - [1.96 \times 0.01881] = 1.3950 - 0.03687 = 1.3161, \text{ and}$$
$$U = \log_e 4.035 + [1.96 \times 0.01881] = 1.3950 + 0.03687 = 1.4319.$$

These are the 95% confidence limits for the OR in logarithmic units. To recover the actual units, the 95% confidence limits are the antilogarithms $e^{1.3161}$ to $e^{1.4319}$, or 3.729 to 4.1866. Because this range does not include 1, there is a difference in proportions between the two treatment groups, and we reject the null hypothesis; this is exactly what the chi-square test concluded.

If any counts are zero, it is not possible to calculate an odds or cross-product ratio, and the standard error of $\widehat{OR}$ is undefined. To overcome this problem, add a small number to each count, commonly 0.5, and the OR and its standard error are calculated with these new increased counts. Thus

$$\widehat{OR} = \frac{(a + 0.5) \times (d + 0.5)}{(b + 0.5) \times (c + 0.5)},$$

and SE $\log_e \widehat{OR} = \sqrt{\frac{1}{a+0.5} + \frac{1}{b+0.5} + \frac{1}{c+0.5} + \frac{1}{d+0.5}}.$

The modification makes little difference to the results when the numbers are large. Online calculations can be performed at http://vassarstats.net/odds2x2.html or http://statpages.org/ctab2x2.html.

For the RR confidence intervals, Morris and Gardner (Gardner and Altman, 1995; Ludbrook and Royse, 2008) recommended using

$$\text{SE}\left(\log_e \text{RR}\right) = \sqrt{\frac{1}{a} - \frac{1}{a+c} + \frac{1}{b} - \frac{1}{b+d}}.$$

Then the $100(1 - \alpha)\%$ confidence interval is given by

$$\text{Log}_e \text{RR} \pm \left(z_{1-\alpha/2} \times \text{SE log}_e \text{RR} \right)$$

From Table 20.3

$$\text{SElnRR} = \sqrt{\frac{1}{2134} - \frac{1}{2134 + 3882} + \frac{1}{16176} - \frac{1}{118703 + 16176}} = 0.01889.$$

Because the RR for the data in Table 20.3 was 3.6811, the 95% confidence limits (equivalent to $\alpha = 0.05$) are ln $3.6811 \pm 1.96 \times 0.01889 = 1.3032 \pm 0.0370 = 1.2662$ to 1.3402. Taking antilogarithms $e^{1.2662}$ and $e^{1.3402}$ gives the 95% confidence limits as 3.5473 and 3.8198.

These confidence limits can be calculated online at http://statpages.org/ctab2x2.html or http://vassarstats.net/odds2x2.html, but these programs give minimally different limits.

To determine the significance of the difference between two different RR values, use

$$z = \frac{R_1 - R_2}{\sqrt{\frac{R_1(1-R_1)}{n_1} + \frac{R_2(1-R_2)}{n_2}}}.$$

Sample Size and Power

To detect the RR of a rare disease in a prospective (cohort) study, the sample size N for each of the exposed and the unexposed groups (R_1 and R_2 as set out in Table 20.1) that gives Type I error $\alpha = 0.05$ and power $1 - \beta = 0.8$ is given by (van Belle, 2002)

$$N = \frac{4}{p_u \left(\sqrt{\text{RR}} - 1 \right)^2},$$

where $R_2 = c + d$ and $p_u = \frac{c}{R_2}$. Multiplying each side by p_u gives

$$p_u R_2 = c = \frac{4}{\left(\sqrt{\text{RR}} - 1 \right)^2}.$$

The first equation allows us to calculate R_2, the number of unexposed subjects and the second equation allows us to calculate the number of events that occur in the unexposed population.

Figure 20.1 shows the relationship between the number of events in the unexposed group and the RR.

The number of events needed in the unexposed group rises sharply as the RR becomes smaller. To determine the number needed in the exposed group, multiply the above numbers by the RR. To translate these numbers into the total numbers required in each group (assuming similar numbers) examine Figure 20.2.

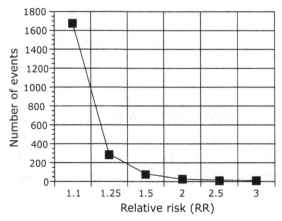

Figure 20.1 Relative risk versus number of events in the unexposed group.

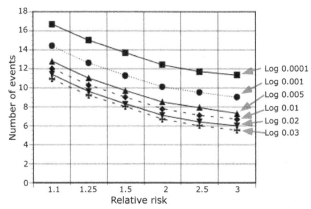

Figure 20.2 Relative risk versus logarithm of the number needed in exposed group. The values for Y (right-hand scale) are the population incidences, ranging from 3/100 to 1/10,000.

The numbers required for a very low population incidence of the disease in the unexposed group are huge. Thus if the incidence is 0.0001 (highest curve), the required numbers range from 55,968 for an RR of 3 to 16,790,471 for an RR of 1.1. This is why the prospective study is seldom used for very rare diseases, and is replaced by the cross-sectional study.

Such calculations allow us to decide if the number of subjects required can be recruited for the study in the allotted time, or given the early results how many more will be needed.

To determine if the results from a completed study had adequate power of 0.8 and $\alpha = 0.05$, use the formulas given above. For the data in Table 20.5(c), the proportion unexposed was $33/1293 = 0.0255$ and the RR was 1.87. The estimated sample size would be

$$N = \frac{4}{0.0255\left(\sqrt{1.87} - 1\right)^2} = 1162.$$

This was the approximate size of the samples used in that study. An approximation to these results can be obtained online at http://www.stat.ubc.ca/~rollin/stats/ssize/caco. html. This calculator gave 1268 for the above problem with a power of 0.80, good enough for practical purposes.

To determine the desired number of events needed in the unexposed group with an RR of 1.87, we need $N = \frac{4}{0.0255(\sqrt{1.87}-1)^2} = 1162$ unexposed subjects and $1.87 \times 33 = 62$ events in the exposed subjects.

What if, before the study, there was a predicted RR of 3? Then we would have needed about 8 events in the unexposed subjects and about 24 in the exposed subjects.

An alternative formula for determining the required number in the unexposed group is

$$N = \frac{\frac{8(RR+1)}{RR}}{p_u(\ln RR)^2}.$$

For the data of Table 20.5(c), the total number in the unexposed group should be

$$N = \frac{\frac{8(1.87+1)}{1.87}}{0.0255(\ln 1.87)^2} = 1229,$$

similar to the results from the previous formula and the online calculator.

A graph for estimating power for a given RR and sample size is provided on page 77 in the book by Selvin (1991).

To make a similar estimate for an OR, in which the population prevalence is unknown, approximate it from the following formula (Laupacis et al., 1988)

$$R_2 = \frac{8\text{var}(\ln OR)}{(\ln OR)^2}$$

where the variance of the OR is determined by

$$\text{varOR} = \frac{1}{a/R_1} + \frac{1}{b/R_1} + \frac{1}{c/R_2} + \frac{1}{d/R_2}.$$

These variances can also be used to assess the public health benefits of removing a putative factor responsible for diseases.

Not all clinical entities have an RR. It is not possible for a person to get pneumonic plague unless there is exposure to the plague *bacillus*, so that although it is possible to calculate the attack rate of the disease as $\frac{\text{number with disease}}{\text{number exposed}}$, there is no way to calculate an RR because unexposed people cannot get the disease.

Problem 20.2

Calculate sample size if the risk ratio is 1.5 and p_u is 0.03, if the risk ratio is 2.7 and p_u is 0.3, and if the risk ratio is 2.7 and p_u is 0.8.

When an RR can be estimated, it must be interpreted with caution. An RR of 2.0 might occur if $p_e = 0.2$ and $p_u = 0.1$, or $p_e = 0.000002$ and $p_u = 0.000001$, where p_e and p_u refer to exposed and unexposed incidence rates, respectively. In the first example disease is potentially preventable in 1 out of 10 people, but in the second example only 1 in 1 million might be helped. The different public health implications of these two different absolute figures are concealed in the single RR number. RR should never be referred to without also referring to the absolute risk.

Attributable Risk (AR)

To derive a more interpretable magnitude, use attributable risk (AR), sometimes referred to as the population attributable risk (PAR), the attributable fraction (Boslaugh and McNutt, 2007), the etiologic fraction λ, or the RR difference (Sinclair, 2003). The field is clouded by a variety of terms for the same calculation, a variety of calculations for the same term, and a variety of symbols for the same entities (Levin, 1953; Miettinen, 1974; Markush, 1977; Schlesselman, 1982; Greenland and Robins, 1988). All the different formulas use the same few numbers, and so are interrelated. The term attributable risk is used below to refer to the excess incidence of disease in those exposed to a given (causal) factor, and AR% is the percentage of the incidence of a disease in the exposed that would be eliminated if exposure were eliminated; it is sometimes expressed as a proportion. The corresponding index for the whole population is PAR, referring to the excess incidence of disease in the whole population, and PAR% is the percentage of the incidence of a disease in the whole population that would be eliminated if exposure were eliminated; it is sometimes expressed as a proportion (Kaelin and Bayona, 2004).

The attributable fraction indicates how many excess diseased subjects were due to exposure, given that there usually is a baseline incidence of the disease in the absence of exposure to a particular factor. We argue that in any group of patients with a given disease the total incidence rate of the disease (p_t) is a function of the incidence rate not due to exposure to a suspected causal factor (p_u) and the superimposed incidence rate due to exposure (p_e). Table 20.1 gives the basic data used in the calculations.

The AR is the excess risk due to the factor as measured by $AR = p_e - p_u$. The proportion of the incidence rate due to association with the risk factor is $(p_e - p_u)/p_e$, either as a fraction (proportional AR) or multiplied by 100 as percent (AR%).

Applying these concepts to the data in Table 20.3, $p_e = 2134/18,310 = 0.1165$, $p_u = 3822/122,612 = 0.0317$, and $p_t = 6016/140,922 = 0.0427$. Then $\widehat{RR} = 0.1165/0.0317 = 3.6751$, $\widehat{AR} = 0.1165 - 0.0317 = 0.0848$, and $\widehat{AR}$%, the percentage of diseased subjects that are associated with exposure, is $(0.0848/0.1165) \times 100 = 72.79\%$ (or 0.7279). Exposure is associated with excess disease in about 73/100 patients. There are other ways of determining AR that may be used if some of the primary data are not available.

Because $\widehat{RR} = p_e/p_u$, then $\widehat{RR}p_u = p_e$.

Therefore $\widehat{AR} = p_e - p_u = \widehat{RR}p_u - p_u = p_u(\widehat{RR} - 1)$.

Using the above numbers, $\widehat{AR} = 0.0317 \times (3.6751 - 1) = 0.0848$ as before (slight difference due to rounding off).

Dividing the numerator and denominator of the expression for proportional AR by p_u gives

$$\text{proportional } \widehat{AR} = \frac{\left(\frac{p_e}{p_u} - \frac{p_u}{p_u}\right)}{\frac{p_u}{p_u}} = \frac{\widehat{RR} - 1}{\widehat{RR}}, \quad \text{as long as } \widehat{RR} \geq 1.$$

Using the data from Table 20.3, proportional $AR = (3.6811 - 1)/3.6811 = 0.7283$ (or 72.83%) as before.

The incidence rate due to the risk factor among those with the risk factor is

$$p_e\left(\frac{\widehat{RR} - 1}{RR}\right) \text{as long as } \widehat{RR} \geq 1.$$

From the data in Table 20.3, this becomes $0.1165 \times 0.7283 = 0.0848$, as before. These alternative formulations require a cohort study that allows RR to be calculated, or require the assumption that the OR and the RR are similar.

Population Attributable Risk (PAR)

The PAR can be determined by the difference between the incidence in exposed subjects and the incidence in the whole study population:

$$PAR = p_t - p_u, \quad \text{and}$$
$$\text{proportional PAR} = (p_t - p_u)/p_t.$$

From the data of Table 20.3

$$\widehat{PAR} = 0.0427 - 0.0317 = 0.011,$$

and proportional $\widehat{PAR} = \frac{0.0427 - 0.0317}{0.0427} \times 100 = 0.2576$ (or 25.76%).

An alternative calculation mentioned by Schlesselman (1982) is the relative difference between the number of exposed people developing the disease (C_1) and the number who would have developed the disease had there been no exposure (Np_t):

$$\lambda_p = \frac{C_1 - Np_u}{C_1} = \frac{6016 - 140922 \times 0.0317}{6016} = 0.2574.$$

Comparing $\widehat{AR}$ and $\widehat{PAR}$ shows that removing the exposure might reduce the incidence of the disease by 73% in the exposed population and 26% in the whole population. Finally, PAR can be calculated easily from

$$\left(\frac{a}{a+c}\right)\left(\frac{\widehat{RR}-1}{\widehat{RR}}\right).$$

where $a = P(D+|E+)$ and $c = P(D+|E-)$.

From Table 20.3,

$$\text{proportional } \widehat{PAR} = \left(\frac{2134}{21343882}\right)\left(\frac{3.6811-1}{2.6811}\right) = 0.2584.$$

Another formula giving the same results is

$$\text{proportional } \widehat{PAR} = \frac{\text{Prevalence}(RR-1)}{1+\text{Prevalence}(RR-1)} = \frac{\frac{a+c}{N}(RR-1)}{1+\frac{a+c}{N}(RR-1)}.$$

For a given value of AR, PAR changes as the proportion of exposed subjects in the population changes (Schlesselman, 1982).

Relative Risks Below 1; Number Needed to Treat (NNT)

The RR can be <1 if the exposure is protective, for example, with an effective treatment, and then it allows the calculation of how many patients are needed in a clinical trial (Boslaugh and McNutt, 2007). For example, Sinclair (2003) asked the question: "Based on existing data in the literature about the possible effect of using steroids to prevent chronic lung disease at 36 weeks in a premature 900 g infant, how many patients will we need to treat to demonstrate one success?"

He used the following empirical data.

RR = 0.69 (69%);

Risk reduction = $1 - RR = 0.31$ (31%);

Risk difference (RD) = $p_e - p_u = 0.09$ (9%). This is what others have termed attributable risk and has to be calculated from the primary data.

Then NNT, the number of patients needed to treat in order to prevent chronic lung disease in 1 patient = $1/RD = 1/0.09 \approx 11$ (Laupacis et al., 1988). That is, given the known effect of steroids on these immature lungs, we would have to treat 11 patients in order to see 1 improved patient. This concept is important in terms of cost but even more so in terms of risks. From the database it is possible to determine how often a given complication would occur. If the NNT for complications is lower than for improvement, the risk might be unacceptable. If it is much larger, then the risk might be tolerable. Sinclair describes how to determine risk—benefit ratios. Online calculations can be performed at http://graphpad.com/quickcalcs/NNT2.cfm, http://araw.mede.uic. edu/cgi-bin/nntcalc.pl, http://www.calctool.org/CALC/prof/medical/NNT, http:// easycalculation.com/medical/treat-number.php, http://statpages.org/ctab2x2.html, or http://ktclearinghouse.ca/cebm/practise/ca/calculators/statscalc. The NNT concept allows us to attach concrete numbers to concepts of RR and AR (or RD). For example, the RR might be 2 for each of two different diseases. For disease A, the AR might be $0.2 - 0.1 = 0.1$, with NNT being $1/0.1 = 10$, whereas for disease B the AR might be $0.002 - 0.001 = 0.001$, so that NNT is $1/0.001 = 1000$. For disease A, we need to treat 10 patients for one to benefit, and for disease B we need to treat 1000 for one to benefit. A simple nomogram for determining NTT is available (Chatellier et al., 1996).

If a new treatment turns out to be harmful, then the AR $p_e - p_u$ is negative. Altman (1998) proposed that instead of using the term NNT we should use the terms NNTB, where B = benefit, and NNTH, where H = harm. NNTB is a positive number, and NNTH is a negative number. This concept is of value when calculating confidence limits (see below).

When applying the NNT calculation, all members of the intended treatment group must be homogeneous with respect to the RR. If several strata are used for the trial, then the RR should be similar in each stratum if it is to be used to calculate a single number or NNTB. If one person or subgroup has a different baseline risk, say f times as high, then the number to treat based on the rest of the study needs to be divided by f to obtain a realistic NNTB (Cook and Sackett, 1995).

Some investigators have criticized the NNT concept for emphasizing the benefit to one patient while ignoring the lack of benefit or even harm to the remainder of the group (Bogaty and Brophy, 2005). To stress this point, they recommended (perhaps with tongue in cheek) the use of a new index—NTN, the number treated needlessly. Thus if NNT was 250, NTN would be 249, and the investigator must be sure that the benefit to one patient is sufficiently important to justify treating the remaining patients with no benefit.

As with all summary numbers there are subtleties to consider. If, for example, control (c) and treatment (t) groups are observed then there will be an NNT_c and an NNT_t, and it is the difference between these that demonstrates the value of the treatment (Curiel and Rodriguez-Plaza, 2005). Some problems that occur with the NNT concept were discussed by Walter (2005). Furthermore, if two groups are to be compared, they need to be followed for similar periods if NNT is to have meaning (Suissa et al., 2012).

Example 20.1

Plint et al. (2009) treated patients who came to the Emergency Room with bronchiolitis, and compared the effectiveness of placebo versus nebulized epinephrine + oral dexamethasone as judged by what percentage in each group were admitted to hospital in the next 7 days. They found the following results:

	Placebo	Epinephrine + steroid
Readmitted	53	34
Not readmitted	148	166

Calculate the NNT from the formula cited above.

$$\text{NTT} = \frac{1}{\frac{53}{201} - \frac{34}{200}} = \frac{1}{0.2639 - 0.17} = 10.64, \text{ or } 11 \text{ to the nearest integer.}$$

An online calculator http://graphpad.com/quickcalcs/NNT2/ gave 11 as the answer, as well as confidence limits.

Problem 20.3

Assume that the Plint data table above had the following data:

	Placebo	Epinephrine + steroid
Readmitted	53	34
Not readmitted	148	165

Calculate the odds and risk ratios with confidence limits, and NNT by using http://statpages.org/ctab2x2.html and the formula.

ADVANCED CONCEPTS

Confidence Limits for Attributable Risk

Approximate limits can be set in several ways, depending on whether we examine the difference between proportions or some ratio of proportions.

Differences Between Proportions

Because AR is the difference between two proportions p_e and p_u, use the formula for the difference between two proportions

$$\left(p_e - p_u\right) \pm 1.96 \sqrt{\frac{p_e\left(1 - p_e\right)}{n_1} + \frac{p_u\left(1 - p_u\right)}{n_2}},$$

where n_1 is the total number exposed and n_2 is the total number unexposed. Thus for the data of Table 20.3,

$$(0.1165 - 0.0317) \pm 1.96\sqrt{\frac{0.1165(1 - 0.1165)}{18310} + \frac{0.0317(1 - 0.0317)}{122162}}$$

$$= 0.0848 \pm 0.004749.$$

This produces 95% confidence limits of 0.0801–0.0895. These limits can be calculated online from http://vassarstats.net/prop2_ind.html that gives limits of 0.0802–0.0897 with or without a continuity correction; the continuity correction should be used for small sample sizes. Another program http://in-silico.net/statistics/ztest/two-proportion gives limits of 0.0792–0.0904, and allows for unequal sample variances. The differences between test results depend on the specific method used, with http://vassarstats.net/prop2_ind.html using Wilson's method that has been shown to be more accurate than most (Miettinen, 1974).

Similar calculations can be done for PAR, using p_t and p_u as the proportions.

Difference Between Proportional Ratios (Proportional AR and Proportional PAR)

A method developed by Walter for confidence limits for the proportional PAR λ_p (Walter, 1975, 1978) depends on the finding that the distribution of $1 - \lambda_p$ is asymptotically log normal. In the form depicted by Armitage et al. (2002)

$$SE \ln\left(1 - \lambda_p\right) = \sqrt{\frac{a}{c(a + c)} + \frac{b}{d(b + d)}}$$

$$= \sqrt{\frac{P(D^+|E^+)}{P(D^+|E^-)[(P(D^+|E^+) + P(D^+|E^-))]} + \frac{P(D^-|E^+)}{P(D^-|E^-)[P(D^-|E^+) + P(D^-|E^-)]}}$$

$$SE \ln\left(1 - \lambda_p\right) = \sqrt{\frac{2134}{3882(3882 + 2134)} + \frac{16176}{118730(118730 + 16176)}} = 0.009612.$$

$$\ln\left(1 - \lambda_p\right) = \ln(1 - 0.2576) = -0.2979.$$

95% limits are $-0.2979 \pm 1.96 \times 0.009612 = -0.3167$ to -0.2791.

Taking antilogarithms gives 0.7285 to 0.7565.

Subtracting these from 1 gives 95% limits of 0.2715 to 0.2435.

Finally, a simplified method involves substituting the lower and upper 95% confidence limits for $\widehat{RR}$ in the relevant equation to obtain the corresponding confidence limits for $\widehat{PAR}$ (Daly, 1998).

Then the lower confidence limit is

$$\text{lower limit proportional } \widehat{PAR} = \frac{2134}{(2134 + 3882)}\left(\frac{3.5473 - 1}{3.5473}\right) = 0.2547.$$

Similarly the upper confidence limit is

$$\text{upper limit proportional } \widehat{\text{PAR}} = \frac{2134}{(2134 + 3882)} \left(\frac{3.8198 - 1}{3.8198}\right) = 0.2619$$

Calculations involving RR must be done cautiously in cross-sectional studies, and designs such as pairing may need special approaches. Statistical consultation is advised.

Confidence Limits for NNT

These have conventionally been determined from the reciprocals of the confidence limits for the AR (Cook and Sackett, 1995). Thus if the AR is 0.09 and the 95% confidence limits are 0.06 and 0.14, then the NNTB is $1/0.09 = 11$, with confidence limits of $1/0.06 = 17$ and $1/0.14 = 7$. This method, however, works only if the AR is significantly above zero and both confidence limits are positive. Altman (1998) raised a conceptual difficulty if the AR is not significant because then the confidence limits range from positive to negative. If, as in his example, the AR is 10% with 95% confidence limits of -5% to 25%, then the number to treat is $1/0.1 = 10$, and those limits imply numbers to treat of $-1/0.05 = -20$ to $1/0.25 = 4$. Apart from not making any sense to have a negative number to treat, these numbers do not include the point estimate of NNT. In addition, the limits include the possibility that the AR is zero, which would lead to $NNT = 1/0 = \infty$. Altman pointed out there are two disjoint sets of data, one from -20 to ∞ and one from ∞ to 4. In order to resolve the difficulties he developed a diagram plotting the AR reduction from -4 to 20 on a reversed axis on the left and on a double inverted scale on the right, as in Figure 20.3.

The confidence limits calculated as suggested above are approximate and usually serve their purpose, but may be greatly in error if samples are small. More accurate ways of calculating these limits are available (Newcombe, 1998; Bender, 2001).

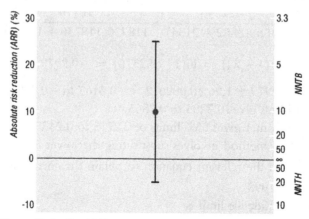

Figure 20.3 *Confidence limits for NNT.* NNTB, number needed to treat—benefit; NNTH, number needed to treat—harm.

Cautionary Tales

A cross-sectional study allows only legitimate calculation of the OR, but this is frequently used as an estimate of the risk ratio. Failure to appreciate the difference between OR and risk ratio, and when the OR can and cannot be a surrogate for the risk ratio, accounts for many serious errors in the medical literature.

Differences between these two ratios were illustrated in Table 20.5(a)–(d). Feinstein (1986) clarified the difference by examining the 2 × 2 table used for calculating the OR in light of the known risk ratio $\frac{p_e}{p_u}$ when the proportion of people exposed to the risk factor was e. He then displayed the data as in Table 20.6.

Table 20.6 Expected proportions of patients in each cell

	Disease	No disease	Incidence rate
Exposed	ep_e	$e(1 - p_e)$	p_e
Not exposed	$(1 - e)p_u$	$(1 - e)(1 - p_u)$	p_u

The OR is calculated from $\frac{ep_e(1-e)(1-p_u)}{e(1-p_e)(1-e)p_u} = \frac{p_e(1-p_u)}{p_u(1-p_e)} = \frac{p_e}{p_u} \times \frac{1-p_u}{1-p_e} \approx \frac{p_e}{p_u}$ as long as p_e and p_u are both very small so that $\frac{1-p_u}{1-p_e}$ is close to 1. The proportional error in estimating RR from OR $\left(\frac{OR-RR}{RR}\right)$ can be shown to be

$$= \frac{RRp_u}{1 - RRp_u}.$$

Therefore the error rises for large values of RR or p_u, and can be considerable (Figure 20.4)

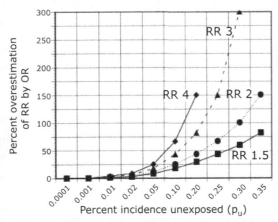

Figure 20.4 *Relation of RR, OR and incidence.* Percent overestimation of relative risk (RR) by the odds ratio (OR) for different combinations of RR and incidence in the unexposed population (based on Feinstein formula). For an unexposed incidence under 0.02%, OR and RR are similar. With increasing population incidence the OR overestimates the RR, and for any population incidence the overestimate increases as RR increases.

(Continued)

Cautionary Tales—cont'd

RR and ORs are similar only if the probability of an event is low. Zhang and Yu (1998) developed a formula relating OR to RR,

$$RR = \frac{OR}{(1 - P_0) + (P_0 + OR)}.$$

and this was rearranged further by Shrier and Steele (2006):

$$OR/RR = (OR - 1)Po + 1.$$

Here Po is the prevalence of the disease in the population. If Po and OR are both small, then $OR/RR \approx 1$ and OR is a good estimate of RR, but if either OR or Po are large, the close relationship breaks down. They provided appropriate graphs for examining these relationships.

Example 20.2

Use the data from Problem 20.3 (data of Plint et al.) to calculate RR from the OR:

The OR for readmission while taking epinephrine plus steroids is

$$OR = \frac{34 \times 148}{53 \times 166} = 0.5719.$$

Then using the Zhang and Yu formula, the RR is

$$RR = \frac{0.5719}{\left(1 - \frac{53}{201}\right) + \left(\frac{53}{201} \times 0.5719\right)} = 0.6446.$$

There is often confusion between OR and RR in practice. Katz (2006) analyzed a report from Nijsten et al. (2005) who found that 89.3% of National Psoriasis Foundation members reported having heard of treatment with calcipotriene compared with 25.3% of nonmembers. They reported an OR of 24.41 and concluded that "members were more than 20-fold more likely than non-members to have heard of calcipotriene." On the face of it, this result appears to be unlikely. The ratio of members to nonmembers who had heard of the drug was 89.3/25.3 = 3.53, and this is the RR. Where did the error occur? It was due to ignoring the difference between OR and RR when prevalence is very low (Katz, 2006).

A second more serious error entered the medical literature when Schulman et al. (1999) reported that both race and gender influenced the way in which physicians managed chest pain, and concluded that blacks and women were 40% less likely than whites and men to be referred for cardiac testing (cardiac catheterization) when they presented with chest pain. These conclusions were given prominence by newspapers and television commentaries. Schulman et al. based this conclusion on finding in their study that blacks had an OR of 0.6 for referral, but in reality, as pointed out by Schwartz et al. (1999) the RR was 0.93, a relatively trivial difference compared to whites. Schwartz et al. did not discount the possibility of bias in referrals, but did not find good evidence for this in the reported study.

REFERENCES

Altman, D.G., 1998. Confidence intervals for the number needed to treat. BMJ 317, 1309–1312.

Armitage, P., Berry, G., Matthews, J.N.S., 2002. Statistical Methods in Medical Research. Blackwell.

Bender, R., 2001. Calculating confidence intervals for the number needed to treat. Controlled Clin. Trials 22, 102–110.

Bogaty, P., Brophy, J., 2005. Numbers needed to treat (needlessly?). Lancet 365, 1307–1308.

Boslaugh, S., McNutt, L.A., 2007. Encyclopedia of Epidemiology. Sage Publications, California.

Chatellier, G., Zapletal, E., Lemaitre, D., Menard, J., Degoulet, P., 1996. The number needed to treat: a clinically useful nomogram in its proper context. BMJ 312, 426–429.

Cook, R.J., Sackett, D.L., 1995. The number needed to treat: a clinically useful measure of treatment effect. BMJ 310, 452–454 (correction p. 1056).

Curiel, R., Rodriguez-Plaza, L., 2005. Basal NNT and interventional NNT. J. Clin. Epidemiol. 58, 1074.

Daly, L.E., 1998. Confidence limits made easy: interval estimation using a substitution method. Am. J. Epidemiol. 147, 783–790.

Feinstein, A.R., 1986. The bias caused by high values of incidence for p1 in the odds ratio assumption that 1-p1 approximately equal to 1. J. Chronic Dis. 39, 485–487.

Gardner, M.J., Altman, D.G., 1995. Statistics with Confidence—Confidence Intervals and Statistical Guidelines. British Medical Journal, London.

Greenland, S., Robins, J.M., 1988. Conceptual problems in the definition and interpretation of attributable fractions. Am. J. Epidemiol. 128, 1185–1197.

He, Y., Lam, T.H., Jiang, B., Wang, J., Sai, X., Fan, L., Li, X., Qin, Y., Hu, F.B., 2008. Passive smoking and risk of peripheral arterial disease and ischemic stroke in Chinese women who never smoked. Circulation 118, 1535–1540.

Kaelin, M.A., Bayona, M., 2004. Attributable Risk Applications in Epidemiology. College Entrance Examination Board.

Katz, K.A., 2006. The (relative) risks of using odds ratios. Arch. Dermatol. 142, 761–764.

Kelly, T.N., Gu, D., Chen, J., Huang, J.F., Chen, J.C., Duan, X., Wu, X., Yau, C.L., Whelton, P.K., He, J., 2008. Hypertension subtype and risk of cardiovascular disease in Chinese adults. Circulation 118, 1558–1566.

Kleinbaum, D.G., Kupper, L.L., Morgenstern, H., 1982. Epidemiologic Research. Principles and Quantitative Methods. Lifetime Learning Publications, Wadsworth, Inc., Belmont, CA.

Laupacis, A., Sackett, D.L., Roberts, R.S., 1988. An assessment of clinically useful measures of the consequences of treatment. N. Engl. J. Med. 318, 1728–1733.

Levin, M.L., 1953. The occurrence of lung cancer in man. Acta Unio Int. Contra Cancrum 19, 531–541.

Ludbrook, J., Royse, A.G., 2008. Analysing clinical studies: principles, practice and pitfalls of Kaplan-Meier plots. ANZ J. Surg. 78, 204–210.

Markush, R.E., 1977. Levin's attributable risk statistic for analytic studies and vital statistics. Am. J. Epidemiol. 105, 401–406.

Miettinen, O.S., 1974. Proportion of disease caused or prevented by a given exposure, trait or intervention. Am. J. Epidemiol. 99, 325–332.

Newcombe, R.G., 1998. Interval estimation for the difference between independent proportions: comparison of eleven methods. Stat. Med. 17, 873–890.

Nijsten, T., Rolstad, T., Feldman, S.R., Stern, R.S., 2005. Members of the National Psoriasis Foundation: more extensive disease and better informed about treatment options. Arch. Dermatol. 141, 19–26.

Pearce, N., 1993. What does the odds ratio estimate in a case-control study? Int. J. Epidemiol. 22, 1189–1192.

Plint, A.C., Johnson, D.W., Patel, H., Wiebe, N., Correll, R., Brant, R., Mitton, C., Gouin, S., Bhatt, M., Joubert, G., Black, K.J., Turner, T., Whitehouse, S., Klassen, T.P., Pediatric Emergency Research Canada, 2009. Epinephrine and dexamethasone in children with bronchiolitis. N. Engl. J. Med. 360, 2079–2089.

Schlesselman, J.J., 1982. Case Control Studies. Design, Conduct, Analysis. Oxford University Press, Oxford.

Schulman, K.A., Berlin, J.A., Harless, W., Kerner, J.F., Sistrunk, S., Gersh, B.J., Dube, R., Taleghani, C.K., Burke, J.E., Williams, S., Eisenberg, J.M., Escarce, J.J., 1999. The effect of race and sex on physicians' recommendations for cardiac catheterization. N. Engl. J. Med. 340, 618–626.

Schwartz, L.M., Woloshin, S., Welch, H.G., 1999. Misunderstandings about the effects of race and sex on physicians' referrals for cardiac catheterization. N. Engl. J. Med. 341, 279–283 discussion 286–7.

Selvin, S., 1991. Statistical Analysis of Epidemiologic Data. Oxford University Press, Oxford.

Shrier, I., Steele, R., 2006. Understanding the relationship between risks and odds ratios. Clin. J. Sport Med. 16, 107–110.

Sinclair, J.C., 2003. Weighing risks and benefits in treating the individual patient. Clin. Perinatol. 30, 251–268.

Suissa, D., Brassard, P., Smiechowski, B., Suissa, S., 2012. Number needed to treat is incorrect without proper time-related considerations. J. Clin. Epidemiol. 65, 42–46.

van Belle, G., 2002. Statistical Rules of Thumb. Wiley Interscience, New York.

Walter, S.D., 1975. The distribution of Levin's measure of attributable risk. Biometrika 62, 371–374.

Walter, S.D., 1978. Calculation of attributable risks from epidemiological data. Int. J. Epidemiol. 7, 175–182.

Walter, S.D., 2005. Is NNT now the number needed to traumatize? J. Clin. Epidemiol. 58, 1075–1076.

Woolf, B., 1955. On estimating the relation between blood group and disease. Ann. Hum. Genet. 19, 251–253.

Zhang, J., Yu, K.F., 1998. What's the relative risk? A method of correcting the odds ratio in cohort studies of common outcomes. JAMA 280, 1690–1691.

CHAPTER 21

Probability, Bayes' Theorem, Medical Diagnostic Evaluation, and Screening

Contents

BAYES' THEOREM APPLIED

Almost all of us use a Bayesian approach to medical diagnosis, even if we do not realize it. Consider a 3-day-old patient with a transposition of the great arteries who is referred to a hospital. If the receiving doctor knows nothing more than the age, the list of possible diagnoses is enormous: congenital anomalies of the bowel, urinary tract infections, seizures, aspiration pneumonia, heart disease, and so on. If the patient is known to be cyanotic, then heart and lung diseases go to the head of the list of possible diagnoses. If the baby is breathing normally, then heart disease is more likely than lung disease. If there is no cardiac murmur, then transposition of the great arteries goes to the head of the list. Almost all diagnoses go through this procedure, often so quickly that we do not realize that we are using a sequential logical process. What Bayes' theorem does is to formalize and quantify the process?

Diagnosing a neural tube defect prenatally is a practical example of the use of Bayes' theorem. Some children are born with neural tube defects, that is, the skin and vertebrae have not closed completely over the lower end of the spinal cord. These anomalies are associated with an increased concentration of alpha-fetoprotein in the blood. Therefore, a high concentration of the protein suggests that there might be a neural tube defect, but because there are other causes of these high concentrations, they do not diagnose the defect with certainty. The other variable to be considered is that if one child has already

For a list of all websites referred to in this chapter, as clickable links, see the book companion website: www.booksite.elsevier.com/9780128023877.

Biostatistics for Medical and Biomedical Practitioners
http://dx.doi.org/10.1016/B978-0-12-802387-7.00021-4

been born with a neural tube defect, there is an increased tendency for subsequent children to have the abnormality. In order to give some diagnostic help to the perinatologist in attempting to diagnose neural tube defects in utero, turn to Bayes' theorem. The following primary data are needed:

D^+ is the presence of the disease and T^+ is a positive test, here an increased concentration of alpha-fetoprotein. If the family history suggests that the mother is at risk of having children with neural tube defects, then $P(D^+) = 0.05$. If the mother is not at risk, then $P(D^+) = 0.001$. These are the prior probabilities. Then there are two conditional probabilities that are the same whether the mother is at risk or not. $P(T^+|D^-) = 0.001$ and $P(T^+|D^+) = 1$; if the fetus has the disease, the alpha-fetoprotein concentration is always high, and if the fetus is normal, the probability of a false-positive test is very low.

The simple form of Bayes' theorem (Chapter 5) can be rewritten in several forms.

Bayes' theorem is $P(D^+|T^+) = \frac{P(T^+|D^+)P(D^+)}{P(T^+)}$.

The denominator can be written $P(T^+) = P(T^+\cap D^+) + P(T^+\cap D^-)$, where D^- indicates those with no disease.

The two right-hand components can be written

$$P(T^+\cap D^+) = P(T^+|D^+)P(D^+) \text{ and}$$
$$P(T^+\cap D^-) = P(T^+|D^-)P(D^-)$$

Now we can rewrite Bayes' theorem as

$$P(D^+|T^+) = \frac{P(T^+|D^+)P(D^+)}{P(T^+|D^+)P(D^+) + P(T^+|D^-)P(D^-)}$$

Because $P(T^+|D^-) = 1 - P(T^-|D^-)$ and $P(D^-) = 1 - P(D^+)$ we can also write the theorem as

$$P(D^+|T^+) = \frac{P(T^+|D^+)P(D^+)}{P(T^+|D^+)P(D^+) + [1 - P(T^-|D^-)(1 - P(D^+)]}$$

The advantage of this formula is that it can be related to the well-known concepts of sensitivity and specificity (see below).

If the mother is at risk, then Bayes' theorem gives

$$P(D^+|T^+) = \frac{1 \times 0.05}{(1 \times 0.05) + (0.001 \times \{1 - 0.05\})} = \frac{0.05}{0.05095} = 0.9813.$$

If the mother is not at risk, then the theorem gives

$$P(D^+|T^+) = \frac{1 \times 0.001}{(1 \times 0.001) + (0.001 \times \{1 - 0.001\})} = \frac{0.001}{0.001999} = 0.5002.$$

For the mothers not at risk, the prior (pretest) probability of having a child with a neural tube defect is 0.001. The posterior probability if there is a positive test for an abnormal concentration of alpha–fetoprotein has risen to just over 50%, so that the test has given a great deal of information. If the mother has already had a child with a neural tube defect, then the prior probability of having another child with this defect is 0.05, but a positive test makes it almost certain that the fetus is affected. (In practice, other tests are done to make the diagnosis more certain.)

Cautionary Tale

The failure to apply Bayes' theorem has had devastating consequences in some criminal cases. One striking example was the case of Sally Clark (Joyce). She had a child who died in infancy from what was initially diagnosed as sudden infant death syndrome (SIDS), but when a second infant died from presumed SIDS she was charged with infanticide. She was convicted of murder largely because of testimony from an expert pediatrician who testified that the chances of two infants in the same family dying from SIDS were one in 73 million, and therefore extremely unlikely.

There were numerous factual errors in this testimony.

1. The probability of 1/73,000,000 was derived from two misconceptions. Information available at that time was that SIDS occurred in 1/1300 live births, but the expert witness chose to use a probability of 1/8543 births because of information showing that SIDS was less likely in families who were affluent and nonsmoking. This is an example in which the posterior probability is less than the prior probability. On the other hand, he ignored the fact that both infants were boys, who have a greater risk of dying from SIDS; the prior probability of dying from SIDS is less than the posterior probability of dying from SIDS if the child is a boy, symbolized by $P(SIDS) < P(SIDS|boy)$.

   If the witness had used the figure of 1/1300 instead of 1/8543, then the chances of two successive deaths from SIDS would have been estimated as 1/1,690,000 instead of 1/72,982,849.

2. The second error was assuming that the two consecutive events were independent, so that $P(SIDS_2) = P(SIDS_1)$. At that time, it was known that if one child had died from SIDS the risk was 5–10 times higher for the next child (Hill, 2004). The two risks are not independent, and $P(SIDS_2) < P(SIDS_2|SIDS_1)$. Therefore, instead of estimating the probability of two consecutive deaths from SIDS as $1/1300 \times 1/1300 = 1/1,690,000$, the probability should have been 5- to 10-fold greater, namely 1/169,000 to 1/338,000, a far cry from 1 in 73 million.

3. A more important conceptual error, however, was failing to consider the alternative hypothesis, namely the probability of two infants being murdered in the same family. By conservative estimates from a study group, this was about 5 times less likely than two consecutive SIDS deaths (Hill, 2004). Therefore, in the absence of direct evidence of murder, on probability two consecutive SIDS deaths were about 5 times as likely as two consecutive infanticides in the same family. This error is sometimes termed the

(Continued)

Cautionary Tale—cont'd

prosecutor's fallacy, namely the tendency to state that a person is guilty because he or she is associated with some very rare event (Goldacre, 2006; Thompson and Schumann, 1987). Thompson and Schumann (1987) described this fallacy simply:

Suppose you are asked to judge the probability a man is a lawyer based on the fact that he owns a briefcase. Let us assume all lawyers own a briefcase but only one person in ten in the general population owns a briefcase. Following the prosecutor's logic, you would jump to the conclusions that there is a 90% chance the man is a lawyer. But this conclusion is obviously wrong. We know that the number of non-lawyers is many times greater than the number of lawyers. Hence lawyers are probably outnumbered by briefcase owners who are not lawyers (and a given briefcase owner is more likely to be a non-lawyer than a lawyer). To draw conclusions about the probability that the man is a lawyer based on the fact he owns a briefcase, we must consider not just the incidence rate of briefcase ownership, but also the a priori likelihood of being a lawyer. Similarly, to draw conclusions about the probability a criminal suspect is guilty based on evidence of a "match", we must consider not just the percentage of people who would match but also the a priori likelihood that the defendant in question is guilty.

These issues are described clearly in a Wikipedia article (Wikipedia, 2011).

Many pediatricians and statisticians pointed out the fallacies, and eventually after 4 years the sentence was reversed on a second appeal. Unfortunately, the tragedy of her children's deaths and 4 years unjustified imprisonment were too much for Sally Clark, who died a few years later of alcoholism. Failure to consider posterior probabilities in the light of (correct) prior probabilities caused a grave miscarriage of justice.

An explanatory article with other examples has recently been published (Skorupski and Wainer, 2015).

SENSITIVITY AND SPECIFICITY

There is another way of looking at diagnostic tests that is often used and is closely related to Bayes' theorem. A new test for a given disease should ideally detect all instances of the occurrence of that disease. In common language, the test should be sensitive to the presence of that disease. Perfect sensitivity of 100% would occur if the test were always positive when the disease was present; sensitivity below 100% would occur if the tests were negative in some people who had that disease, that is, if there were false-negative tests. Furthermore, ideally the test should be highly specific for that disease, and not to be positive if other diseases were present. If this occurred, then the test could be said to be 100% specific for that disease. If, however, the test was positive in some people who had other diseases, then that would be a false-positive result, and the test would be less than 100% specific.

Table 21.1 shows data published by Rubin (1992) about evaluating fever in a young child who has no obvious focus of infection. The causes of such a nonspecific symptom range from a self-limiting viral illness that needs no specific treatment to a serious bacterial infection that requires urgent antibiotic treatment. At issue are the facts that it is expensive

Table 21.1 Data from children with occult bacteremia

Neutrophil count/mm^3	Sensitivity %	Specificity %
>10,000	100	88
>15,000	100	97
>20,000	40	99

and frequently unnecessary to perform many laboratory tests; furthermore, decisions about treatment may have to be made before test results return.

All children with bacteremia have more than 10,000 neutrophils per cubic millimeter, so that for this test the sensitivity is 100%. However, for this cell count the specificity is only 88%; children with fever not due to bacteremia can often have neutrophil counts of this magnitude. If a positive test requires a neutrophil count of over 20,000 per mm^3, then the sensitivity is only 40%, that is, only 40% of bacteremic children have such high neutrophil counts. On the other hand, the specificity has risen to 99%, because few children with febrile viral illnesses have such high counts.

Table 21.2a shows results concerning a prostatic acid phosphatase (PAP) test for prostate cancer (Watson and Tang, 1980).

Table 21.2a Prostate cancer data

Test	Disease		Total
	Cancer	Normal	
PAP positive	79	13	92
PAP negative	34	204	238
Total	113	217	330

Assume that the diagnosis of cancer has been established with certainty by another test ("the gold standard"). Then each of the four cells in which the coincidence of a test result and a disease result can be labeled as shown in Table 21.2b:

Table 21.2b Generalized sensitivity and specificity table

Test	Disease		Total
	Present	Absent	
Positive	**True positive TP**	**False positive FP**	Total positive
Negative	**False negative FN**	**True negative TN**	Total negative
Total	Total disease	Total normal	Total

Sensitivity = probability that a test result is positive when the disease is present

$$= \frac{True\ positive}{True\ positive + False\ negative} = \frac{79}{79 + 34} = 0.699.$$

Specificity = probability that a test result is negative when the disease is not present

$$= \frac{True\ negative}{True\ negative + False\ positive} = \frac{204}{204 + 13} = 0.940.$$

Sensitivity as a percentage is termed the true positive rate, and specificity as a percentage is termed the true negative rate.

The complements of these terms can also be defined:

$1 -$ Sensitivity is also termed the false-negative rate, and is the probability that the test is negative when the disease is present:

$$1 - Sensitivity = \frac{False\ negative}{True\ positive + False\ negative} = \frac{34}{34 + 79} = 0.301,$$

$1 -$ Specificity is also termed the false-positive rate, and it is the probability that the test is positive when the disease is absent:

$$1 - Specificity = \frac{False\ positive}{True\ negative + False\ positive} = \frac{13}{13 + 204} = 0.060.$$

Three more terms need to be defined.

Positive predictive value = proportion of times that a positive test will detect a diseased person:

$$= \frac{True\ positive}{True\ positive + False\ positive} = \frac{79}{79 + 13} = 0.859,$$

Negative predictive value = proportion of times that a negative test will detect a person without that disease:

$$= \frac{True\ negative}{True\ negative + False\ negative} = \frac{204}{204 + 34} = 0.857.$$

Population prevalence = proportion of positive tests in the total population:

$$Prevalence = \frac{True\ positive}{Total\ population}.$$

This is also sometimes referred to as the pretest probability, that is, the rate in the population before any diagnostic tests have been done. Online calculators for these various ratios are found at http://statpages.org/ctab2x2.html, and http://vassarstats.net/clin1.html (all of which provide confidence limits as well), http://www.hutchon.net/Bayes.htm, and http://ktclearinghouse.ca/cebm/practise/ca/calculators/statscalc.

Some investigators use the terms predictive value or accuracy (as defined above) as equivalent. Most investigators use the terms predictive value for these ratios, and reserve the term predictive accuracy for the ratio of all the correct tests to all the tests $\frac{True\ positive + True\ negative}{True\ positive + True\ negative + False\ positive + False\ negative}$. Therefore, the definition used by any investigator should be checked before trying to interpret the data.

The true prevalence rate cannot be calculated from the data given in Table 21.2a, because patients were selected because they did or did not have prostatic cancer and there is no reason to believe that these represent the true ratios in the population.

Because these ratios give point estimates for one particular set of data, it is also valuable to calculate the 95% confidence intervals. For sensitivity these are

$$sensitivity \pm 1.96\sqrt{\frac{sensitivity(1 - sensitivity)}{N}}$$

where N is the number of people with the disease. For specificity these limits are

$$specificity \pm 1.96\sqrt{\frac{specificity(1 - specificity)}{N}},$$

where N is the number of people without the disease. These confidence limits can be obtained online at http://vassarstats.net/clin1.html.

From these results, the PAP test is only 70% sensitive; it misses 30% of those with prostatic cancer, but it is 94% specific because only rarely is it positive in someone who does not have prostatic cancer. The ability of the test to detect the disease, that is, its positive predictive accuracy, has a probability of 86%. (This PAP test is not the same as the Pap test used to diagnose uterine cancer. Furthermore, the PAP test has been replaced by another test, the prostate-specific antigen (PSA) test.)

These probabilities have their exact equivalents in the probability symbols used in Bayes' theorem. The probability that defines sensitivity involves a marginal subtotal, and so concerns a conditional probability. The probability of having a true positive test is $\frac{79}{330} = 0.239$ and the probability of having prostatic cancer is $\frac{113}{330} = 0.342$. The conditional probability of having a true positive test in someone with prostatic cancer is therefore $\frac{\frac{79}{330}}{\frac{113}{330}} = \frac{79}{113} = 0.699$. This ratio, $\frac{79}{113}$, is the definition of the probability that we term sensitivity.

Therefore,

Sensitivity $= P(T^+|D^+)$, and by similar reasoning

Specificity $= P(T^-|D^-)$,

$1 -$ Sensitivity $= P(T^-|D^+)$, and

$1 -$ Specificity $= P(T^+|D^-)$.

Based on these identities, rewrite Bayes' theorem as:

$$P(D^+|T^+) = \frac{P(T^+|D^+)P(D^+)}{P(T^+)} = \frac{P(T^+|D^+)P(D^+)}{P(T^+|D^+)P(D^+) + P(T^+|D^-)}$$

$$= \frac{P(T^+|D^+)P(D^+)}{P(T^+|D^+)P(D^+) + [1 - P(T^-|D^-) + (1 - P(D^+))]}$$

So $P(D^+|T^+) = \dfrac{\text{Sensitivity} \times \text{Prevalence}}{(\text{Sensitivity} \times \text{Prevalence}) + (1 - \text{Specificity})(1 - \text{Prevalence})}$.

By similar manipulations,

$$P(D^-|T^-) = \frac{\text{Specificity} \times (1 - \text{Prevalence})}{\text{Specificity}(1 - \text{Prevalence}) + \text{Prevalence}(1 - \text{Sensitivity})}.$$

Problem 21.1

Testing for bowel cancer by a fecal blood test gave

		Bowel cancer	
		Present	**Absent**
Occult blood in stool	Present	25	187
	Absent	14	1947

Calculate sensitivity, specificity, positive, and negative predictive values. What do the results tell you?

We are not restricted to evaluating sensitivity and specificity one test at a time, whether done simultaneously or sequentially. For example, consider two independent tests A and B for a disease. Assume that our observed results are shown in Table 21.3.

The two most common rules for combined testing are "either positive," in which the combined test is positive if either test is positive, or "both positive" in which the combined test is positive only if both tests are positive. With the "either positive" rule, the sensitivity of the combined test will be no less than the higher sensitivity of each component test but the specificity will be no greater than the lower specificity of each of component tests. The opposite occurs under the "both positive" rule (Macaskill et al., 2002; Marshall, 1989).

Sensitivity and specificity apply to groups of patients, and are seldom useful in confirming or excluding a diagnosis in a single patient. However, a highly sensitive test

Table 21.3 Combining test results

Test	Sensitivity %	Specificity %
A	70	90
B	90	45
A or B	97.5	41
A and B	67.5	93.5

that is negative argues strongly against a particular diagnosis (Sensitivity out or **Sn**out), and a highly specific test that is positive strongly supports the diagnosis (Specificity in or **Sp**in) (Akobeng, 2007a).

Cautionary Tales
Practical Issues of Screening Tests

Whereas we can obtain values for sensitivity and specificity from a table such as Table 18.3a, this does not provide a value for prevalence; that value has to come from other observations. The importance of prevalence may be illustrated by an editorial by Redwood et al. that appeared in Circulation in 1976 (Redwood et al., 1976). They discussed the discrepancy between two sets of studies of the relationship of abnormal ST segments on electrocardiograms taken during an exercise test to the subsequent diagnosis of significant coronary arterial disease. In one set of studies, the positive predictive value of an abnormal ST segment response was high, and in the other it was low. Both sets of studies appeared to have been done carefully and adequately. In order to explain this discrepancy, the authors showed how the predictive value of a test depended on the population under study, and in particular on the prevalence of the disease. To illustrate this concept, they assumed that a given diagnostic test was both 95% sensitive and 95% specific for a particular disease, but that the prevalence of the disease could be either 90% or 2%. The data for each of these are set out in Tables 21.4a and 21.4b.

Table 21.4a Disease prevalence 90%

Subjects	Positive test	Negative test	Total
Diseased	855	45	900
Normal	5	95	100
Total	860	140	1000

$$\text{Positive Predictive Value} = \frac{855}{860} = 0.994 \text{ or } 99.4\%.$$

$$\text{Negative Predictive Value} = \frac{95}{140} = 0.679 \text{ or } 67.9\%.$$

Table 21.4b Disease prevalence 2%

Subjects	Positive test	Negative test	Total
Diseased	19	1	20
Normal	49	931	980
Total	68	932	1000

$$\text{Positive Predictive Value} = \frac{19}{68} = 0.279 \text{ or } 27.9\%.$$

(Continued)

Cautionary Tales—cont'd

$$\text{Negative Predictive Value} = \frac{931}{932} = 0.999 \text{ or } 99.9\%.$$

High positive predictive value was obtained in studies of groups of males over 50 years old with chest pain, and this is a population with a high prevalence of coronary arterial disease that would lead to a positive electrocardiographic stress test. On the other hand, low positive predictive value was found in studies of asymptomatic subjects, most of whom could be expected to be normal so that the prevalence (prior risk or pretest probability) of coronary arterial disease would be low. Because most people the latter group would not have coronary arterial disease, even a low false-positive rate of 5% produces a large absolute number (49) of false positives compared to the smaller number of true positives (19).

Redwood et al. also showed the relationship of predictive value to disease prevalence for different sensitivities and specificities. Figure 21.1 shows a modification of their figure:

The curves are numbered from 1 to 9, based initially on decreasing sensitivities and, within a given sensitivity, based on decreasing specificities. Combinations 1 and 5 are almost identical, and are not displayed separately. For all the combinations of sensitivity and specificity, the higher the prevalence, the higher the positive predictive value; if almost all of a population have a disease, all tests are likely to confirm the presence of that disease. However, in practice, high prevalences are seen only in selected subpopulations known from current medical information to be at high risk; for examples, obese, smoking, inactive, stressed diabetic males with chest pain have a high prevalence of coronary arterial disease, and middle-aged women with

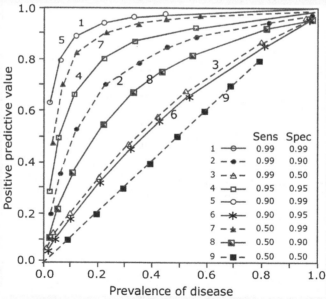

Figure 21.1 Relationship between positive predictive value, sensitivity (Sens), specificity (Spec), and prevalence.

Cautionary Tales—cont'd

an extremely high family history of breast cancer are at high risk for breast cancer. Therefore screening whole populations, in which no disease has a high prevalence, is likely to produce low predictive value with many false positives, thus causing distress to the subjects and substantial costs in following up the tests. Thus, Watson and Tang (1981), using a reasonable figure for the prevalence of prostatic cancer of 35 per 100,000 population, pointed out that if the PAP test was 70% sensitive and 94% specific, based on previously described data, the predictive value of a positive test used as a routine screening examination would be only 0.41%; that is, only 1 out of 244 people with a positive test would have prostatic cancer. They pointed out also that for predictive value to be 50% the prevalence of prostatic cancer would have to be 7894 per 100,000 population, an unrealistic figure.

The best predictive values at any prevalence come with sensitivities and specificities both of 0.99 (curve 1) but decreasing sensitivity to 0.90 makes little difference to positive predictive value (curve 5). In fact, decreasing sensitivity to 0.50 (curve 7) decreases positive predictive value only slightly at any prevalence. On the other hand, decreasing specificity to 0.90 materially lowers the positive predictive value, as can be seen by comparing curves 1 and 2, 5 and 6, and 7 and 8. A specificity of 0.50 produces low positive predictive value, no matter what the sensitivity.

Taking the values for sensitivity, specificity, and prevalence from Tables 21.4a and 21.4b gives:

$$P(D^+|T^+) = \frac{0.95 \times 0.90}{(0.95 \times 0.90) + (0.05 \times 0.10)} = \frac{0.855}{0.860} = 0.994 \text{ (high prevalence)},$$

and

$$P(D^+|T^+) = \frac{0.95 \times 0.02}{(0.95 \times 0.02) + (0.05 \times 0.98)} = \frac{0.019}{0.068} = 0.279 \text{ (low prevalence)}.$$

Similarly:

$$P(D^-|T^-) = \frac{0.95 \times 0.90}{(0.95 \times 0.90) + (0.90 \times 0.05)} = 0.95 \text{ (high prevalence)},$$

and

$$P(D^-|T^-) = \frac{0.95 \times 0.02}{(0.95 \times 0.02) + (0.02 \times 0.05)} = 0.95 \text{ (low prevalence)}.$$

Therefore, positive predictive value is merely another term for the conditional probability of a disease, given a positive test. Similarly, negative predictive value (the probability that a negative test means no disease) is another term for the conditional probability of no disease, given a negative test. The posterior probability that is required may be calculated by Bayes' theorem, as above. This form of the expression for predictive value also shows why, in Figure 18.5, specificity is a more important determinant of positive predictive value than is sensitivity. If sensitivity is below 100% and prevalence is low, there will be only a small number

(Continued)

Cautionary Tales—cont'd

of false-negative tests, so that the numerator of the expression will be small. On the other hand, even a small decrease in specificity from 100% with a large number of normal people will give a large number of false-positive tests, so that the denominator of the expression will be large and the ratio will be low.

Dichotomous Test and Range

With a dichotomous test, the sample from which the test data come needs careful assessment. In a large series of studies to determine whether fractional flow reserve (FFR) is useful in deciding whether an intermediate coronary artery stenosis is the cause of the patients' symptoms, a critical value of 075 was established (Pijls et al., 1995). Taking the whole range of patients with narrowed coronary arteries might produce a table such as shown in Table 21.5a:

Table 21.5a Hypothetical table using the FRR cutoff of 0.75 with disease being verified by a thallium uptake test

	Positive test <0.75	Negative test ≥0.75
Disease present	100 TP	5 FN
Disease absent	15 FP	100 TN

From this table, sensitivity is $\frac{100}{105}$ = 95.2% and specificity is $\frac{100}{115}$ = 86.0%. Positive predictive value is $\frac{100}{115}$ = 87.0%.

By angiography, some coronary arteries will be widely dilated and therefore not a cause of symptoms whereas others will be so narrowed that there is no doubt about their harmful effect. Including more of these obvious positives and negatives might produce data such as shown in Table 21.5b.

Table 21.5b Hypothetical table with many more true positives and true negatives present in the sample

1000	Positive test <0.75	Negative test ≥0.75
Disease present	1000 TP	5 FN
Disease absent	15 FP	1000 TN

From these data, sensitivity is $\frac{1000}{1005}$ = 99.5%, specificity is $\frac{1000}{1015}$ = 98.5%, and positive predictive value is 99.5%.

Merely increasing the numbers of subjects in whom the diagnosis is obvious has increased the values of sensitivity, specificity, and positive predictive accuracy. If those subjects with an obvious diagnosis are excluded and only those with borderline constrictions are included, then results shown in Table 21.5c might be produced.

Cautionary Tales—cont'd

Table 21.5c Hypothetical table in which only subjects with borderline lesions are included. These data should not be taken to represent the actual data, but are used to illustrate the possible error

	Positive test <0.75	Negative test ≥0.75
Disease present	20 TP	5 FN
Disease absent	15 FP	10 TN

Sensitivity is $\frac{20}{25} = 80\%$, specificity is $\frac{10}{25} = 40\%$, and positive predictive value is $\frac{20}{35} = 57.1\%$.

Therefore the values for sensitivity, specificity, and predictive accuracy depend on the prevalence of the disease and how we select our sample from the population.

LIKELIHOOD RATIOS

A likelihood ratio (LR) is the probability of a given test result in those with disease compared to the probability of the same test result for those without the disease. By definition, a positive LR (LR+) is:

$$\frac{\text{True positive rate}}{\text{False positive rate}} = \frac{\frac{TP}{TP+FN}}{\frac{FP}{FP+TN}} = \frac{Sensitivity}{1 - Specificity}, \text{ also symbolized by } \frac{P(T^+|D^+)}{P(T^+|D^-)}.$$

The definition of a negative LR (LR−) is:

$$\frac{\text{False negative rate}}{\text{True negative rate}} = \frac{\frac{FN}{TP+FN}}{\frac{TN}{FP+TN}} = \frac{1 - Sensitivity}{Specificity}, \text{ also symbolized by } \frac{P(T^-|D^+)}{P(T^-|D^-)}.$$

These ratios are not independent of prevalence (Brenner and Gefeller, 1997; Willis, 2012), and this can be allowed for by multiplying each expression by the odds, represented by $\frac{\text{Prevalence}}{1-\text{Prevalence}}$. If prevalence is close to 0.5 the correction is not needed, but becomes important at lower prevalence.

The ratio can be refined by dividing LR+ by LR− to give a diagnostic odds ratio (Sackett et al., 1985; Lijmer et al., 1999). This is identical to the odds ratio (cross–product ratio) obtained from a fourfold table. It has the merit of using all the data that help to differentiate true positives from true negatives.

Approximate 95% confidence limits for the LR of a given test result are: (Simel et al., 1991)

$$\exp\left(\ln\frac{p_1}{p_2} \pm 1.96\sqrt{\frac{1-p_1}{p_1 N_1} + \frac{1-p_2}{p_2 N_2}}\right)$$

where N_1 is the number with the disease, N_2 the number without the disease, p_1 the proportion of subjects with the disease who have test result X (sensitivity), and p_2 the proportion of subjects without the disease who have test result X (1 − specificity). Online calculators include http://ktclearinghouse.ca/cebm/practise/ca/calculators/statscalc, http://www.hutchon.net/Bayes.htm, http://easycalculation.com/statistics/Bayesian-analysis.php, http://statpages.org/ctab2x2.html, http://araw.mede.uic.edu/cgi-bin/testcalc.pl, and http://vassarstats.net/clin2.html.

What does LR+ indicate? $TP/(TP+FN)$ is the proportion of people with a disease who have a positive test, and $FP/(FP+TN)$ is the proportion of people without the disease who have a positive test. The ratio therefore indicates the likelihood that a person with a positive test has the disease. From the data in Table 18.3a, $TP/(TP+FN)$ is $79/113 = 0.6991$, and $FP/(FP+TN)$ is $13/217 = 0.05991$. The ratio of these two is 11.7, showing that a person with a positive test has 11.7 times the risk of having the disease than not having it.

An LR >1 indicates an association between a positive test and the disease, whereas a ratio <1 indicates that a test result is not associated with the disease. Ratios over 10 and under 0.1 are strong arguments for or against the diagnosis (Deeks and Altman, 2004). A useful simplification was reported by McGee (2002). LR of 2, 5, and 10 increase the probability of the disease by approximately 15%, 30%, or 45%, respectively, and ratios of 1/2, 1/5, and 1/10 decrease the probability of the disease by approximately 15%, 30%, and 45%, respectively.

Posttest odds can be shown to equal Pretest odds × LR. The pretest odds is the ratio of the probability of having the disease divided by the probability of not having the disease, and is

$$\frac{P(D^+)}{P(1-D^+)}.$$

The posttest probability is defined by

$$\frac{Post\ test\ odds}{1 + Post\ test\ odds}.$$

The posttest probability can be derived by rearranging the original equation, but to avoid cumbersome calculations use the nomogram developed by Fagan (1975). This nomogram and some of the associated calculations are provided online by http://araw.mede.uic.edu/cgi-bin/testcalc.pl?DT=0&Dt=0&dT=0&dt=0&2x2=Compute, http://www.hsl.unc.edu/services/tutorials/ebm/nomogram.pdf and https://mclibrary.duke.edu/sites/mclibrary.duke.edu/files/public/guides/nomogram.pdf. Results without the nomogram are provided online by http://www.medcalc.com/bayes.html and http://www.dokterrutten.nl/collega/LRcalcul.html. These nomograms can be used with the primary sensitivity and specificity data by referring to articles by Moller-Petersen (1985) and Caraguel and Vanderstichel (2013). The latter authors devised an elegant extension of the Fagan nomogram that allows the physician to start with known sensitivity, specificity, and pretest probability (Figure 21.2). There is an excellent accompanying Web site at http://www.adelaide.edu.au/vetsci/research/pub_pop/2step-nomogram/,

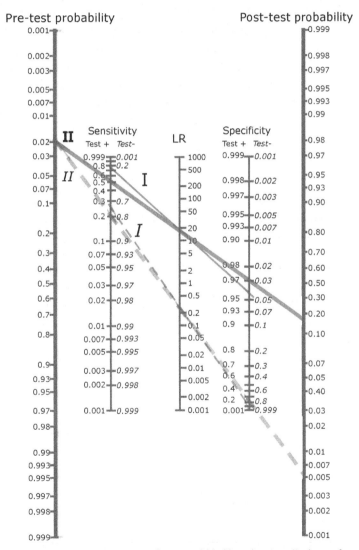

Figure 21.2 Nomogram for sensitivity, specificity, and likelihood ratios. *(Redrawn from Caraguel and Vanderstichel (2013) by permission of the publisher and the authors.)*

and a very useful free application for the iPhone, iPad, and iPod touch obtainable from iTunes as DocNomo app at https://itunes.apple.com/us/app/docnomo/id901279945? mt=8.

Because a test is usually either positive or negative, their combined probability is 1. Therefore, in both the sensitivity and the specificity scales, a value of 0.4 for test+ is the same as the value 0.6 for test−.

To use this nomogram, if the test is positive and has a sensitivity of 0.8 and a specificity of ~0.06, the thin solid line (I) indicates a LR of about 20. If we know the pretest probability (prevalence) is 0.02, then the thick solid line (II) passing from 0.02 through the LR of 20 intercepts the posttest probability at about 0.18, suggesting that the patient does have the disease. (In the total population, most pretest probabilities are low. In selected populations, e.g., middle-aged obese diabetic male smokers with sudden onset chest pain, the pretest probability of coronary artery disease is high.) If the test is negative with a known sensitivity of 0.28 and a specificity of 0.9 (dashed line I), it crosses the LR scale at about 0.22. Given the same prevalence of 0.02, extending this through the LR of 0.22 intersects the posttest probability scale at about 0.005 (thick dashed line II), indicating that the disease is very unlikely to be present.

Problem 21.2

For the fecal blood data, calculate the posttest probability and comment on the results.

An excellent discussion of LR and an online calculator are provided by Tape. Hayden and Brown (1999) have emphasized the value of using LRs rather than sensitivity and specificity because LRs of necessity lead to a Bayesian approach that takes prior probabilities into consideration. On the other hand, posttest probabilities cannot be calculated if no pretest probability is available.

LR can be applied to a complete data set, or to subgroups within it. Table 21.6 shows the sensitivity, specificity, and LR+ for different threshold concentrations of procalcitonin (PCT) in diagnosing septic shock (Hatherill et al., 1999).

Table 21.6 Effect of using different PCT concentrations to differentiate patients with and without septic shock of bacterial origin. As the critical concentration is increased, sensitivity decreases, but specificity and LR increase. If all the data were lumped to regard all patients with an elevated PCT concentration, the averaged LR+ would be lower than the maximum

PCT concentration (ng/ml)	Sensitivity	Specificity	LR+
>2	100	62	2.63
>5	99	78	4.50
>10	88	84	5.50
>20	83	92	10.37

Problem 21.3
Calculate the LRs for the data in Problem 21.1.

Discussing sensitivity and specificity assumes that when we calculate $P(T^+|D^+)$ we are certain about the presence of the disease. This may not always be true, and we may end up comparing a new test T^+ with a standard test ("D^+") that may not always be positive when the disease is present. If, for example, the false-positive rate of the standard test is assumed to be zero, but is not, then the false-negative rate of the new test is overestimated. Also, if the standard test is assumed to have no false negatives, but this is wrong, then the false-positive rate of the new test will be overestimated (Buck and Gart, 1966; Gart and Buck, 1966; Greenberg and Jekel, 1969; Line et al., 1997). Improved results may be obtained by using maximum likelihood methods.

CUTTING POINTS

The data presented in the decision matrix in 21.4a are dichotomous; a test is assumed to be either positive or negative, with no overlap. However, this may not occur with measurements of continuous variables. What is much more likely is that the higher (or lower) some test measurement is, the more likely is that the person has the disease.

Thyroid hormone is essential for development of the nervous system, and children born with thyroid hormone deficiency develop mental retardation unless replacement therapy is started soon after birth. Therefore in many countries, it is mandatory to test for thyroid deficiency at birth. A drop of blood from the umbilical cord is placed on filter paper, dried, and then sent to a laboratory for measurement of thyroid hormones. Morissette and Dussault (1979) found that in a large population of infants without hypothyroidism, the distribution of thyroxine (T4) was log normal with a mean of 1.73 ng/spot and a standard deviation of 1.35 ng/spot. In a group of 72 hypothyroid infants, the mean T4 was 0.52 ng/spot with a standard deviation of 0.188 ng/spot, and the distribution was approximately normal (Figure 21.3).

In this figure, the normal and hypothyroid distributions are drawn overlapping; the means are put in, but the curves are not drawn to scale. A vertical line is drawn where the two lines cross. The shaded area to the left of this vertical line is the proportion α of the normal population ($=TN$) that lies below the cutoff point and would be regarded as abnormal; this shaded area therefore represents false positives. The cross-hatched area to the right of the vertical line indicates the proportion β of the hypothyroid distribution ($=TP$) that lies above the cutoff point and would be regarded as normal; this shaded area therefore represents false negatives.

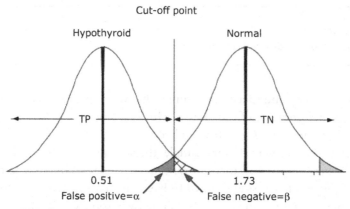

Figure 21.3 Congenital hypothyroid data. TP, true positive; TN, true negative.

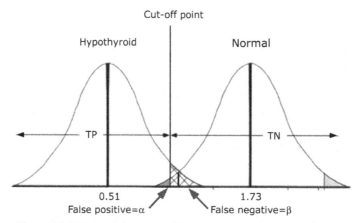

Figure 21.4 New cutting point. TP, true positive; TN, true negative.

What happens if the cutting point is moved to the left (Figure 21.4)?

The proportion of false positives is decreased, but the proportion of false negatives is increased. Conversely, if the cutoff points were moved to the right, the proportion of false negatives is decreased, but the proportion of false positives is increased. From the values for means and standard deviations, Morissette and Dussault computed the proportions of false negatives and false positives for several cutting points and also computed the probability of missing an infant with hypothyroidism by multiplying β, the proportion of false negatives, by the prevalence of the disease in the population. Thus for β equal to 0.016 and prevalence equal to 1/5000, the probability of missing a patient with disease is $0.016 \times 1/5000 = 0.0000032 = 3.2$ per million infants screened. Changing the cutting point altered these values. Thus, moving the cutting point to the left (more standard deviation units below the normal mean, lower T4 concentrations) decreased the false positives almost 10-fold from the highest to the lowest cutting points, but at the same

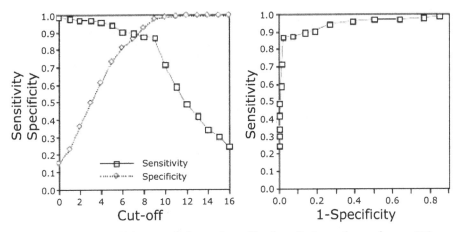

Figure 21.5 Sensitivity, specificity, and cutoff points. *(Redrawn from reference 32.)*

time increased the false negatives and the chances of missing a hypothyroid infant about 240-fold. Where the cutting point should be placed is debatable, and depends to some extent on the penalty (in human suffering or cost) to be paid on failing to diagnose a disease or in diagnosing too many normal subjects as having disease. Some consequences of varying the cutting point have been discussed (Cheetham, 2011; Krude and Blankenstein, 2011).

One way of examining the relationship of the cutoff point to sensitivity and specificity is to plot both of these against various cutoff points. To illustrate this, Figure 21.5 shows the data in which scores are obtained from the Early Motor Pattern Profile (EMPP) at 6 months of age in an attempt to predict which children will have cerebral palsy (Morgan and Aldag, 1996).

The left-hand panel shows that the sensitivity and specificity curves cross near a cutoff point of 7, where both sensitivity and specificity are high.

RECEIVER OPERATING CHARACTERISTIC CURVES

One approach to the problems imposed by variations in cutting points is to construct receiver operating characteristic (ROC) curves. A graph is constructed by plotting the false-positive fraction (1 − specificity) on the horizontal axis against the true positive fraction (sensitivity) on the vertical axis (Figure 21.6(a) and (b)) at each cutting point, each cutting point giving one value for true positive and false positive. To produce such a curve, the sensitivity and specificity are calculated for each of several different cutting points, ideally, a large number of cutting points between 0 and 1 with small equal bin sizes. The curve must pass from the lower left-hand corner of the graph if all the tests are negative up to the upper right-hand corner if all the tests are positive. The diagonal

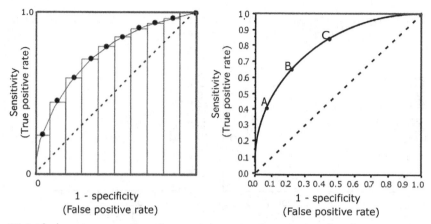

Figure 21.6 Ideal receiver operating characteristic curves. Sometimes only a few cutting points are used (right panel).

dashed line indicates that a positive decision is no more likely if the test is positive than if it is negative, and implies that the test is worthless. If the tests were a perfect marker for the disease, then the curve would run up the left-hand boundary from 0 to 1, and then run horizontally from the upper left- to right-hand corners. In reality, tests give a curve above the diagonal line. The points are joined by a curve that is usually monotonic and often capable of being fitted to some function. In fact, conversion of probabilities into z values and plotting them on a binormal linear plot usually produces reasonably straight lines (Hermann et al., 1986; Rombach et al., 1986). Any point on the line indicates the ratio of positive to negative tests in patients with the disease (Figure 21.6).

In the right panel, point A indicates a test with relatively low sensitivity but with very few false positives; many with the disease will be missed but few normal subjects will be falsely diagnosed as having the disease. Point C, on the other hand, indicates that most of the people with the disease will be detected, but at the cost of a large number of false-positive tests. Point B gives intermediate values.

The data from the thyroid study are plotted as an ROC curve produces Figure 21.7.

The false positive increases as sensitivity is increased to the highest level is well shown, but changing the cutting point to increase sensitivity from 0.928 to 0.984 incurs little increase in the false-positive rate.

Plotting ROC curves for the EMPP data shown in the left panel of Figure 21.5 gives the curve shown in the right-hand panel of that figure. As the cutting point is raised from 0 to 7, there is a great increase in sensitivity with very little increase in false positives. At higher cutoff points, there is little further gain in sensitivity but a big increase in false positives.

ROC curves may be constructed to compare the relative merits of different tests in several ways. A single number that summarizes the curve is the area under the curve

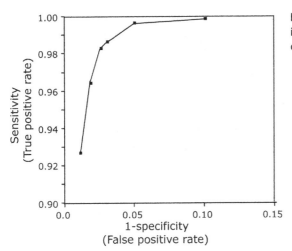

(AUC). This area represents the probability that a random person with the disease has a higher measured value than a random person without the disease (Akobeng, 2007b). For the uninformative diagonal line, the probability is 0.5 and thus is of no diagnostic help.

Some authors have recommended a simple scale to indicate the value of the area (Swets, 1988; Fischer et al., 2003; Tape) (Adapted from Tape).

Excellent: >90%; Good: 80–90%; Fair: 70–80%; Poor: 60–70%; Bad: 50–60%, but simple inspection is probably adequate for deciding if discrimination is good. The area, however, is only a point estimate, and determining 95% confidence limits as $1.96SE$ is useful. A formula for determining these limits was published by Hanley and McNeil (1982):

$$SE = \sqrt{\frac{A(1 - A) + (N_a - 1)(Q_1 - A^2) + (N_n - 1)(Q_2 - A^2)}{N_a N_n}}$$

where A is the AUC, and N_a and N_n are the number of abnormal and normal results, respectively, $Q_1 = A/(2 - A)$, and $Q_2 = 2A^2/(1 + A)$.

If two curves are to be compared, for example, two different tests for the same disease, observation will tell if the two curves are similar or quite different. In a study done on prediction of septic shock in children in which PCT, C-reactive protein, and white cell count were compared (Figure 21.8, based on the study by Hatherill et al. (1999) and used in an explanatory article by Akobeng (2007b).

$$z = \frac{A_1 - A_2}{SE_{A_1 - A_2}}$$

where $SE_{A_1 - A_2} = \sqrt{SE^2 A_1 + SE^2 A_2 - 2rSE(A_1)SE(A_2)}$ (Hanley and McNeil, 1982, 1983; Hopley and Van Schalkwyk, 2007).

Figure 21.8 Receiver operating characteristic curves comparing procalcitonin (PCT), C-reactive protein (CRP), and white blood cell count (WBC) from the same patients. The white cell count was nondiscriminatory because at every value there were about equal numbers of true and false positives. The other two curves, however, did show discrimination, with PCT better than CRP. Was the difference between these two curves due to chance? To assess this, perform a z test.

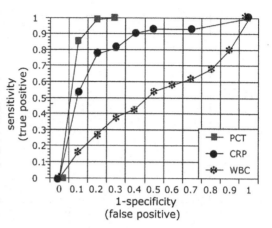

Here r is the correlation coefficient averaged for positive tests and negative tests separately. If the two tests to be compared are done in different groups of patients, the component of the formula involving the correlation coefficient drops out.

Single curves can be fitted to a theoretical distribution online at http://vassarstats.net/index.html, and this will also calculate the AUC. Unfitted curves cannot be drawn, and curves cannot be superimposed. On the other hand, XY plots can be drawn by several programs (Chapter 27).

The power of the test should be determined, preferably in advance. Appropriate numbers can be determined from Table III in the publication by Hanley and McNeil (1982). An online test is available at http://vassarstats.net/index.html for selected data values.

The ROC plot has several advantages. It provides an easy visual compilation of all the data, does not depend on the parameters of any distribution, and is independent of the prevalence of the disease. On the other hand, the graph does not indicate the patient numbers from which the data were derived, does not show the cutting points used, may be unduly influenced by the initial and final parts of the curve that contain little information, and the decision thresholds used in the calculations are not apparent. Furthermore, although the plots give useful information about individual tests, they do not tell us whether better discrimination could be obtained by combining the results from two or more tests (something that can be done with Bayes' theorem applied sequentially). Finally, the curve does not provide an answer about where the best cutoff point is, because the answer to that question is multifactorial. One recommended method is to examine where the separate curves for sensitivity or specificity versus cutting points cross, and set confidence limits around this point (Greiner, 1995, 1996; Greiner et al., 1995, 2000). Another is to calculate the Youden index J, the maximum value of (Sensitivity + Specificity − 1) (Youden, 1950; Fluss et al., 2005).

If it were just a matter of financial cost it would be possible to find an optimal cutoff point by these or similar methods, but some of the human costs cannot be so easily enumerated. It may be more important not to miss early cancer than many other diseases. There is also a difference in cost to a patient versus cost to a community. For example, now that few people are immunized against smallpox, the failure to diagnose a single patient with smallpox would be catastrophic to the community and would outweigh the costs of dealing with false positives. The subject is discussed in Zweig and Campbell (1993). In this context, it is sometimes appropriate to focus on a specific part of the ROC curve; for example, if two curves cross, or if only cutting points with sensitivities over 90% are essential. Special tests are available in these circumstances (Jiang et al., 1996; Obuchowski, 2003).

Another sensible use of ROC curves was provided Bhatt et al. (2009). They investigated the important problem of how to diagnose acute appendicitis in children so as to minimize both false negatives (missed appendicitis) and false positives (unnecessary surgery). They developed a pediatric appendicitis score and applied it to 246 patients aged 4—18 years referred for possible acute appendicitis. The score, based on clinical findings and a white blood cell count, ranged from 1 to 10. By relating the scores to what was found at surgery or, if no surgery was done, to the subsequent course, they were able to calculate specificity and sensitivity for each score, and created an ROC curve (Figure 21.9).

No single score was ideal for discriminating between abdominal pain that was or was not due to appendicitis. What they did, however, was to use two threshold scores, one to recommend discharge home and other to recommend operation. A score of 1—4 allowed

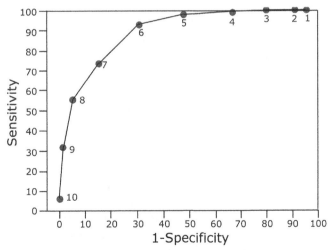

Figure 21.9 Receiver operating characteristic curve based on pediatric appendicitis score (numbers under points on the curve).

then to send home patients without surgery with only 2.4% missed appendicitis, and a score of 8—10 allowed them to operate with a low false-positive rate of 8.8%. Patients with scores of 5—7 had an indeterminate diagnosis, and required further investigation.

SOME COMMENTS ON SCREENING TESTS

The aims of a screening test are to detect asymptomatic disease so that it may be treated early and lead to decreased morbidity and mortality.

A screening test must fulfill certain requirements:

1. It should have high sensitivity, so that as many people as possible with the disease can be detected.
2. It should have high specificity, so that the false-positive rate is kept low. However, even a small false-positive rate when the population incidence is low yields a very large number of people to have follow-up tests.
3. There should be a treatment for the diagnosed disease. Without an effective treatment, the results are useful at best for counseling or research.
4. The results should be cost-effective. Although we cannot put a cost benefit on saving one life, if the costs of the test are so high that they reduce the total pool of money available for other aspects of medical care, then society does not benefit. Certain newborn screening tests for genetic disorders (phenylketonuria and congenital hypothyroidism) have been shown to be cost-effective. For many other neonatal screening tests, the cost—benefit ratio is unknown.
5. Screening for cancer in later life has had a checkered course, and this is nowhere better shown than in screening for breast cancer by mammography, ovarian cancer by transvaginal ultrasonography and cancer antigen-125, or prostatic cancer by blood testing for PSA. These studies have not shown a reduction in deaths. Furthermore, the follow-up testing needed to eliminate false positives may involve potentially harmful radiation, surgery, or invasive biopsies, all of which have substantial cost and may have short- or long-term complications. More importantly, there is now evidence (Hinkley, 1969) that detecting early lesions in the breast or prostate may not reduce the number of late advanced cancers, so that the screening tests may be detecting small, relatively innocuous lesions. Ductal carcinoma in situ may occur in up to 40% of adult women, and most elderly males have histological evidence of prostatic cancer; both of these changes may be so slowly progressive that they do not account for premature death from cancer. If this concept is true, then these screening tests are not detecting the important lesions and are merely causing anxiety in both patient and doctor (Wainer, 2011). An excellent discussion of the advantages and disadvantages of screening mammography for breast cancer recently appeared in the New York Times magazine (Orenstein, 2013). Some issues about screening tests have been highlighted by a recent publication (Wegwarth et al., 2012) in which a survey of primary care

physicians showed that relatively few of them could determine if the evidence supporting a hypothetical screening test was relevant or irrelevant. One of the main errors was in using evidence based on survival statistics rather than cancer mortality. Survival statistics, if not obtained by a randomized trial, contain two potentially serious errors (Welch and Black, 2010; Welch et al., 2000, 2007): lead-time bias and overdiagnosis bias. The lead-time error is displayed in Figure 21.10, redrawn from Welch et al. (2007).

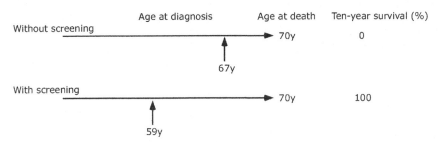

Figure 21.10 Illustration of lead-time bias. Although cancer death has not been prevented, the 10-year survival estimate shows a great improvement.

The overdiagnosis bias is made when a screening test detects small and often innocuous lesions. As a result, the percent survival will be much increased, even if the number dying from the disease has not changed.

REFERENCES

Akobeng, A.K., 2007a. Understanding diagnostic tests 1: sensitivity, specificity and predictive values. Acta Paediatr. 96, 338—341.

Akobeng, A.K., 2007b. Understanding diagnostic tests 3: receiver operating characteristic curves. Acta Paediatr. 96, 644—647.

Bhatt, M., Joseph, L., Ducharme, F.M., Dougherty, G., Mcgillivray, D., 2009. Prospective validation of the pediatric appendicitis score in a Canadian pediatric emergency department. Acad. Emerg. Med. 16, 591—596.

Brenner, H., Gefeller, O., 1997. Variation of sensitivity, specificity, likelihood ratios and predictive values with disease prevalence. Stat. Med. 16, 981—991.

Buck, A.A., Gart, J.J., 1966. Comparison of a screening test and a reference test in epidemiologic studies. I. Indices of agreement and their relation to prevalence. Am. J. Epidemiol. 83, 586—592.

Caraguel, C.G., Vanderstichel, R., 2013. The two-step Fagan's nomogram: ad hoc interpretation of a diagnostic test result without calculation. Evid. Based Med. 18, 125—128.

Cheetham, T., 2011. Congenital hypothyroidism: managing the hinterland between fact and theory. Arch. Dis. Child. 96, 205.

Deeks, J.J., Altman, D.G., 2004. Diagnostic tests 4: likelihood ratios. BMJ 329, 168—169.

Fagan, T.J., 1975. Letter: nomogram for Bayes theorem. N. Engl. J. Med. 293, 257.

Fischer, J.E., Bachmann, L.M., Jaeschke, R., 2003. A readers' guide to the interpretation of diagnostic test properties: clinical example of sepsis. Intensive Care Med. 29, 1043—1051.

Fluss, R., Faraggi, D., Reiser, B., 2005. Estimation of the Youden Index and its associated cutoff point. Biom. J. 47, 458—472.

Gart, J.J., Buck, A.A., 1966. Comparison of a screening test and a reference test in epidemiologic studies. II. A probabilistic model for the comparison of diagnostic tests. Am. J. Epidemiol. 83, 593—602.

Goldacre, B., 2006. Prosecuting and Defending by Numbers. The Guardian England.

Greenberg, R.A., Jekel, J.F., 1969. Some problems in the determination of the false positive and false negative rates of tuberculin tests. Am. Rev. Respir. Dis. 100, 645—650.

Greiner, M., 1995. Two-graph receiver operating characteristic (TG-ROC): a Microsoft-EXCEL template for the selection of cut-off values in diagnostic tests. J. Immunol. Methods 185, 145—146.

Greiner, M., 1996. Two-graph receiver operating characteristic (TG-ROC): update version supports optimisation of cut-off values that minimise overall misclassification costs. J. Immunol. Methods 191, 93—94.

Greiner, M., Pfeiffer, D., Smith, R.D., 2000. Principles and practical application of the receiver-operating characteristic analysis for diagnostic tests. Prev. Vet. Med. 45, 23—41.

Greiner, M., Sohr, D., Gobel, P., 1995. A modified ROC analysis for the selection of cut-off values and the definition of intermediate results of serodiagnostic tests. J. Immunol. Methods 185, 123—132.

Hanley, J.A., McNeil, B.J., 1982. The meaning and use of the area under a receiver operating characteristic (ROC) curve. Radiology 143, 29—36.

Hanley, J.A., McNeil, B.J., 1983. A method of comparing the areas under receiver operating characteristic curves derived from the same cases. Radiology 148, 839—843.

Hatherill, M., Tibby, S.M., Sykes, K., Turner, C., Murdoch, I.A., 1999. Diagnostic markers of infection: comparison of procalcitonin with C reactive protein and leucocyte count. Arch. Dis. Child. 81, 417—421.

Hayden, S.R., Brown, M.D., 1999. Likelihood ratio: a powerful tool for incorporating the results of a diagnostic test into clinical decisionmaking. Ann. Emerg. Med. 33, 575—580.

Hermann, G.A., Sugiura, H.T., Krumm, R.P., 1986. Comparison of thyrotropin assays by relative operating characteristic analysis. Arch. Pathol. Lab. Med. 110, 21—25.

Hill, R., 2004. Multiple sudden infant deaths—coincidence or beyond coincidence? Paediatr. Perinat. Epidemiol. 18, 320—326.

Hinkley, D.V., 1969. Inference about the intersection in two-phase regression. Biometrika 56, 495—504.

Hopley, L., Van Schalkwyk, J., 2007. The Magnificent ROC [Online]. Available: http://www.anaesthetist.com/mnm/stats/roc/Findex.htm.

Jiang, Y., Metz, C.E., Nishikawa, R.M., 1996. A receiver operating characteristic partial area index for highly sensitive diagnostic tests. Radiology 201, 745—750.

Joyce, H. https://plus.maths.org/content/beyond-reasonable-doubt.

Krude, H., Blankenstein, O., 2011. Treating patients not numbers: the benefit and burden of lowering TSH newborn screening cut-offs. Arch. Dis. Child. 96, 121—122.

Lijmer, J.G., Mol, B.W., Heisterkamp, S., Bonsel, G.J., Prins, M.H., van der Meulen, J.H., Bossuyt, P.M., 1999. Empirical evidence of design-related bias in studies of diagnostic tests. JAMA 282, 1061—1066.

Line, B.R., Peters, T.L., Keenan, J., 1997. Diagnostic test comparisons in patients with deep venous thrombosis. J. Nucl. Med. 38, 89—92.

Macaskill, P., Walter, S.D., Irwig, L., Franco, E.L., 2002. Assessing the gain in diagnostic performance when combining two diagnostic tests. Stat. Med. 21, 2527—2546.

Marshall, R.J., 1989. The predictive value of simple rules for combining two diagnostic tests. Biometrics 45, 1213—1222.

McGee, S., 2002. Simplifying likelihood ratios. J. Gen. Intern. Med. 17, 646—649.

Moller-Petersen, J., 1985. Nomogram for predictive values and efficiencies of tests. Lancet 1, 348.

Morgan, A.M., Aldag, J.C., 1996. Early identification of cerebral palsy using a profile of abnormal motor patterns. Pediatrics 98, 692—697.

Morissette, J., Dussault, J.H., 1979. Commentary: the cut-off point for TSH measurement or recalls in a screening program for congenital hypothyroidism using primary T4 screening. J. Pediatr. 95, 404—406.

Obuchowski, N.A., 2003. Receiver operating characteristic curves and their use in radiology. Radiology 229, 3—8.

Orenstein, P., 2013. Our Feel-Good War on Breast Cancer [Online]. Available: http://www.nytimes.com/2013/04/28/magazine/our-feel-good-war-on-breast-cancer.html?adxnnl=1&smid=tw-Share&adxnnlx=1413748974-Q5M+nCSVvqItymShri37Ow.

Pijls, N.H., Van Gelder, B., Van der voort, P., Peels, K., Bracke, F.A., Bonnier, H.J., El Gamal, M.I., 1995. Fractional flow reserve. A useful index to evaluate the influence of an epicardial coronary stenosis on myocardial blood flow. Circulation 92, 3183–3193.

Redwood, D.R., Borer, J.S., Epstein, S.E., 1976. Whither the ST segment during exercise. Circulation 54, 703–706.

Rombach, J.J., Collette, B.J., De Waard, F., Slotboom, B.J., 1986. Analysis of the diagnostic performance in breast cancer screening by relative operating characteristics. Cancer 58, 169–177.

Rubin, L.G., 1992. Occult bacteremia. Curr. Opin. Pediatr. 4, 65–69.

Sackett, D.L., Haynes, R.B., Tugwell, P., 1985. Clinical Epidemiology: A Basic Science for Clinical Medicine. Brown, Boston, Toronto Little.

Simel, D.L., Samsa, G.P., Matchar, D.B., 1991. Likelihood ratios with confidence: sample size estimation for diagnostic test studies. J. Clin. Epidemiol. 44, 763–770.

Skorupski, W.P., Wainer, H., 2015. The Bayesian flip. Correcting the Prosecutor's Fallacy. Significance 12, 16–20.

Swets, J.A., 1988. Measuring the accuracy of diagnostic systems. Science 240, 1285–1293.

Tape, G.T. Introduction to Roc Curves [Online]. Available: http://gim.unmc.edu/dxtests/ROC1.htm.

Thompson, W.C., Schumann, E.L., 1987. Interpretation of statistical evidence in criminal trials. The Prosecutor's Fallacy and the Defense Attorney's Fallacy. Law Hum. Behav. 11, 167–187.

Wainer, H., 2011. How should we screen for breast cancer? Using evidence to make medical decisions. Significance 8, 28–30.

Watson, R.A., Tang, D.B., 1980. The predictive value of prostatic acid phosphatase as a screening test for prostatic cancer. N. Engl. J. Med. 303, 497–499.

Wegwarth, O., Schwartz, L.M., Woloshin, S., Gaissmaier, W., Gigerenzer, G., 2012. Do physicians understand cancer screening statistics? A national survey of primary care physicians in the United States. Ann. Intern. Med. 156, 340–349.

Welch, H.G., Black, W.C., 2010. Overdiagnosis in cancer. J. Natl. Cancer Inst. 102, 605–613.

Welch, H.G., Schwartz, L.M., Woloshin, S., 2000. Do increased 5-year survival rates in prostate cancer indicate better outcomes? JAMA 284, 2053–2055.

Welch, H.G., Woloshin, S., Schwartz, L.M., Gordis, L., Gotzsche, P.C., Harris, R., Kramer, B.S., Ransohoff, D.F., 2007. Overstating the evidence for lung cancer screening: the International Early Lung Cancer Action Program (I-ELCAP) study. Arch. Intern. Med. 167, 2289–2295.

Wikipedia, 2011. Prosecutor's Fallacy [Online]. Available: http://en.wikipedia.org/wiki/Prosecutor's_fallacy.

Willis, B.H., 2012. Empirical evidence that disease prevalence may affect the performance of diagnostic tests with an implicit threshold: a cross-sectional study. Br. Med. J. Open 2, e0076 (6 pages).

Youden, W.J., 1950. Index for rating diagnostic tests. Cancer 3, 32–35.

Zweig, M.H., Campbell, G., 1993. Receiver-operating characteristic (ROC) plots: a fundamental evaluation tool in clinical medicine. Clin. Chem. 39, 561–577.

## PART 6

Comparing Means

CHAPTER 22

Comparison of Two Groups: t-Tests and Nonparametric Tests

Contents

BASIC CONCEPTS

Introduction

One of the most frequent questions asked is if the means of two groups are different enough that they are unlikely to have come from the same population. Did the blood sugar decrease more with drug A than drug B? To evaluate this question with continuous data, we usually use the t-test for comparing the means of two groups. It is the prototype for almost all other statistical inferences, and brings into play most of the considerations involved in making these inferences. The t-test is a version of the more general analysis of variance (ANOVA) restricted to two groups.

For a list of all websites referred to in this chapter, as clickable links, see the book companion website: www.booksite.elsevier.com/9780128023877.

Biostatistics for Medical and Biomedical Practitioners
http://dx.doi.org/10.1016/B978-0-12-802387-7.00022-6

There are two types of t-tests. In one, data are collected in pairs of subjects and the set of differences between each pair is tested to determine if the variation is consistent with the null hypothesis that the set of differences comes from a population with a mean difference of zero, that is, the two groups are not different. This is termed the paired t-test. Its counterpart is where two different groups are compared and the question asked is if the two means could have come from the same or different populations.

Paired t-Test

Paired comparisons are frequent. For example, a blood sample is divided into half and placed in two tubes: one is a control and the other has some chemical added, with the question being whether the chemical causes a change in the concentrations of the substance of interest. Blood from several subjects is examined, each time in pairs. Another type of paired experiment might have one pair of rat littermates from several different litters, with one of each pair being given a standard diet and the other member of the pair being given the same diet with a food additive to determine if the additive affects growth. A third experiment might be to study a group of hypertensive people before and after a given dose of a drug to determine if it lowers blood pressure.

In order to determine if the experimental group differs from the control group or if the drug lowers pressure, examine the *differences* between each pair of data values. For example, a study of the biological value of raw (R) versus roasted (P) peanuts as judged by the weight gain of rat littermates (in grams) produced the data of Table 22.1 (Mitchell et al., 1936).

For each pair of rats the difference D in weight gain is calculated, giving the data in column 3. Now ask: "If there is no average difference between the weight gains on the

Table 22.1 Weight gain of paired littermates fed either raw or roasted peanuts in their diet

Raw peanuts R	Roasted peanuts P	Difference D
61	55	6
60	54	6
56	47	9
63	59	4
56	51	5
63	61	2
59	57	2
56	54	2
44	63	−19
61	58	3
		$\Sigma X_i = 20$
		$\overline{X_D} = 2$

two diets, how likely is it that there would be a difference of as much as 2 g?" That is, Ho: $\mu_D = 0$.

If it is very likely, then we would not consider that roasting affected the nutritional value of peanuts, but if it is an unlikely difference, then we might want to consider that roasting affected their nutritional value. Assess the probability of the null hypothesis by determining how many standard deviations from the mean that difference represents. If the difference is many standard deviations from the mean, then there is reason to reject the null hypothesis. To do the required calculations, calculate the mean and standard deviation of the differences, $\overline{X_D} = 2$, $\sum(X_i - \overline{X})^2 = 536$. Therefore, $s^2 = 59.56$, $s = 7.72$, and $s_{\overline{X}} = 7.72/\sqrt{10} = 2.44$. Then relate the difference to the standard error to determine the probability of observing that difference if the true population difference is zero.

$$t = \frac{2 - 0}{2.44} = 0.82. \ P = 0.43.$$

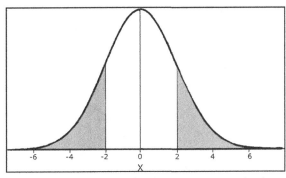

Figure 22.1 Normal curve with shaded areas indicating proportion under the curve beyond the value of t. That is, assuming normality, if the mean difference in the long run was truly 0, at least 43% of similar samples would have a mean difference >2. On this basis, we would not want to reject the null hypothesis.

The 0.05 value of t for 9 degrees of freedom (df) is 2.262, so that the 95 confidence limits of the mean are $2 \pm 2.262 \times 2.44 = -3.52$ to 7.52. Because 0 is included within these limits, the null hypothesis cannot be rejected. The t table can be seen online at http://www.sjsu.edu/faculty/gerstman/StatPrimer/t-table.pdf, the probabilities for the t values can be obtained from http://vassarstats.net/tabs.html, http://in–silico.net/statistics/ttest. The online programs http://www.graphpad.com/quickcalcs/ttest1.cfm, http://www.usablestats.com/calcs/2samplet, and http://easycalculation.com/statistics/ttest-calculator.php allow you to enter the data, and then perform the test.

Problem 22.1

The table below shows the peak flow rates (l/min) in asthmatic patients before and after exertion.

Subject	Before	After
1	320	297
2	235	200
3	322	220
4	376	334
5	286	210
6	254	255
7	381	338
8	397	341
9	299	227

Did exertion cause a decrease in peak flow rate? Would you reject the null hypothesis?

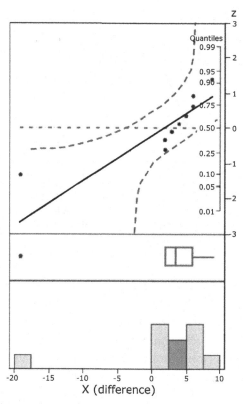

Figure 22.2 Upper panel: normal quantile plot with dashed lines showing 95% confidence limits. Middle panel: box plot. Lower panel: histogram of differences.

There are several points to notice about the paired t-test:

1. The numbers should be ratio or interval numbers, and the distribution of the set of differences should be approximately normal. This is not true here, as shown by observation and Figure 22.2.

There is one extreme outlier shown in all the panels, and the data do not fit a normal quantile plot.

It does not matter if each distribution is not normal; what matters is the distribution of the differences between paired measurements.

2. There must be justification for pairing based on intuitive reasoning or experience. For example, a blood sample divided into two portions should have the same constituents in each portion. Therefore, adding something to one of the pair constitutes the difference to be examined. If theory does not provide the answer, we can turn to experience. Prior work has shown that rat littermates reared on the same diet grow at very similar rates that are more closely matched than are rats from two different litters, or two different species. Patients who are being tested for airway reactivity tend to have the same reactivity when tested on different days, so that testing a patient before and then again after administering a potential airway irritant allows pairing. If, however, previous studies have not shown consistency of response to the same stimulus (diet, airway inhalant, etc.) then pairing should not be used. Any investigator using a paired design (shown below to be more efficient than an unpaired design) must be prepared to justify the use of pairing.

3. The calculated value for t is 0.82, and the probability of t is 0.43 (Figure 22.1).

4. t is a ratio of a difference between an observed mean and a population mean (numerator) to a measure of variability (denominator). The numerator is the signal and the denominator is the noise, so that t represents the signal-to-noise ratio. If the difference is small or the variability is big, t will be small, leading to inability to reject the null hypothesis. On the other hand, if the numerator is big relative to the denominator, t will be big, leading to rejection of the null hypothesis.

5. The numerator indicates the absolute difference between two measurements (the effect size), and its importance has to be judged on the physiological or clinical importance of its magnitude. A difference of 2 mg/dl of serum potassium is huge and potentially serious, whereas a difference of 2 mm Hg of systolic blood pressure is trivial and not clinically important. Whether a difference is big or small is not a statistical question but a matter of judgment by the investigator. The numerator reveals the importance of the measured difference.

6. The denominator, here the standard deviation of the mean, has variability determined by the variability within the population. For a given numerator to yield a high value of t and thus lead to rejection of the null hypothesis the denominator should be as small as possible for that set of measurements. This can sometimes be achieved by making the sampled population as homogeneous as possible. For example, there should be less variability of weight gain in the peanut experiment with rats from the same inbred species rather than from different species. At other

times minimize variability by avoiding outliers because the standard deviation is not a resistant measurement. Sometimes it is appropriate to transform the data by logarithmic or other transformation to avoid having long tails to the distribution and thus inflating the standard deviation. Another way of minimizing the denominator is to increase the sample size. Because variability is a function of $\sqrt{N}$, an increase in sample size decreases the standard deviation of the mean.

7. The probability of t therefore is based on a ratio of an observed difference to its variability. If t is large, so that it is unlikely that the mean difference is zero, then we may wish to reject the null hypothesis. We cannot be certain that the null hypothesis is false; the best we can do is estimate its probability of being false. If we reject the null hypothesis but are wrong (as shown by future work) we commit a Type I error. It is our choice as to what probability to use to minimize a Type I error. Conventionally, the 95% confidence limits are used, giving a 5% chance of making a Type I error, and this is often called "statistical significance."

   a. In normal conversation, significance implies importance, but that is not true in statistics. Its meaning is confined to the chances of making a Type I error, whether or not the observed difference is physiologically or clinically important (see Chapter 10).

   b. The 5% (or 0.05) figure for significance is arbitrary. One percent gives a smaller chance of making a Type I error and rejecting the null hypothesis falsely, 10% has a greater chance of making a Type I error. The 5% level means that a Type I error occurs about 1/20 times, and most people find that psychologically pleasing. On the other hand, if an investigator is doing a number of screening tests on different types of peanut preparation, he or she might well use the 10% cut off value to decide which types to study further.

8. To summarize: If t is significant, that is, we think it reasonable to reject the null hypothesis, we still need to evaluate the absolute magnitude of the difference. If small, we may elect to ignore it. For example, 1 million hypertensive people are tested with a new antihypertensive drug. The mean difference before and after the drug is 2 mm Hg, but because the standard deviation of the mean is incredibly small, t is significant. But that does not mean that the difference is important, and the company manufacturing the drug might elect not to market it.

9. If t is significant, it argues for a difference between the pairs, but does not prove that the difference observed was due to the experiment. There might have been factors outside our control or knowledge that were the causes. Perhaps the 9/10 rats fed raw peanuts and gained more weight than their littermates were kept warm and slept a lot, whereas their littermates were kept cold and made to be active, so that they burned up more calories. We would see a difference that was *associated* with the type of peanuts, but not due to it.

10. If t is small, first examine the numerator—the difference. If it is small and unimportant, then we really do not care that we have not reached statistical significance. Effectively, the difference does not matter to us. If the difference is large enough

to be important, but *t* is too low for significance, then examine the denominator. Is the large variability due to inhomogeneity that can be reduced? Is it due to a non-normal distribution that can be normalized? Is it practical (cost, time, manpower) to increase sample size? If none of these remedies is possible, it may be possible to do a nonparametric analysis (see below). Failure to reject the null hypothesis does not mean that the difference was zero, but merely that you have not proved it is not.

11. The one outlier should have been picked up before the analysis was done. Why did 9/10 rats gain more weight on raw peanuts whereas 1 rat not only lost weight, but lost a great deal of weight? Was there an error in weighing or entering the data? Perhaps whoever weighed that rat misread the scale. Did that rat differ in any way? Rats can get pneumonia or tuberculosis, and if that rat was ill it was not validly a member of the group. The effect of removing the outlying pair from Table 22.1 is shown in Figure 22.3.

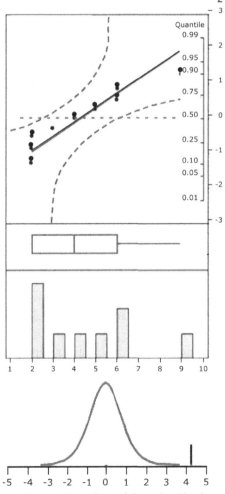

Figure 22.3 Upper panel: quantile plot. Second panel: box plot. Third panel: histogram. Fourth panel: t-test for the nine paired observations.

Removing the outlier has changed the mean difference from 2 to 4.33, standard deviation from 7.72 to 2.40, standard deviation of the mean from 2.44 to 0.80, and t from 0.82 to 5.42. That is, the mean difference is now 5.42 standard deviations of the mean from a hypothesized mean of 0, and this would happen with a probability of only 0.00006. The 95% confidence limits become $4.33 \pm 0.80 \times 2.306 = 2.49$ to 6.17. These limits do not include 0, confirming the statistical significance of the test.

12. If t is significant, it does not matter if the distribution was not normal. Uninformed reviewers often make this error. In fact, if t is significant under these circumstances, it would be even more statistically significant if the distribution were made more normal.

13. Because the normal curve is symmetrical, the tails of the curve that suggest that the null hypothesis can be rejected contain equal areas. If the null hypothesis is true, there is only a 0.025 (2.5%) probability that the sample mean will lie more than $t_{0.05} \, s_{\overline{X}}$ above the mean and another 0.025 probability that it will lie less than $t_{0.05} \, s_{\overline{X}}$ below the mean. The two probabilities together add up to 0.05. Whether to use two areas or only one area depends upon the alternative hypothesis H_A. Remember that if the null hypothesis H_O is rejected, an alternative hypothesis has to be accepted. There are three alternative hypotheses:

$$H_A : \overline{X} \neq \mu;$$

$$H_A : \overline{X} > \mu;$$

$$H_A : \overline{X} < \mu.$$

The first hypothesis states that an excessive deviation from $\mu = 0$ in either direction will lead to rejection of the null hypothesis, the second states that a mean significantly above $\mu = 0$ will lead to rejection of the null hypothesis, and the third states that a mean significantly below $\mu = 0$ will lead to rejection of the null hypothesis. The first is known as the two-tailed test, and the other two each as a one-tailed test. Because the area in a one-tailed test is half that of a two-tailed test, a given value of t will give a probability for a one-tailed test that is half that of a two-tailed test, for example, 0.025 instead of 0.05. It is thus easier to achieve statistical significance for a one-tailed than for a two-tailed test.

When is a one-tailed test permissible? The answer depends in part on what we are looking for. In the raw versus roasted peanut experiment, we might have had no prior guesses as to how the results would turn out, so that a two-tailed test would be appropriate. However, even if we had expected raw peanuts to be better, they could have turned out to be worse. Some proposed treatments are actually harmful, not helpful. Therefore, a two-tailed test is appropriate. An example of how predictions can be wrong can be found by examining the CAST trial (CAST, 1989; Ruskin, 1989). The drug flecainide had been shown to be useful in treating and preventing ventricular arrhythmias in experimental animals and in some humans with a normal myocardium, and was being used extensively in clinical practice to treat ventricular arrhythmias in patients after myocardial infarction. To investigate further and to legitimize an accepted practice, the CAST trial randomized patients to a control group or one of several newer antiar-rhythmic agents, including flecainide. An interim analysis after about one-third of the patients had been admitted to the study showed to everyone's dismay that four times as many patients had died in the flecainide arm than the control arm of the study. The study was abruptly halted.

One-tailed tests are occasionally used. If a peanut producer is testing the growth potential of a new species of peanut, there is interest in producing it commercially only if it is better than the standard type. Therefore, the manufacturer is interested only in a mean growth potential greater than the standard, that is, only in the upper tail. Remember that, it is easier to show significance in a one- than a two-tailed test, because to exceed 5% of the area under the curve in one direction takes a smaller devi-ation from the zero population mean. For example, in a two-tailed test with $N = 10$, the value of t that corresponds to 0.025 of the area under the curve for a total of 0.05 for both tails is 2.262, but for 0.05 in one tail is 1.833 (See Figure 22.4).

There is little use for one-tailed tests in biology or medicine. We can never be sure that an adverse response might not occur, and so should consider a deviation in either direction. There is no justification for using a one-tailed rather than a two-tailed test sim-ply because it is easier to show significance. It may, however, be used when only one alternative hypothesis is of interest, for example, the new treatment will be used only if it does not cause harm. If it is, the decision to use a one-tailed test must be made before the experiment is done to avoid unconscious bias.

14. Although most two-sided tests are symmetrical, with 2.5% of the area under the curve more than 1.96 σ above and below the mean, this is not an absolute

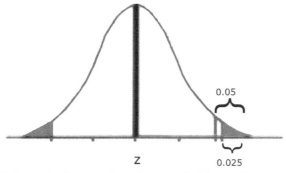

Figure 22.4 The shaded areas in the two tails make up 0.05 of the total area under the curve, as does the area in the upper tail demarcated by the left of the two lines. The second line is closer to the mean, so that for a given value of α, a smaller value of t is needed for a one-tailed test than a two-tailed test.

requirement. A statistical test provides support for a decision, and decisions have consequences. Blind adherence to a standard method may not be effective. As discussed in detail by Moyé (2000), there are times when there is more concern for H_A: $\overline{X} < \mu$ than for H_A: $\overline{X} > \mu$. As an example, he discusses testing a new treatment for diabetes mellitus. There is a current standard treatment that is effective in reducing the risk of cardiovascular disease, and its harmful side effects are uncommon and readily recognized and dealt with. A new treatment is proposed and tested. The investigator might be more concerned with an increase in harmful side effects than in an improvement in treatment effect. If in the planning stage the investigator has decided to make the critical value of the Type I error α 0.05, the decision could be made to apportion 0.03 to the tail that indicates harm and 0.02 to the tail that indicates benefit. The decision then is to reject the null hypothesis in favor of harm if $t \leq -1.88$, and in favor of benefit if $t \geq 2.05$. This concept applies to unpaired t-tests, and to significance tests in general.

There is no reason not to do the test as usual, and then interpret the observed t value differently for the two alternative hypotheses.

15. The P value of a test such as the t-test has a composite origin, depending as it does on the observed difference (effect size), sample size, sample variability, and by implication the shape of the distribution and the presence or absence of outliers.

Sample Size for Paired Test

To determine what sample size is needed to show significance in any paired experiment, we have to specify the standard deviation of the data, usually taken from similar experiments or a pilot study, the effect size (difference from zero) that is required, and the designated value of α, usually 0.05 or 0.01. Sample size may be calculated online at http://www.stat.ubc.ca/~rollin/stats/ssize/n2.html, http://www.dssresearch.com, http://www.maths.surrey.ac.uk/cgi-bin/stats/sample/twomean.cgi, and http://www.sample-size.net.

Unpaired t-Test

To compare two unmatched groups, use an unpaired t-test. The numbers in the two groups may be different, but even if they are the same a paired test cannot be done unless pairing is justified.

Return to the data shown in Table 22.1, and assume that the experiment compared two separate groups of young rats, one group fed with added raw peanuts, the other with added roasted peanuts. No pairing is done. To do the required calculations, first calculate the mean and standard deviation for each group. These values for the means are: Raw 57.9 g, Roasted 55.9 g, and for the standard deviations are: Raw 5.59 g and Roasted 4.75 g.

The t ratio then becomes the difference between the means divided by the measure of variability. The variability is, however, derived from two separate variabilities, one for each group. The variability of the difference between two groups is greater than either one alone, because we have to allow for one mean being unusually low and the other unusually high. To calculate the combined variability, calculate a common or pooled variance s_p^2 that is the weighted average of the two variances (Chapter 3). This can be calculated as $s_p^2 = \frac{\sum (X_{1i}-\overline{X}_1)^2 + \sum (X_{2i}-\overline{X}_2)^2}{N_1+N_2}$.

Then the standard deviation of the difference between two means is

$$S_{\overline{X}_1-\overline{X}_2} = \sqrt{\frac{s_p^2}{N_1} + \frac{s_p^2}{N_2}}.$$

(This formula implies no correlation between the members of the two groups. If there is correlation, the formula needs to be modified.)

Therefore, $t = \dfrac{\overline{X}_1-\overline{X}_2}{\sqrt{\left(\frac{s_p^2}{N_1} + \frac{s_p^2}{N_2}\right)}}$.

(Strictly speaking, the numerator should be $\left|\overline{X}_1 - \overline{X}_2\right| - \mu$, because the hypothesis is that the difference between the two means is not significantly different from the population mean difference of zero. It is simpler to omit μ from the formula.)

The value obtained for t is tested against $N - 2$ df, because two groups are involved.

For the data in Table 22.1, the difference between the means is 2. The argument is that if in the long run there is no difference between the means of the two groups, then the mean difference will be zero. If this null hypothesis is true, how often will a difference of 2 arise? The way to determine this is to relate the difference between the means to a measure of variability. If variability is such that a difference of 2 can arise frequently, then we will not reject the null hypothesis. If, however, a difference is unlikely to occur with that population, then we can reject the null hypothesis. For the data in Table 22.1 tested as an unpaired experiment, $t = \frac{2}{2.32} = 0.8621$, df $= 18$, and P $= 0.40$. About 40% of the time if we drew two samples with $N = 10$ from this population, the means would differ by 2 or more. We therefore do not reject the null hypothesis.

The unpaired t-test can be done online at http://www.graphpad.com/quickcalcs/ttest1.cfm, http://www.usablestats.com/calcs/2samplet, and http://easycalculation.com/statistics/ttest-calculator.php.

Problem 22.2

Reanalyze the peak flow rate data as if they were two different groups of subjects. How do the results differ from a paired test on the same data? Explain why the results are so different.

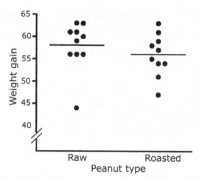

Figure 22.5 Distribution of data from raw peanuts (left) and roasted peanuts (right).

Requirements for unpaired t-test:

1. First consider if the data meet the requirements for an unpaired t-test. Two of these are similar to the requirements for a paired test, namely that the numbers are ratio numbers and each distribution is normal. As seen in Figure 22.5, the second requirement has not been met, but for the moment ignore that.

   Another requirement not needed for the paired test is that the variances should be similar in the two data sets. The way of determining this will be described later.

2. Once again, the 44 g weight gain for the rat fed raw peanuts in the 10th pair is unduly low. Exclude this measurement and repeat the unpaired t-test with 9 in the raw group and 10 in the roasted group. The means become 59.44 g (raw) and 55.90 g (roasted), with respective standard deviations of 2.88 and 4.74, respectively. Now $t = 1.939$ with 17 df, and $P = 0.0693$. The P value for rejecting the null hypothesis is much bigger than when the paired test was done—0.0693 versus 0.0006—attesting to the greater sensitivity of the paired test *provided it is legitimate to do it*.

3. The remaining considerations about importance versus significance, how to interpret the numerator and the denominator, and what to do about a nonsignificant P value are the same as for the paired test.

   We always need to ask if the observed difference, whether significant or not, is important. This is a value judgment made by workers in that field who ought to know if a difference of 3.54 g weight gain is important. It is possible to quantitate this difference by assessing what contribution the diet makes to total variability. If we take the total variability of the 19 weight gains (excluding the aberrant value), we can ask how much this is reduced if we allow for differences due to the diet. This subject will be taken up more fully in Chapter 25 on ANOVA, but we can estimate the relative reduction, termed ω^2, as (Hays, 1973)

$$\omega^2 = \frac{t^2 - 1}{t^2 + N_1 + N_2 - 1}.$$

Thus for the unpaired peanut data,

$$\omega^2 = \frac{1.939^2 - 1}{1.939^2 + 10 + 9 - 1} = 0.1268$$

which can be interpreted as showing that about 13% of the variability of weight gains can be accounted for by differences in diet.

Unequal Variances

The logic of the t-test requires a pooled variance from the two groups with comparable variances as a way of obtaining a more representative variance from a larger total sample. If the variances are very different, then their weighted average represents neither sample, with the potential for distorting the value for the standard deviation of the mean that is the denominator for the t-test. If the sample sizes and the variances are very different, the smaller sample has a disproportionate effect on the pooled value because we are dividing by the square root of N. To test the hypothesis of equal variances, divide the larger variance by the smaller variance to obtain the variance ratio termed F (Chapter 8). This will be discussed fully in the Chapter 25 on Analysis of Variance. Suffice it to state that it is possible to determine whether the observed F ratio is far enough removed from the population ratio of 1 that the hypothesis of equal variances can be rejected.

If the variances are significantly different, use a modified t-test or a non-parametric test. If a nonparametric test, it should not be the Mann–Whitney U test (see below) because if the group variances are very different, Type I error rates may be too high or too low; if too low, the risk of inflating the Type II error is increased (Kasuya, 2001; Neuhäuser, 2002; Ruxton, 2006). Modified t-tests appear in statistics programs as the Welch or the Satterthwaite test, the latter being preferable. In both tests, first determine the ratio d (analogous to t) by

$$d = \frac{\overline{X_1} - \overline{X_2}}{\sqrt{\frac{s_1^2}{N_1} + \frac{s_2^2}{N_2}}}.$$

In the Welch test, the value d is assessed by a distribution that depends on the values for the F ratio $\frac{s_1^2}{s_2^2}$, N_1, and N_2, as determined by tables (see Pearson and Hartley, 1966) or provided by the computer program. It may be performed online at http://www.graphpad.com/quickcalcs/ttest1.cfm.

The Satterthwaite method uses the same value of d, but uses the t distribution with the df being not $N_1 + N_2 - 2$ but rather

$$\nu = \frac{\left(\frac{s_1^2}{N_1} + \frac{s_2^2}{N_2}\right)^2}{\frac{\left(\frac{s_1^2}{N_1}\right)^2}{N_1 - 1} - \frac{\left(\frac{s_2^2}{N_2}\right)^2}{N_2 - 1}}.$$

Because this will usually not be an integer, the next smallest integer is used. There is no need to compare the two variances before doing the test, and many authorities prefer to perform the test routinely.

As an example, return to the peanut data tested in unpaired groups. The two means are 57.9 and 55.9, and the variances are 31.21 and 22.48, with $N = 10$ in each group. Then d becomes

$$d = \frac{57.9 - 55.9}{\sqrt{\left(\frac{31.21}{9} + \frac{22.48}{9}\right)}} = \frac{2}{2.44} = 0.82 \text{ (as before)}.$$

$$\nu = \frac{\left(\frac{31.21}{10} + \frac{22.48}{10}\right)^2}{\frac{\left(\frac{31.21}{10}\right)^2}{9} - \frac{\left(\frac{22.48}{10}\right)^2}{9}} = \frac{28.83}{1.08 + 0.56} = 17.57 \text{ and so } P = 0.40.$$

The probability of rejecting the null hypothesis of 0.40 is not very different from the value of 0.43 obtained when the differences between the variances were ignored. That is because these two variances are not significantly different; the one aberrant measurement had more effect on the mean difference than on the variances. Some online tests provide the option for using unequal variances: http://studentsttest.com/, http://in-silico.net/statistics/ttest, http://graphpad.com/quickcalcs/ttest1.cfm, http://vassarstats.net/, and http://www.quantitativeskills.com/sisa/statistics/t-test.htm.

In general, the t-test is robust and tolerates moderate departures from the basic requirements. Nonnormality of the distribution is more serious than differences in variances, and it is worse to have the larger variance associated with the smaller group than with the larger group. Finally, lack of normality or inequality of variances is much worse for small than large samples, and, if practical, samples with over 15 in each group are needed to minimize Type I errors (Ramsey, 1980). In addition, nonnormality and unequal variances greatly diminish the power of the t-test (Rosner, 1995).

Sample Size for Unpaired Test

Arguments similar to those used in Chapter 11 apply to the two-sample t-test. Online calculations may be done at http://www.stat.ubc.ca/~rollin/stats/ssize/n2.html, http://www.graphpad.com/quickcalcs/ttest1.cfm, http://www.danielsoper.com/statcalc3/calc.aspx?id=47, and http://www.sample-size.net.

Conclusion

Statistical testing is valuable in emphasizing the variability of the measurements. We can cautiously draw conclusions from the tests as long as we use them in support of reasonable biological hypotheses, allow for the possibility of Type II errors, and make sure that any experiment has sufficient power to allow sensible conclusions to be drawn. This does not mean that we discard unexpected results, but merely that these need stronger confirmation.

Nonparametric or Distribution Free Tests

Parametric tests such as the t–test lose efficiency, sometimes drastically, when the distributions are severely nonnormal because of skewing, outliers, kurtosis, or grossly unequal variances. They can be replaced by several robust tests that are referred to as distribution free or nonparametric tests. The two tests to be described below, when applied to normal distributions, are very efficient. The relative efficiency of two tests is determined by the ratio of the sample sizes needed to achieve the same power for a given significance level and a given difference from the null hypothesis (Healy, 1994). When the two distributions are normal, the distribution free tests are about 95% as efficient as the t–test (Wilcox, 1996; Siegal and Castellan, 1988). When the distributions are grossly abnormal, then the distribution free tests have greater efficiency. The main nonparametric test to replace the paired t–test is the Wilcoxon-signed rank test, and the major replacement for the unpaired t–test is the Mann—Whitney U test.

The Wilcoxon-Signed Rank Test

As for the paired t–test, the paired values for each group are set out, and the difference between each pair is calculated. Then these differences are ranked from the smallest (1) to the biggest (N), ignoring the sign of the difference; **differences of zero are not ranked**. Any tied ranks are averaged. Once the ranking has been done, the negative signs are put back, and the sums of the negative and the positive ranks are calculated.

The basic theory is that if the paired sets are drawn from the same population, then there will be some small, some medium, and some large positive differences, and approximately the same number of small, medium, and large negative differences. Therefore, the sums of the negative and positive ranks should be about the same. If we can calculate the sampling distribution of T, the smaller of these two sums (positive vs negative) for any value of N, then we can determine if one of those sums is so much smaller than the other that the null hypothesis should be rejected. Although the test is part of statistical computer packages, an example to illustrate the principle is shown in Table 22.2.

The three smallest differences are each 2. Because these account for the first 3 ranks, in the fourth column average them $\frac{1+2+3}{3}$ and assign each a rank of 2. The next value, 3, occupies the next rank, the fourth rank. Similarly the two 6 differences occupy ranks 7 and 8, but being equal are each assigned a rank of 7.5. The fifth column shows the same ranks, but now the positive and negative ranks are identified. The sums of the positive and negative ranks are different. If the null hypothesis were true, the two sums should be similar. Calculations or tables show that the probability of such a

Table 22.2 Wilcoxon-signed rank test used for paired peanut data

Raw peanuts R	Roasted peanuts P	Difference D	Rank	Signed rank
61	55	6	7.5	+7.5
60	54	6	7.5	+7.5
56	47	9	9	+9
63	59	4	5	+5
56	51	5	6	+6
63	61	2	2	+2
59	57	2	2	+2
56	54	2	2	+2
44	63	−19	10	−10
61	58	3	4	+4
		$\Sigma X_i = 20$ $\overline{X_D} = 2$		$\Sigma+ = 45$ $\Sigma- = 10$

difference in signed rank sums based on listing all the possible combinations of the signed ranks for the sample size studied is 0.082. This is not at the conventional level of statistical significance, but is much closer to it than the probability of 0.43 obtained by the paired test. If the Wilcoxon test is done for the nine pairs after excluding the one aberrant pair, the probability from the Wilcoxon test is 0.0039, not as striking as the 0.0006 from the paired t-test but still a good reason to reject the null hypothesis.

The Wilcoxon-signed rank test does not give any result if N is ≤ 5.

If the number of pairs is >10, T approximates a normal distribution and we do not need special tables to test the null hypothesis. Because the sum of the first N numbers is $\frac{N(N+1)}{2}$, if the sums of the negative and positive ranks were equal, each would be $\frac{N(N+1)}{4}$. Therefore, test the difference between the observed and expected value of T $\left(T - \frac{N(N+1)}{4}\right)$ by dividing by the standard deviation of T

$$\sigma_T = \sqrt{\frac{N(N-1)(2N+1)}{24}}$$

Therefore, use the z table to test.

$$z = \frac{T - \frac{N(N+1)}{4}}{\sqrt{\frac{N(N-1)(2N+1)}{24}}}$$

Pratt (1959) pointed out that ignoring the zeros may produce paradoxical probabilities, and proposed ranking the differences including the zeros, then dropping the zeros when summing the negative and positive ranks, and using the tables of probabilities for the total number of observations, including the zeros.

Online calculations can be done at http://www.socscistatistics.com/tests/signedranks/ Default2.aspx, http://www.sdmproject.com/utilities/?show=Wilcoxon, and http:// vassarstats.net/wilcoxon.html.

Problem 22.3

Perform a Wilcoxon test on the data from Problem 22.1.

The Sign Test

This is a simpler and less powerful version of the Wilcoxon test. It is used when the data are ordinal or nominal (or categorical). For example, 11 observers rate two different bacteriological stains A and B for clarity. Each observer records a preference: if A is better than B, the result is +, and if B is better than A, the result is −. On the null hypothesis that there is no difference between the two stains, there should be as many negative results as positive results. If there are more of one sign than the other, then the departure from the null hypothesis can be tested using the binomial distribution for $p = 0.5$. Hypothetical data are presented in Table 22.3.

The results show a preference for A in 9 out of 11 trials. On the null hypothesis of no difference between the stains we expect 5 or 6. The question then is to determine if 9 is an unusual event if the null hypothesis is true. To see how this decision is reached, examine Figure 22.6.

Adding 9, 10, and 11 together gives a probability of 0.0328, and we would probably reject the null hypothesis. This is the probability of one tail of the distribution. However, a finding of 0, 1, or 2 would also lead to a rejection of the null hypothesis. Because the designation of + or − is arbitrary, finding either 0, 1, 2, 9, 10, or 11 + would occur with a probability of $2 \times 0.0328 = 0.0656$. This is still evidence against the null hypothesis, although not quite as strong.

Table 22.3 Sign test

Observer	Result
1	+
2	+
3	−
4	+
5	+
6	+
7	−
8	+
9	+
10	+
11	+

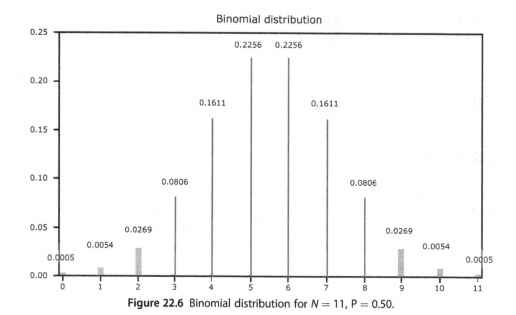

Figure 22.6 Binomial distribution for $N = 11$, $P = 0.50$.

Using this test in place of the Wilcoxon-signed rank test loses the information provided by the size of the differences and so produces a less powerful test. The test can be done easily with online programs http://www.graphpad.com/quickcalcs/binomial1.cfm, and http://www.fon.hum.uva.nl/Service/Statistics/Sign_Test.html.

The Mann–Whitney U Test

In 1945, Wilcoxon developed a ranking test for comparing the positions of two distributions; he called the statistic T that was the sum of the ranks in the smaller group. Two years later, Mann and Whitney extended the theory and they called their statistic U. The two statistics are interconvertible.

$$U = N_1 N_2 - \frac{1}{2} N_1 (N_1 + 1) - T$$

Requirements

1. Each sample is drawn at random from its own population.
2. The values are independent of each other within each sample, and the two samples are independent of each other.
3. The measurement scale is at least ordinal.

The test can be done easily. Consider two groups, A with n_1 members and B with n_2 members, each drawn at random from the same distribution. Because the two sets of measurements come from the same distribution, pool them into a single set and then rank them from the smallest, with a rank of 1, to the largest with a rank of $n_1 + n_2$. Then add up the ranks in each group separately. Intuitively, each group should have similar proportions of low ranks, medium-sized ranks, and high ranks, so that if n_1 and n_2 are equal the sums of the ranks in the two groups should be equal or nearly so. If n_2 is twice as big as n_1, for example, then the sum of the ranks of n_2 should be about twice as large as the sum of ranks from n_1. The more the sums of ranks in the two groups differ from the expected proportion, the less likely is it that the null hypothesis that they come from the same distribution is true. The possible combinations can be enumerated and the probability of any discrepancy between the sums in the two data sets can be ascertained.

The critical values of rank sums for possible combinations of n_1 and n_2 have been calculated, are given in standard tables, and are available in standard computer programs.

If N is >20 in either group use the normal approximation

$$z = \frac{U - \frac{N_1 N_2}{2}}{\sqrt{\frac{N_1 N_2 (N_1 + N_2 + 1)}{12}}}.$$

This test is available in computer programs, but an example will clarify the method (Table 22.4).

The probability of such a discrepancy is 0.2240, and suggests that we cannot reject the null hypothesis. For the unpaired t-test, the probability of rejecting the null hypothesis was 0.4336. The Mann–Whitney test is closer to rejecting the null hypothesis.

When two or more values are tied, the sum of ranks is modified by averaging the tied ranks. For example, the fourth and fifth measurements are each 54, so allocate them each a rank of 4.5. (If the tied measurements are in the same group, it does not matter if we average their ranks or not, because the sum of ranks 4 and 5 is the same as the sum of ranks 4.5 and 4.5. If the tied ranks are in different groups, then the ranks must be averaged.) Average all the sets of tied measurements. The value of T is usually corrected for ties

Table 22.4 Mann–Whitney test using peanut data

Raw peanuts R	Rank R	Roasted peanuts P	Rank P
61	16	55	6
60	14	54	4.5
56	8	47	2
63	19	59	12.5
56	8	51	3
63	19	61	16
59	12.5	57	10
56	8	54	4.5
44	1	63	19
61	16	58	11
	$\Sigma R = 121.5$		$\Sigma P = 88.5$

but the correction factor is usually unimportant; there are several types of correction possible (Conover, 1980; Krauth, 1988; Rosner, 1995). The whole test can be done online at http://www.socscistatistics.com/tests/mannwhitney/Default2.aspx, http://www.wessa.net/rwasp_Reddy-Moores%20Wilcoxon%20Mann-Witney%20Test.wasp, and http://vassarstats.net/utest.html. A clear description of how these tests are derived and used appears in several publications (LaVange and Koch, 2006; Noether, 1976; Bland, 1995).

Problem 22.4

Perform a Mann–Whitney test on the data from Problem 22.1.

ADVANCED CONCEPTS

Comparing Two Coefficients of Variation

Sometimes we are interested in comparing the coefficients of variation of two groups. This can be done in two ways. If the logarithms of the data are normally distributed, then the ratio

$$F = \frac{s^2_{\log X_1}}{s^2_{\log X_2}}$$

can be evaluated from standard F tables. If the data are normally distributed, however, their logarithms will not be normally distributed, so use

$$Z = \frac{CV_1 - CV_2}{\sqrt{\left(\frac{CV_p^2}{N_1 - 1} + \frac{CV_p^2}{N_2 - 1}\right)\left(0.5 + CV_p^2\right)}},$$

where $CV_p = \frac{CV_1(N_1 - 1) + CV_2(N_2 - 1)}{N_1 + N_2 - 1}$ is the weighted mean of the two coefficients of variation CV_i (Zar, 2010).

The Paired t-Test Implies an Additive Model

The paired t-test implies the model

$$X_{i2} = X_{i1} + \alpha + \varepsilon_i \text{ or } X_{i2} - X_{i1} = \alpha + \varepsilon$$

where X_{i1} and X_{i2} are the two members of each pair, α is the mean difference between them (the effect of the treatment), and ε_i is the error associated with each difference. On the other hand, in any given study the relationship might be multiplicative:

$$X_{i2} = \alpha X_{i1} + \varepsilon_i.$$

In this model, the effect of the treatment is to increase each value for X by a factor α. The difference between these two models is unimportant if all the X_i values are close together, but assumes importance if X_i varies widely. For example, Table 22.5 shows data based on hypothetical norepinephrine concentrations (pg/ml) before and after dialysis.

The initial data are in the first column, and the final values for the additive model are in the second column. The differences between the two are similar for each pair (column 3), with a mean difference of 31.11 and a narrow standard deviation; it is reasonable to reject the null hypothesis that this difference is not significantly different from a mean difference of zero. If we postulate a multiplicative model with about a 10% decrease, as shown in column 5, then the actual decreases vary widely, with a mean of 36.22 but a standard deviation of 32.03, which suggests a skewed distribution as well as a difficulty in rejecting the null hypothesis. On the other hand, taking the ratio of the two gave a mean of 0.896 with a very small standard deviation and standard error, making it easier to reject the null hypothesis that the ratio was 1.

Motulsky (2009) recommended that instead of setting out the data to display proportional differences, as shown in Table 22.5, the two members of the pair should be set out as a ratio of $\frac{treated}{control}$. The disadvantage to working with ratios is that they are asymmetric; below 1 the range can be only from 1 to 0, where above 1 the ratio can in theory be

Table 22.5 Effects of additive and multiplicative models

		Fixed additive model		Fixed multiplicative model		
Initial	Final	Fixed difference	Final proportional difference	Proportional % difference	Actual difference	Final/ initial ratio
1	2	3	4	5	6	7
847	817	30	762	10	85	0.90
794	766	28	699	12	95	0.88
439	400	39	399	9	40	0.91
254	220	34	231	9	23	0.91
245	218	27	218	11	27	0.89
174	143	31	151	13	23	0.87
140	112	28	129	8	11	0.92
119	87	32	105	12	14	0.88
81	50	31	73	10	8	0.90
		Mean 31.11 sd 3.69 se 1.23		Mean 10.44	Mean 36.22 sd 32.03 se 10.68	Mean 0.896 sd 0.017 se 0.0056

any value >1. To overcome this, he recommended using the logarithms of the ratios. A zero value means no change, a negative value means a decrease, and a positive value means an increase. If this is done for the initial and final data in Table 22.6, the results in the final column are reproduced, and are interpreted as showing that the ratio is significantly below 1 so that there has been a consistent decrease from initial to final measurements.

Confidence Limits for Medians

We usually perform nonparametric tests either for ordinal data or for nonnormally distributed ratio numbers. For the latter, the descriptive summaries include the median. Sometimes we may want to determine the confidence limits for the median, or the difference between two medians. Gardner and Altman (1995) describe a conservative method for these calculations.

The $100(1-\alpha)\%$ confidence interval for the population interval requires calculating the lower (R_L) and upper (R_U) ranks, assuming the data are arranged in order from smallest to largest:

$$R_L = \frac{N}{2} - \left(z_{1-\alpha/2} \sqrt{\frac{N}{2}} \right)$$

$$R_U = 1 + \frac{N}{2} + \left(z_{1-\alpha/2} \sqrt{\frac{N}{2}} \right).$$

For the data presented in Tables 3.3, 3.4, and 3.16, there were $N = 53$ measurements. Then for 95% confidence limits,

$$R_L = \frac{53}{2} - \left(1.96 \sqrt{\frac{53}{2}} \right) = 16.4$$

$$R_U = 1 + \frac{53}{2} + \left(1.96 \sqrt{\frac{53}{2}} \right) = 37.6.$$

Return to the array of measurements and locate the 16th and the 38th measurements as the nearest integers. These are 1.18 and 1.32, which are the required limits of the median.

To set limits for a percentile, modify the above equation to

$$R_L = N_p - \left(1.96 \sqrt{N_p(1 - p)} \right)$$

$$R_U = 1 + N_p + \left(1.96 \sqrt{N_p(1 - p)} \right),$$

where p is the percentile. Thus for the 75th percentile, $p = 0.75$, and the 95% confidence limits are

$$R_L = 53 \times 0.75 - \left(1.96\sqrt{53 \times 0.75(1 - 0.75)}\right) = 33.6$$

$$R_U = 1 + 53 \times 0.75 + \left(1.96\sqrt{53 \times 0.75(1 - 0.75)}\right) = 46.93.$$

The measurements corresponding to ranks 34 and 47 are 1.20 and 1.53, respectively.

Online calculations can be performed at http://www.mountaingoatsoftware.com/tools/velocity-range-calculator.

Calculating the confidence limits of the difference between two medians is not often wanted, but can be done by the bootstrap technique (Chapter 37) or by the online program at http://www.wessa.net/rwasp_bootstrapplot1.wasp.

Ranking Transforms

If the measurements in the two groups are ranked but then a classical parametric t-test is done on the ranks, a robust test results that can be used for abnormal distributions (Iman, 1974). This approach is supported by Healy (1994).

The Meaning of the Mann–Whitney Test

An issue that causes confusion is what the Mann–Whitney test indicates. Because the measurements have been turned into ranks, the test cannot allow us to compare the means of the two distributions. Does it compare medians? Consider two groups A and B of equal size with the following measurements (Table 22.6):

The sum of ranks for group A is $1 + 2 + 3 + 10 + 11 + 12 = 39$, and the sum of ranks for B is $4 + 5 + 6 + 7 + 8 + 9 = 39$. The null hypothesis of equality of the sums of ranks of the two groups is obvious, but what is equal? The median of group A is 8.55 and the median of group B is 7.85. These are fairly close to each other. If, however, we make the three largest measurements in group A 127, 158, and 192, the sums of ranks are unaltered, but the median of group A becomes 65.7, much greater than the median of group B. Therefore, the test does not compare medians, although with less dispersed distributions it does serve this purpose. What the test actually does is to compare the equality of mean ranks, and thus, by inference, of the distributions. However, like all tests it must not be used without thought, as the example above shows. Many texts point

Table 22.6 Two distributions compared

A: 1.3, 2.7, 4.4,		12.7, 15.8, 19.2
B:	5.9, 7.0, 7.2, 8.5, 9.0, 11.4	

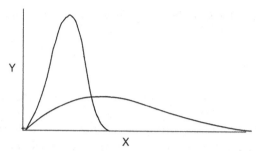

Figure 22.7 Comparison between two distributions.

out that the Mann–Whitney test is most useful when the only difference between the two groups is a measure of location. More formally, that the unspecified distributions of two groups X and Y differ only in location, such that $X = Y + d$, where d is a constant. This may be true for some distributions, but not for others. For example, Healy (1994) has pointed out that many biochemical and endocrine distributions share a common start, for example, a low or zero value, but then the control and experimental groups differ in shape (Figure 22.7).

Under these circumstances, the curves differ by more than location.

APPENDIX

1. Often a publication provides the data as the mean $(\overline{X})$, standard deviation (s), and number of observations (N), but does not give the individual measurements. You may want to perform an unpaired t-test that compares your own data set with the published data, but how can you do this without having all the data? Let us assume that the published data for cerebral arterial pulsatility in normal neonates has mean 34.3, standard deviation 4.1, and 37 observations. Your own data in neonates with heart disease have values of 51.6, 9.2, and 22, respectively.

To calculate t we need the differences between the two means, which we have, and the standard deviation of that difference which we need to obtain. To derive the required values, you can make use of known relationships:

a. $s^2 = \dfrac{\sum (X_i - \overline{X})^2}{N-1}$ and so $\sum (X_i - \overline{X})^2 = (N-1)s^2$ (Columns 3 and 6 below)

b. Then the pooled variance can be calculated from Eqn (19.13), using total in column 7: $s_p^2 = \dfrac{2382.57}{57} = 41.80$

1	2	3	4	5	6	7
Group	N	N − 1	$\overline{X}$	s	s^2	$(N - 1)s^2$
1	37	36	34.3	4.1	16.81	605.16
2	22	21	51.6	9.2	84.64	1777.44
Total	59	57	Difference = 17.3			2382.6

Based on these calculations,

$$s_{\overline{X_1} - \overline{X_2}} = \sqrt{\frac{41.8}{37} + \frac{41.8}{22}} = 1.74, \text{ and}$$

$$t = \frac{51.6 - 34.3}{1.74} = 9.94. \text{ Degrees of freedom } 57, \text{ P} < 0.0001.$$

As you will realize, this simple arithmetic can be automated, and it can be obtained by entering the means, standard deviations, and number of measurements in a computer program. A simple online program can be obtained at http://graphpad.com/quickcalcs/ttest1.cfm?Format=SD. Should you wish to calculate values for $\sum X_i$, multiply the mean by N, and to obtain $\sum X_i^2$ just add $\frac{\left(\sum x_i\right)^2}{N}$ to $(N-1)s^2$.

Problem 22.5

To make sure that you understand the unpaired t-test, try the following problem, and then check the results with the online application.

Group	Number	Mean	Standard Deviation
1	197	14.7	2.9
2	39	19.3	3.3

You should get $t = 6.92$.

REFERENCES

Bland, M., 1995. An Introduction to Medical Statistics. Oxford University Pess, Oxford.

CAST, 1989. Preliminary report: effect of encainide and flecainide on mortality in a randomized trial of arrhythmia suppression after myocardial infarction. The Cardiac Arrhythmia Suppression Trial (CAST) investigators. N. Engl. J. Med. 321, 406−412.

Conover, W.J., 1980. Practical Nonparametric Statistics. John Wiley & Sons, New York.

Gardner, M.J., Altman, D.G., 1995. Statistics with Confidence—Confidence Intervals and Statistical Guidelines. British Medical Journal, London.

Hays, W.H., 1973. Statistics for the Social Sciences. Holt, Rinehart and Winston, Inc., New York.

Healy, M.J.R., 1994. Statistics from the Inside. 12. Non-normal data. Arch. Dis. Child. 70, 158−163.

Iman, R.L., 1974. Use of a t-statistic as an approximation to the exact distribution of the Wilcoxon signed ranks test statistic. Commun. Stat. 3, 795−806.

Kasuya, E., 2001. Mann−Whitney U test when variances are unequal. Anim. Behav. 61, 1247−1249.

Krauth, J., 1988. Distribution-free Statistics. An Application-oriented Approach. Elsevier, Amsterdam.

Lavange, L.M., Koch, G.G., 2006. Rank score tests. Circulation 114, 2528−2533.

Mitchell, H.H., Burroughs, W., Beadles, H.P., 1936. The significance and accuracy of biological values of proteins computed from nitrogen metabolism data. J. Nutr. 11, 257−274.

Motulsky, H.J., 2009. Statistical Principles: The Use and Abuse of Logarithmic Axes [Online]. Available: http://www.graphpad.com/faq/file/1487logaxes.pdf.

Moyé, L.A., 2000. Statistical Reasoning in Medicine. The Intuitive P-Value Primer. Springer-Verlag, New York.

Neuhäuser, M., 2002. Two-sample tests when variances are unequal. Anim. Behav. 63, 823−825.

Noether, G.E., 1976. Introduction to Statistics. A Nonparametric Approach. Houghton Miflin Co., Boston.

Pearson, E.S., Hartley, H.O., 1966. Biometrika Tables for Statisticians. Cambridge University Press, Cambridge.

Pratt, J.W., 1959. Remarks on zeros and ties on the Wilcoxon signed rank procedures. J. Stat. Assoc. 54, 655—667.

Ramsey, P.H., 1980. Exact type I error rates for robustness of student's t test with unequal variances. J. Educ. Stat. 5, 337—349.

Rosner, B., 1995. Fundamentals of Biostatistics. Duxbury Press, New York.

Ruskin, J.N., 1989. The cardiac arrhythmia suppression trial (CAST). N. Engl. J. Med. 321, 386—388.

Ruxton, G.D., 2006. The unequal variance t-test is an underused alternative to student's t-test and the Mann—Whitney U test. Behav. Ecol. 17, 688—690.

Siegal, S., Castellan Jr., N.J., 1988. Nonparametric Statistics for the Behavioral Sciences. McGraw-Hill, New York.

Wilcox, R.R., 1996. Statistics for the Social Sciences. Academic Press, San Diego.

Zar, J.H., 2010. Biostatistical Analysis. Prentice Hall, Upper Saddle River, NJ.

CHAPTER 23

t-Test Variants: Crossover Tests, Equivalence Tests

Contents

CROSSOVER TRIALS

The main requirement for a paired t-test is that if both members of the pair are given the same treatment, the results would on average be the same. One form of paired trial, often used, is to give some subjects treatment A, and then after a waiting period give the same subjects treatment B. The null hypothesis is that the two treatments have the same effect, and if we reject the null hypothesis there is some basis for concluding that one treatment is better than the other. An example might be giving a group of hypertensive subjects drug A for a few days, recording the change in blood pressure, and then a week later give the same subjects drug B for a few days to determine which drug caused the greater fall in pressure. For each subject there will be a pressure difference Δi. This difference would not be identical in each subject, and for each subject $\Delta i = \overline{\Delta} + \varepsilon_i$, where ε_i is the individual error term. These error terms have a mean of zero, and their variability allows the calculation of the standard deviation and standard error.

The concern with this design is that the effects of the first treatment might still be present when the second treatment is given. There might be residual blood levels of the drug, some receptors might still be occupied, psychological effects might alter responses, or some long-term physiological changes might have been caused. Some diseases get better or worse with time. If there is any such carryover effect, then any difference between treatments A and B is a function of a possible real effect of the drugs plus an unknown effect of time, and these cannot be separated. To solve some of these problems, the crossover design can be used, as described by Hills and Armitage, 1979.

Patients are randomized into two similar groups A and B: group A is given treatment X and group B is given treatment Y. One of the treatments can be a placebo. After an

For a list of all websites referred to in this chapter, as clickable links, see the book companion website: www.booksite.elsevier.com/9780128023877.

Biostatistics for Medical and Biomedical Practitioners
http://dx.doi.org/10.1016/B978-0-12-802387-7.00023-8

Table 23.1 Basic 2 × 2 crossover trial

Period	Group A	Group B
1	Treatment X Result Washout	Treatment Y Result Washout
2	Treatment Y Result	Treatment X Result

appropriate time to allow for washout of the effects of the treatment, the groups are reversed, so that group A gets treatment Y, and group B gets treatment X (Table 23.1).

The trial is designed to test two hypotheses: the mean values of treatments X and Y are significantly different, and there is no effect of time on the results. Among the assumptions required are similarity between patient groups, attained by randomization, and a response that is on average the same for the two periods on the same treatment; that is, the results of the treatments should not be affected by the order in which they were given (Brown, 1980; Hills and Armitage, 1979; Jones, 2008, 2010; Jones and Haughie, 2008; Jones and Kenward, 2003). For any given subject in group A, the response in period 1 is Y_1, and can be considered to be the sum of the fixed effect of the treatment T_X and a response that is due to the passage of time ε_{1A}. For that same subject, the response Y_2 in period 2 is $T_Y + \varepsilon_{2A}$. Similarly, a subject in the B group has responses in periods 1 and 2, respectively, $T_Y + \varepsilon_{1B}$ and $T_X + \varepsilon_{2B}$ (Table 23.2).

Table 23.2 Individual responses

Period	Group A subject	Group B subject
1	$Y_1 = T_X + \varepsilon_{1A}$	$Y_1 = T_Y + \varepsilon_{1B}$
2	$Y_2 = T_Y + \varepsilon_{2A}$	$Y_2 = T_X + \varepsilon_{2B}$

Based on the assumptions, the values of T_X and T_Y are fixed, but all the other values can change from subject to subject. The effect of treatment (the difference between X and Y) in a group A subject is determined from $d_A = Y_1 - Y_2 = (T_X - T_Y) + (\varepsilon_{1A} - \varepsilon_{2A})$, and in a group B subject it is $d_B = Y_2 - Y_1 = (T_X - T_Y) - (\varepsilon_{1B} - \varepsilon_{2B})$. If there is no effect of time, then the average values for $\varepsilon_{1A} - \varepsilon_{2A}$ and $\varepsilon_{1B} - \varepsilon_{2B}$ are zero; if there is an effect of time, then $\varepsilon_{1A} - \varepsilon_{2A} =$ some mean value δ, with standard error of $\frac{\sigma}{\sqrt{N_A}}$ for group A and $\frac{\sigma}{\sqrt{N_B}}$ for group B. Calculate the mean values for each group as $\overline{d_A}$ and $\overline{d_E}$, and then the average of the difference between these means is

$$\frac{\overline{d_A} - \overline{d_B}}{2} = \frac{\left\{\overline{(T_X - T_Y)_A} + \overline{(\varepsilon_1 - \varepsilon_2)_A}\right\} - \left\{\overline{(T_X - T_Y)_B} - \overline{(\varepsilon_1 - \varepsilon_2)_B}\right\}}{2}$$

$$= \frac{\left\{\overline{(\varepsilon_1 - \varepsilon_2)_A} + \overline{(\varepsilon_1 - \varepsilon_2)_B}\right\}}{2}$$

because the sums of $T_X - T_Y$ for each group cancel out. The standard error of this difference, as in the unpaired t-test, is $\frac{1}{2}\sqrt{\left(\frac{s_p^2}{N_A} + \frac{s_p^2}{N_B}\right)}$, and this can be used to determine whether it is possible to reject the hypothesis that $\overline{d_A} - \overline{d_B} = 0$, that is, that there is no average effect of time. If the null hypothesis is not rejected, then test the average effects of the two treatments as

$$\frac{\overline{d_A} + \overline{d_B}}{2} = \frac{\left\{\overline{(T_X - T_Y)_A} + \overline{(\varepsilon_1 - \varepsilon_2)_A}\right\} + \left\{\overline{(T_X - T_Y)_B} - \overline{(\varepsilon_1 - \varepsilon_2)_B}\right\}}{2}$$

$$= \frac{\overline{(T_X - T_Y)_A} + \overline{(T_X - T_Y)_B}}{2}$$

because time has been shown to have no effects. This difference is tested for significant difference from zero by the same standard error. An alternative set of calculations and a simple explanation are provided by Wellek and Blettner (2012).

If there is a significant effect of time, then it might not be useful to proceed with the analysis. Various alternatives have been proposed, but care is needed in applying them (Jones et al., 1996). Some designs include three or more periods, for example, group A is given three successive treatments X, Y, Y and group B is given treatments Y, X, X (Ebbutt, 1984; Jones and Haughie, 2008; Laska et al., 1983). If the second and third identical treatments in each group are similar, it is unlikely that there is a carryover effect from the first treatment. As an example, Ramsey et al. (1993) studied the effect of aerosolized tobramycin in treating patients with cystic fibrosis who had pneumocystis infection. Group I was given aerosolized tobramycin for 28 days, followed by aerosolized half-normal saline for two 28-day periods. Group II was given aerosolized half-normal saline, followed by two periods of aerosolized tobramycin. The primary outcomes were based on tests of forced vital capacity, forced expiratory volume (FEV), and forced expiratory flow (FEF). Approximate differences from control values of FEF are shown in Table 23.3.

Table 23.3 Three period crossover trial

	Period 1	Period 2	Period 3
Group I	Placebo	Tobramycin	Tobramycin
	−7	+5	+4
Group II	Tobramycin	Placebo	Placebo
	+8	+1	+2

As shown, the duplicate values in periods 2 and 3 are almost identical, suggesting no carryover from period 1 to period 2. In this study, however, there was carryover for FEV.

Crossover designs can have more groups and can deal with ordinal numbers or binary categories (Brown, 1980). What are the advantages of the crossover design? Using each subject as his or her own control minimizes variability as compared with a parallel design with two groups, just as a paired t-test has less variability than an unpaired test because it does not have to allow for differences among subjects. Therefore the total number of subjects is less, often considerably less, for the crossover design. This is particularly important when studying treatments for a rare disease. Furthermore, unlike the paired test at two different times, the effect of time can be estimated.

Some key assumptions must be met for the crossover design to be useful (Brown, 1980; Jones, 2008; Hills and Armitage, 1979). (1) The two groups must be equally matched at the onset; it would be futile to have thin, nonhypertensive subjects in one group and obese hypertensive subjects in the other. (2) The subjects should be in the same clinical state at the beginning of the second period as they were at the beginning of the first period; that is, the first treatment should not leave the subject in a different state, and the disease process has not changed. (3) The effect of the agent used in the first treatment should not carry over to the beginning of the second period; that is, the drug or treatment activity should have a short half-life. (4) The order in which the treatments are given should not affect the results. Therefore crossover designs are best used for chronic diseases such as chronic obstructive pulmonary disease or rheumatoid arthritis. The design is not restricted to these chronic diseases, though. It has been used to test the ability of acetazolamide to prevent or modify mountain sickness, all of the above criteria being met (Greene et al., 1981). It has even been used to study the effect of sumatriptan on acute cluster headaches (Ferrari, 1991). Crossover designs are often used in equivalence studies.

As an example, treatment with acetazolamide in preventing acute mountain sickness was studied (Greene et al., 1981). Twenty-four amateur mountain climbers were divided at random into two groups. Before climbing Mt Kilimanjaro (5895 m) one group was given acetazolamide and the other a placebo. After descending, there was a 5-day rest period, and then the treatments were switched when the climbers ascended Mt Kenya (5186 m). Each climber made daily notes of symptoms, and a scoring system was used; the more symptoms, the higher the score. The results are given in Tables 23.4a and b.

The average effect due to time is

$$\frac{(4.83 - 1.91) - (2.5 - 14.25)}{2} = 7.34.$$

The average effect of the drug (difference between scores with acetazolamide and placebo) is

$$\frac{(4.83 - 1.91) + (2.5 - 14.25)}{2} = -4.42.$$

Table 23.4a Scores

	Group 1			Group 2		
	Acetazolamide Kilimanjaro (Period 1)	Placebo Mt Kenya (Period 2)	Period 1−2	Placebo Kilimanjaro (Period 1)	Acetazolamide Mt Kenya (Period 2)	Period 2−1
	7	0	7	25	−1	−26
	13	7	6	19	5	−14
	3	3	0	17	9	−8
	4	−	−	7	1	−6
	5	−1	6	9	3	−6
	6	−1	7	12	2	−10
	0	0	0	18	2	−16
	1	0	1	12	0	−12
	3	0	3	5	4	−1
	5	2	3	12	−1	−13
	9	9	0	18	−2	−20
	2	2	0	17	8	−9
ΣX	58	21	33	171	30	−141
$\overline{X}$	4.83	1.91	3	14.25	2.5	−11.75
N	12	11	11	12	12	12
s	3.61	3.30	3	5.74	3.50	6.7
$s_{\overline{X}}$			0.9			1.94

Data adapted from Greene et al. (1981).

Table 23.4b Summary of high-altitude trial results (see text)

Group	Treatment	Period	Mean score
I	A. Acetazolamide	1	4.83
	B. Placebo	2	1.91
II	A. Acetazolamide	2	2.5
	B. Placebo	1	14.25

From the data, the standard error was

$$\frac{1}{2}\sqrt{(0.9^2 + 1.94^2)} = 1.07.$$

Therefore to test the null hypothesis that time had no effect calculate $t = \frac{7.34}{1.07} = 6.86$. P < 0.00001, and we can safely reject the null hypothesis. This conclusion is reasonable because of the known effect of acclimatization to altitude. The effect of treatment can be tested by $t = \frac{4.42}{1.07} = 4.13$. P < 0.00001, also a reason to reject the null hypothesis. Many reports of crossover studies in the literature have ignored requirements (Baer et al., 2010).

N of 1 trials

These are variations of the cross-over trials in which treatments are given in random order to a single patient. All the issues about carry over pertain. If, for example, two medications for back pain are given and symptoms are recorded accurately, it might be possible to show that one treatment is better than the other *for that particular patient*. This avoids the "one size fits all" approach of randomized clinical trials with a gain in efficiency. (Lillie et al., 2011).

EQUIVALENCE AND NONINFERIORITY TESTING

One type of test that compares two samples seems to be the antithesis of a statistical test, and that is the equivalence or noninferiority test. Equivalence implies that the new mean is only slightly better or worse than the old mean, whereas noninferiority means that the new mean is not significantly worse than the old mean. These tests are aimed at introducing a new treatment that is cheaper, less invasive, has fewer side effects, or has other advantages (Pocock, 2003). A pharmaceutical company might want to establish the merits of a new preparation of a vaccine, or a new combination of vaccines. The advantages of the new preparation might be that it can be stored for longer times, or may save costs. What is important for the company is to show that the new preparation is not less effective than the old vaccine. If the new item is more effective than the old one that would be advantageous, but all that is required for the company to be licensed to produce the new vaccine is to show equivalent effectiveness with the previous one. This type of testing was found in 2% of vaccine studies reported in several major medical journals (Jacobson and Poland, 2005), but the principles apply widely. Other examples are examining the incidence of infective endocarditis before and after changing the guidelines for antibiotic prophylaxis (no difference was found) (Thornhill et al., 2011), comparing two different types of coronary stents (Hofma et al., 2012) or two types of stem cell transplantation (da Silva et al., 2008). The two latter references describe the methods of testing clearly.

Performing a standard t-test and finding that it does not disprove the null hypothesis is not a substitute for equivalence testing because it may merely reflect a low power. "Absence of evidence is not evidence of absence" (Altman and Bland, 1995). On the other hand, even a trivial difference between two means can be significant if the sample size is huge. What is important to consider is not significance but the effect size Δ. In noninferiority tests the investigator decides on what sized Δ is acceptable. For example, if drug A lowers blood pressure by a mean of 30 mm Hg, and drug B lowers blood pressure by a mean of 27 mm Hg, then drug B would be regarded as satisfactory. Many regulatory agencies accept a difference of as much as 15% of the mean, that is, if the new treatment is not more than 15% worse than the old treatment, then noninferiority (accepting the null hypothesis) may be asserted. One Federal standard accepts a 20% difference (Food and Drug Administration, 1977). It would be preferable to have a smaller deviation, for example, 5%, but this may demand an impractically large number of subjects.

Often the two one-sided test (TOST) is done to test the joint null hypothesis.

$$H_{01} : \mu_1 - \mu_2 \geq \Delta$$
$$H_{02} : \mu_1 - \mu_2 \leq -\Delta$$

Rejection of H_{01} implies that $\mu_1 - \mu_2 \leq \Delta$, and rejecting H_{02} implies that $\mu_1 - \mu_2 \geq -\Delta$. Rejecting both hypotheses implies that the difference lies within the range Δ to $-\Delta$ and hence that for practical purposes the two drugs have equivalent effects. Therefore do TOSTs.

$$t_1 = \frac{\left(\overline{X_1} - \overline{X_2}\right) - \Delta}{S_{\overline{X_1} - \overline{X_2}}} \quad \text{and} \quad t_2 = \frac{\left(\overline{X_1} - \overline{X_2}\right) - (-\Delta)}{S_{\overline{X_1} - \overline{X_2}}}.$$

If neither t-test shows significance, then the observed difference lies within the permissible difference so that the two drugs have equivalent effects.

A variant of this test is to calculate confidence limits for the difference between the two means. If this lies within the limits $\pm\Delta$, which demarcates a zone of scientific or clinical indifference, equivalence is demonstrated. Figure 23.1, based on a similar figure by Jones et al. (1996), shows the principle.

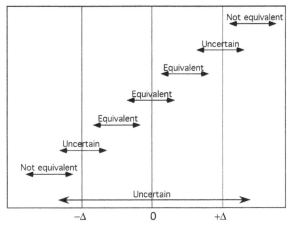

Figure 23.1 Range from $-\Delta$ to $+\Delta$ within which equivalence is assumed (zone of indifference).

Lines labeled "Equivalent" are within this range, so that studies producing these limits are equivalent to existing products. Lines labeled "Not-equivalent" are outside this range so that the two groups are not equivalent. Lines labeled "Uncertain" are inconclusive, and may call for further studies. Two of the lines showing confidence limits that demonstrate equivalence do not cross zero, so that they argue for rejecting the null hypothesis, but equivalence is still postulated because the observed difference is not meaningful. The European Agency for the Evaluation of Medicinal Products has set out criteria for making these decisions at http://www.ema.europa.eu/docs/en_GB/document_library/Scientific_guideline/2009/09/WC500003519.pdf and at http://www.tga.gov.au/pdf/euguide/ewp048299en.pdf. The confidence limits are calculated from $(\overline{X_1} - \overline{X_2}) \pm t_{0.10} S_{\overline{X_1} - \overline{X_2}}$, and $t_{0.10}$ is chosen so that the chances of rejecting the null hypothesis are 0.05 at each end of the limits. Tryon (2001) developed a method of inferential confidence intervals that slightly reduces the lengths of the confidence limits by about 10—20%.

One problem with equivalence testing is that it often requires large numbers of subjects because small differences are being examined. One estimate of numbers required is based on the formula

$$N \geq \frac{(z_\beta + z_\alpha)^2 s^2}{\Delta^2}.$$

Because twice z is squared, four times as many subjects are required as for a simple t- or z-test. Jacobson and Poland (2005) recommended a modified approach, based on a suggestion by Feinstein. This eliminates consideration of very small differences by setting two thresholds, one for an insignificant difference, designated i, and the other for the threshold of an important difference, Δ. Then it is possible to calculate

$$N \geq \frac{z_\alpha^2 s^2}{(\Delta - i)^2}.$$

What this does is to eliminate the need to consider trivial differences less than i (Deeks et al., 2005), with consequent reduction in the required numbers. A calculator for sample size can be found online at http://www.sealedenvelope.com/power/binary-noninferior.

A simple explanation of this subject can be found at http://www.graphpad.com/support/faqid/1061/.

REFERENCES

Altman, D.G., Bland, J.M., 1995. Absence of evidence is not evidence of absence. BMJ 311, 485.
Baer, H.J., Tworoger, S.S., Hankinson, S.E., Willett, W.C., 2010. Body fatness at young ages and risk of breast cancer throughout life. Am. J. Epidemiol. 171, 1183—1194.
Brown Jr., B.W., 1980. The crossover experiment for clinical trials. Biometrics 36, 69—79.
Deeks, J.J., Macaskill, P., Irwig, L., 2005. The performance of tests of publication bias and other sample size effects in systematic reviews of diagnostic test accuracy was assessed. J. Clin. Epidemiol. 58, 882—893.
Ebbutt, A.F., 1984. Three-period crossover designs for two treatments. Biometrics 40, 219—244.
Ferrari, M.D., 1991. Treatment of migraine attacks with sumatriptan. The subcutaneous sumatriptan international study group. N. Engl. J. Med. 325, 316—321.
Food and Drug Administration, 1977. The bioavailability protocol guideline for ANDA and NDA submission. Division of Biopharmaceutics, D. M. B. O. D., Food and Drug Administration.
Greene, M.K., Kerr, A.M., Mcintosh, I.B., Prescott, R.J., 1981. Acetazolamide in prevention of acute mountain sickness: a double-blind controlled cross-over study. Br. Med. J. (Clin. Res. Ed.) 283, 811—813.

Hills, M., Armitage, P., 1979. The two-period cross-over clinical trial. Br. J. Clin. Pharmacol. 8, 7–20.

Hofma, S.H., Brouwer, J., Velders, M.A., van't Hof, A.W., Smits, P.C., Queré, M., de Vries, C.J., van Boven, A.J., 2012. Second-generation everolimus-eluting stents versus first-generation sirolimus-eluting stents in acute myocardial infarction. 1-year results of the randomized XAMI (XienceV Stent vs. Cypher Stent in Primary PCI for Acute Myocardial Infarction) trial. J. Am. Coll. Cardiol. 60, 381–387.

Jacobson, R.M., Poland, G.A., 2005. Studies of equivalence in clinical vaccine research. Vaccine 23, 2315–2317.

Jones, B., 2008. The cross-over trial: a subtle knife. Significance 5, 135–137.

Jones, B., 2010. The waiting game: how long is long enough? Significance 2, 40–41.

Jones, B., Haughie, S., 2008. Cross-over trials in practice: tales of the unexpected. Significance 5, 183–184.

Jones, B., Jarvis, P., Lewis, J.A., Ebbutt, A.F., 1996. Trials to assess equivalence: the importance of rigorous methods. BMJ 313, 36–39.

Jones, B., Kenward, M.G., 2003. Design and Analysis of Cross-over Trials. Chapman & Hall/CRC, Boca Raton, FL.

Laska, E., Meisner, M., Kushner, H.B., 1983. Optimal crossover designs in the presence of carryover effects. Biometrics 39, 1087–1091.

Lillie, E.O., Patay, B., Diamant, J., Issell, B., Topol, E.J., Schork, N.J., 2011. The n-of-1 clinical trial: the ultimate strategy for individualizing medicine? Per. Med. 8, 161–173.

Pocock, S.J., 2003. The pros and cons of noninferiority trials. Fundam. Clin. Pharmacol. 17, 483–490.

Ramsey, B.W., Dorkin, H.L., Eisenberg, J.D., Gibson, R.L., Harwood, I.R., Kravitz, R.M., Schidlow, D.V., Wilmott, R.W., Astley, S.J., McBurnie, M.A., et al., 1993. Efficacy of aerosolized tobramycin in patients with cystic fibrosis. N. Engl. J. Med. 328, 1740–1746.

da Silva, G.T., Logan, B.R., Klein, J.P., 2008. Methods for equivalence and noninferiority testing. Biol. Blood Marrow Transpl. 15.

Thornhill, M.H., Dayer, M.J., Forde, J.M., Corey, G.R., Chu, V.H., Couper, D.J., Lockhart, P.B., 2011. Impact of the NICE guideline recommending cessation of antibiotic prophylaxis for prevention of infective endocarditis: before and after study. BMJ 342, d2392.

Tryon, W.W., 2001. Evaluating statistical difference, equivalence, and indeterminacy using inferential confidence intervals: an integrated alternative method of conducting null hypothesis statistical tests. Psychol. Methods 6, 371–386.

Wellek, S., Blettner, M., 2012. On the proper use of the crossover design in clinical trials: part 18 of a series on evaluation of scientific publications. Dtsch. Arztebl. Int. 109, 276–281.

CHAPTER 24

Multiple Comparisons

Contents

INTRODUCTION

A population has a mean of 50 units and a standard deviation of 10 units. Draw 10 random samples with $N = 25$ from this population. The central limit theorem indicates that the means of the 10 samples are distributed normally about a mean of 50 with a standard error of the mean estimated from $\frac{10}{\sqrt{25}} = 2$. Therefore the 95% confidence limits for these means are $50 \pm t_{0.05} \times 2 = 50 \pm 2.262 \times 2 = 45.476$ to 54.524. If the highest and lowest means from these 10 samples are compared by an unpaired t-test, they will be significantly different, with t being about 3.199, $P = 0.005$.

What is wrong with this scenario? Only about 5% of means of such samples drawn from the same population will be more than two standard errors from the population mean, so that only about 1 time in 20 would we incorrectly reject the null hypothesis. Note that this is the conventional argument. As discussed in Chapter 8, the type I error is more in the order of 30% (Colquhoun, 2014) However, by selecting the highest and lowest means from such a series, the difference between them has caused us to reject the null hypothesis. In fact, rejecting the null hypothesis for a mean in the lower tail of the distribution implies rejecting it for comparison between that mean and any mean that is above the population mean.

More realistic scenarios are frequent in the scientific literature. Consider Figure 24.1 that illustrates figures and comparisons commonly shown in the literature.

The left panel shows seven sequential time periods with significant differences. The right panel shows significant differences for all pairs of comparisons.

Short vertical lines are standard errors, and asterisks indicate $P < 0.05$ (*) or 0.01 (**).

For a list of all websites referred to in this chapter, as clickable links, see the book companion website: www.booksite.elsevier.com/9780128023877.

Biostatistics for Medical and Biomedical Practitioners
http://dx.doi.org/10.1016/B978-0-12-802387-7.00024-X

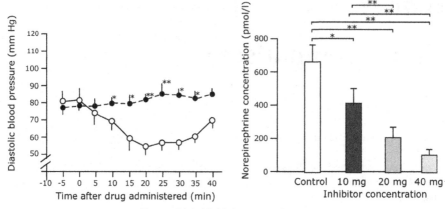

Figure 24.1 Multiple comparisons.

The questions raised by these multiple comparisons are whether they are legitimate because multiple t-tests have been done. The arguments to follow apply equally to other multiple tests, such as chi-square tests. The subject is controversial with some asserting that there is no need to correct for the multiple comparisons and others that correction is always necessary. Most statisticians occupy the middle ground and use correction selectively.

To clarify this issue Tukey (1977) provided the following argument. Consider drawing at random two samples of the same size from the same population. The logic of the t-test tells us that there is a 0.05 probability of rejecting the null hypothesis falsely (α, Type I error), and therefore a $1 - \alpha = 1 - 0.05 = 0.95$ chance of correctly accepting the null hypothesis. If we draw another two samples from that population, then by the same argument there is a 0.95 chance of correctly accepting the null hypothesis. What then is the chance of correctly accepting the null hypothesis both times? By the product rule for probabilities, it is $(1 - \alpha)^2 = 0.95 \times 0.95 = 0.95^2 = 0.9025$. Therefore, the probability of rejecting the null hypothesis incorrectly is $1 - (1 - \alpha)^2 = 1 - 0.9025 = 0.0975$, even though we use the conventional 0.05 level of α. Draw a third set of samples from that population. Then the probability of correctly accepting the null hypothesis all three times is $(1 - \alpha)^3 = 0.95^3 = 0.8574$. Similarly, drawing 10 pairs of samples, the chance of correctly accepting the null hypothesis in all 10 comparisons is $(1 - \alpha)^{10} = 0.95^{10} = 0.5987$. Therefore, the probability of incorrectly rejecting the null hypothesis at least once is $1 - (1 - \alpha)^{10} = 1 - 0.5987 = 0.4013$, even though the 0.05 value for α is what we should get. The value of α has thus been inflated. A similar example illustrated by Bland and Altman (1995) involved 20 comparisons, and then the chance of finding at least one comparison significant at the 0.05 level is 0.64. For 100 comparisons, the probability of incorrectly rejecting the null hypothesis at the 0.05 level is $1 - (1 - \alpha)^{100} = 1 - (1 - 0.05)^{100} = 0.9941$.

BONFERRONI CORRECTION AND EQUIVALENT TESTS

One way to correct for this inflation factor is attributed to the Italian mathematician Carlo Bonferroni (1892–1960), although the concept had been known for centuries (Bland and Altman, 1995). To keep the value of α at 0.05 for the whole set of comparisons (call this α_F indicating the value of α for the whole family of experiments), then we have to solve the equation for the value of α_c (c indicating the individual comparison) for each independent comparison:

$1 - (1 - \alpha_c)^k = 0.05$ for different values of k, the number of tests conducted.

The expression $\alpha_F = 1 - (1 - \alpha_c)^k$ is sometimes written $\alpha_c = 1 - (1 - \alpha_F)^{1/k}$. In either form it is known as the Dunn–Sidak equation.

Thus if k is 10, then $\alpha_c = 0.005116$. For k = 20, 50, and 100, and for $\alpha_e = 0.05$ and 0.01, the values of α_c are given in Table 24.1. These values of α_c are close to what we would get by dividing α by k. This is known as the Bonferroni equation, and its results are only very slightly different from the Dunn–Sidak test (Abdi, 2007). Therefore the Bonferroni correction for k t-tests requires that each individual comparison be declared significant only if P is less than α/k. The approximation works because if with k independent t-tests, each with $\alpha = 0.05$ then the probability of getting no significant differences is $(1 - \alpha)^k$. Because α is small, expanding the expression approximates $1 - k\alpha$, because all the higher powers of α are tiny. Then if the null hypothesis is true, for one of the k comparisons to have a probability <0.05, $k\alpha$ must be less than 0.05, so that α must be less than 0.05/k (Bland and Altman, 1995).

Table 24.1 Results of Bonferroni correction

k	$\alpha = 0.05$		$\alpha = 0.01$	
	α_c	$\alpha_F = \alpha/n$	α_c	$\alpha_F = \alpha/n$
10	0.005116	0.005	0.00100453	0.001
20	0.002561	0.0025	0.00050239	0.0005
50	0.001025	0.001	0.00020099	0.0002
100	0.000513	0.0005	0.0001005	0.0001

As initially stated, Bonferroni defined an inequality that states that if several events are considered, the probability that at least one of the events will occur cannot exceed the sum of the probabilities of the individual events; the experiment-wise error rate can never exceed the sum of the comparison-wise error rates (CWERs) (see below for definition of terms). Thus if for five groups each CWER is 0.05, the experiment-wise error rate cannot exceed $5 \times 0.05 = 0.25$. This leads us directly to the correction described above, because by making the CWER 0.05/5 = 0.01, the experiment-wise error rate can never exceed $0.01 \times 5 = 0.05$.

Table 24.1 shows that with a large number of comparisons, the corrected value of α is so small that it may be difficult to achieve. By being very conservative in trying to avoid Type I errors, the Type II error becomes larger, with the risk of failing to reject the null hypothesis falsely too many times. There is thus loss of statistical power. More efficient procedures were described by Holm (1979) and by Hochberg and Benjamini (1990). For the Holm test, rank all the P values from all the k comparisons from smallest to biggest. Then test the smallest against 0.05/k, the number of comparisons. If that is not significant, accept the null hypothesis for all the comparisons. If it is significant, test the second smallest P value against $0.05/(k - 1)$, and so on. Assume that the P values are 0.005, 0.020, 0.026, and 0.09. Then test 0.005 against $0.05/4 = 0.0125$. Because it is smaller, reject the null hypothesis for that comparison. Then test the second smallest P value, 0.020, against $0.05/3 = 0.017$. Because it is bigger, accept the null hypothesis for this and all remaining comparisons. An online calculator using Excel is at http://www.researchgate.net/publication/236969037_Holm-Bonferroni_Sequential_Correction_An_EXCEL_Calculator.

For the Hochberg test, rank all the P values from largest to smallest. Assume that these values are 0.09, 0.026, 0.020, and 0.005. Because the first P value exceeds 0.05, do not reject the null hypothesis. Then compare the next P value with $0.05/2 = 0.025$. Because $P = 0.026$ exceeds this, do not reject the null hypothesis for this comparison. For the third comparison the critical P value is $0.05/3 = 0.017$. Because $P = 0.020$ exceeds this critical value, do not reject the null hypothesis for the third comparison. The fourth P value is compared with the critical value of $0.05/4 = 0.0125$. Because $P = 0.005$ is less than the critical value, reject the null hypothesis for the fourth comparison. If the second comparison had had a P value of 0.021, then this would have been less than the critical value of 0.025, and we would have rejected the null hypothesis for this and *all subsequent comparisons*. Both of these tests keep the error rate for the whole set of tests at 0.05, but greatly reduce the Type II error. The Hochberg test is more powerful than the Holm test, and both improve considerably on the original Bonferroni correction (Aickin and Gensler, 1996; Levin, 1996). An online but complex program for this test is at http://www.ncbi.nlm.nih.gov/pmc/articles/PMC3263024/. Variations of these methods are used when the various end points are correlated with each other, for example, different symptoms in a disease are often correlated (Wright, 1992; Yao and Wei, 1996). A good comparison of these tests appears in a publication by Wright (1992). Several statistical programs, including R, implement these tests. An excellent discussion of these tests with examples is given by Walsh at http://nitro.biosci.arizona.edu/workshops/Aarhus2006/pdfs/Multiple.pdf

The Bonferroni correction is often misused. In 1980, Glantz (1980) and Wallenstein et al. (1980) wrote editorials to address some common statistical errors in the journals Circulation and Circulation Research, one of the errors being the use of multiple t-tests. They recommended the Bonferroni correction. Similar conclusions were reached by Pocock et al. (1987) who examined the reports of 45 comparative trials published in the British Medical Journal, the Lancet, and the New England Journal of Medicine. Unfortunately, the Bonferroni correction is needed for only a subset of multiple t-tests, and there has been a tendency to apply it to all such tests, whether or not they require the correction (Kusuoka and Hoffman, 2002).

Error Rates

Some statisticians reject the Bonferroni adjustment (Rothman, 1990) and others restrict its use to certain types of experiments (Perneger, 1998). An important distinction is between *experiment-wise* and *comparison-wise* error rates. Creasy et al. (1972) embolized the placenta in pregnant sheep with microspheres and compared the resultant runted lambs with control lambs. They measured body and organ weights and organ blood flows, as well as hematocrit, blood glucose concentrations, and arterial pH and oxygen and carbon dioxide tensions. In all, 14 t-test comparisons were made. Figure 24.2 shows some of their data. Was it correct to do so many t-tests, and did they have to use the Bonferroni correction?

There are two main types of error rates (Dunnett, 1970; O'Neill and Wetherill, 1971; O'Brien and Shampo, 1988a). One is the CWER, defined as:

$$\frac{Number \ of \ comparisons \ leading \ to \ erroneous \ rejection \ of \ the \ null \ hypothesis}{Total \ number \ of \ comparisons}$$

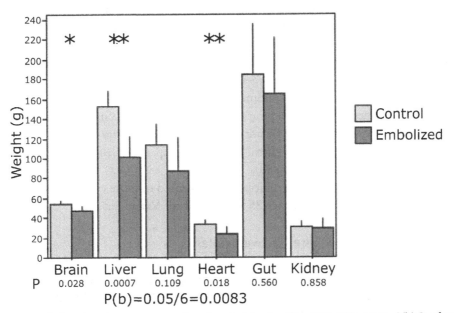

Figure 24.2 Comparison between control and runted lambs. *P < 0.05; **P < 0.01. P(b) Bonferroni adjustment. Vertical lines are standard errors.

The second is the *experiment-wise (or family-wise)* error rate, defined as:

$$\frac{\textit{Number of families with one or more erroneous rejection of the null hypothesis}}{\textit{Total number of families}}$$

The term "family" refers to a set or a subset of experiments. The main distinction is that the experiment-wise error rate considers that the risk of one false rejection of the null hypothesis over an entire set of experiments should be kept to 0.05; in other words, the two groups are identical in all the tested variables. Thus in the Creasy experiment, rejection of the null hypothesis for any one of the several comparisons leads to rejection of the null hypothesis that placental embolization does not change fetal lamb development. This needs protection by the Bonferroni or other methods. By contrast, the CWER is separate for each comparison, and may legitimately be set at 0.05 for each comparison. After all, why should the Type I error for any one organ comparison depend upon the other comparisons? It would not make sense to change the value of α if more organs were compared, or if serum sodium and potassium were measured as well. Furthermore, what should we do if we measure three sets of organs now, and a year later do another experiment and measure another three organs? It would make no sense to go back and change the value of α for the first experiment in the light of the second set of data. To complicate matters more, if one investigator did the experiment with 6 comparisons, and another investigator used 12 comparisons, both should detect the same significant differences, but this might not happen with the Bonferroni correction (O'Brien, 1983).

The issue of whether or not to make corrections is still hotly debated. There are also variations of the definitions given above. Most statisticians agree that the Bonferroni adjustment should be used if the universal null hypothesis of no differences in any variable is used. For example, doing a battery of biochemical tests on a presumed normal subject.

There are many scenarios on the theme of simultaneous multiple comparisons. For example, making consecutive measurements over time such as Figures 24.1 (left panel) (O'Brien and Shampo, 1988b) using multiple statistical tests to examine possible heterogeneity of response (O'Brien and Shampo, 1988c), or combining the results of several different end points to provide a global measure of superiority of one treatment over another (O'Brien and Shampo, 1988d).

The controversies about doing multiple t-tests extend to more complex analyses, and will be discussed in detail in Chapter 25 on Analysis of Variance.

Extreme Multiplicity and False Discovery Rates

Multiplicity problems become extreme when large scale sets of hundreds or thousands of data points are examined, most notably in examining microarrays used to evaluate gene or protein expression (Pawitan et al., 2005; Karp et al., 2007; Elo et al., 2009; Elo and Schwikowski, 2012) or voxels used in imaging (Genovese et al., 2002; Nichols and Hayasaka, 2003). In these types of studies the test object (e.g., blood for genes and proteins, organs such as brain or heart for imaging) is divided into thousands of samples, each of which is compared with control normal values. These normal values have their own variability, and some threshold is needed to determine if any one locus differs between test and control.

The CWER with $\alpha = 0.05$ examines each comparison separately. For any single comparison there is a 5% chance of falsely rejecting the null hypothesis. Therefore standard t-tests on 10,000 spots in a microarray chip would provide 500 false positive "significant" differences even if the test and control material were identical. Family-wise error rates (FWERs) reduce this potential error and keep the total error rate for the whole array below 5%. An example of such a test is the Bonferroni inequality in which the null hypothesis for each spot is rejected only with a value of α/k, where k is the number of spots. With $k = 10,000$ the power of the test is very low, and the Type I error is controlled at a given value for α at the cost of an inflated Type II error. Consequently, many differences that might be important would not be detected.

In 1995, Benjamini and Hochberg (1995) proposed the concept of the false discovery rate (FDR) to deal with these problems. Results of testing a large number of samples are given in Table 24.2.

Table 24.2 Type I and Type II errors applied to microarrays

	Do not reject H_0 (Non-DE)	Reject H_0 (DE)	Total
H_0 true (non-DE)	U = true negative	V = false positive (Type I error)	m_0
H_0 false (H_A true; DE)	T = false negative (Type II error)	S = true positive	$m - m_0$
	$m - R$	R	m

DE = differential expression (difference between test and control value); m = total number of hypotheses tested; m_0 = number of true null hypotheses; $m - m_0$ = number of true alternative hypotheses. m is known in advance and R is an observed random variable, but none of the other values are known. S, T, U, and V are rates.

The CWER is stipulated to be E(V/m), where E indicates the expectation of the ratio in the long run. Testing each hypothesis at level α guarantees that $E(V/m) \leq \alpha$. Setting a value for α sets a limit for the value of V/m. Testing each hypothesis at level α/m gives the FWER that keeps the Type I error for the whole data set $\leq \alpha$. The false discovery error rate is represented by the random variable $Q = V/(V + S)$ or V/R, and indicates the proportion of rejected null hypotheses that are erroneously rejected. If all the null hypotheses are true, then Q is zero, and the FDR and FWERs are the same. If not, then the FDR is much lower.

Given that the FDR decreases both Type I and Type II errors, how is it possible to calculate FDR when the values for S, T, U, and V are unknown? One approach (Karp and Lilley, 2007; Storey, 2002; Storey and Tibshirani, 2003) has been to plot the histogram of the relative frequency with which each P value (for the individual t-tests) occurs (Figure 24.3).

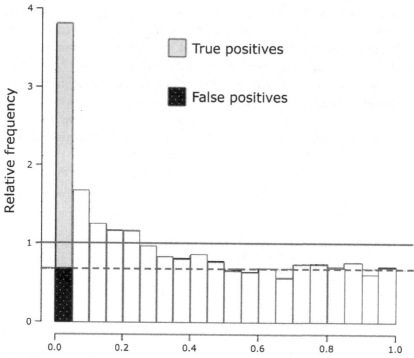

Figure 24.3 Diagram to illustrate one approach to calculating FDR, based on published figures by Karp and Lilley (2007) and by Storey and Tibshirani (2003). If there were no differences between test and control materials, then the relative frequency of each P value (the number of times it occurred relative to what is expected from a normal distribution) would be constant, as indicated by the horizontal solid line. On the reasonable assumption that high p values indicate that the null hypothesis is likely and that there is no difference between the control and the test material, the relatively uniform part of the histogram with P > 0.5 provides an estimate of the true background level, as shown by the dashed line. Portions of the columns above this dashed line indicate the true positives (shaded area for the lowest P values) as compared to the baseline false positives shown in dark dotted area.

A simple technique is to set a value Q for the FDR. Assume we choose 0.2. List the P values from smallest (rank 1) to largest (rank N) and calculate $(i/m)Q$. Thus for the 4th ranked P value out of 17, $(i/m)Q = 4/17 \times 0.2 = 0.0471$. If the P value is less than 0.0471, reject the null hypothesis; if it is greater then it is unsafe to reject the null hypothesis. As an example, consider the data in Table 24.3.

Table 24.3 Example of serial testing for significance

Rank	P value	(i/m)Q	Comment
1	0.010	0.0118	Reject H_0
2	0.022	0.0235	Reject H_0
3	0.029	0.0353	Reject H_0
4	0.043	0.0471	Reject H_0
5	0.11	0.0588	Do not reject H_0
6	0.16	0.0706	Do not reject H_0
7	0.27	0.0824	Do not reject H_0
8	0.31	0.0941	Do not reject H_0
9	0.38	0.1059	Do not reject H_0
10	0.49	0.1176	Do not reject H_0
11	0.55	0.1294	Do not reject H_0
12	0.61	0.1412	Do not reject H_0
13	0.63	0.1529	Do not reject H_0
14	0.69	0.1647	Do not reject H_0
15	0.75	0.1765	Do not reject H_0
16	0.83	0.1882	Do not reject H_0
17	0.98	0.2000	Do not reject H_0

There are numerous approaches to computing FDR, and numerous complications such as the fact that often several genes or proteins rise or fall together, so that consultation with an expert in the field is essential. Different methods of setting the threshold for declaring a difference significant give different results. There is a trade-off between sensitivity and specificity, and the results should not be accepted blindly without realizing their limitations.

Another approach to minimizing FDRs that is especially useful in genomic studies was proposed by Broer et al. (2013) who showed that, depending on the prior probability of an association, the Type I error could be kept low by requiring $P < 0.00001 - 0.0000001$.

GROUP SEQUENTIAL BOUNDARIES

It is common in clinical trials to plan a study involving many subjects for a long time, but to check the results at intervals to determine if the study should be ended prematurely because of unexpectedly bad or good results in one group. It would be unethical to continue the study when one group receives a less good treatment. In this context, the multiple comparisons problem is invoked (Armitage et al., 1969; McPherson, 1974). The approach depends in part on how the trial is likely to proceed. In some trials, many subjects are readily available and unambiguous results are obtained early for each patient. The trial supervisors then estimate how many are needed in each group, what the primary outcome will be, and how long the trial is expected to continue. At the other extreme is a trial when patient accrual is slow and irregular, the time to completion of the trial is uncertain, and the outcome may not be known for several years. These two extremes need different analyses. Furthermore, because most clinical trials test treatments that will produce only modest improvements, the patient numbers required can be very large (Mehta et al., 2009).

One of the most often used methods for interim checks was devised by O'Brien and Fleming (O'Brien and Fleming, 1979; O'Brien and Shampo, 1988e). The number of interim tests is defined in advance. Because earlier interim tests involve smaller numbers of patients, they have large standard errors and confidence limits, and therefore demand a higher level of significance before the trial should be stopped. With each succeeding interim examination the criterion for accepting the null hypothesis becomes less strict, until for the final test at the end of the trial the conventional predetermined value of α is achieved. O'Brien and Fleming calculated the critical values of α for a predetermined per experiment error rate of 0.05 for 2, 3, 4, or 5 interim tests (Table 24.4, column 2).

Table 24.4 column 2 shows critical P values for a final Type I error rate of 0.05, based on tables from O'Brien and Shampo (1988e) and Pocock (2006). The final test on the completed trial has a critical value close to the designated 0.05. If the final error rate is to be 0.01, then the O'Brien–Fleming method requires critical P values of 0.0000001,

Table 24.4 Critical values for interim checks

Test number	Critical P value	
	O'Brien–Fleming	Haybittle–Peto
One interim test		
1	0.005	0.001
2	0.049	0.050
Two interim tests		
1	0.0006	0.001
2	0.0151	0.001
3	0.0471	0.0495
Three interim tests		
1	0.00005	0.001
2	0.004	0.001
3	0.018	0.001
4	0.042	0.0492
Four interim tests		
1	0.000005	0.001
2	0.0013	0.001
3	0.009	0.001
4	0.023	0.001
5	0.042	0.0489

0.00001, 0.001, and 0.004 for the first to fourth interim analyses respectively. Column 3 shows alternative critical values (see below).

As an example, Jamerson et al. (2008) conducted a clinical trial to compare the effects of benazepril with amlodipine or hydrochlorothiazide for treating hypertension in high-risk patients. After determining sample size based on expected results, they began the trial, but terminated early after 36 months when the advantages of the benazepril—amlodipine combination were shown to be manifestly superior during an interim examination. A trial can also end early if there is no reasonable chance that a statistically significant difference will appear. Some trials have built-in futility rules that stipulate when early termination is appropriate (Karp and Lilley, 2007).

Another popular method was developed by Haybittle (1971) and Peto et al. (1976). These authors use a constant boundary for the interim analyses but retain the α value of 0.05 if early termination does not occur (Table 24.4).

Finally, one other type of test has been proposed to deal with the problem that preliminary data may suggest the need to change the times at which interim analyses are made, or due to slow recruitment the trial has to be extended so that more interim analyses may be needed. The adaptive procedures used were developed by Lan and DeMets (Lan and DeMets, 1983; Lan and Wittes, 1988; DeMets and Lan, 1994), and are variants of the O'Brien and Fleming method. They proposed an "alpha spending function" that controlled how much of the false positive error can be used at each interim analysis as a function of the proportion of total information available for the whole test. This proportion is usually based on the fraction of total patients enrolled or the proportion of expected events that had occurred. Internet programs for doing these calculations may be found at https://www.biostat.wisc.edu/content/lan-demets-method-statistical-programs-clinical-trials, or some specialized computer programs such as PASS or Cytel will perform the calculations.

A simple rough test was advocated by Pocock (2006) when examining interim results. With the reasonable assumptions that the two groups being compared had approximately equal numbers and that the incidence of events was small and therefore fitted a Poisson distribution, the ratio $z = \frac{a-b}{\sqrt{a+b}}$, where a and b are the numbers of events in the two groups, has an approximately normal distribution. If z is 1.96, then P = 0.05. The P values of 0.01, 0.001, and 0.0001 are equivalent to z values of 2.68, 3.29, and 3.89, respectively. This method does not eliminate the need for more accurate interim analyses, but serves as a check on the arithmetic and provides a more easily understandable figure to evaluate. The reasons for early termination, however, are not affected by this calculation.

The issue of prematurely stopping a clinical trial is complex, and data monitoring committees must take more into account than a P value that refers to the primary end point. Complications need to be taken into account, so does the possibility of late occurring results, and the importance of that particular trial. Pocock discussed these issues in detail (Pocock and White, 1999; Pocock, 2006). He pointed out that most reported trials that were terminated early for significant benefit were based on limited data and showed unrealistically and unexpectedly large treatment effects. In fact, in some trials that were continued after apparent interim significance had been reached, subsequent results indicated a less marked difference between the treatments, and Pocock termed this effect "regression to the truth" (Pocock and White, 1999).

The decision to correct for multiplicity is often complicated, and factors such as who benefits by the lack of correction may need to be invoked (O'Brien and Shampo, 1988c). The problem is intensified in clinical trials where multiple end points may be involved (O'Brien and Shampo, 1988c).

SEQUENTIAL ANALYSIS

The ultimate form of interim analysis is sequential analysis, performed after each pair of data points is accrued, whether the data are measured values or preferences (Armitage, 1975). As an example, for comparing preferences (e.g., A is better than B or worse than B) a grid is prepared (Figure 24.4). To construct the figure, the α and β errors are designated, usually $\alpha = 0.05$ and $\beta = 0.1 - 0.2$, and the magnitude of the expected difference θ is selected (often 0.85). Based on these three numbers, the appropriate tables are consulted to determine how to draw the boundary lines.

Left panel: For the first pair of preferences (two subjects, two forearms, two cough remedies, etc.), if A is better than B then a diagonal line is drawn upwards in the first square. In the above example, this is true of the second preference set, so another diagonal line is drawn upwards. If the next preference is for B to be better than A, the next diagonal line passes downwards, as in the third box. Eventually one of three patterns will occur. The jagged preference line crosses the upper boundary, indicating that A is significantly better than B with the stated α and β errors; or it crosses the lower boundary which means that B is significantly better than A; or it crosses the middle boundary which means that the trial has failed to show a difference of the expected magnitude.

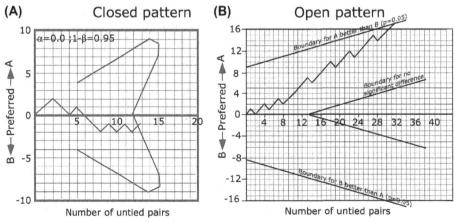

Figure 24.4 Closed pattern with treatment A being no better than treatment B, and open pattern with A being better than B.

The figure shows a closed pattern because the middle boundaries are set. It is also possible to have an open design (right panel) for which the tables provide pairs of parallel lines that serve the same function as the boundaries above. This design has some advantages except that with unbounded parallel lines it is possible for the observed data preference line to meander forever without crossing a boundary. A good example was published by Lewis et al. (1983) on the use of aspirin in angina pectoris.

Cautionary Tale

It is important to graph correctly. One study (Hellier, 1963) published results comparing the effects of trimeprazine versus amylobarbitone in controlling pruritus. A preference for trimeprazine over amylobarbitone produced a line going up at 45°, and a preference for amylobarbitone over trimeprazine produce a line going down at 45°. This graph also showed horizontal lines that indicated no preference. These should not be part of the figure construction, and drawing horizontal portions has the effect of decreasing the mean angle and making the preference line cross the null boundary, giving a false sense of no difference between the treatments. It is, of course, possible for the vast majority of comparisons to result in ties. If that happened, the correct conclusion would be that for most subjects there was no difference between the two treatments, but that for the few who expressed a difference A was preferred more often than B.

Sequential analysis can also be done for measured values. For example, if paired differences are examined, then for each pair calculate a ratio $z = \frac{(\Sigma d)^2}{\Sigma d^2}$, where d is the difference (A − B) between the pairs, and may be positive or negative. Σd is the result obtained by accumulating successive values for d. If the null hypothesis is true, then Σd will remain small, and become a smaller and smaller fraction of the expression. If there is a meaningful difference, z will increase and eventually reach significance. The data are plotted on a figure (Figure 24.5) in which the boundaries are set by tables available in Armitage's book (Armitage, 1975).

Several variations of these designs are possible (Armitage, 1975).

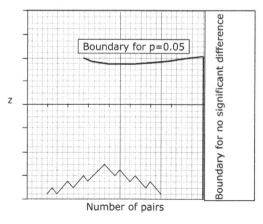

Figure 24.5 Sequential trial of paired measurements that do not show a significant difference.

Sequential analyses offer the possibility of minimizing the number of patients involved in a trial, although the method may sometimes not reduce numbers (Armitage, 1975). All the precautions needed in thinking about early termination of a grouped sequential clinical trial discussed above apply here too.

ADAPTIVE METHODS

Randomized sampling of the type described here is the hallmark of good clinical trials (Chapter 38) but apart from practical problems of designing an impeccable trial, such trials have a major ethical issue, namely is it ethical to give one group of patients what will turn out to be an inferior treatment? (Royall et al., 1991). This cannot be known beforehand because that is why the trial is being done, but is there a way to shorten the time of use of the less effective treatment? One method described above is to examine the results at different times after starting the trial, but this cannot be done too often. A second method, sequential sampling, on the average decreases the needed sample size, but is sometimes difficult to implement. An interesting variant is an adaptive strategy termed randomized play-the-winner that can be used if there are binary outcomes detectable soon after treatment has started. As described by Rosenberger (1999) for two treatments A and B, an urn (actual or theoretical) is set up to contain α_A balls of type A and α_B balls of type B. For the null hypothesis that A and B are equally good, $\alpha_A = \alpha_B$. After the first few patients are selected at random, the adaptive strategy begins. Any success with A or failure with B causes another α_A type ball to be added to the urn; conversely, any success with B or failure with A causes another α_B type ball to be added to the urn. In this way, if treatment A tends to produce better results, the number of α_A type balls grows faster than the number of α_B type balls, and the next patient has a greater chance of receiving the apparently better treatment, and only a minimum number of patients will have received inferior treatment. The theory and practice of this technique have been well described (Rosenberger, 1999; Yao and Wei, 1996).

In the first reported clinical trial with this method (Bartlett et al., 1985), the value of extracorporeal membrane oxygenation (ECMO) was assessed in moribund infants with respiratory failure and no response to optimal therapy; their mortality risk was estimated to be 80–100%. The first patient was randomized to receive ECMO and survived. The next patient was assigned to no ECMO and died. The next patient was assigned to ECMO and survived, and all subsequent patients were assigned to ECMO and survived. Eventually there were 11 survivors of ECMO and 1 death of a patient who did not receive ECMO. Unfortunately there were problems in that trial, not the least of which were that only one subject did not receive ECMO, and that none of the infants not in the trial who did not receive ECMO died (Paneth and Wallenstein, 1985; Ware and Epstein, 1985). Subsequently, more extensive trials confirmed the value of ECMO (1996).

Care is needed when selecting adaptive designs, and power is difficult to determine. Nevertheless, sometimes such a design might give a clear answer using the minimum number of subjects. In a conventional trial of azidothymidine (AZT) in preventing the vertical transmission of HIV from mother to infant, 239 women received AZT and 238 received placebo; 60 infants in the placebo group had HIV as against 20 in the treated group (Connor et al., 1994). An analysis of this study using an adaptive design suggested that a similar significant result could have been attained with only seven failures in the placebo group, and thus would have involved a much smaller trial (Yao and Wei, 1996).

REFERENCES

Abdi, H., 2007. O'Brien test for homogeneity of variance. In: Salkind, N. (Ed.), Encyclopedia of Measurement and Statistics. Sage, Thousand Oaks, CA.

Aickin, M., Gensler, H., 1996. Adjusting for multiple testing when reporting research results: the Bonferroni vs Holm methods. Am. J. Public Health 86, 726–728.

Armitage, P., 1975. Sequential Medical Trials, p. 194.

Armitage, P., McPherson, C.K., Rowe, B.C., 1969. Repeated significance tests on accumulating data. J. R. Stat. Soc. A 132, 235–244.

Bartlett, R.H., Roloff, D.W., Cornell, R.G., Andrews, A.F., Dillon, P.W., Zwischenberger, J.B., 1985. Extracorporeal circulation in neonatal respiratory failure: a prospective randomized study. Pediatrics 76, 479–487.

Benjamini, Y., Hochberg, Y., 1995. Controlling the False Discovery Rate: a practical and powerful approach to multiple testing. J. R. Stat. Assoc. Ser. B Methodol. 57, 289–300.

Bland, J.M., Altman, D.G., 1995. Multiple significance tests: the Bonferroni method. BMJ 310, 170.

Broer, L., Lill, C.M., Schuur, M., Amin, N., Roehr, J.T., Bertram, L., Ioannidis, J.P., Van Duijn, C.M., 2013. Distinguishing true from false positives in genomic studies: p values. Eur. J. Epidemiol. 28, 131–138.

Colquhoun, D., 2014. An investigation of the false discovery rate and the misinterpretation of P values. Royal Society Open Science, 1:10.1098/rsos.140216.

Connor, E.M., Sperling, R.S., Gelber, R., Kiselev, P., Scott, G., O'Sullivan, M.J., Vandyke, R., Bey, M., Shearer, W., Jacobson, R.L., et al., 1994. Reduction of maternal-infant transmission of human immunodeficiency virus type 1 with zidovudine treatment. Pediatric AIDS Clinical Trials Group Protocol 076 Study Group. N. Engl. J. Med. 331, 1173–1180.

Creasy, R.K., Barrett, C.T., De Swiet, M., Kahanpaa, K.V., Rudolph, A.M., 1972. Experimental intrauterine growth retardation in the sheep. Am. J. Obstet. Gynecol. 112, 566–573.

DeMets, D.L., Lan, K.K., 1994. Interim analysis: the alpha spending function approach. Stat. Med. 13, 1341–1352 discussion 1353–6.

Dunnett, C.W., 1970. Multiple comparisons. In: Mcarthur, J.W., Colton, T. (Eds.), Statistics in Endocrinology. The MIT Press, Cambridge, MA.

UK collaborative randomised trial of neonatal extracorporeal membrane oxygenation. UK Collaborative ECMO Trail Group. Lancet 348, 1996, 75–82.

Elo, L.L., Hiissa, J., Tuimala, J., Kallio, A., Korpelainen, E., Aittokallio, T., 2009. Optimized detection of differential expression in global profiling experiments: case studies in clinical transcriptomic and quantitative proteomic datasets. Brief. Bioinform. 10, 547–555.

Elo, L.L., Schwikowski, B., 2012. Mining proteomic data for biomedical research. WIREs Data Min. Knowl. Discov. 2, 1–13.

Genovese, C.R., Lazar, N.A., Nichols, T., 2002. Thresholding of statistical maps in functional neuroimaging using the false discovery rate. Neuroimage 15, 870–878.

Glantz, S.A., 1980. Biostatistics: how to detect, correct, and prevent errors in the medical literature. Circulation 61, 1–7.

Haybittle, J.L., 1971. Repeated assessment of results in clinical trials of cancer treatment. Br. J. Radiol. 44, 793—797.

Hellier, F.F., 1963. A comparative trial of trimeprazine and amylobarbitone in pruritus. Lancet 1, 471—472.

Hochberg, Y., Benjamini, Y., 1990. More powerful procedures for multiple significance testing. Stat. Med. 9, 811—818.

Holm, S., 1979. A simple sequentially rejective multiple test procedure. Scand. J. Stat. 6, 65—70.

Jamerson, K., Weber, M.A., Bakris, G.L., Dahlof, B., Pitt, B., Shi, V., Hester, A., Gupte, J., Gatlin, M., Velazquez, E.J., 2008. Benazepril plus amlodipine or hydrochlorothiazide for hypertension in high-risk patients. N. Engl. J. Med. 359, 2417—2428.

Karp, N.A., Lilley, K.S., 2007. Design and analysis issues in quantitative proteomics studies. Proteomics 7 (Suppl. 1), 42—50.

Karp, N.A., McCormick, P.S., Russell, M.R., Lilley, K.S., 2007. Experimental and statistical considerations to avoid false conclusions in proteomics studies using differential in-gel electrophoresis. Mol. Cell. Proteomics 6, 1354—1364.

Kusuoka, H., Hoffman, J.I., 2002. Advice on statistical analysis for Circulation Research. Circ. Res. 91, 662—671.

Lan, K.K., Wittes, J., 1988. The B-value: a tool for monitoring data. Biometrics 44, 579—585.

Lan, K.K.G., DeMets, D.L., 1983. Discrete sequential boundaries for clinical trials. Biometrika 70, 659—663.

Levin, B., 1996. On the Holm, Simes, and Hochberg multiple test procedures. Am. J. Public Health 86, 628—629.

Lewis Jr., H.D., Davis, J.W., Archibald, D.G., Steinke, W.E., Smitherman, T.C., Doherty 3rd, J.E., Schnaper, H.W., Lewinter, M.M., Linares, E., Pouget, J.M., Sabharwal, S.C., Chesler, E., Demots, H., 1983. Protective effects of aspirin against acute myocardial infarction and death in men with unstable angina. Results of a Veterans Administration Cooperative Study. N. Engl. J. Med. 309, 396—403.

McPherson, K., 1974. Statistics: the problem of examining accumulating data more than once. N. Engl. J. Med. 290, 501—502.

Mehta, C., Gao, P., Bhatt, D.L., Harrington, R.A., Skerjanec, S., Ware, J.H., 2009. Optimizing trial design: sequential, adaptive, and enrichment strategies. Circulation 119, 597—605.

Nichols, T., Hayasaka, S., 2003. Controlling the familywise error rate in functional neuroimaging: a comparative review. Stat. Methods Med. Res. 12, 419—446.

O'Brien, P.C., 1983. The appropriateness of analysis of variance and multiple-comparison procedures. Biometrics 39, 787—788.

O'Brien, P.C., Fleming, T.R., 1979. A multiple testing procedure for clinical trials. Biometrics 35, 549—556.

O'Brien, P.C., Shampo, M.A., 1988a. Statistical considerations for performing multiple tests in a single experiment. 1. Introduction. Mayo Clin. Proc. 63, 813—815.

O'Brien, P.C., Shampo, M.A., 1988b. Statistical considerations for performing multiple tests in a single experiment. 3. Repeated measures over time. Mayo Clin. Proc. 63, 918—920.

O'Brien, P.C., Shampo, M.A., 1988c. Statistical considerations for performing multiple tests in a single experiment. 4. Performing multiple statistical tests on the same data. Mayo Clin. Proc. 63, 1043—1045.

O'Brien, P.C., Shampo, M.A., 1988d. Statistical considerations for performing multiple tests in a single experiment. 5. Comparing two therapies with respect to several endpoints. Mayo Clin. Proc. 63, 1140—1143.

O'Brien, P.C., Shampo, M.A., 1988e. Statistical considerations for performing multiple tests in a single experiment. 6. Testing accumulated data repeatedly over time. Mayo Clin. Proc. 63, 1245—1250.

O'Neill, R., Wetherill, G.B., 1971. The present state of multiple comparison methods. J. R. Stat. Soc. Ser. B 33, 218—241.

Paneth, N., Wallenstein, S., 1985. Extracorporeal membrane oxygenation and the play the winner rule. Pediatrics 76, 622—623.

Pawitan, Y., Michiels, S., Koscielny, S., Gusnanto, A., Ploner, A., 2005. False discovery rate, sensitivity and sample size for microarray studies. Bioinformatics 21, 3017—3024.

Perneger, T.V., 1998. What's wrong with Bonferroni adjustments. BMJ 316, 1236—1238.

Peto, R., Pike, M.C., Armitage, P., Breslow, N.E., Cox, D.R., Howard, S.V., Mantel, N., McPherson, K., Peto, J., Smith, P.G., 1976. Design and analysis of randomized clinical trials requiring prolonged observation of each patient. I. Introduction and design. Br. J. Cancer 34, 585−612.

Pocock, S., White, I., 1999. Trials stopped early: too good to be true? Lancet 353, 943−944.

Pocock, S.J., 2006. Current controversies in data monitoring for clinical trials. Clin. Trials 3, 513−521.

Pocock, S.J., Hughes, M.D., Lee, R.J., 1987. Statistical problems in the reporting of clinical trials. N. Engl. J. Med. 317, 426−432.

Rosenberger, W.F., 1999. Randomized play-the-winner clinical trials: review and recommendations. Control. Clin. Trials 20, 328−342.

Rothman, K.J., 1990. No adjustments are needed for multiple comparisons. Epidemiology 1, 43−46.

Royall, R.M., Bartlett, R.H., Cornell, R.G., Byar, D.P., Dupont, W.D., Levine, R.J., Lindley, F., Simes, R.J., Zelen, M., 1991. Ethics and statistics in randomized clinical trials. Stat. Sci. Rev. J. Inst. Math. Stat. 6, 52−88.

Storey, J.D., 2002. A direct approach to false discovery rates. J. R. Stat. Soc. Ser. B Stat. Methodol. 64, 479−498.

Storey, J.D., Tibshirani, R., 2003. Statistical significance for genomewide studies. Proc. Natl. Acad. Sci. U.S.A. 100, 9440−9445.

Tukey, J.W., 1977. Some thoughts on clinical trials, especially problems of multiplicity. Science 198, 679−684.

Wallenstein, S., Zucker, C.L., Fleiss, J.L., 1980. Some statistical methods useful in circulation research. Circ. Res. 47, 1−9.

Ware, J.H., Epstein, M.F., 1985. Extracorporeal circulation in neonatal respiratory failure: a prospective randomized study. Pediatrics 76, 849−851.

Wright, S.P., 1992. Adjusted P-values for simultaneous inference. Biometrics 48, 1005−1013.

Yao, Q., Wei, L.J., 1996. Play the winner for phase II/III clinical trials. Stat. Med. 15, 2413−2423 discussion 2455−8.

CHAPTER 25

Analysis of Variance I. One-Way

Contents

BASIC CONCEPTS

Basic Test

The discussion about multiple comparisons introduces the most effective way of comparing the means of several groups—analysis of variance (ANOVA). The one-way ANOVA is simple conceptually and computationally, but has powerful extensions that underlie more complex analyses. When comparing the means of several groups, several replicate determinations are made for each independent variable, and measurements within each data set will vary. The independent variables are termed factors. For example, different drugs that might lower blood pressure are tested, using 10 different subjects for each drug. The drugs therefore are factors. In some experiments, different concentrations of each drug might be used, for example, a low dose and a high dose. These subdivisions of the factors are termed levels. The set of levels and factors is termed a treatment.

One requirement for the unpaired t-test was that the variances in the two groups should be homogeneous, and this applies if >2 groups are compared. To see why this is important, examine the problem of determining the variance of a population. Twelve random measurements are selected from a population, and the sum of squares of

For a list of all websites referred to in this chapter, as clickable links, see the book companion website: www.booksite.elsevier.com/9780128023877.

Biostatistics for Medical and Biomedical Practitioners
http://dx.doi.org/10.1016/B978-0-12-802387-7.00025-1

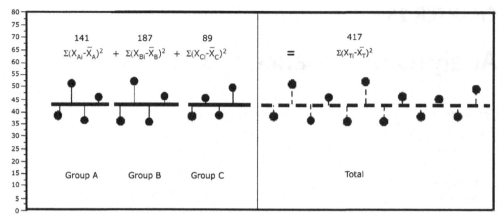

Figure 25.1 Diagram to illustrate basis of ANOVA. See text.

deviations from the mean is calculated. This term is shortened to "sum of squares" and abbreviated to SS, with a subscript to indicate the group. Here the subscript is T to indicate the total group. Calculate SS_T (right hand panel, Figure 25.1). Dividing SS_T by degrees of freedom $N_T - 1$ gives the variance. In ANOVA the variance is usually called the mean square (MS), which is what it is.

Assume that there are 3 data sets A, B, and C with 4 measurements in each, each set taken at random from the same population as used for the total group of 12. As shown in Figure 25.1, the subgroup means might be equal—an unlikely occurrence. If that occurred, then there would be no difference by adding up the sums of squared deviations from the means in sets of 4 for the 3 subgroups separately, or by adding up all 12 squared deviations as in the total group on the right. The two SS are equal.

It is more likely that there will be three different means: $\overline{X}_A$, $\overline{X}_B$, and $\overline{X}_C$, as in Figure 25.2. In this example the mean for group A has been increased by 9 and the

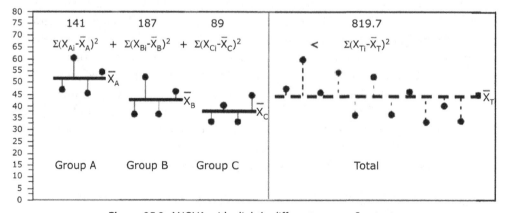

Figure 25.2 ANOVA with slightly different means. See text.

mean for group C has been decreased by 5. The variability of points about the means has not been changed.

The thin solid vertical lines show the deviations of each point from its own mean. Squaring these deviations and adding them up gives the respective SS for each group shown in the formula above each data set: these are SS_A (141), SS_B (187), and SS_C (89). When these are added together, their total remains 417 because the variability about each mean has not changed. This sum is, however, much smaller than the SS for the total group because now many of the deviations from the mean of the total group have increased, as shown by the dashed vertical lines in the right hand panel. This is due to the Principle of Least Squares (Chapter 4); the sum of squared deviations is always least about the mean of its own data set. As a result, if we add the three subgroup SS, that total will be less than the SS for the total group.

This increased total SS therefore reflects differences among the means. If the means are close to each other then the difference will be small, and if the means differ markedly then the difference will be large.

Dividing each subgroup SS by its own degrees of freedom (here $4 - 1 = 3$) gives the MS (or variance) for each group, and we can average these three MSs to obtain another estimate of the population MS. (Although the example has equal numbers in each subgroup, this is not a requirement for ANOVA. If the numbers in each subgroup were different, derive a weighted MS by adding up all the SS and dividing by the total degrees of freedom, namely $N_T - k$, where k is the number of subgroups.) There is a third way to estimate the population variance. The means of the three subgroups are averaged to give an overall mean $\overline{X}_T$, and we can calculate the SS of deviations from these means (SS_B) as $\sum (\overline{X}_i - \overline{X}_T)^2$. The subscript B indicates that the SS is derived from differences between the means. Divide this sum by $k - 1$ degrees of freedom ($3 - 1 = 2$ because there are 3 subgroups) to obtain the variance of the mean, and the square root of this is the standard deviation of the mean. But the standard deviation of the mean can also be estimated from $s_{\overline{X}} = \frac{s}{\sqrt{N}}$, where N is the sample size. Square this expression to get $s_{\overline{X}}^2 = \frac{s^2}{N}$. Therefore multiplying the variance of the mean $s_{\overline{X}}^2$ by N, the subgroup sample size (here $N = 4$), gives another estimate of the population variance.

There are thus three ways of estimating the population MS or variance: one from the total group (MS_T), one by averaging the subgroup variances (MS_W), and one from the means (MS_B). (In many texts, the SS within groups is referred to as SSE, where E stands for error, and the SS between groups is referred to as SST, where T refers to treatment. In reading about statistics, it pays to make sure what the abbreviations mean.)

ANOVA calculations are best done by computer, with free online programs available at http://www.physics.csbsju.edu/stats/anova_NGROUP_NMAX_form.html, http://vassarstats.net/anova1u.html, http://web.mst.edu/~psyworld/anovacalculator.htm; all

Table 25.1 Vitamin B_{12} data

	Litter A	Litter B	Litter C	Litter D	Total
Daily weight	1.30	1.26	1.29	1.38	
gain (lbs)	1.19	1.21	1.23	1.27	
	1.08	1.19	1.23	1.22	
ΣX	3.57	3.66	3.75	3.87	14.85
N	3	3	3	3	12
$\overline{X}$	1.19	1.22	1.25	1.29	1.2375
$\sum (X_i - \overline{X})^2$	0.0242	0.0026	0.0024	0.0134	0.059025
MS	0.0121	0.0013	0.0012	0.0067	0.005366
$(\sum X_i)^2$	12.7449	13.3956	14.0625	14.9769	220.5225
$\dfrac{(\sum X_i)^2}{N}$	4.2483	4.4652	4.6875	4.9923	18.3769

of these allow entry of all the data points. Other programs such as http://danielsoper. com/statcalc3/calc.aspx?id=43 and http://statpages.org/anova1sm.html allow entry of sample size, mean, and standard deviation of groups when the primary measurements are unavailable. The discussion to follow shows what the computations do, and helps to clarify the method.

Table 25.1, from an experiment by Richardson et al. (1951) on the requirement of weanling pigs for vitamin B_{12}, shows the average daily weight gain (in lbs) of three animals in each of four litters, each litter receiving a different amount of vitamin B_{12}.

The last two rows are inserted to show an alternative calculation for the between group SS, discussed below.

The table shows for each litter in columns 2–5 the sums ΣX, the number N, and the mean value $\overline{X}$. The last column shows the sum of weights, number of pigs, and mean value for the total set of 12 pigs. The next row shows the SS for each litter separately $\left(\sum (X_i - \overline{X})^2 \right)$, and for the total group; the four litter SS do not add up to the total SS, for the reason shown in Figure 25.2. Divide the SS for each litter and for the total group by the corresponding degrees of freedom ($N - 1$) to obtain the MS in the next line. These values do vary, and whether this is sampling variation or not will be described later. Finally, estimate the population MS from the group means:

$$s_{\overline{X}}^2 = \frac{(1.19 - 1.2375)^2 + (1.22 - 1.2375)^2 + (1.25 - 1.2375)^2 + (1.29 - 1.2375)^2}{3}$$

$$= 0.001825.$$

Therefore estimate s^2 as $s_{\overline{X}}^2 N = 0.001825 \times 3 = 0.005475$.
Summary of results are shown in Table 25.2.

Table 25.2 Basic ANOVA

Source of variation	SS	Df	MS	F
Total (SS_T)	0.059025	11	0.005366	
Within (SS_W)	0.0426	8	0.005325	
Between (SS_B)	0.016425	3	0.005475	1.028
				$P = 0.4109$

The value of SS_B calculated directly is 0.016425, but this is also the same as $SS_T - SS_W$: 0.059025 − 0.0426. Similarly, the degrees of freedom for SS_B is 4 − 1 = 3, but this is also the same as total degrees of freedom minus within degrees of freedom = 11 − 8 = 3. These are identities. We have partitioned the total SS and total Df into two components: one due to the within group SS and Df, and one due to the between group SS and Df. Divide each SS by its own Df to obtain the within group and between group MSs. (These are **not** additive.) In the example above, both MSs are similar. What would happen if the means were very different? Adding 9 to each member of group A and subtracting 5 from each member of group C gives (Figure 25.3).

In this figure, the within group SS has not changed, because each SS is calculated from its own mean. As shown by the dashed vertical lines in the right panel, however, the SS_T has become very large because the mean of the total set is now very different from the individual group means. The MS estimated from the SS_B would be much greater than the MS estimated from SS_W, and we might consider rejecting the null hypothesis that

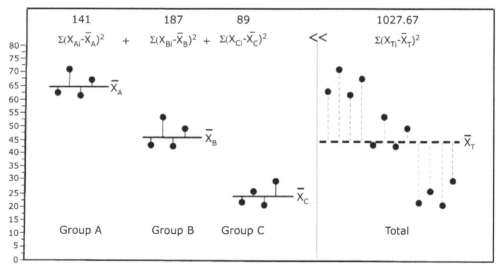

Figure 25.3 Diagram to show effect of large differences among means. A, B, and C are the same data sets used in Figure 25.1 but with their means made to be very different. Note the large increase in α_i ($= \bar{X}_i - \bar{\bar{X}}$, where $\bar{X}_i$ is the mean of subgroup i, and $\bar{\bar{X}}$ is the mean of the whole population) when compared with Figure 25.2.

all the group means come from the same population. Because the SS_W is the smallest estimate of variation available, being based on deviations of points from their own means, any marked increase from this value indicates a component due to differences among the means. The between groups MS is an unbiased estimate of σ^2 + component due to differences among means. This is formally

$$\sigma^2 + \frac{n \sum (\mu_1 - \bar{\mu})^2}{k - 1},$$

where σ^2 is the population variance, k is the number of groups, and n is the number in each group (Snedecor and Cochran, 1989). If the subgroup means are very close to each other, then the numerator of the second part of the expression is very small, and SS_B is only slightly larger than SS_W. If differences among the means are large, then $SS_B \gg SS_W$, and F, the ratio of MS_B to MS_W, will be large enough to reject the null hypothesis.

The between group SS can be obtained directly by calculating $\frac{\left(\sum X_1\right)^2}{N_1} + \frac{\left(\sum X_2\right)^2}{N_2} + \dots \frac{\left(\sum X_k\right)^2}{N_k} - \frac{\left(\sum X_T\right)^2}{N_T}$ (see last two rows of Table 25.1).

That is, square each subgroup sum of X and divide by the number in that subgroup, add all these subgroup values together, and subtract the square of the total measurements divided by the total number of items. This result is important, because in more complex forms of ANOVA, it is always possible to calculate the between-group SS in this way, but may be difficult to calculate the within-group SS directly.

How do we determine a probability of accepting or rejecting the null hypothesis? R. A. Fisher determined the distribution of the ratio MS_B/MS_W, and Snedecor subsequently termed it F. Just as for the t-test, ANOVA estimates the probability of obtaining any given F ratio if the null hypothesis is true. This ratio depends on two different degrees of freedom, one for the between-group SS and one for the within-group SS. In this example, $F = 1.028$ with Df 3, 8, and $P = 0.43$ (Chapter 8). The probabilities of given F ratios can be determined online at http://stattrek.com/online-calculator/f-distribution.aspx, http://www.danielsoper.com/statcalc3/calc.aspx?id=7, http://easycalculation.com/statistics/f-test-p-value.php, http://www.appliedregression.com/statistical-calculators/fdistribution.

Some programs do not include the row for total values, inasmuch as these are used only to obtain the other two rows.

The term "error" for the within-group refers to the minimal natural variation of the data, independent of any differences among the means. SS_W is also termed the residual SS. Other programs may use the term "treatment" for between-groups, because what distinguishes the groups is often the application of different treatments or levels; in the pig data, the four groups represent four different doses of vitamin B_{12}. This type of ANOVA is known as a one-way or one-factor ANOVA, because there is one independent variable being studied. In the example above, the factor was vitamin B_{12} added to the diet in one of four levels.

Problem 25.1

Here is a simple set for practice, based on the blood pressure response (area under the curve) after drinking 480 ml water rapidly in four groups of subjects: MSA-multiple system atrophy (Shy–Drager syndrome), PFA-pure autonomic failure (Bradley-Eggleston syndrome), older controls, and younger controls (Jordan et al., 2000).

MSA	PFA	Older controls	Younger controls
3750	6330	1209	−40
4879	4234	786	−60
3145	3346	826	20
2681	2762	524	20
2580	1875	544	121
2278	1774	444	−504
1935	1854	363	
1774	1552	423	
1572	1431	605	
1230	1310	544	
1350	1169	181	
1512	1048	60	
1310	1230	161	
1190	826	0	
907	604		
665	665		
544	−262		
423			
927			
1048			
645			
464			
262			
161			
−40			
20			
80			

Perform an ANOVA, and think carefully about the results.

Requirements for Test

What are the requirements for a one-way ANOVA? These are similar to those for the unpaired t-test that is equivalent to an ANOVA with two groups. (For two groups, the critical 0.05 value of F is 3.84, and this is the square of 1.96, the critical value of t for large numbers.)

1. The numbers must be ratio or interval numbers.
2. The distributions should be approximately normal.

3. The variances should be homogeneous.
4. There is no need for the numbers in the groups to be the same.
5. The measurements must be independent of each other.

An example with a bigger F value is presented in Table 25.3 and Figure 25.4.

Table 25.3 ANOVA table for stellate ganglion study. There were 26 total measurements, so that the total degrees of freedom are $26 - 1 = 25$. There were 4 groups so that the between group degrees of freedom were $4 - 1 = 3$. The F ratio is high, but not quite at the 0.05 level. Is this because we have not met the requirements? The data appear to be fairly normally distributed, and the numbers are too small to be worth further normality testing. However, we can try to assess the homogeneity of variances.

Source of variation	SS	Df	MS	F
Total (SS_T)	110.4250	25		
Within (SS_W)	83.1652	22	3.7802	
Between (SS_B)	2.2598	3	9.0866	2.4037
				$P = 0.0948$

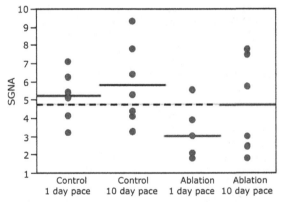

Figure 25.4 Stellate ganglion nerve activity. Dashed line is mean of all data; solid lines are group means.

In this study by Tan et al. (2008), nerve activity in the stellate ganglion (SGNA) was measured after pacing the left atrium in control dogs for 1 day (group A) and 10 days (group B) and 1 day (group C) and 10 days (group D) after cryoablation of sympathetic nerves. Analyze this first as if it were an unplanned experiment. (The term "unplanned" implies that the authors had no specific hypotheses about which groups would differ from the others; this is sometimes referred to as a fishing expedition. The alternative is a planned experiment in which even before the study is performed the authors intend to compare selected groups. Tan et al. actually performed a planned experiment, and the unplanned analysis is used merely for illustration.)

The basic ANOVA is shown in Table 25.3.

Homogeneity of Variance

This is a contentious subject that needs discussion because readers will see these tests mentioned frequently.

How do we tell if the variances are homogeneous, and what difference does it make? (Homogeneous variances are termed "homoscedastic" and heterogeneous variances are termed "heteroscedastic".) Recall that ANOVA compares the average subgroup variance with the total variance, the difference being a function of the differences among the means. If the subgroup variances are very different themselves, they are no longer good estimates of the population variance. More practically, one or a few large variances among several subgroups inflate the value of SS_W, and make it more difficult to achieve a critical F ratio. Various tests are used to assess homogeneity, but they are imperfect.

In the t-test, homogeneity of variances is tested by dividing the larger by the smaller variance to obtain an F ratio, and determining the probability of that ratio for 1 and $N - 2$ degrees of freedom. In ANOVA, it is more complicated. In particular, the frequent combination of big differences in variance, sample size, and departure from normality makes it difficult to develop a single effective statistical test for homogeneity of variance that minimizes Type I and II errors. The literature has references to tests by Levene, Bartlett, Brown and Forsythe, Hartley, O'Brien, Cochrane, and several others, attesting to the unsatisfactory nature of these tests (Zhang, 1998).

There are two main types of tests. One uses the subgroup variances in several ways:

$$\text{calculating Fmax} = \frac{s^2_{max}}{s^2_{min}} \text{ (Hartley)}, \quad C = \frac{s^2_{max}}{\sum^N_{i=1} s^2_i} \text{ (Cochrane)}, \quad or$$

$$z = \frac{\ln s^2_{max} - \ln s^2_{min}}{\sqrt{\frac{N}{2}}},$$

where N is the subgroup size, or an average size if subgroup sizes are not very different (Bartlett and Kendall, 1946), or Bartlett's χ^2 test that involves logarithms of all the subgroup variances (see pages 251–2 (Snedecor and Cochran, 1989)), and which can be implemented online at http://home.ubalt.edu/ntsbarsh/Business-stat/otherapplets/BartletTest.htm. Some of these tests require special tables (see, for example, http://www.stat.ufl.edu/~winner/tables/hartley.pdf for Hartley's test). All are inefficient when the distributions are markedly asymmetrical.

The second type of test examines deviations from the mean. These are typified by Levene's test (Levene, 1960), in which the absolute deviation from the mean is obtained from each subgroup, and an ANOVA is done on these deviations. If one or more subgroups have abnormally large variances, their mean deviations will also be large, and a significant F value will be obtained. A second form of Levene's test is to use the squared deviations, although this exaggerates the effect of outliers. More robust versions of Levene's test are performed by taking deviations either from the median of each subgroup or from a 10% trimmed mean (Brown and Forsythe, 1974). Another variation was recommended by O'Brien (O'Brien and Fleming, 1979).

Unfortunately, all these tests become unreliable when the distributions are very abnormal, and most of them do not give any information about how many variance differences there are.

In the example of nerve activity used above, JMP gives the results of several of these tests of homogeneity of variance (Table 25.4).

Table 25.4 Variance homogeneity tests

Test	F ratio	Df	Prob > F
O'Brien (0.5)	2.5555	3	0.0814
Brown—Forsythe	2.1793	3	0.0602
Levene	3.4274	3	0.0348*
Bartlett	1.1484	3	0.3279

* = p < 0.05.

In addition, Hartley's maximal to minimal variance ratio was $7.3940/1.7036 = 4.3402$, and this was much above the 0.05 value of 3.27. Note the discrepancies: some tests (e.g., Bartlett's) give no indication of heterogeneity and others (Brown—Forsythe, Levene, and Hartley) suggesting the strong possibility of heterogeneity.

The consensus among statisticians is that ANOVA is robust despite considerable heterogeneity of variances as long as the groups have similar sizes. If group sizes are very unequal, then if the larger variances are associated with the larger samples, the Type I error is $<\alpha$, and if they are associated with the smaller sizes the Type I error is $>\alpha$, sometimes by a large amount (see Zar (2010), page 185, Myers and Well (2003), page 221, and Maxwell and Delaney (1990), pages 723—4). The more important question is what should be done if the variances are inhomogeneous. One approach is to carry out the ANOVA, and if it is significant under these circumstances it would be more significant had the variances been homogeneous. If there appear to be samples differing in size, variance, and with severe abnormality (especially with long tails), Lix and Keselman (1998) found by simulation studies that using a trimmed mean and Winsorized variances almost always controlled the Type I error within narrow limits. Given that Type I errors can be as high as 50% under some circumstances, their approach should be considered whenever there is severe abnormality of distributions.

A third approach is to transform the data by, for example, logarithmic or square root transformation (the latter most useful for counts) and then perform an ANOVA.

Although the transformed means are not the same as the original means, the ANOVA still tests for differences in location. Methods of finding the correct transformation are available (Emerson and Stoto, 1983; Sokal and Rohlf, 1995). A fourth approach is to use a test such as the Welch or the Games and Howell test that allows for inhomogeneity of variance (Games and Howell, 1976; Games et al., 1981). In the example used above, the F ratio was higher with the Welch than the regular ANOVA (3.34 vs 2.43, respectively) with a reduction in the value of α from 0.0925 to 0.0574. A fifth approach is to use a nonparametric or distribution-free test. The test most often used in the Kruskal–Wallis test that is an extension of the Mann–Whitney test to more than two groups.

Kruskal–Wallis Test

All the data are pooled and ranked from smallest (1) to largest (N), then the sums of ranks in each subgroup are added up, and the probability is calculated. The statistic H is

$$ H = \frac{12}{N(N+1)} \sum \frac{R_i^2}{n_i} - 3(N+1), \quad \text{or} \quad H = \frac{12}{N(N+1)} \sum n_i \overline{r_i^2} - 3(N+1) $$

where N is the total number, n_i is the number in the ith group, and R_i is the total sum of ranks in the ith group; in the second equation $\overline{r_i^2} = \frac{\sum R_i^2}{n_i^2}$. Either equation can be used. The value of H is tested against the chi-squared distribution for $k - 1$ degrees of freedom, where k is the number of groups. If there are tied ranks a correction is used, but makes very little difference.

Example: the stellate nerve ganglion data from Figure 25.3 are ranked (Table 25.5).

Table 25.5 Kruskal–Wallis test. The ranks are in parentheses

A	B	C	D
7.19 (5)	9.38 (1)	5.47 (9)	7.89 (2)
6.25 (7)	7.81 (3)	3.91 (17)	7.66 (4)
5.39 (10)	6.48 (6)	2.97 (20.5)	5.86 (8)
5.23 (13)	5.31 (11.5)	1.72 (25.5)	2.97 (20.5)
5.31 (11.5)	4.53 (14)	1.80 (24)	2.50 (22)
4.14 (15.5)	4.14 (15.5)	2.11 (23)	1.72 (25.5)
3.20 (19)	3.28 (18)		
$\Sigma R_i = 81$	69	119	82
$\overline{r_i} = 11.37$	9.86	19.83	13.67

Therefore, $H = \frac{12}{26 \times 27} \left(\frac{81^2}{7} + \frac{69^2}{7} + \frac{119^2}{6} + \frac{82^2}{6} \right) - 3 \times 27 = 6.1498$, with 3 degrees of freedom, so that $P = 0.1045$. This was no better than the original ANOVA.

Both tests suggest differences among the group means, but with small sample sizes the power of the ANOVA was low (0.53). Standard computer programs perform the analysis, and online calculators are available: (http://faculty.vassar.edu/lowry/kw4.html, or http://www.swogstat.org/stat/public/freqstat.htm), and at http://www.mathcracker.com/kruskal-wallis.php. The Kruskal—Wallis test is also used when data sets are composed of ordinal values.

If the Kruskal—Wallis test shows significance, which means are different? Of the several recommended tests, Dunn's is the most useful because it allows for different sample sizes (Dunn, 1964). To perform the test, calculate the statistic Q as

$$Q = \frac{R_i - R_j}{\sqrt{\frac{N(N+1)}{12}\left(\frac{1}{n_i} + \frac{1}{n_j}\right)}},$$

where R_i and R_j are the average ranks for the two groups being compared, with n_i and n_j their respective sample sizes, and N the total sample size.

The critical values for Q depend on the number of groups. It is a Bonferroni type correction in which a critical value to hold the family wide comparison rate at 0.05 is a z value equivalent to $\frac{0.05}{\frac{k(k-1)}{2}}$. The denominator is the number of possible comparisons that can be made with k groups. The critical value can be determined online at http://www.graphpad.com/faq/viewfaq.cfm?faq=1156.

The Kruskal—Wallis test with only two groups is equivalent to the Mann—Whitney U test.

Problem 25.2

Savman et al. (Savman, et al., 1998. Cytokine response in cerebrospinal fluid after birth asphyxia. Pediatr. Res. 43 (6), 746—751) studied newborns who were normal or else had grades I—III of hypoxic-ischemic brain injury (HIE). They measured interleukin-6 (IL-6) concentrations in the cerebrospinal fluid and found the following results:

Raw data for sample

A	B	C	D
0	26	0	28
0	27	33	79
0	56	42	261
0	247	171	292
0		236	538
35		247	551
43		549	624
		574	640

Problem 25.2—cont'd

IL-6 concentrations in pg/ml. A is the control group, and B, C, and D are grades I, II, and III, respectively, of HIE.

The differences in sample size and ranges are large enough to suggest that ANOVA might not be the best choice to analyze these data. Use the Kruskal–Wallis test instead. Then compare the mean ranks of groups A and C by Dunn's test.

Conover and Iman (1981) developed a rank test by performing ANOVA on the ranks. The rank statistic F_R is evaluated with degrees of freedom $k - 1$ and $N - k$. F_R and H are equivalent. Unlike a classical ANOVA that requires normality of distributions (but certainly tolerates quite wide departures from normality) these rank tests do not require any specific form of distribution, but do require that each group has a similar distribution.

No one method for dealing with heteroscedasticity is ideal (Grissom, 2000), and caution is needed in interpreting the results of ANOVA when it is present.

Independence of Observations

An assumption is that when successive measurements of a variate are made, the errors are independent of each other, without any correlation due to space or time. When sequential errors are examined they should be random, not a series of positive errors and other series with negative errors. Because uniformity and independence of errors is an essential part of ANOVA, failure of independence makes the test less sensitive.

Several ways of testing for independence of errors are mentioned in Chapter 31. Another simple one was developed in 1941 by von Neumann et al. (1941), who computed the square of each difference $d^2 = (X_{i+1} - X_i)^2$ and added all these differences up to get Σd^2. (The X_i values indicate each successive value.) Divide this sum by $\sum (X_i - \overline{X})^2$. If the measurements are independent the ratio $\eta = \dfrac{\sum d^2}{\sum (X_i - \overline{X})^2}$ should equal 2. Values other than near 2 can be assessed from tables (Sokal and Rohlf, 1995) or, if $N > 25$, from the normal approximation

$$t = \frac{\left|1 - \frac{\eta}{2}\right|}{\sqrt{\frac{N-2}{N^2-1}}}.$$

Lack of independence suggests some bias in making the measurements, and indicates the need to redesign the experiment. Values $\ll 2$ suggest some correlation between the measurements. The test can be performed online at http://www.wessa.net/slr.wasp.

Independence may be more important than homogeneity of variance or normality when testing hypotheses (van Belle, 2002). Correlation between successive measurements increases the true over the calculated standard error and increases the chances of a Type I error, sometimes considerably.

Effect Size

In the t-test the effect size is evaluated not only by the absolute difference between the means, but also by the relative difference, namely absolute difference/standard deviation. Similarly in ANOVA, we need a relative difference. Several statistics have been recommended. One of them is the coefficient of multiple determination, R^2.

$$R^2 = \frac{SS_{Between}}{SS_{Total}}$$

This indicates what proportion of the total SS the between group SS makes. To correct for a slight overestimation, an adjusted formula is usually used:

$$R_{adj}^2 = 1 - \left(\frac{N-1}{N-k}\right)(1 - R^2)$$

For the example in Table 25.2, this gives

$$R^2 = \frac{0.016425}{0.059025} = 0.2783,$$

so that

$$R_{adj}^2 = 1 - \frac{11}{8}(1 - 0.2783) = 0.0077.$$

This result suggests that differences between the group means contribute little to the total variability, and is consistent with the lack of significance in the ANOVA. It shows too the importance of the adjustment.

An alternative approach based on the contribution of the treatment variability to the total variability (effect size) (Cohen, 1992; Keppel et al., 1992) is

$$\omega_B^2 = \frac{\sigma_B^2}{\sigma_B^2 + \sigma_W^2},$$

where $\sigma_B^2 = \frac{DF_B(MS_B - MS_W)}{kn}$, k is the number of groups and n the number per group (assumed equal). If they are unequal, an average of N can be substituted.

Another way of calculating ω_B^2 is

$$\omega_B^2 = \frac{(k-1)(F-1)}{(k-1)(F-1) + kn},$$

and yet another way (Maxwell et al., 1981) is

$$\omega_B^2 = \frac{SS_B - (k-1)MS_W}{SS_T + MS_W}.$$

Which formula is used depends upon which of the required values are readily available.

Sample Size

There are different formulas when all the subsample sizes are the same ($n_i = n_j$) and if they differ ($n_i \neq n_j$), and if all the means but one are similar versus all the means appear to be different versus the highest and lowest means are different but the rest are bunched in the middle versus the means are fairly evenly scattered from highest to lowest. The basic principle is to calculate a standardized difference, sometimes termed ϕ, the noncentrality parameter, as

$$\phi = \frac{\delta}{\sigma}\sqrt{\frac{n}{2k}},$$

where δ is the difference between the one mean and the average of the others (the effect size), σ is the common within group standard deviation, n is the common sample size, and k is the number of groups. Alternatively, if sample sizes are the same and the means are all different, then use

$$\phi = \sqrt{\frac{n \sum \left(\overline{X}_i - \mu\right)^2}{k\sigma^2}},$$

where $\overline{X}$ refers to each individual expected mean and μ is the mean of the whole set. These two formulas are described by Glantz (2005), who gives tables that are entered with the estimates of ϕ and the degrees of freedom for the between group SS and the within group SS.

Cohen (1988) rearranges the formula so that $f = \frac{\phi}{\sqrt{n}}$. The calculation of f depends on the distributions of the means and whether sample sizes are same or not the same. He provides extensive tables.

A small effect is $\omega_B^2 \leq 0.01$, a medium effect is $0.01 \leq \omega_B^2 \leq 0.15$, and a large effect is $\omega_B^2 > 0.15$. Based on estimated effect sizes, formulas are available for estimating sample size. The programs can be used also to calculate the power of a completed ANOVA. Into the program put values for alpha, total sample size N, the number of groups k, and the calculated value of Cohen's f (see above).

Calculations can be done for simple analyses online at https://www.statstodo.com/ SSizAOV_Pgm.php, by interpolation in the simple online program, http://www. divms.uiowa.edu/~rlenth/Power/, and with the program G*Power found at http://www.psycho.uni-duesseldorf.de/abteilungen/aap/gpower3/. Because of all the variables concerned, any results obtained should be regarded as conservative.

ADVANCED CONCEPTS

Multiple Comparisons

This section is necessary to any study of ANOVA, but should be omitted at a first reading until the reader is satisfied about how to perform an ANOVA. There are numerous tests available, no one test is ideal, and there is no consistency in their use. Standard statistics programs implement most of these tests, but readers need to know what the tests do and how reliable they are. I will describe the preferred ones at the end of this section, but because the biomedical community still uses the older tests, readers need to be aware of what they are and how they perform in making statistical inferences. Inferences based on these tests are even less secure if sample sizes differ greatly, variances are very heterogeneous, or distributions are grossly abnormal.

Although ANOVA is recommended for comparing the means of several groups, if the null hypothesis of equality of means is rejected the problem is to decide how many subgroups there are. If the F test allows us to reject the null hypothesis for 6 groups, are there 6 different groups, or does 1 group differ from the other 5, or are there 3 sets of 2 groups, and so on? The approach to this subject depends on what type of experiment is being done. There are two main types of experiments—*planned* and *unplanned*. The planned experiment is one in which a specific hypothesis is being tested. For example, if we prepare a batch of dough to make doughnuts, we might hypothesize that more unsaturated than saturated fat is taken up by the dough during the frying process. It is convenient to make one large batch of dough and test many different types of fats at the same time in one experiment. In the analysis, however, the primary interest is in comparing saturated with unsaturated fat uptake. The unplanned experiment is one with no specific hypothesis and is referred to as data dredging, data mining, or fishing. The experiments are performed, the means of each group are determined, and then all the means are inspected to find out if any large differences exist. As another example, an investigator may do a screening experiment to determine the effect on white blood cells of many different types of anesthetic agents. Those found worthy of more detailed study enter a second more focused round of experiments. The planned study is termed an a *priori* study, one in which the important comparisons to be made are designated ahead of time. The unplanned study is termed an a *posteriori* experiment in which, based on the mean values observed, we try to decide which groups are different and worth further study. The latter approach is less efficient, and often precedes a more focused study.

Evaluating unplanned comparisons in an a posteriori study involves striking a balance between keeping the Type I error low without inflating the Type II error. In 2000, Curran-Everett reported that in 1997 about 40% of the articles published in the *American Journal of Physiology* used multiple comparison procedures (Curran-Everett, 2000). The tests most often used were the Student—Newman—Keuls (SNK), Fisher's least significant difference (LSD), and the Bonferroni tests, but other tests such as Duncan, Dunnett, Scheffé's, Tukey, and unnamed procedures formed 45% of the tests used. Tests vary with philosophy, and may differ if there are variations in sample size, variances, or shape of the distribution. The tests may be classified as single step (Tukey, Fisher, Scheffé) and multiple step (SNK, Duncan, Dunnett, Holm, Hochberg, Ryan). The single-step tests use a single factor in a formula to calculate an "allowance"; if the difference between the means exceeds that allowance then the means are regarded as significantly different at a selected level of α, the Type I error. The multiple step methods change the value of the factor depending on the number of means being examined; they start by comparing the two means that show the greatest difference, then select the next smaller difference, and so on.

Studentized Range Test

Multiple comparisons for ANOVA are usually performed with a modified t-test based on the studentized range that allows for several groups. The studentized range, attributed to Gosset, is symbolized by q or Q: $q_{ar} = \frac{\overline{X}_{max} - \overline{X}_{min}}{s}$ or $\frac{\overline{X}_{max} - \overline{X}_{min}}{\sqrt{\frac{MS_W}{n}}}$, where the independent X variates come from a normal distribution, $\overline{X}_{min}$ and $\overline{X}_{max}$ are the smallest and largest of the means, n is the number in each subgroup (assumed equal), s is the standard deviation, r is the number of groups, and MS_W is the within group, residual or error MS. This formula is very similar to the formula for t that is $t = \frac{\overline{X}_1 - \overline{X}_2}{\sqrt{\frac{2MS_W}{n}}}$. The only difference is $\sqrt{2}$ in the denominator. In both tests, the difference between the means (absolute effect size) is compared to a measure of variability that is standardized to 1 unit standard deviation.

The distribution of q is available from tables or statistics programs. This distribution for mean values depends on r, the number of means (or groups), k, the within group degrees of freedom, v, and the desired value of α. The value of q is shown for selected values of k and v for $\alpha = 0.05$ (Table 25.6).

These critical values can be interpreted as follows. If there are 10 independent means from a normal distribution, and 20 Df, then the ratio q as defined above exceeds 5.008, only 5% of the time.

Table 25.6 0.05 one-sided values of the studentized range value q for selected numbers of groups and degrees of freedom. More complete tables or calculations can be found online at http://vassarstats.net/tabs.html#q, http://cse.niaes.affrc.go.jp/miwa/probcalc/s-range/, and http://academic.udayton.edu/gregelvers/psy216/tables/qtab.htm

	Within group degrees of freedom		
r = **Number of means**	**10**	**20**	**∞**
2	3.151	2.950	2.772
5	4.654	4.232	3.858
10	5.599	5.008	4.474

The pooled value of the variance is calculated from MS_W. The use of q as related to the number of groups is like the Bonferroni adjustment that requires a bigger value of t for any critical probability value.

There are two ways of utilizing the q test. One is just like the t-test. The ratio of the difference between the means to the estimate of variability is calculated and compared with the value of q for $\alpha = 0.05$, or 0.01. If the ratio exceeds the critical value of q,

$$q_{\alpha,r} \leq \frac{\overline{X_i} - \overline{X_j}}{\sqrt{\frac{MS_W}{n}}}$$

then the null hypothesis may be rejected at the given probability. The second way of performing the test is to multiply both sides of the equation by the estimate of variability $\sqrt{\frac{MS_W}{n}}$ to give $q_r\sqrt{\frac{MS_W}{n}} \leq \overline{X_i} - \overline{X_j}$. In this form, the difference between the means is known as the minimum significant difference or MSD or the allowance. Therefore, if the MSD is greater than the critical value of q multiplied by the estimate of variability, the null hypothesis may be rejected at that level.

Single-Step Tests

Fisher introduced the LSD method in which each pair of means is compared by simple t-test, the only difference being that the pooled variance is derived from SS_W. Because the LSD test is performed only after a significant F ratio allows one to reject the universal null hypothesis, this test is sometimes called the protected LSD test. The number of groups does not affect the results, and the critical value is the same as that used for the ANOVA. It is symbolized by $LSD = t_\alpha \sqrt{\frac{2MS_W}{n}}$, where n is the number per subgroup (assumed equal) or if unequal, the harmonic mean of n_i and n_j, the two groups being compared. Any difference >LSD is significant at the specified value of α. This test loses power if there are >3 groups, and is not recommended for more groups.

Similarly, the number of groups does not change the results in the honest significant difference (HSD) method, introduced by Tukey:

$$\text{HSD} = q_\alpha \sqrt{\frac{MS_W}{n_h}},$$

where i and j are the two groups being compared and n_h is the harmonic mean of n_i and n_j. That is, the HSD is the studentized t-test for the two groups being compared. (The factor of 2 that appears in the LSD formula is included in the value of q.) If the difference between the two means exceeds the HSD, then it is significant at that level of alpha. This test can be done online at http://web.mst.edu/~psyworld/virtualstat/tukeys/tukeycalc.html and http://vassarstats.net/anova1u.html. The test, like the Bonferroni adjustment, keeps the experiment-wise error rate at the specified level, for example, 0.05, but at the cost of loss of power. If the sample sizes of the two groups compared are so different that averaging them is of concern, then the Tukey–Kramer test is used. In this variation, the standard error of the difference is calculated as

$$\sqrt{\left[\frac{s^2}{2}\left(\frac{1}{n_j}+\frac{1}{n_k}\right)\right]}.$$

If the variances are very inhomogeneous, then the Welch or Games and Howell test (Games and Howell, 1976; Games et al., 1981) can be used. The Games and Howell cri-

terion is $\left(\sqrt{\frac{s_i^2}{n_i}+\frac{s_j^2}{n_j}}\right)\left(\frac{q_{\alpha k v_{ij}}}{\sqrt{2}}\right)$, where $v_{ij} = \dfrac{\left(\frac{s_i^2}{n_i}+\frac{s_j^2}{n_j}\right)^2}{\dfrac{\left(\frac{s_i^2}{n_i}\right)^2}{n_i-1}+\dfrac{\left(\frac{s_j^2}{n_j}\right)^2}{n_j-1}}$. Here k is the number of

subgroups and v_{ij} is the degrees of freedom, similar to the Welch and Satterthwaite formulas.

Looking at the data for the stellate ganglion activity example (Figure 25.3), the means of groups A, B, and D seem to be similar and higher than the mean of group C. The results of Fisher's LSD test are given in Table 25.7. The 0.05 critical value of t was 2.074.

Thus the mean of group B is significantly different from the mean of C, the mean of group A is almost significantly different from the mean of group C, but remaining mean differences are not significantly different. Looking at the confidence limits rather than P values in such tables is useful. For example, although the A versus C comparison has a P value >0.05, there is a strong trend for A to exceed C such that if the difference is important a modest increase in sample size might allow us to reject the null hypothesis.

The results of the Tukey–Kramer test are shown in Table 25.8. The 0.05 critical value of q was 2.777.

Table 25.7 Fisher's LSD test

	Level	Mean
B	A	5.8471429
A	AB	5.2442857
D	AB	4.7666667
C	B	2.9966667

Levels not connected by same letter are significantly different

Level	−Level	Difference	Lower CL	Upper CL	P Value
B	C	2.850476	0.56589	5.135064	0.0168*
A	C	2.247619	−0.03697	4.532207	0.0535
D	C	1.770000	−0.60083	4.140829	0.1358
B	D	1.080476	−1.20411	3.365064	0.3373
B	A	0.602857	−1.59210	2.797819	0.5747
A	D	0.477619	−1.80697	2.762207	0.6688

* = P < 0.05

Table 25.8 Tukey–Kramer test

Level	−Level	Difference	Lower CL	Upper CL
B	C	2.850476	−0.20850	5.909453
A	C	2.247619	−0.81136	5.306596
D	C	1.770000	−1.40445	4.944450
B	D	1.080476	−1.97850	4.139453
B	A	0.602857	−2.33611	3.541827
A	D	0.477619	−2.58136	3.536596

With this more conservative test, none of the differences were significant. (The power of the test was low.)

The JMP program has an ingenious way of showing the results of testing multiple comparisons with a circle diagram based on studies by Hsu (Figure 25.5).

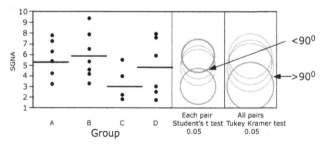

Figure 25.5 Circle tests.

Each circle has its center at the mean for the distribution, and radius corresponding to 95% confidence limits. Where two circles overlap, if the angle between the two overlapping arcs is >90° (lower arrow), the two groups are not significantly different (as shown by the two lowest red (gray in print versions) circles in either column). If the angle is 90°, the difference is borderline, and if the angle is <90° (upper arrow), the difference is significant. Furthermore, selecting a circle reveals color differences. All circles of the same color are not significantly different, as shown for the Tukey−Kramer test. Two circles that indicate a significant difference have different colors, and heavy lines, as shown for the highest and lowest circles in the t-test panel. The lower confidence limits for the t-test (LSD) than the Tukey HSD test are well shown.

The Scheffé test determines the critical value of the minimal studentized difference (MSD) not from the studentized range but from the value of $\sqrt{(k-1)F_{\alpha,(k-1)(N-k)}}$. Thus for $\alpha = 0.05$, $k = 4$, and $N = 25$, and F is the variance ratio, the MSD is 3.005. This MSD is kept constant for all the comparisons, and is not adjusted for different numbers of groups in that particular experiment. In the stellate ganglion example, the MSD exceeds the largest difference between the means, so that none of them are significantly different from each other. These are the same conclusions as reached by the Tukey test. The Scheffé test is excellent for complex comparisons (e.g., the average of means of groups 1 and 2 vs the average of means of groups 3, 4, 5), but is less powerful than the other tests for paired comparisons. The Scheffé test can be performed online at https://www.statstodo.com/LSDScheffe_Pgm.php.

Multiple-Step Tests

The loss of power was partly addressed by the Newman−Keuls method, also known as the SNK method. Rank the means in order of size and compare the largest and smallest means of the k groups. If these are not significantly different by the studentized range test (HSD test), then any lesser differences are also not significant. If, however, the two means with the greatest difference are significantly different, then compare two means that differ by a range of $k - 1$. For example, if the means are 10, 11, 14, 18, 25, each with $n = 5$, and $s = 30$, then compare 10 and 25 over a range of 5 groups. With 20 Df for the within group MS the value of q is 6.12, and the 0.05 level is 4.23, so the difference is significant. Then compare two pairs of means over the range of 4 groups: 11 with 25, and 10 with 18. Each of these is compared with the critical value that is now 3.96. These critical values are based on tables that relate degrees of freedom to the size of the range. As the range gets bigger, so does the critical value, ensuring that the Type I error is not exceeded.

For the stellate ganglion example, the means were in order 5.847 (B), 5.376 (D), 5.244 (A), and 2.997 (C). Test first B versus C, with difference 2.850. The studentized range table for degrees of freedom 4, 21 gives a critical MSD of 3.944. Because this exceeds the observed difference, the difference is not significant, and there is no need to test smaller differences. The SNK test has relatively low power, and is no longer favored.

A similar test by Duncan uses different critical values, and according to some authorities gives too many Type I errors.

To show an example where several pair-wise significant differences are shown, take the stellate ganglion data of Figure 25.3 and add a hypothetical fifth group E (Figure 25.6).

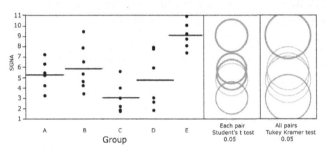

Figure 25.6 Stellate ganglion data with one added group.

The ANOVA is shown in Table 25.9.

Table 25.9 ANOVA with added group

Source of variation	SS	Df	MS	F
Total (SS_T)	211.0440	31		
Within (SS_W)	94.8825	27	3.5412	
Between (SS_B)	116.1615	4	29.0404	8.2638
				$P = 0.0002$

Now the F ratio is highly significant. The results of the LSD and HSD tests are shown in Tables 25.10 and 25.11.

For the LSD test, group E is different from all the other groups (as intended by the artificial construction) but now both groups A and B differ from group C. Adding new data has altered some of the values used in the comparison. For the HSD test, again group E differs from all the other groups, and no other comparisons are significant.

What does the SNK test indicate? The means in order of size are 9.017 (E), 5.847 (B), 5.244 (A), 4.767 (D), and 2.997 (C). Compare first groups E and C, having the greatest difference and a span of 5. If that is significant (as it will be from the Tukey test), then compare E with D, the second smallest, and then B, the second largest, with C, the smallest; each of these comparisons with a span of 4. Then compare means with a span of 3: E versus A, B versus D, and A versus C. The values of $q_{0.05}$ vary with the span and the within group degrees of freedom, which here are 27. For a span of 5 $q = 4.134$, for a

Table 25.10 LSD tests

Level	−Level	Difference	Lower CL	Upper CL	P value
E	C	6.020000	3.79929	8.240711	<0.0001*
E	D	4.250000	2.02929	6.470711	0.0005*
E	A	3.772381	1.63245	5.912312	0.0012*
E	B	3.169524	1.02959	5.309455	0.0052*
B	C	2.850476	0.71055	4.990407	0.0109*
A	C	2.247619	0.10769	4.387550	0.0402*
D	C	1.770000	−0.45071	3.990711	0.1136
B	D	1.080476	−1.05945	3.220407	0.3094
B	A	0.602857	−1.45312	2.658836	0.5524
A	D	0.477619	−1.66231	2.617550	0.6506

* = P <0.05

Table 25.11 HSD tests

Level	−Level	Difference	Lower CL	Upper CL
E	C	6.020000	2.85892	9.181078
E	D	4.250000	1.08892	7.411078
E	A	3.772381	0.72629	6.818472
E	B	3.169524	0.12343	6.215615
B	C	2.850476	−0.19561	5.896567
A	C	2.247619	−0.79847	5.293710
D	C	1.770000	−1.39108	4.931078
B	D	1.080476	−1.96561	4.126567
B	A	0.602857	−2.32373	3.529447
A	D	0.477619	−2.56847	3.523710

span of 4 it is 3.873, and for a span of 3 it is 3.509. Calculate the standard error if $n_i = n_j$ as

$\sqrt{\frac{MS_W}{n_i}}$, and if they are not equal as $\sqrt{\frac{MS_W}{2}\left(\frac{1}{n_i}+\frac{1}{n_j}\right)}$. With these considerations, set up

Table 25.12.

It makes no difference if we compare the MSD with the difference between the means or, as in some texts, compare the critical value of q with the difference divided by the standard error.

Therefore with this test, reject the null hypothesis for comparisons E versus C, E versus D, E versus B, and E versus A. None of the other differences are significant.

The differences among the various multiple comparison methods are shown in Figure 25.7.

The Tukey HSD and the Fisher LSD tests are fixed range tests. (So is the Scheffé test, but its factor changes with the total number of groups tested.) The Tukey test is the most conservative and holds the experiment-wise error rate constant. The Fisher LSD test is

Table 25.12 Student–Newman–Keuls results. DNR; do not reject H_0 at $\alpha = 0.05$. R; reject H_0 at $\alpha = 0.05$. MSD $= SE \times q_{0.05,k,27}$

Comparison	$\overline{X}_i - \overline{X}$	SE	k	$q_{0.05,k,27}$	MSD	H_0
E vs C	6.02	0.7653	5	4.134	3.164	R
E vs D	4.25	0.7653	4	3.873	2.964	R
B vs C	2.85	0.7375	4	3.873	2.856	DNR
E vs A	3.773	0.7375	3	3.509	2.588	R
B vs D	1.08	0.7375	3	3.509	2.588	DNR
A vs C	2.247	0.7375	3	3.509	2.588	DNR
E vs B	3.17	0.7375	2	2.903	2.141	R
B vs A	0.603	0.7085	2	2.903	2.057	DNR
A vs D	0.477	0.7375	2	2.903	2.141	DNR
D vs C	1.77	0.7653	2	2.903	2.222	DNR

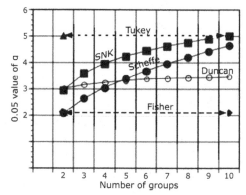

Figure 25.7 Relation of 0.05 value of q to the number of groups for 5 multiple comparison tests when the error degrees of freedom are 20.

the most liberal of all these tests and is intended to keep the comparison-wise error rate constant. However, if there are >3 groups, the LSD test sometimes allows the Type I error rate to rise well above 0.05. To abolish this risk, Hayter (1986) used the studentized range q value for $k - 1$ means or all paired comparisons. Because q is bigger than t, the Type I error rate is lower. The SNK and Scheffé tests start at small values for q and then increase toward the Tukey value as the number of groups increases. They both hold the experiment-wise error rate constant. Duncan's test also has an increased value of q at higher group numbers but the increase is small and regarded by many statisticians as too liberal, that is giving too many Type I errors.

Recommendations

The best advice was given by Dallal (2008). If a difference between means is significant by Tukey's HSD test, then it probably is significant. If it is not significant by Fisher's

LSD test, then it does not warrant further investigation. Anything between the two limits should be investigated further. This is one of the penalties paid for doing unplanned tests.

One possibility to be considered is the Hochberg test (Chapter 24) that has good power. An even better test is the extension of the Ryan test. The SNK test is more powerful than the Tukey test, but does not keep the family-wise error rate low as the number of groups increases. To overcome this, Ryan introduced a way to keep the error rate low and constant by entering the SNK tables with $\alpha_r = \frac{\alpha_{0.05}}{k/r}$, where k is the number of groups and r is the span of the means being compared. Thus, if there are 6 groups and we are comparing the 3rd and 5th means, $k = 6$ and $r = 2$. This basic method was modified to provide the Ryan–Einot–Gabriel–Welsch (R-E-G-W) test in which $\alpha_r = 1 - (1 - \alpha)^{r/k}$. Note the similarity between these corrections and the Bonferroni and Dunn–Sidak approaches. The test is best done by a computer program. Tables for different combinations of k and r (r is termed p in the tables) are given at http://cse.niaes.affrc.go.jp/miwa/probcalc/ryan/ryan_tbl.html#fivepercent.

To show the difference between the SNK and the R-E-G-W tests, Table 25.12 is repeated as Table 25.13 with the addition of the Ryan factors.

Linear Combinations

By definition, a linear combination L is

$$L = \lambda_1 \overline{X_1} + \lambda_2 \overline{X_2} + ... \lambda_n \overline{X_n},$$

where the λs are fixed numbers. The linear combination is called a comparison or contrast if $\sum \lambda_i = 0$.

L has a standard error $\sqrt{\sum \lambda_i^2 \left(\frac{S_W^2}{n} \right)}$.

Here n is the number of observations per group. To see how this information can be used, consider the unpaired t-test that examines the difference between $\overline{X_i}$ and $\overline{X_j}$. This compares one whole part of $\overline{X_i}$ with one whole part of $\overline{X_j}$ for the null hypothesis $\overline{X_i} - \overline{X_j} = 0$, so that the coefficients are $+1$ and -1. Because $1 - 1 = 0$, this is a contrast in which the standard error is $\sqrt{2 \left(\frac{S_W^2}{n} \right)}$, and this is the same as the denominator in the standard t-test (assuming that $n_1 = n_2$).

The advantage of this concept is that it allows us to explore contrasts among more than two groups. For example, in an experiment on yields of different wheat varieties (discussed in detail in Chapter 26), assume that there were three varieties of winter wheat (W) with mean yields of 22.5, 18.83, and 20.62 bushels/acre, and that the summer wheat

Table 25.13 Comparison of SNK and Ryan factors. Column headed $q_{0.05,4,27}$ shows the factors from the SNK table; Column headed Ryan q' gives $q_{0.05}$ values modified for total number of groups and is a better way of keeping the family-wise error rate near 0.05. $MSD = SE \times q_{0.05,k,27}$; $MSD' = SE \times q'$. The Ryan factors increase the size of the MSD when subgroups closer together are compared. H_0; null hypothesis, R; reject, DNR; do not reject

Comparison	$\overline{X}_i - \overline{X}_j$	SE	k	$q_{0.05,k,27}$	MSD	Ryan q'	MSD'	H_0
E vs C	6.02	0.7653	5	4.134	3.164	4.13	3.16	R
E vs D	4.25	0.7653	4	3.873	2.964	3.87	2.96	R
B vs C	2.85	0.7375	4	3.873	2.856	3.87	2.85	DNR
E vs A	3.773	0.7375	3	3.509	2.588	3.828	2.82	R
B vs D	1.08	0.7375	3	3.509	2.588	3.828	2.82	DNR
A vs C	2.247	0.7375	3	3.509	2.588	3.828	2.82	DNR
E vs B	3.17	0.7375	2	2.903	2.141	3.487	2.57	R
B vs A	0.603	0.7085	2	2.903	2.057	3.487	2.47	DNR
A vs D	0.477	0.7375	2	2.903	2.141	3.487	2.57	DNR
D vs C	1.77	0.7653	2	2.903	2.222	3.487	2.67	DNR

(S) yielded 32.83 bushels/acre. How different is the summer yield from the average of the three winter yields? The null hypothesis is

$$\overline{S} - \frac{\overline{W_1} + \overline{W_2} + \overline{W_3}}{3} = 0.$$

From the ANOVA (Chapter 26), the within group or residual MS was 76.225, so that its square root was 8.73; there were 20 degrees of freedom. Then the standard error of the linear contrast is

$$\sqrt{1^2 + \left(\frac{-1}{3}\right)^2 + \left(\frac{-1}{3}\right)^2 + \left(\frac{-1}{3}\right)^2 \left(\frac{8.73}{6}\right)} = 1.68.$$

The observed difference was $32.83 - \frac{22.5 + 18.83 + 20.62}{3} = 12.18$.

Therefore $t = \frac{12.18 - 0}{1.68} = 7.25$, $P < 0.0001$, and we can safely reject the null hypothesis.

Why not use the Bonferroni adjustment to make these multiple comparisons? The maximal Bonferroni adjustment for k groups involves $\frac{k(k-1)}{2}$ comparisons if all pair-wise comparisons are to be tested, even if after inspecting the data fewer comparisons are actually performed, and even if initially a subset of comparisons was planned but more comparisons were done after the results were obtained. This makes the Bonferroni adjustment less powerful than the alternative methods used above (Maxwell and Delaney, 1990).

Planned Experiments

In planned experiments, certain comparisons are designated before the experiment is done. The investigator tests certain specific hypotheses. For these a priori hypotheses, and only for these, once a significant F ratio has been found, t-tests may be done. Returning to the stellate ganglion ablation experiment of Tan et al. (2008), the investigators a priori wanted to compare stellate ganglion activity on day 1 in dogs with and without ablation, on day 10 in dogs with and without ablation, and on day 1 versus day 10 in dogs after ablation. By t-test, these differences had respective probabilities of 0.0157, 0.4527, and 0.1998.

Why not designate every possible pair-wise combination a priori, and do t-tests on all the pairs of means, thus avoiding all the problems discussed above for unplanned experiments? Such a suggestion is illegal because it negates all the well-established arguments that multiple comparisons inflate the Type I error. Second, comparing every mean against every other mean reuses information. If we compare A with B and A with C, we have used the information in all three groups, and then comparing B with C is repetitious. How then do we know how many t-tests may legitimately be done?

Formally, if we want to know if two comparisons are orthogonal (independent), we consider the coefficients of each comparison. In an example about the growth of sugar beets planted at four different combinations of times and ways (Snedecor and Cochran, 1989, page 229), there were two sets of comparisons. The first one compared the average of combinations 2 and 3 with the average of combinations 1 and 4: $\frac{1}{2}X_2 + \frac{1}{2}X_3 - \frac{1}{2}X_1 - \frac{1}{2}X_4$ that provided the coefficients for calculating L. The second comparison was the average of combinations 2 and 3 against combination 4 alone: $\frac{1}{2}X_2 + \frac{1}{2}X_3 - 1X_4 + 0X_1$, in which the yield with no fertilizer (X_1) had a zero coefficient because it was not part of the comparison. Now multiply the corresponding coefficients, and add up the results: $\left(\frac{1}{2} \times \frac{1}{2}\right) + \left(\frac{1}{2} \times \frac{1}{2}\right) - \left(\frac{1}{2} \times 1\right) - \left(\frac{1}{2} \times 0\right) = 0$. Because these products sum to zero, the two comparisons are orthogonal and both can safely be tested. If an experiment includes several groups, there may be many ways in which an orthogonal set can be constructed. The experimenter must decide which set to choose.

Often an experiment is done in which several groups are compared with a control individually. For example, an investigator may wish to find out if BNP (brain natriuretic peptide) is elevated in a number of different forms of heart disease. Each subgroup—rheumatic, several forms of congenital heart disease, ischemic, cardiomyopathic, etc—has BNP measured and compared with the normal controls. Thus the a priori plan is to make certain selected comparisons. After a significant F ratio, each group is compared with the control by Dunnett's test. This is essentially a form of t or q test in which the critical values are determined by a special set of numbers that are in between t and q. For example, with 5 groups and 20 degrees of freedom within groups, the 0.05 value is 4.232 for q, 2.65 for Dunnett's test, and 2.086 for t. By restricting the comparisons to a specific subset, Dunnett was able to increase the sensitivity of the test without paying the penalty incurred by making an all pairs comparison. Critical values for Dunnett's test may be found online at http://www.watpon.com/table/dunnetttest.pdf, http://davidmlane.com/hyperstat/table_Dunnett.html and http://www.stat.ufl.edu/~winner/tables/dunnett-2side.pdf.

In any form of a priori test, including Dunnett's test, the investigator may be struck by some unexpected differences between the means of two groups that were not involved in the a priori planning. For example, in comparing each subgroup with a control group, the original purpose of the study, the investigator may note a large difference between the mean values for BNP in, for example, patients with a large ventricular septal defect and with a large atrial septal defect. These two means can validly be compared by one of the post hoc tests mentioned above for a posteriori experiments. The same applies to those components of an a priori experiment that are not orthogonal and therefore cannot be compared validly by t-test.

In planning a study with one control and several treatment groups, the control sample must be large enough to reflect the control population because that control sample is to be used in all the subsequent comparisons, and if the control group is unrepresentative, all comparisons with the treatment groups will be in jeopardy. Given enough time and money, the control group can be made very large, but often the total number of subjects in the experiment is limited. Assume that there are N total subjects to be divided into k treatment groups, each replicated r times, and one control group replicated ar times: $N = ar + kr$. Then the lowest residual error is produced if $a = \sqrt{k}$ so that the number of control replicates is $\sqrt{k}r$ (Ridgman, 1975). As an example, with $N = 30$ subjects, and $k =$ four treatment groups and a control, then $\sqrt{k} = 2$, and we need twice as many replicates in the control as in each treatment group. Therefore, we need 10 control replicates and 5 replicates in each treatment group.

As shown above, it is possible (and desirable) to calculate confidence limits for the differences between pairs of means. This allows more careful interpretation of the data.

Computation of power is necessary when planning an ANOVA, and can also be done post hoc when the results are available. This computation is more complicated than when comparing two groups, and is best done by computer programs.

REFERENCES

Bartlett, M.S., Kendall, D.G., 1946. The statistical analysis of variances-heterogeneity and the logarithmic transformation. J. R. Stat. Soc. Suppl. 8, 128–138.

Brown, M.B., Forsythe, A.B., 1974. Robust tests for equality of variances. J. Am. Stat. Assoc. 69, 364–367.

Cohen, J., 1988. Statistical Power Analysis for Behavioral Sciences. Lawrence Erlbaum Associates, Hillsdale, NJ.

Cohen, J., 1992. A power primer. Psychol. Bull. 112, 155–159.

Conover, W.J., Iman, R.L., 1981. Rank transformations as a bridge between parametric and nonparametric statistics. Am. Stat. 35, 124–129.

Curran-Everett, D., 2000. Multiple comparisons: philosophies and illustrations. Am. J. Physiol. Regul. Integr. Comp. Physiol. 279, R1–R8.

Dallal, G.E., 2008. Multiple Comparison Procedures (Online). Available: http://www.jerrydallal.com/LHSP/mc.htm.

Dunn, O.J., 1964. Multiple comparisons using rank sums. Technometrics 6, 241–252.

Emerson, J.D., Stoto, M.A., 1983. Transforming data. In: Hoaglin, D.C., Mosteller, F., Tukey, J.W. (Eds.), Understanding Robust and Exploratory Data Analysis. John Wiley & Sons, New York.

Games, P.A., Howell, J.F., 1976. Pairwise multiple comparison procedures with unequal N's and/or variances: a Monte Carlo study. J. Educ. Stat. 1, 113–125.

Games, P.A., Keselman, H.J., Rogan, J.C., 1981. Simultaneous pairwise multiple comparison procedures for mean when sample sizes are unequal. Psychol. Bull. 90, 594–598.

Glantz, S.A., 2005. Primer of Biostatistics. McGraw-Hill, New York.

Grissom, R.J., 2000. Heterogeneity of variance in clinical data. J. Consult. Clin. Psychol. 68, 155–165.

Hayter, A.J., 1986. The maximum familywise error rate of Fisher's least significance difference test. J. Am. Stat. Assoc. 81, 1000–1004.

Jordan, J., Shannon, J.R., Black, B.K., Ali, Y., Farley, M., Costa, F., Diedrich, A., Robertson, R.M., Biaggioni, I., Robertson, D., 2000. The pressor response to water drinking in humans: a sympathetic reflex? Circulation 101, 504–509.

Keppel, G., Saufley Jr., W.H., Tokunaga, H., 1992. Introduction to Design and Analysis. A Student's Handbook. W.H. Freeman and Company, New York.

Levene, H., 1960. In: Olkin, I. (Ed.), Contributions to Probability and Statistics: Essays in Honor of Harold Hotelling. Stanford University Press, Stanford, CA.

Lix, L.M., Keselman, H.J., 1998. To trim or not to trim: tests of location equality under heteroscedasticity and nonnormality. Educ. Psychol. Meas. 58, 409–429.

Maxwell, S.E., Camp, C.J., Arvey, R.D., 1981. Measures of strength of association: a comparative examination. J. Appl. Psychol. 66, 525–534.

Maxwell, S.E., Delaney, H.D., 1990. Designing Experiments and Analyzing Data. A Model Comparison Perspective. Wadsworth Publishing Company, Belmont, CA.

Myers, J.L., Well, A., 2003. Research Design and Statistical Analysis. Lawrence Erlbaum Associates.

von Neumann, J., Kent, R.H., Bellinson, H.R., Hart, B.I., 1941. The mean square successive difference. Ann. Math. Stat. 12, 153–162.

O'Brien, P.C., Fleming, T.R., 1979. A multiple testing procedure for clinical trials. Biometrics 35, 549–556.

Richardson, D., Catron, D.V., Underkofler, L.A., Maddock, H.M., Friedland, W.C., 1951. Vitamin B_{12} requirement of male weanling pigs. J. Nutr. 44, 371–381.

Ridgman, W.J., 1975. Experimentation in Biology. An Introduction to Design and Analysis. Halsted Press/ John Wiley & Sons, New York.

Snedecor, G.W., Cochran, W.G., 1989. Statistical Methods. Iowa State University Press, Ames, Iowa.

Sokal, R.R., Rohlf, F.J., 1995. Biometry. The Principles and Practice of Statistics in Biological Research. W.H. Freeman and Company, New York.

Tan, A.Y., Zhou, S., Ogawa, M., Song, J., Chu, M., Li, H., Fishbein, M.C., Lin, S.F., Chen, L.S., Chen, P.S., 2008. Neural mechanisms of paroxysmal atrial fibrillation and paroxysmal atrial tachycardia in ambulatory canines. Circulation 118, 916–925.

van Belle, G., 2002. Statistical Rules of Thumb. Wiley Interscience, New York.

Zar, J.H., 2010. Biostatistical Analysis. Prentice Hall, Upper Saddle River, NJ.

Zhang, S., 1998. Fourteen homogeneity of variance tests: when and how to use them. In: Annual Meeting of the American Educational Research Association. San Diego, CA, April 13–17, 1998.

CHAPTER 26

Analysis of Variance II. More Complex Forms

Contents

BASIC CONCEPTS

Introduction

The one-factor analysis of variance (ANOVA) type of analysis is termed model I, or fixed effects analysis, because the different treatments have potentially different effects. The study of the amount of four different levels of vitamin B12 on piglet growth tested the hypothesis that one or more of these levels has a greater effect than the others. Increasing the sample size in each group assumes that the treatment effects remain the same with the means remaining similar in each group but with larger samples giving smaller standard errors and hence making it easier to detect differences among the means. Model II is discussed later in this chapter.

The one-way ANOVA of Chapter 25 is analogous to the unpaired t-test. What, then, is the ANOVA analog of the paired t-test? In its simplest form it is the two-way (or two-factor) analysis of variance, two-way because two different categories of

For a list of all websites referred to in this chapter, as clickable links, see the book companion website: www.booksite.elsevier.com/9780128023877.

Biostatistics for Medical and Biomedical Practitioners
http://dx.doi.org/10.1016/B978-0-12-802387-7.00026-3

treatments (or factors) are tested simultaneously. The standard two-factor analysis is the randomized complete block design, based on the agricultural studies of R.A. Fisher. Soils in which crops are grown often have different growth potentials that may affect the conclusions of experiments on, for example, different fertilizers. There are two ways of dealing with this problem. One is to randomize the plots of ground so that each treatment (fertilizer) is given to soils with many different growth potentials. This is the standard one-factor ANOVA. The other way is to select blocks of ground with similar growth potential (based on prior knowledge) and allocate the treatments at random to smaller plots within the block. This is equivalent to pairing in the *t*-test, and has the same effect of reducing variability. The gain in efficiency can be large (see pp. 409—410 in Glantz and Slinker, 2001). The term blocking is used not in the sense of obstructing but in the sense of creating homogeneous sets (blocks).

In biomedical research similar considerations apply. To design a study on the effect of four different agents for lowering blood sugar in diabetics, a one-factor ANOVA procedure might be to select at random from a large database of diabetic patients 20 patients for each of the four agents, that is, each of the 80 patients receives an agent once, and the next day fasting blood sugar is measured. Alternatively, a two-factor ANOVA can be performed by testing the same four agents on four different groups of diabetics: young men, older men, young women, older women, so that each patient is tested once, but with this design any differential response of one group will be disclosed by the analysis, and differences among the agents can be tested more sensitively.

Little new is needed for such a test. Graybill (1954) used data from a wheat varietal test performed by the Oklahoma Agricultural Experimental Station. Part of the data is used here. Four varieties of wheat are grown in six different locations (Table 26.1).

Our object is to answer the following questions:

1. Does the mean yield (bushels/acre) differ for different types of wheat?

Table 26.1 Partial data from experiment with different wheat varieties (factor 1) and different locations (factor 2)

	Wheat A	Wheat B	Wheat C	Wheat D	ΣX_r	N	$\bar{X}$
Location 1	44	24	19	19	106	4	26.5
Location 2	40	22	17	24	103	4	25.75
Location 3	18	14	17	16	65	4	16.25
Location 4	20	19	18	18	75	4	18.75
Location 5	55	34	19	25	133	4	33.25
Location 6	20	22	23	22	87	4	21.75
ΣX_c	197	135	113	124	569	24	23.7803
N	6	6	6	6	24		
$\bar{X}$	32.83	22.5	18.83	20.67	23.7083		

2. Does the mean yield differ for different locations?

3. Do the two factors interact, that is, is the yield of a particular wheat increased for one location but decreased for another?

Although these calculations are done best with statistical programs, they are described here to show what the programs are doing.

Online programs for performing two-way ANOVA may be found at http://vassarstats.net/, http://home.ubalt.edu/ntsbarsh/Business-stat/otherapplets/ANOVATwo.htm (without replications), http://home.ubalt.edu/ntsbarsh/Business-stat/otherapplets/ANOVA2Rep.htm (with replications), http://www.wessa.net/rwasp_Two%20Factor%20ANOVA.wasp, http://www.ltcconline.net/greenl/courses/201/regression/twowayanova.htm, and http://www.mccauslandcenter.sc.edu/mricro/ezanova/index.html.

Two-Way ANOVA

Table 26.1 displays the data.

For the moment, ignore factor 2 (locations), and perform a one-way ANOVA on the wheats (Figure 26.1).

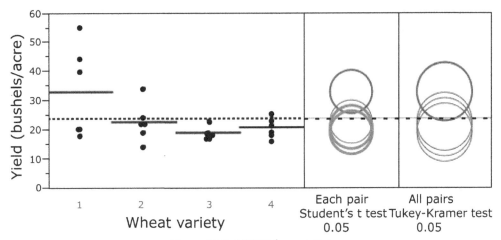

Figure 26.1 ANOVA for varieties.

The ANOVA table is shown in Table 26.2.

Table 26.2 ANOVA table for varieties

Source of variation	SS	DF	MS	F
Total (SS$_T$)	2230.9583	23		
Within (SS$_W$)	1524.5	20	76.225	
Between (SS$_B$) (Variety)	706.4583	3	235.486	3.0894 $P = 0.0504$

The ANOVA confirms that there were some differences among the means. The difference was slightly greater than P = 0.05. The residual error SS or SS$_W$ was 1524.5.

Now take the same data, ignore factor 1 (yield) and do a one-way ANOVA for the different locations (factor 2) (Figure 26.2).

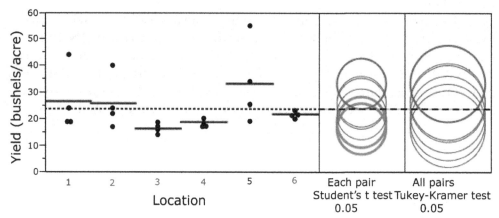

Figure 26.2 ANOVA for locations.

The ANOVA table is presented in Table 26.3.

Table 26.3 ANOVA table for locations

Source of variation	SS	DF	MS	F
Total (SS$_T$)	2230.9583	23		
Within (SS$_W$)	1482.75	18	82.375	
Between (SS$_B$) (Location)	748.2083	5	149.642	1.8166
				P = 0.1603

The results do not allow rejection of the null hypothesis, and the means of the locations could well have come from the same population. The data allow us to calculate the residual sum of squares (SS$_W$ = 1482.75) from the same total sum of squares, although this is not the same as the SS$_W$ for varieties because the differences among the means for varieties are not the same as for the means among locations. Both these sets of calculations are done on the same 24 measurements.

The model for a two-way or two-factor ANOVA is that the value of any measurement X_{ij} depends only on the mean value of X_i, the mean value of X_j (i.e., on the means of each factor), and the residual error ε_{ij}:

$$X_{ij} = \mu + \alpha_i + \beta_j + \varepsilon_{ij},$$

where $\alpha_i = \overline{X}_i - \mu$ and $\beta_j = \overline{X}_j - \mu$.

The residuals are assumed to be normally distributed, and the two factors to be independent. In other words, if wheat variety 1 has a large yield in location 2, all the other varieties should produce a large yield at location 2. A test of this assumption, known as additivity, is given below.

Now partition the total SS into a component due to differences between locations (SS_{BL}), a component due to differences between varieties (SS_{BV}), and the residual SS_W (Table 26.4).

Table 26.4 Two-way ANOVA

Source of variation	SS	DF	MS	F
Total (SS_T)	2230.9583	23		
Between (SS_{BL}) (Location)	748.2083	5	149.642	2.8914
				P = 0.0505
Between (SS_{BV}) (Variety)	706.4583	3	235.486	4.5502
				P = 0.0185
Within (SS_W)	776.2917	15	51.7528	

Out of the total sum of squares of 2230.9583 with 23 degrees of freedom, we have accounted for $748.2083 + 706.4583 = 1454.6666$ from the contributions of varieties and locations. Therefore, this leaves $2230.9583 - 1454.6666 = 776.2917$ as the residual unexplained variation (SSw). We have used $5 + 3 = 8$ degrees of freedom for the two known entities, leaving 15 for the within group sum of squares. Note how removing components related to both varieties and locations has reduced the within group sum of squares.

The conclusion is that we can safely reject the null hypothesis for differences between varieties, but differences between location are borderline.

The two-way ANOVA has considerable value. Not only does it reduce the residual (nonspecific) variability, thereby making the F test more sensitive, but it reduces the amount of work involved. If we just tested four varieties of wheat, each with six replicates, that comes to 24 plots. If we studied just locations, each with four replicates, that comes to another 24 plots. Combining the two into one analysis halves the work, and makes the comparisons more sensitive. Furthermore, it avoids an expensive and unethical use of more animals or patients than needed for the experiment.

The two-way ANOVA has similar requirements to the paired t-test.

1. Ratio or interval numbers
2. Normal distributions (hard to tell if sample sizes are small)

3. Homogeneous variances (hard to tell if sample sizes are small)

4. Justification for pairing.

This last point leads us to another requirement, namely additivity, the cardinal feature of the model described above.

Additivity

To test additivity, calculate the value of ε_{ij} for each value of X_{ij} (Tukey, 1977).

The model is, $X_{ij} = \mu + \alpha_i + \beta_j + \varepsilon_{ij}$, where α_i is the difference between the grand mean μ and the mean of the first factor and β_j is the difference between the grand mean μ and the mean of the second factor.

Return to the original data (Table 26.1), and subtract the row mean value from each of the four measurements in that row for each location separately (Table 26.5).

Table 26.5 Additivity stage 1

	Row mean $\overline{X}_r$	Variety A	Variety B	Variety C	Variety D
Location 1	26.5	$26.5 - 44 = -17.5$	2.5	7.5	7.5
Location 2	25.75	-14.25	3.75	8.75	1.75
Location 3	16.25	-1.75	2.25	-0.75	-0.25
Location 4	18.75	-1.25	-0.25	0.75	0.75
Location 5	33.25	-21.75	-0.75	8.25	8.25
Location 6	21.75	1.75	-0.25	-1.25	-0.25
$\overline{X}_i$		-3.00	1.21	3.875	2.96

This procedure removes the mean variability for locations from each measurement, leaving residual error and the effect of each given variety on this residual. Then calculate the means of these new values for each variety (as shown in the table) and subtract these from the residual values (Table 26.6).

Table 26.6 Additivity stage 2. Final table of residuals

	Variety A	Variety B	Variety C	Variety D
Location 1	$-17.5 - (3) = -20.5$	1.29	3.625	4.54
Location 2	-11.25	1.54	4.625	-1.21
Location 3	1.25	1.04	-4.625	-3.21
Location 4	1.75	-1.46	-3.125	-2.21
Location 5	-18.75	-1.96	4.375	5.29
Location 6	4.75	-1.46	-5.125	-3.21

Ideally, there should be as many positive as negative differences; in the table there are 13 negatives and 11 positives. Furthermore, most difference should be small, and this is not true here. The distribution can be checked on a quantile plot (Figure 26.3).

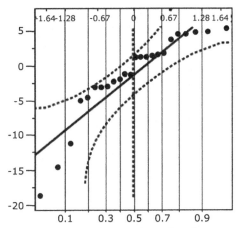

Figure 26.3 Double residual quantile plot. All points lie within then 95% confidence limits (curved dashed lines) but although negative and positive residuals are about equal in number, there are some very large negatives. The two-way ANOVA, however, is robust and there is no reason to reject the conclusions.

Additivity can be checked formally by Tukey's test (Myers and Well, 2003; Tukey, 1949) that is implemented by some commercial programs. It is tedious but not difficult to do by hand (see Appendix), and alternative ways of performing the test have been described (Berenson et al., 1983).

What if the additivity assumption is unlikely? Check the residuals to determine where the discrepancies might be (outliers), and also consider a transformation, possibly logarithmic or square root. One general type of transformation is the Anscombe—Tukey transformation (Anscombe and Tukey, 1963; Myers and Well, 2003), a power function $X' = X^{power}$ that frequently produces acceptable additivity without having to eliminate outliers.

Sometimes, we may want to make serial measurements on one of the factors. It is common in research to take several subjects and then measure a given variable, for example blood pressure, at different times after each subject is given a particular drug. Thus subject 1 is given amlodipine, at another time atenolol, at another time losartan, and so on. The other subjects are also given each of these agents. The benefit to such a design is that each subject acts as his or her own control, thereby making this equivalent to a paired t-test with the gain in sensitivity that a paired test has over an unpaired test. The subjects are the blocks, and we know that different subjects react differently to these agents. In addition, for a 4×6 two-factor design, with 4 drugs, we need only 6 patients and not 24 patients. If such a design is used, care must be taken to avoid a carryover effect of a previous treatment or any effect related to a given order of treatments. Apart from pharmacological carryover, order effects can occur for psychological reasons, so that treatments should therefore be given in random order to different patients.

These calculations for repeated measures samples can be done online for three groups at http://faculty.vassar.edu/lowry/corr3.html, for four groups at http://faculty.vassar.edu/lowry/corr4.html, and for three groups of up to 40 in each group at http://home.ubalt.edu/ntsbarsh/Business-stat/otherapplets/ANOVADep.htm.

To summarize, instead of comparing treatments with a one-way ANOVA, allocate subjects (patients, animals) at random to subgroups (or blocks) that are expected to be homogeneous. For example, several litters of animals may be chosen, and within each litter, four animals are selected at random to receive one of the treatments. The calculations show differences between treatments, differences between litters (blocks), and residual variability. This makes testing the differences among treatments more sensitive. The differences among blocks may or may not have meaning. Often, as in the example of different litters, the differences are random variables with a mean of zero and a given mean square (see below for model II). On the other hand, it would be possible to do an experiment in which each block represented a different strain or breed, and then differences among blocks may be of interest.

Multiple Factors

More than two factors can be analyzed by using Latin squares. The name (based on the name of an early mathematical puzzle) was introduced into statistical analysis for use in agricultural experiments. To allow for possible underlying differences in soil fertility, the plot of land is divided into smaller blocks to which seeds and treatments (fertilizers) are allocated at random, but in such a way that each treatment occurs once in each row and each column, and each seed occurs once in each row and each column. This principle can be applied to biological experiments as well. In an experiment with testicular spreading factor (now known to be hyaluronidase), Bacharach et al. (1940) injected it subcutaneously in six different sites on each of six rabbits. This example appears in the book by Finney (Finney, 1955). The study was done so that each site and each rabbit had the injection in a different order. As a result, each site (symbolized by A to F) occurred once with each rabbit and once with each order of injection, each rabbit occurred once with each order and each site; and each order occurred once with each rabbit and each site. (Individual data are in the original publication.) Then a three-factor ANOVA was performed (Table 26.7).

Table 26.7 Three-factor ANOVA

Source of variation	SS	DF	MS	F	P
Total	30.36	35			
Between animals	12.83	5	2.566	3.91	0.0123
Between order	0.56	5	0.112	0.17	0.9707
Between sites	3.83	5	0.766	1.17	0.3582
Within (residual)	13.14	20	0.657		

There are three factors that contribute to the total sums of squares: order, animal, and site. Adding up their contributions and subtracting that sum from the total produces a residual error independent of site, order, or animal. The contribution of each factor is compared with the residual mean square to provide an F ratio. In Table 26.7, there are significant differences among animals, with rabbit number 2 having the largest bleb and thus the slowest fluid absorption. Neither site nor order had any major effect, so that in planning future experiments site and order can be ignored, but precautions are needed to allow for interanimal variability.

It is possible to do an ANOVA with four factors, by allocating the fourth factor (symbolized by Greek letters) once to each of the other three factors. This is known as a Graeco-Latin square, and is analyzed in similar fashion. Latin squares must have the same number of cells for each factor. The requirements for ratio numbers, normality, and homogeneity of variance apply equally to these more complex ANOVA.

Friedman Test

If there is concern about the normality or variability of the distributions, or if ordinal numbers are involved, then a straightforward two-way ANOVA might yield misleading results. Then a distribution-free test, the Friedman test (developed by Milton Friedman, the economist), can be used. The data table is setup with the columns representing the j factors and the k rows representing the subjects. The measurements for each subject are then ranked 1, 2, 3, etc., and the mean rank for each factor is calculated. Then a modified ANOVA is done to calculate the SS between ranks. The theoretical mean rank with a random distribution is $(j + 1)/2$; for 3 factors this is 2.0. Then for each factor calculate k (observed mean rank $-$ theoretical mean rank)^2, and the sum of these is the SS between ranks. This is then referred to the chi-square table with $j - 1$ degrees of freedom.

An alternative formulation involves summing the ranks in each column (S_i) and the Friedman statistic is calculated as,

$$T = \frac{12 \sum S_i^2}{jk(j + 1)} - 3k(j + 1).$$

This is then assigned a probability from a table or program. With 3 treatments and >7 subjects, or 4 treatments and >4 subjects, then the distribution of T is similar to that of chi-square for 2 or 3 degrees of freedom, respectively. Online calculations for 3 or 4 factors (columns) can be found at http://vassarstats.net/ under the ordinal data heading, or at http://socr.ucla.edu/htmls/SOCR_Analyses.html.

Once overall significance is obtained, which groups are different? There are nonparametric equivalents of the Student–Newman–Keuls (SNK) and Dunnett's tests. The SNK equivalent for all the pairwise comparisons is

$$q = \frac{R_i - R_j}{\sqrt{\frac{kN(k+1)}{12}}},$$

where k is the number of groups, N is the total number, and R_i and R_j are the rank sums for the groups being compared; critical values can be found at http://cse.niaes.affrc.go.jp/ miwa/probcalc/s-range/srng_tbl.html. For Dunnett's test, replace R_i by $R_{control}$ in the above formula, and divide by 6 instead of 12. The critical values are presented online at http://davidmlane.com/hyperstat/table_Dunnett.html, http://www.graphpad.com/ faq/images/337CriticalDunettTables.pdf.

Cochrane's Q Test

This is a nonparametric test to answer the question about whether two or more treatments are equally effective when the data are dichotomous (Binary: yes, no) in a two-way randomized block design. It is equivalent to the Friedman test with dichotomous variables. The results are set out as in Table 26.8.

Table 26.8 Cochrane's Q test

	Treatment 1	Treatment 2	...	Treatment m	Sum
Block 1	X_{11}	X_{12}	...	X_{1m}	$\sum X_1.$
Block 2	X_{21}	X_{22}	...	X_{2m}	$\sum X_2.$
...	...	...	...	...	...
Block n	X_{n1}	X_{n2}	...	X_{nm}	$\sum X_n.$
Sum	$\sum X._1$	$\sum X._2$	...	$\sum X._m$	N

m = number of treatments; n = number of blocks; N = grand total; $X._j$ is the column total for the jth treatment; $X_i.$ is the row total for the ith block.

H_0: All treatments are equally effective.
H_A: There is a difference between some of the treatments.
The test formula is

$$Q = m(m-1)\frac{\sum \left(X._j - \frac{N}{m}\right)^2}{\sum X_i.\left(m - X_i.\right)}.$$

The critical value of Q is

$$Q > \chi^2_{1-\alpha,m-1}$$

If H_0 is rejected, then pairwise comparisons of treatment can be done.

As an example, consider testing three different medications (treatments) in six different patients, and recording the results as improved (0) and unimproved (1) (Table 26.9).

Table 26.9 Example of Cochrane's Q test

	Treatment 1	Treatment 2	Treatment 3	Sum
Patient 1	1	0	0	1
Patient 2	0	0	1	1
Patient 3	0	0	0	0
Patient 4	1	0	1	1
Patient 5	0	1	1	2
Patient 6	0	0	1	2
Sum	2	1	4	7

$$Q = 3(3-1)\frac{\left(1-\frac{7}{3}\right)^2 + \left(1-\frac{7}{3}\right)^2 + \left(0-\frac{7}{3}\right)^2 + \left(1-\frac{7}{3}\right)^2 + \left(2-\frac{7}{3}\right)^2 + \left(2-\frac{7}{3}\right)^2}{[2(3-2)] + [1(3-1)] + [4(3-4)]}$$

$$= 6\frac{1.78 + 1.78 + 5.44 + 1.78 + 0.11 + 0.11}{2 + 2 + 4} = 1.375.$$

With $3 - 1 = 2$ degrees of freedom, this chi-square of 1.375 has a probability of 0.5028, so that there is no evidence provided against the null hypothesis that the treatments are similar.

Because all the results are either 1 or 0, the arithmetic is trivial.

Interaction

In the wheat study, there is a possibility that wheat number 2 might grow more in one location than another, so that there would not have been additivity. This form of dependence is termed interaction. To illustrate the effect of interaction, Figure 26.4 shows results of a hypothetical experiment to determine the effects of two drugs

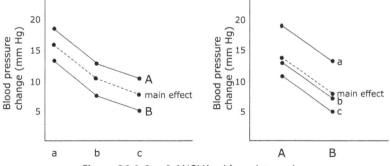

Figure 26.4 3 × 2 ANOVA with no interaction.

(A and B) for lowering blood pressure on 20 patients in each of three different racial groups (a, b, and c).

The left-hand panel shows that group a has a larger change in blood pressure than does group b and this in turn exceeds the change in group c. The average change of blood pressure for the two drugs is shown by the dashed line labeled "main effect." Therefore, in group a, the average decrease in pressure is about 16 mm Hg, in group b about 11 mm Hg, and in group c about 8 mm Hg. The right-hand panel shows a larger change in blood pressure for drug A than for drug B. The main effect that averages out differences due to the racial group is about 14 mm Hg for drug A and about 8 mm Hg for drug B. There is no interaction between drugs and racial groups.

Figure 26.5, however, shows interaction between drugs and racial groups.

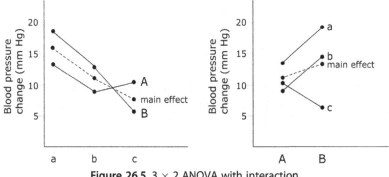

Figure 26.5 3 × 2 ANOVA with interaction.

In the left panel, groups a and b have the same relative response to drugs, with A < B, but now group c has the effect of drug A > B. In the right-hand panel, drug A has its order of effects a > c > b, whereas the order for drug B is a > b > c. It therefore makes no sense to examine main effects because these are not the same across all classes. Therefore, when a two-way ANOVA with replications is done to test interaction, first examine the significance of the interaction. If it is not significant, then it is reasonable to proceed to examine the main effects to find out if A > B or if a > b > c. On the other hand, if interaction is significant, testing main effects is unrealistic, because drug A is better than B in some racial groups but not others.

Interaction can be determined for a three-way (and higher) ANOVA by making use of replications. There will now be three main effects to calculate, but the interactions are more complex. If the main factors are A, B, and C, then there are first order interactions: A × B, A × C, and B × C, as well as a second order interaction: A × B × C. With more factors, higher order interactions occur.

How can we test for interaction? As an example, an experiment is done in which subjects classified as having high or low anxiety were divided into two groups, one untreated and one given a serotonin reuptake inhibitor, and their norepinephrine concentrations were measured after being given a problem-solving test (Table 26.10).

Table 26.10 Effects of treatment

Agent	High anxiety	Low anxiety
Untreated	180	122
	190	87
	140	65
	163	104
	122	63
	187	55
ΣX	982	496
N	6	6
$\overline{X}_i$	163.67	82.67
Treated	63	107
	47	96
	24	97
	44	98
	27	63
	13	115
ΣX	218	576
N	6	6
$\overline{X}_i$	36.33	96

Inspection of the means suggests that, whereas treatment decreases mean catecholamine concentrations in high-anxiety patients (163.67 vs 36.33), it has little effect in low-anxiety patients (82.67 vs 96).

Begin the analysis as a one-way ANOVA on the smallest subgroups: high anxiety untreated, high anxiety treated, low anxiety untreated, and low anxiety treated (Figure 26.6).

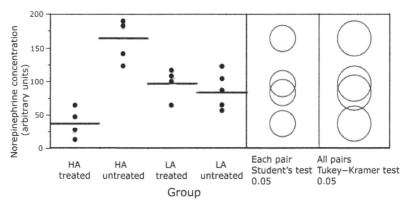

Figure 26.6 ANOVA for all anxiety and treatment data. HA = high anxiety; LA = low anxiety.

There are significant differences, with high-anxiety untreated patients having the highest catecholamine concentrations.

Now combine the groups into larger sets (treated and untreated, or high and low anxiety) and do a one-way ANOVA for each of the combined groups. The results are shown in Figure 26.7.

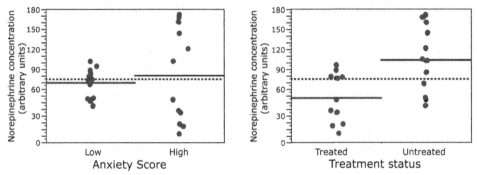

Figure 26.7 ANOVA for high versus low anxiety, and treated versus untreated.

(When measurements are superimposed, the points on the graph may be staggered out of alignment; this is termed "jittering.") Dashed line is grand mean of all measurements.

Tables 26.11A and 26.11B give the ANOVA calculations for anxiety score and treatment status. They are used not for themselves but for the next stage of the calculation.

Table 26.11A ANOVA for anxiety score

Source of variation	SS	DF	MS	F	P
Total	60,387.33	23			
Between groups	682.67	1	682,67	0.2515	0.6210
Within (residual)	59,074.67	22	2713.85		

Table 26.11B ANOVA for treatment status

Source of variation	SS	DF	MS	F	P
Total	60,387.33	23			
Between groups	19,494.00	1	19,494.00	10.4875	0.0038*
Within (residual)	40,893.33	22	1858.8		

* = p < 0.05.

Assemble these results into the standard ANOVA format (Table 26.12).

Table 26.12 ANOVA table for all four groups. The value 49,857.33 is the value for groups in Figure 26.7

Source of variation	SS	DF	MS	F	P
Total	60,387.33	23			
Between groups	49,857.33	3	16,619.10	31.56	<0.0001
Within (residual)	10,530.00	20	526.5		

The four groups, however, are not merely four different groups with one factor, but that there are actually two factors—anxiety level and treatment. Therefore, partition the between group sum of squares (Table 26.13).

Table 26.13 Partitioned ANOVA

Source of variation	SS	DF	MS	F	P
Between groups	49,857.33	3	16,619.10		
Between anxiety level	682.67	1	682.67		
Between treatments	19,494.00	1	19,494.00		
Sum	20,176.67	2			
Between groups—sum	29,680.66	1	29,680.66		

From the between group SS of 49,857.33 with 3 degrees of freedom, 682.67 SS is between anxiety levels with 1 df and 19,494.00 SS between treatments with 1 df; these are referred to as main effects. Therefore, there are 29,680.66 SS and 1 df unaccounted for, and these are termed the interaction SS and df. The full ANOVA table is shown in Table 26.14. Each of the between subgroups is tested against the error term.

Table 26.14 Full ANOVA

Source of variation	SS	DF	MS	F	P
Total	60,387.332	23			
Between groups	49,857.33	3	16,619.10		
Between anxiety levels	682.67	1	682.67	1.30	0.2677
Between treatments	19,494.00	1	19,494.00	37.03	0.000,01
Interaction	29,680.66	1	29,680.66	5637.35	<0.000,01
Within groups (residual)	10,530.00	20	526.5		

Therefore, the experiment has shown a significant difference due to treatments, but no significant difference related to anxiety levels (treatment and no treatment combined) and a significant interaction effect with treatment having a large effect in high-anxiety patients but none in the low-anxiety patients.

As long as there are replications, interaction effects can be assessed, no matter how many groups there are. If testing 3 hypnotic agents against 4 different strains of rats, with three replicates in each group, start with 12 small subgroups of 3 each which are used to determine the within group SS with 24 df and the general between group SS with 11 df. Then pool all the agent data within each strain group and determine the between strain SS with 3 df, and then pool all the strain data within each agent group to determine the between agent SS with 2 df. That leaves 6 df over for the interaction (Table 26.15).

Table 26.15 ANOVA setup

Source of variation	SS	DF	MS	F	P
Total		35			
Between groups		11			
Between strains		3			
Between agents		2			
Interaction		6			
Within groups (residual)		24			

Interaction can be tested by online programs at http://home.ubalt.edu/ntsbarsh/ Business–stat/otherapplets/ANOVA2Rep.htm, http://vassarstats.net/anova2u.html, and http://www.wessa.net/rwasp_Two%20Factor%20ANOVA.wasp#output.

Problem 26.1

Because a two-way ANOVA with replication is an efficient design, this problem involves testing for interaction.

	Low	Medium	High
Male	4	7	10
	5	9	12
	6	8	11
	5	12	9
Female	6	13	12
	6	25	13
	4	12	10
	4	12	13

Weight gain (g) after eating breakfast with high, medium, or low carbohydrate content. Did the carbohydrate content affect energy, and did males and females respond in the same way?

ADVANCED AND ALTERNATIVE CONCEPTS

Missing Data or Unequal Cell Sizes

More complex forms of ANOVA have symmetry. All Latin square designs have equal numbers for each factor. A two-way ANOVA need not have the same number of factors for factor 1 as for factor 2, but all the cells should contain data. In replicated experiments, too, ideally there should be equal numbers of replications in each cell for maximal efficiency. This may not always be possible. For example, if factor 1 involves three diseases, one might be rare so that finding enough measurements is difficult or impossible. It is still possible to carry out the ANOVA if there is equal representation within rows and proportional representation within columns, for example, row 1 has 3, 3, 3, and 3 measurements (one in each column). Row 2 has 4, 4, 4, and 4, and row 3 has 2, 2, 2, and 2 measurements. Alternatively, there can be proportional representation within rows and columns, for example, 3, 6, 9, and 6 in row 1; 4, 8, 12, and 8 in row 2; and 2, 4, 6, and 4 in row 3. The ANOVA is carried out with slight modifications (see Zar (2010), p. 247).

In practice, though, sometimes data are lost: an animal may die, a test tube is broken, a patient decides to leave the trial. There will thus be missing data and the symmetry of cells is lost. To deal with this, the missing values can be estimated in various ways that to some extent depend upon why the data are missing. Some data are missing for random reasons, for example, dropping a test tube. If only a few cells have one missing datum that prevents proportional representation, the missing value can be replaced by the mean value for that cell, and the calculations are done with one less degree of freedom for each missing datum. More complex ways of estimating the missing value can also be used, but in each instance with loss of degrees of freedom in the final analysis. Only a limited number of missing values can be tolerated.

On the other hand, some missing data may be related to the dependent variable. For example, in a trial of two treatments for a disease, some subjects who get little perceived benefit from one of the treatments might drop out, with the result that the outcomes for those who remain are on the average improved. This makes comparison of the two groups more difficult to evaluate. Several approaches have been used in these situations, maximum likelihood estimates and multiple imputation being two effective but computer intensive solutions. Statistical consultation is required, but a readable explanation by Howell can be found at www.uvm.edu/~dhowell/StatPages/Missing_Data/Missing-Part-Two.html.

Nested Designs

In the two-way ANOVA described above, every member of factor 1 is associated with every member of factor 2; each type of wheat is represented for each location, and each location is represented for each wheat. By contrast, the nested design does not have every member of factor 1 associated with every member of factor 2, as shown in Figure 26.8.

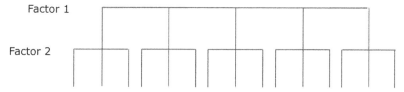

Figure 26.8 Nested design. Here there are 5 members of factor 1, each associated with 3 members of factor 2. However, the first member of factor 2, group 1 is not related to the first member of factor 2, group 2, and so on.

How similar are different laboratories in measuring blood LDL cholesterol in a standard blood sample? To analyze this, the blood sample is split into four equal portions, and one portion is given to each of four laboratories in a city. In each laboratory, three technicians measure cholesterol independently, each with replicate measurements (Table 26.16).

Table 26.16 Nested data

Laboratory	A			B			C			D			Total
Technician	a	b	c	d	e	f	g	h	i	j	k	l	
Replication	108	109	107	113	110	112	108	107	105	114	113	117	
	106	110	108	112	112	113	108	108	105	115	115	113	
	106	109	107	111	111	114	110	111	108	116	117	114	
ΣX (tech)	320	328	322	336	333	337	326	343	318	345	345	344	3997
ΣX (lab)	970			1006			987			1034			3997

The technicians are not crossed with laboratories. This would happen only if each technician made measurements in each laboratory. However, the first technician in laboratory A is not the same as the first technician in laboratory B, and so on. The main question is whether laboratories get the same results. They should, but it is possible that differences in reagents used, type of measuring equipment, and conditions such as temperature may cause differences. Another question is how much technicians differ from each other or, to put it another way, is there more variability between technicians than can be accounted for by variability of the method of measurement. It is of no value to compare technicians with each other, because then differences among laboratories might be responsible.

Looking at the 12 sums (ΣX) for each technician, there are certainly differences, sometimes marked; for example, 320 versus 345. On the other hand, the sums for the four laboratories ΣX (lab) have equally great variations. How much of the variation among technicians is due to the differences among laboratories?

Begin by considering the 12 smallest groups, that is 3 replications in each of 12 technicians, and do a one-way ANOVA (Figure 26.9; Table 26.17).

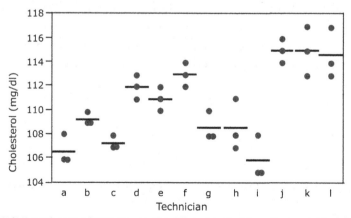

Figure 26.9 ANOVA on the most basic groups, the different technicians. Horizontal lines indicate means.

Table 26.17 ANOVA between technicians

Source of variation	SS	DF	MS	F	P
Total	404.55	35			
Between technicians	358.55	11	32.60	17.01	<0.0001
Within groups (residual)	46	24	1.92		

There are significant differences among technicians, but how much of the difference is due to the laboratories? To evaluate this, pool the data from each laboratory, and do another one-way ANOVA (Figure 26.10; Table 26.18).

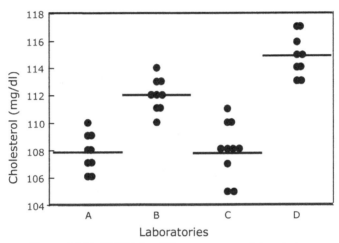

Figure 26.10 ANOVA for differences among laboratories.

Table 26.18

Source of variation	SS	DF	MS	F	P
Total	404.5556	35			
Between laboratories	326.5556	3	108.852	44.6572	<0.0001
Within groups (residual)	78	32	2.437		

There are differences among laboratories too. The interaction among laboratories and technicians is shown in Tables 26.19–26.20.

Table 26.19 ANOVA between technicians and between laboratories

Source of variation	SS	DF	MS	F	P
Total	404.55	35			
Between technicians	358.55	11	32.60		
Between laboratories	326.55	3	108.85		
	(32)	(8)			
Within groups (residual)	46	24	1.92		

Table 26.20 Complete nested design ANOVA

Source of variation	SS	DF	MS	F	P
Total	404.55	35			
Between technicians	358.55	11	32.60		
Between laboratories	326.55	3	108.85	27.21	0.0002
Between technicians in laboratories	32	8	4.00	2.08	0.079
Within groups (residual)	46	24	1.92		

Underneath the line for the between technician data in Table 26.19, there is a line for the between laboratory data. The SS_B for technicians is greater than the SS_B for laboratories by $358.55 - 326.55 = 32$, and the degrees of freedom for technicians is greater than that for laboratories by $11 - 3 = 8$. These discrepancies are due to the variability of technicians within laboratories (Table 26.20).

What has been done is to partition the differences among technicians (part of which is due to differences among laboratories) into a component due to differences among laboratories and a component due to differences between technicians within laboratories. The testing of significance in a nested design differs from the usual two-way or three-way ANOVA in which each between group MS is compared to the within group MS. In the nested design start by comparing the between technicians in laboratories MS to the within group MS; there is no significant difference over and above the variability of replicates (although perhaps a larger sample with more replicates might disclose such a difference). Then to test the difference among laboratories, divide the between laboratory MS by the MS between technicians in laboratories, and not by the residual MS. The reason for this is that we are no longer estimating the population variability due to replication, but instead want to know if the difference among laboratories is greater than expected from the combined variability of replicates and differences among technicians. Therefore, divide 108.85 by 4 to get an F ratio of 27.21, and assess this with degrees of freedom in numerator and denominator, respectively, of 3 and 4.

To understand the technicians within laboratories component, alter the data to make each technician within a laboratory have similar results (Table 26.21).

Table 26.21 Revised data table

Laboratory	A			B			C			D			Total
Technician	a	b	c	d	e	f	g	h	i	j	k	l	
Replication	108	107	106	113	113	111	108	107	108	114	114	117	
	106	107	108	112	113	113	108	108	110	115	117	113	
	106	106	106	111	110	112	110	111	108	116	114	115	
ΣX (tech)	320	320	320	336	336	336	326	326	326	345	345	345	3978
ΣX (lab)	960			1008			978			1035			3978

The ANOVA between technicians is in Figure 26.11; Table 26.22, that between laboratories is in Figure 26.12, and the final table is in Table 26.23.

The contribution of differences among technicians within laboratories is now very small and almost all the variability is associated with the laboratories.

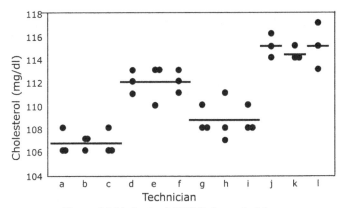

Figure 26.11 Revised ANOVA for technicians.

Table 26.22 ANOVA for technicians. Almost all the variability observed is between technicians

Source of variation	SS	DF	MS	F	P
Total	388.9722	35			
Between technicians	348.3056	11	31.6641	186,870	<0.0001
Within groups (residual)	40.6667	24	1.6944		

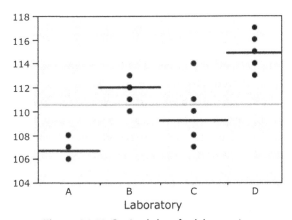

Figure 26.12 Revised data for laboratories.

Table 26.23 Revised ANOVA

Source of variation	SS	DF	MS	F	P
Total	388.97	35			
Between technicians	348.31	11	31.66		0.0007
Between laboratories	322.50	3	107.50	33.49	<0.0001
Between technicians in laboratories	25.81	8	3.21	1.54	0.18
Within groups (residual)	6.48	32	2.08		

Transformations

Although ANOVA is usually performed on ratio numbers, it can be used for counts or proportions with some modifications. This is clarified by Snedecor and Cochran (1989), pp. 287−291 and by Zar (2010), Chapter 13.

Counts often come from Poisson distributions. If there is a large variation in counts from cell to cell, then there will be a correspondingly large variation in cell variances because in a Poisson distribution, the variance is similar to the mean. The effect of this is to make ANOVA less sensitive in detecting differences because the residual variance is inflated. One way of dealing with this problem is to use the square root transformation that stabilizes the variance and makes the distribution of data more normal. If the counts are very small, for example most <10, then $\sqrt{X} + \sqrt{X+1}$ is more effective.

If the standard deviation is proportional to the mean, so that the coefficient of variation is constant, then a logarithmic transformation not only stabilizes the variance but also restores additivity.

Proportions must be handled differently. If, for example, the data set consists of percentages (equivalent to coming from a binomial population), the arc sine transformation is recommended. The proportion p_{ij} is replaced by the angle whose sine is $\sqrt{p_{ij}}$. Various methods of compensating for proportions of 0% or 100% are also described by Snedecor and Cochran (Snedecor and Cochran, 1989).

Model II ANOVA

Model I ANOVA is the fixed effects model. The factors represent groups that might have different means, such as different fats, or different weight gains on different diets. Even without hypotheses about the outcomes, in the wheat experiment there were selected four *specific* wheats to be tested. Each member of the group has a mean value (that may or may not be different), and taking more samples makes the estimates of the means more accurate. Model II ANOVA is the random effects model, and it is designed to reveal different components of variability without placing any importance on mean values. For example, what is the variability in making replicate determinations of endothelin concentrations or how much do different technicians vary in making measurements? The technicians are not specified, but are merely random representatives of the class of technicians.

In a study of the iron content of baboon livers, there are two sources of variability: how much iron content/g varies from one piece of liver to the next, and how much iron content varies from one baboon to the next. The baboons are random selections from the class of baboons. We do not really care if the mean iron contents vary from baboon to baboon (in fact, we expect the null hypothesis $H_0: \overline{X_1} = \overline{X_2} = \overline{X_N}$ to be untrue) but the amount of variation among animals is important in planning experiments. Unlike the wheat example, where we can repeat measurements on wheat number 1 indefinitely, repetition may not be an important question in model II. After all, one particular baboon might be used in a particular experiment but never used again.

The ANOVA is performed as usual, but the analysis of the results is altered. To illustrate this, consider measuring a rare growth factor in three random parts of the liver taken from four randomly selected baboons ($a = 4$). The hypothetical data are given in Table 26.24.

Table 26.24 Growth factor concentration study

Baboon	Growth factor (pmoles/kg wet weight)			ΣX	$\overline{X_i}$
1	2.82	2.38	3.18	8.38	2.79
2	2.33	2.30	2.88	7.51	2.50
3	1.67	1.77	2.44	5.88	1.96
4	1.68	1.53	2.06	5.27	1.76

The ANOVA results are shown in Table 26.25.

Table 26.25 ANOVA for growth factor data

Analysis of variance

Source	DF	Sum of squares	Mean square	F ratio	Prob > F
Baboon	3	2.060 4667	0.686 822	5.3129	0.0263
Error	8	1.034 2000	0.129 275		
C. Total	11	3.094 6667			

The differences among baboons are significant, but their mean values are of no interest. Those baboons might never be used again. Furthermore, liver samples from another baboon have no more reason to provide information about baboon 1 than about baboon 4. What the measurements provide are some estimates of error related to different animals and to different parts of the liver. The error mean square s_W^2 is 0.129275, and is an estimate of the population variability σ^2 of the estimates of growth factor concentrations of baboon livers. The between group mean square s_B^2 is composed of the population variance σ^2 plus a component due to differences among the baboons $n\sigma_A^2$ (Snedecor and Cochran, 1989).

Thus $\sigma_B^2 = \sigma^2 + n\sigma_A^2$ and so $\sigma_A^2 = \frac{\sigma_B^2 - \sigma^2}{n}$.

Therefore, an unbiased estimate of σ_A^2 is

$$s_A^2 = \frac{s_B^2 - s_W^2}{3} = \frac{0.686822 - 0.129275}{3} = 0.185849.$$

There are now two variances, one associated with replicate determinations of growth factor in baboon livers and one associated with differences among baboons.

What is the interest in knowing these two components of variance? If there is only enough money and reagents to do only 30 measurements of some complex growth factor in the liver, should we take one baboon and make 30 measurements on its liver? That is inefficient because baboons will differ in how much hepatic growth factor they have. Should we take one piece of liver from each of 30 baboons? That is also inefficient. Baboons are expensive, there are ethical questions about their use, and besides growth factor may vary in different parts of the liver. If we knew how much variability was associated with differences in baboons and how much with differences in parts of the liver, and the relative costs of baboons and growth factor measurements, we could work out an optimal strategy (Snedecor and Cochran, 1989).

Some experimental designs include both fixed and random effects, and are sometimes referred to as model III ANOVA. In general, biologists and medical investigators use model I most of the time, and more complex designs should be done only with statistical consultation.

Repeated Measures Designs

The examples discussed above all had a single observation of the dependent variable for each subject and each treatment, and are often referred to as *between-subjects* designs. It is, however, common to use a number of subjects and then make a series of measurements on each of them; this is referred to as a *within-subjects* design. The different measurements might be different treatments or different times. These results cannot be analyzed by the usual ANOVA, because the results within each subject are likely to be correlated. If the repeated measurements have a correlation ρ (Chapter 29), then the variance of the treatment mean is not σ^2/n, but is $\frac{\sigma^2[1+(n-1)\rho]}{n}$, and the estimate of the mean square is not σ^2, but is $\sigma^2(1 - \rho)$ (Cochran and Bliss, 1970). This distorts the true variance of the treatment mean. Furthermore, the treatments are fixed effects, that is, there are possible differences between treatment effects, something the experiment is designed to assess. On the other hand, if the subjects are randomly selected, a different set of subjects might have different responses.

What is important is that each subject might have different mean responses independent of the treatments or, to put it another way, averaged across all the treatments. We need a method of removing the intrasubject variability that is not of direct interest to us and has the result of making the experiment less sensitive. The subject is complex, and only outlines will be given here (Glantz and Slinker, 2001; Maxwell and Delaney, 1990, Sullivan 2008).

In a repeated measures design, the effect of treatment (the dependent variable) is measured in continuous interval or ratio numbers, and the independent variable (for example, the subjects) is either nominal or ordinal. The independent variable is also termed the within-subjects factor. The within subjects error sum of squares, derived by subtracting the between subjects sum of squares from the total sum of squares, can then be partitioned into a subject sum of squares and a residual or error sum of squares. This decreases the residual sum of squares and makes the ANOVA more sensitive. Two different approaches have been used—the mixed model univariate approach or the multivariate approach. Each has strengths and weaknesses, although they tend to give similar results (Myers and Well, 2003).

APPENDIX

Tukey's test for additivity separates the residual error into a component due to "pure" error and a component due to nonadditivity, and involves calculating a nonadditivity sum of squares as

$$SS_{NA} = \frac{\left\{ \sum_{i=1}^{r} \sum_{j=1}^{c} X_{ij} \left(\overline{X_{i\cdot}} - \overline{X_{\cdot\cdot}} \right) \left(\overline{X_{\cdot j}} - \overline{X_{\cdot\cdot}} \right) \right\}^2}{\sum_{i=1}^{r} \left(\overline{X_{i\cdot}} - \overline{X_{\cdot\cdot}} \right)^2 \sum_{j=1}^{c} \left(\overline{X_{\cdot j}} - \overline{X_{\cdot\cdot}} \right)^2}$$

$$= \frac{\left\{ \sum_{i=1}^{r} \sum_{j=1}^{c} X_{ij} \left(\overline{X_{i\cdot}} - \overline{X_{\cdot\cdot}} \right) \left(\overline{X_{\cdot j}} - \overline{X_{\cdot\cdot}} \right) \right\}^2}{SS_A SS_B}.$$

Calculate this numerator by taking each value X_{ij} and multiplying it successively by the difference between the corresponding row mean and the grand mean and then by the difference between the column mean and the grand mean. Table 26.26 shows the principles.

The body of data from Table 26.3 is supplemented by a column for the deviation of each row mean from the grand mean and a row for the deviation between each column mean and the grand mean. For each cell, for example, the upper left cell (circled), multiply its value by the product of the corresponding row and column deviations (shown in ovals): $64 \times -1.75 \times -5.75$. Repeat for each cell and sum the results. This when squared gives the numerator of the nonadditivity equation above. (The

Table 26.26 Data table for additivity test

	Fat A	Fat B	Fat C	Fat D	ΣXi	$\overline{X}_{i.}$	$\overline{X}_{i.} - \overline{X}_{..}$
Dough	64	78	75	55	272	68	−5.75
Dough	83	101	103	76	363	90.75	17.00
Dough	68	97	78	49	292	73	−0.75
Dough	77	82	71	64	294	73.5	−0.25
Dough	45	75	53	60	233	58.25	−15.50
Dough	95	77	76	68	316	79	5.25
ΣXj	432	510	456	372	1770		
$\overline{X}_{.j}$	72	85	76	62		73.75 $= \overline{X}_{..}$	
$\Sigma X_{.j}$	−1.75	11.25	2.25	−11.75			0.00

row or column deviations must sum to zero; if they do not, make small adjustments to the numbers until they do.) The denominator is the product of the two between group sums of squares, calculated as

$$\left(-1.75^2 \times 11.25^2 \times 2.25^2 \times -11.75^2 \right)\left(-5.75^2 \times 17^2 \times -0.75^2 \times -0.25^2 \right.$$
$$\left. \times -15.5^2 \times 5.25^2 \right)$$
$$= 161058.875.$$

Then the nonadditivity sum of squares (SS_{NA}) is $\frac{1071.5^2}{161058.875} = 7.1285$. The ANOVA is shown in Table 26.27.

Table 26.27 Nonadditivity ANOVA

Source	DF	SS	MS	F	P
Fat	3	1636.50	545.5	5.15	0.0132
Dough	5	2362.00	472.4	4.46	0.0122
Nonadditivity	1	7.13	7.13	0.067	0.7995
Residual	14	1482.87	105.92		
Total	23	5488.50			

Intuitively, if one or more X values are unusually high or low, thus belying additivity, then the products of the row and column mean deviations from the grand mean will be large, and the numerator of the above equation will be large. This value is then scaled by the product of the two between group sums of squares SS_A and SS_B. This component of the residual SS is then tested for significance.

This test can also be performed by the free program BrightStats http://www.brightstat.com/.

REFERENCES

Anscombe, F.J., Tukey, J.W., 1963. The examination and analysis of residuals. Technometrics 5, 141–160.

Bacharach, A.L., Chance, M.R., Middleton, T.R., 1940. The biological assay of testicular diffusing factor. Biochem. J. 34, 1464–1471.

Berenson, M.L., Levine, D.M., Goldstein, M., 1983. Intermediate Statistical Methods and Applications. A Computer Package Approach. Prentice-Hall, Inc., Englewood Cliffs, NJ.

Cochran, W.G., Bliss, C.F., 1970. In: Mcarthur, J.W., Colton, T. (Eds.), Statistics in Endocrinology. The MIT Press, Cambridge, MA.

Finney, D.J., 1955. Experimental Design and its Statistical Basis. Cambridge University press, London.

Glantz, S.A., Slinker, B.K., 2001. Primer of Applied Regression and Analysis of Variance. McGraw-Hill, Inc., New York.

Graybill, F.A., 1954. Heterogeneity in a randomized block design. Biometrics 10, 516–520.

Maxwell, S.E., Delaney, H.D., 1990. Designing Experiments and Analyzing Data. A Model Comparison Perspective. Wadsworth Publishing Company, Belmont, CA.

Myers, J.L., Well, A., 2003. Research Design and Statistical Analysis. Lawrence Earlbaum Associates.

Snedecor, G.W., Cochran, W.G., 1989. Statistical Methods. Iowa State University Press, Ames, Iowa.

Sullivan, L.M., 2008. Repeated measures. Circulation 117, 1238–1243.

Tukey, J.W., 1949. One degree of freedom for non-additivity. Biometrics 5, 232–242.

Tukey, J.W., 1977. Exploratory Data Analysis. Addison-Wesley Publishing Co., Menlo Park, CA.

Zar, J.H., 2010. Biostatistical Analysis. Prentice Hall, Upper Saddle River, NJ.

## PART 7

Regression and Correlation

CHAPTER 27

Linear Regression

Contents

BASIC CONCEPTS

Introduction

Previous chapters concerned single variables. Now it is time to consider how two variables (X, Y) can be related. Many problems involve relationships between two (X, Y) or more (X, Y, Z…) variables, such as height and weight, or age, blood pressure, and blood cholesterol. If there is a causal relationship between these variables, it is possible to predict the value of one variable (the explained, response, or dependent variable) from the value of the other variables (explanatory or independent variables). One question to ask is if the relationship between two variables is linear, as described in this chapter, or nonlinear as described in Chapter 30. If it is linear, then we can determine the slope of the relationship, that is, how much does Y increase or decrease for a one-unit change in X.

For a list of all websites referred to in this chapter, as clickable links, see the book companion website: www.booksite.elsevier.com/9780128023877.

Biostatistics for Medical and Biomedical Practitioners
http://dx.doi.org/10.1016/B978-0-12-802387-7.00027-5

It is everyone's experience that as a child gets older it gets bigger, that as people become more obese their fasting blood glucose levels rise, or that as incomes decrease more people become homeless. There are two types of ways of examining such relationships. One is to ask how closely a change in one variable is associated with a change in the other variable; this concerns the subject of correlation. The other is to ask not how closely the two are associated, but how much on the average one variable Y changes as the other variable X changes; this concerns the subject of regression. The two subjects are closely related.

The term regression was introduced by Francis Galton who studied the heights of 930 adult children in relation to the heights of 205 of their respective parents (Galton, 1886). He observed that tall parents usually had tall children and that short parents usually had short children, but that tall parents usually had children a little shorter than they were, whereas short parents had children a little taller than they were. He entitled his article "Regression towards Mediocrity in Hereditary Stature," and the term "regression" has been used to denote the relationship between two or more variables ever since that time. More generally, regression has been defined as the analysis of relationships among variables (Chatterjee and Price, 1977).

There is no *necessary* implication of causality in an X—Y relationship. The increase in age of a child is a factor in its increase in height, although the connection between the two is complex. An increase in time of a car traveling at constant speed is a direct causative factor in the distance it goes. An increase in temperature causes a direct increase in the amount of the product of a chemical reaction. On the other hand, some variates are associated indirectly; this is referred to as confounding, and is a common trap in scientific inference. One study showed a linear relationship between the annual birth rate in Oldenburg in Germany and the number of storks observed annually in the city (Box et al., 1978). A high birth rate caused the population to increase and so more houses were needed, and with more nesting sites more storks came to the city. The storks were definitely not the cause of the increased numbers of babies! Numerous striking examples of this fallacious inference are provided online by Vigen on YouTube at http://tylervigen.com. For example, there are almost perfect correlations between US spending on space and technology and suicides by hanging, strangulation, or suffocation, or between the divorce rate in Maine and the per capita consumption of margarine. Obviously these variables are unlikely to be related in any meaningful way.

Another example of association without causality is when X is a measurement of a process (e.g., cardiac output) measured one way and Y is another way of measuring the process. As cardiac output changes both X and Y will change with it, but neither one causes the other.

If X does cause Y, in whole or in part, then X is called an independent, predictor, or explanatory variable and Y is the dependent, response, or explained variable, but that classification can be made only from other considerations. With this convention, the

X values are **always** measured along the horizontal axis (or abscissa) and the Y values **always** along the vertical axis (or ordinate).

The data for regression analysis may be obtained either by bivariate random sampling, the investigator selecting subjects at random from a population and then measuring X and Y, or by regression or selected sampling in which the investigator specifies the values of X (e.g., ages 1—10 in yearly intervals) and then draws a random sample of each of these samples and measures Y. Both these data sets are calculated as set out below, with differences to be discussed later. In general, bivariate sampling is more applicable to observational studies and regression sampling to experimental studies where X (e.g., age, temperature) may be specified in advance.

Exploratory Data Analysis

Just as exploratory data analysis should be done for univariate measurements before launching into calculations and judgments, so should it be done for bivariate analysis. First plot the X and Y data pairs on a *scattergram* in which paired XY values are put into a Cartesian coordinate graph. Each pair of associated values, for example X_i and Y_i, produces one point on the plot, as indicated by the dashed lines in Figure 27.1.

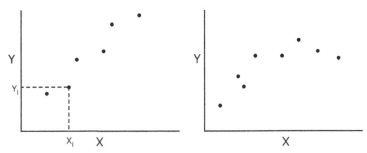

Figure 27.1 Two scattergrams. Left panel: roughly linear relationship between X and Y. Right panel: roughly curvilinear relationship between X and Y. Dashed lines indicate the two coordinates for the point X_1Y_1.

Sometimes there is no regularity, and XY points wander up and down, for example, as in the daily Dow-Jones index. Because it is easier to demonstrate the principles of regression analysis with a simple linear relationship than with any other form, the rest of this chapter will be restricted to linear regression with two variables.

Transforming Curves

Although there are statistical procedures for dealing with curvilinear regression (Chapter 30), often it is simpler to transform the data so that linearity is achieved. A line is the expression of a relationship $Y = c + bX^p$, where c is the intercept on the Y-axis, b is a coefficient, and p is the power to which X is raised (Mosteller and Tukey, 1977).

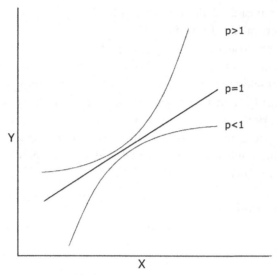

Figure 27.2 Power curves.

If the power of X is 1, the line is straight and b is its slope; if power is >1, then the curve is concave upward; and if it is <1, the curve is concave downward (Figure 27.2).

If the points show decreasing curvature (concave down), taking the square root or the logarithm of X, which shortens the X-axis, or squaring or cubing Y, which lengthens the Y-axis, tends to straighten the points. If the points display an increasing curvature (concave up), then squaring or cubing X, or taking the square root or logarithm of Y may straighten out the points. A range of possible transformations termed the ladder of powers is frequently used (Table 27.1).

Table 27.1 Ladder of powers

Power	Transformation	Name
3	X^3	Cube
2	X^2	Square
1	X	Raw
1/2	$\sqrt{X}$	Square root
0	Log X	Logarithm, usually to base 10
−1/2	$-1/\sqrt{X}$	Reciprocal root
−1	$-1/X$	Reciprocal
−2	$-1/X^2$	Reciprocal square

Anything to the power 0 is 1, logarithms are used.

Higher, lower, or intermediate powers are rarely needed.

Sometimes the underlying process is known to be exponential or logarithmic, and then appropriate procedures can be used. Depending on the approximate curvature of the points, Mosteller and Tukey (1977) recommended general methods of reexpression (transformation) that they termed the bulging rule (Figure 27.3).

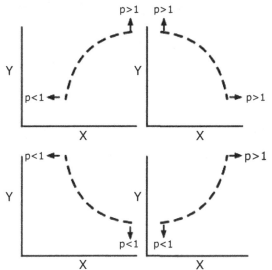

Figure 27.3 Direction of reexpression needed to straighten out the dashed line, based on diagram by Mosteller and Tukey (1977). Horizontal arrows indicate direction of needed change in X values, vertical arrows indicate direction of needed change in Y values. p > 1 indicates increasing power above 1, p < 1 indicates decreasing power below 1. For any quadrant, one or a combination of both indicated transformations tend to straighten the line.

Whether to reexpress X, Y, or both depends upon the effect that reexpression has on the variability of Y. Mosteller and Tukey (1977) described simple methods for deciding what was the most appropriate power. In brief, the slope from a low value of X to a value near the middle of the X array is compared to the slope from that middle value to a high value of X. If the ratio of these slopes is near 1, then the line is approximately straight. Any nonlinear model that can be transformed into a linear model is called "intrinsically linear," and transformation is likely to provide more normally distributed residuals with constant variance than fitting a more complex nonlinear model (Montgomery and Peck, 1982). This produces an improvement that shows up as smaller standard errors and therefore more precise prediction of the model parameters.

Figure 27.4 gives examples of several transformations of data until linearity is achieved.

These transformations are merely made to achieve linearity, and more than one may be suitable. Whether the transformation has an underlying mechanistic interpretation cannot be judged from the information presented.

We summarize X–Y relations by the mean slope of the relationship (does Y increase a lot or a little for a unit increase in X?) and a measure of variability called the standard deviation from regression.

Model I Linear Regression Basics

The requirements for performing a simple linear (model I) regression are as follows:
1. Y must be linearly related to X.
2. The numbers must be ratio or interval numbers.

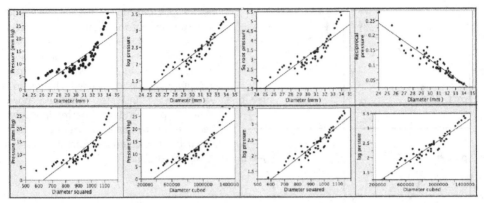

Figure 27.4 Data taken from Senzaki et al. (2000) on pressure—diameter relations of failing dog hearts. Upper row: Left panel shows original data with curved relationship between diameter (X) and pressure (Y). The next three panels show reexpression of the Y variable: natural logarithm, square root, and reciprocal. Only the reciprocal of pressure shows a good linear relationship. Bottom row: First two panels show transformation of the X variate—square and then cube. Neither straightens the set of points. Next two panels show reexpression of both X and Y variates, plotting the square and then the cube of X against the natural logarithm of Y. The cube of diameter against the logarithm of pressure gives good linearity.

3. The X values should be measured with no or little error.
4. The distribution of Y values at any X value is normal. That is, if there are several measurements of reaction products at each of several specified temperatures of 35–39 °C, then at each temperature (X value) the amount of reaction product (Y value) would be normally distributed.
5. The Y values are statistically independent of one another (see below and Chapter 31).
6. At each value of X, the variance of the Y values is constant (homoscedasticity).

Some of these requirements are indicated in Figure 27.5.

The requirement that X is measured with little error is poorly defined. Measurements of temperature, height, age, and so on are never exact, but are usually reproducible with very small standard deviations. This requirement is usually not tested, but if there is reason to be concerned, alternative tests can be done (see below).

The distribution of Y at any X can be seen clearly only when several values of Y are measured at each value of X. It is more usual for there be one Y value with each value, as shown in Figure 27.1, but the scatter of points above and below the line gives a rough estimate of normality. Fortunately, testing of normality is rarely required, and regression analysis is robust in this respect.

Homogeneity of variance is often absent (Figure 27.6).

The increase in variability as X increases is expected, because large measurements usually vary more than small measurements do. Remember from Chapter 4 that the

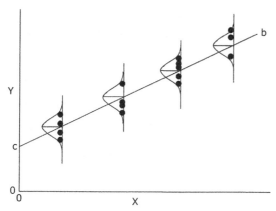

Figure 27.5 Basic linear regression concepts. The line does not pass through zero. The sets of values of Y at each X value are approximately normal, have similar variances, and the short solid horizontal lines indicate the mean of each Y set. If the relationship of Y to X is linear, then the means of each set of Y values lie on a straight line with a slope indicated by *b* and an intercept on the Y-axis of *c*.

coefficient of variation is often constant for a particular set of measurements. This means that if the ratio of standard deviation to mean is constant, then as X increases the standard deviation of Y increases proportionally. If the inhomogeneity of variance (heteroscedasticity) is not marked by eye, the standard regression methods are adequate. If the change in variance is very marked, then although the estimates of slope and intercept are unbiased, the variability is excessive and reduces the efficiency of the test. Methods of testing heteroscedasticity and transforming the Y values are discussed below. (Transforming the X variate only changes its placement on the horizontal axis, and does not alter the variability of the Y variate.)

Whether the line passes through zero, that is, the intercept on the Y-axis is zero, does not affect the ability to perform classical regression analysis. However, if the intercept truly is zero, there are sometimes easier ways of doing the calculations (see Chapter 28).

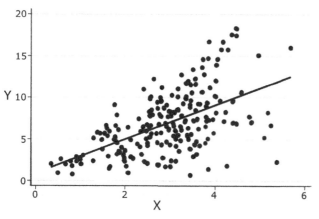

Figure 27.6 The increasing variability of Y as X increases is obvious.

Linear regression, if the requirements are met, answers the questions:

How much does Y increase for a unit increase in X? In other words, what is the slope of the line? and

What is the variability of the Y values at each X value?

If all the points fall exactly on a line, there is no difficulty in defining the line, but what if they do not fall on a line, as in Figure 27.1? Then use what is termed "the line of best fit" that can have several definitions. Most often the line of best fit used is one that minimizes the vertical deviations of the Y values from the line (Figure 27.7).

The principle states that the line of best fit minimizes the sum of the squared deviations of the points from the regression line. As shown in Figure 27.7, the deviations are usually less from the regression line than from the mean. It is essential that in the scattergram the X (independent) values are plotted on the horizontal axis and the Y (dependent) values are plotted on the vertical axis so that the vertical deviations of Y from the regression line will be minimized. If the X and Y axes are interchanged, it is the deviations of X from the regression line that are minimized, giving a different line of best fit and a different interpretation.

How do we calculate the slope of the line of best fit? Although this is done easily in computer programs, it is important that readers understand how this is done, because the elements of the resulting formulas appear frequently, and because understanding the process leads to greater insights. Online calculations can be done at http://vassarstats.net/ under the Correlation and Regression heading; XY data can be entered either one by one in a table or by copying data from a spreadsheet. Other programs online are http://www.easycalculation.com/statistics/regression.php, http://www.wessa.net/slr. wasp, http://www.alcula.com/calculators/statistics/linear-regression/, and http://www. xycoon.com/simple_linear_regression.htm (which also plot the scattergram) and http:// home.ubalt.edu/ntsbarsh/Business-stat/otherapplets/Regression.htm (which gives some

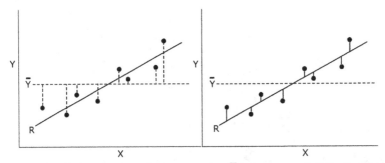

Figure 27.7 Principle of least squares in linear regression. $\bar{Y}$ is the mean of all the Y values (horizontal dashed line), and the regression line is shown as a solid diagonal line. The vertical dashed lines in the left panel are deviations from the mean, and the solid vertical lines in the right panel are deviations from the regression line.

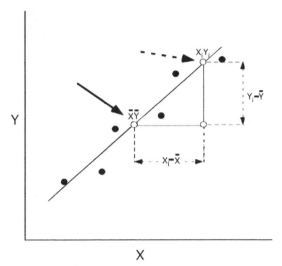

Figure 27.8 Basis of slope calculation. Solid circles are data points. Open circles are hypothetical points, two on the regression line, with their XY coordinates.

additional statistics), and http://bcs.whfreeman.com/ips4e/cat_010/applets/twovarcalcIPS. html, http://people.hofstra.edu/Stefan_Waner/newgraph/regressionframes.html and http://www.xuru.org/rt/PowR.asp. Regression apps for iPhone and iPad can be found at iTunes under "Regression calculators".

Figure 27.8 shows the beginnings of the calculations.

One of the advantages of the least squares principle is that the regression line passes through a point that is the mean of X and the mean of Y, indicated by the solid arrow. Consider any point on the regression line $X_i Y_i$ indicated by the dashed arrow (see figure). Construct a right-angled triangle from these two points, as shown; designate the right angle by the point $X_1 \overline{Y}$. By trigonometry, the slope of the line, b, is the tangent. Therefore,

$$b = \frac{Y_i - \overline{Y}}{X_i - \overline{X}}.$$

Multiply both sides by the denominator:

$$b\left(X_i - \overline{X}\right) = Y_i - \overline{Y},$$

$$\therefore\ b\left(X_i - \overline{X}\right) + \overline{Y} = Y_i,\ \text{ and by rearrangement}$$

$$Y_i = bX_i - b\overline{X} + \overline{Y} = bX_i + \left(\overline{Y} - b\overline{X}\right) = bX_i + c,\ \text{ where } c = \left(\overline{Y} - b\overline{X}\right).$$

Because this is not any Y_i, but the hypothetical Y_i that lies on the regression line, characterize it as $\widehat{Y}_i$ (termed Y hat) where the hat indicates a theoretical point. c, the intercept on the Y-axis, is composed of two portions: the mean of Y and b times the mean of X. Depending on the values for $\overline{Y}$ and $\overline{X}$, c may be positive or negative.

(In pure mathematics texts, this equation is usually written as $Y = aX + b$. Some use a or β_0 instead of c. The meaning is identical.)

The remaining step is to find out how to compute b, the slope.

As in univariate statistics, compute $\sum X_i, \sum Y_i, \sum(X_i^2), \sum(Y_i^2)$ and then for X and Y separately derive the sum of squared deviations from the mean

$$\sum(X_i - \overline{X})^2 = \sum(X_i^2) - \frac{(\sum X_i)^2}{N} \text{ and } \sum(Y_i - \overline{Y})^2 = \sum(Y_i^2) - \frac{(\sum Y_i)^2}{N},$$

as described in Chapter 4. All that remains is to compute the sum of the product deviations from the mean, also known as the covariance. To understand covariance, examine Table 27.2.

Table 27.2 Product deviation from the mean. For each X_i calculate its deviation from mean X, and for each Y_i calculate its deviation from mean Y. Then multiply each deviation from the mean of X by the corresponding deviation from the mean of Y, and add up all the products

X	$X_i - \overline{X}$	Y	$Y_i - \overline{Y}$	$(X_i - \overline{X})(Y_i - \overline{Y})$	XY
7	−2	13	−4	$-2 \times -4 = 8$	91
6	−1	11	−2	$-1 \times -2 = 2$	66
5	0	9	0	0	45
4	1	7	2	$1 \times 2 = 2$	28
3	2	5	4	$2 \times 4 = 8$	15
$\Sigma X = 25$ $\overline{X} = 5$		$\Sigma Y = 45$ $\overline{Y} = 9$		$\sum(X_i - \overline{X})(Y_i - \overline{Y}) = 20$	$\Sigma XY = 245$

To avoid this lengthy procedure with large samples and noninteger deviations from the mean, use the identity

$$\sum(X_i - \overline{X})(Y_i - \overline{Y}) = \sum X_i Y_i - \frac{\sum X_i \sum Y_i}{N}.$$

Thus for the above example, this would be

$$245 - \frac{25 \times 45}{5} = 20, \text{ as shown above.}$$

As shown in Table 27.1, if X and Y are related, then the product deviations from the mean tend to be all positive (or all negative, if the slope is downward) and they will sum to some reasonable value. If X and Y are not associated, then the product deviations from the mean will not be all positive or all negative, and their sum will be small, as shown in Table 27.3.

Therefore a large product deviation from the mean indicates an association between X and Y, and a small product deviation from the mean indicates little or no such

Table 27.3 Rearrangement to show lack of association between X and Y

X	$X_i - \overline{X}$	Y	$Y_i - \overline{Y}$	$(X_i - \overline{X})(Y_i - \overline{Y})$
8	3	13	4	$3 \times 4 = 12$
1	-4	11	2	$-4 \times 2 = -8$
6	1	9	0	0
1	-4	7	-2	$-4 \times -2 = 8$
9	4	5	-4	$4 \times -4 = -16$
$\Sigma X = 25$ $\overline{X} = 5$		$\Sigma Y = 45$ $\overline{Y} = 9$		$\sum(X_i - \overline{X})(Y_i - \overline{Y}) = -4$

association. Is the product deviation from the mean is large or small? Relate it to the variability of the X array as assessed by the sum of squared deviations:

$$b = \frac{\sum(X_i - \overline{X})(Y_i - \overline{Y})}{\sum(X_i - \overline{X})^2}.$$

With this calculation, the line of best fit has the equation:

$$\widehat{Y}_i = bX_i + (\overline{Y} - b\overline{X}).$$

To draw the line by hand, select two values of X_i, calculate the values of the corresponding values of $\widehat{Y}$, and join them by a straight line.

Next calculate the variability of the points about the regression line (Figure 27.9).

For any data point X_iY_i, the deviation of Y_i from the mean of Y can be divided into the difference between Y_i and the corresponding point on the regression line, $(Y_i - \widehat{Y}_i)$, and the difference between the point on the regression line and the mean of Y, $(\widehat{Y}_i - \overline{Y})$. Then the sum of the squared deviations of all the Y values from their mean is:

$$\sum(Y_i - \overline{Y})^2 = \sum[(Y_i - \widehat{Y}_i) + (\widehat{Y}_i - \overline{Y})]^2.$$

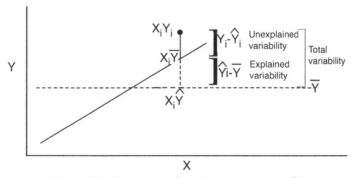

Figure 27.9 Diagram to show the components of Y.

Therefore,

$$\sum (Y_i - \overline{Y})^2 = \sum (Y_i - \widehat{Y}_i)^2 + 2\sum (Y_i - \widehat{Y}_i)(\widehat{Y}_i - \overline{Y}) + \sum (\widehat{Y}_i - \overline{Y})^2.$$

But $2\sum (Y_i - \widehat{Y}_i)(\widehat{Y}_i - \overline{Y}) = 0$ because it involves the sum of deviations from the mean, so that

$$\sum (Y_i - \overline{Y})^2 = \sum (Y_i - \widehat{Y}_i)^2 + \sum (\widehat{Y}_i - \overline{Y})^2.$$

Therefore, the sum of squared deviations from the mean of the Y values can be partitioned into a component due to regression $\sum (\widehat{Y}_i - \overline{Y})^2$ and the residual variation from the regression line $\sum (Y_i - \widehat{Y}_i)^2$. These are the counterparts, respectively, of the between-group sum of squares and the within-group sum of squares in analysis of variance (ANOVA) (Table 27.4).

Table 27.4 ANOVA format for linear regression

Source of variation	Sum of squares	Degrees of freedom	Mean square	F ratio
Total	$\sum (Y_i - \overline{Y})^2$	$N-1$		
Due to regression	$\sum (\widehat{Y}_i - \overline{Y})^2$	1	$\sum (\widehat{Y}_i - \overline{Y})^2$	
Residual	$\sum (Y_i - \overline{Y})^2 - \sum (\widehat{Y}_i - \overline{Y})^2$	$N-2$	$\frac{\sum (Y_i-\overline{Y})^2-\sum (\widehat{Y}_i-\overline{Y})^2}{N-2}$	

Therefore, information about the association of Y with X has reduced the total variability of Y by an amount related to the relationship between X and Y.

For the total variation calculate

$$\sum (Y_i - \overline{Y})^2 = \sum Y_i^2 - \frac{\sum (Y_i)^2}{N}.$$

For the component of variation due to the regression line calculate

$$\sum (\widehat{Y}_i - \overline{Y})^2 = \frac{\sum \left(X_i Y_i - \frac{\sum X_i \sum Y_i}{N}\right)^2}{\sum (X_i - \overline{X})^2}.$$

Many of these additional statistics can be calculated online at http://home.ubalt.edu/ntsbarsh/Business-stat/otherapplets/Regression.htm and http://www.wessa.net/slr.wasp.

As an example, Harker and Slichter (1972) studied the relationship of platelet count to bleeding time (Table 27.5).

The first thing to do is to plot these data on an X–Y plot (Figure 27.10). Because bleeding time depends on platelet count, the platelet count is plotted on the X-axis.

Table 27.5 Bleeding time and platelet count for each patient

▼	Bleeding time (min)	Platelet count x10,000/μL	▼	Bleeding time (min)	Platelet count x10,000/μL
1	7.1	10.5	27	17	6
2	5.1	10.3	28	17	4.9
3	4.6	10.1	29	16	4.7
4	4	9.9	30	15.5	4.5
5	5.6	9.9	31	15.9	4.3
6	4.1	9.5	32	17	4.2
7	5.1	9.2	33	17.9	4.3
8	6.1	9.3	34	18	4
9	6.6	9.2	35	19.1	4.3
10	6.5	8.9	36	19	4
11	7	8.6	37	19	3.7
12	8.5	9	38	20.1	3.5
13	9.6	8.6	39	23	3.4
14	9.1	7.8	40	23.1	2.3
15	7.7	7.5	41	24.1	1.8
16	10	6.9	42	25	2.3
17	10.1	6.5	43	25	2.1
18	11.1	6.9	44	25	1.9
19	12	7.2	45	26.1	1.7
20	13	7.3	46	25.4	1.5
21	14.1	6.5	47	28	2
22	14	5.8	48	28.9	1.2
23	14.6	5.3	49	30	0.8
24	14	5.2	50	20.9	4.2
25	15.9	5.3	51	18.9	2.9
26	16.9	5.6			

The figure shows reasonable linearity and homogeneity of variance. The line slopes downward because as platelet count decreases the bleeding time increases.

Calculate the basic features of regression (Table 27.6).

This gives the line of best fit: the intercept on the Y-axis at X = 0 is 29.41 and the slope is −2.52. The ANOVA shows that the total variability of bleeding time (Y) has been reduced from 2709.24 to 151.73 (residual, error, or within-group SS, also termed s_{res}^2) by virtue of the regression (model) accounting for 2557.51. The F ratio that, as usual, divides MS_B by MS_W is $2557.51/3.1 = 825.90$ and is highly significant. In a univariate distribution, the sum of squared deviations from the mean divided by degrees of freedom

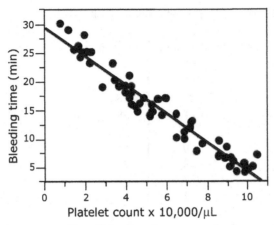

Figure 27.10 Plot of bleeding time versus platelet count.

Table 27.6 Basic regression results

Summary

R square	0.9440
R square adjusted	0.9429
Root mean square error	1.7597
Number of observations	51

ANOVA

Source	DF	Sum of squares	Mean square	F ratio
Model	1	2557.5092	2557.51	825.90
Error	49	151.7343	3.10	Prob>F
Total	50	2709.2435		P<0.0001

Parameter estimates

Term	Estimate	Standard error	t ratio	Prob>t
Intercept	29.41	0.5512	53.36	<0.0001
Slope	−2.52	0.0875	−28.74	<0.0001

Equation: Bleeding time (min) = 29.41−2.52 × platelet count (×10,000 μL)

was termed the variance s^2, and the comparable value in regression analysis is the within-group error, or residual sum of squares (SS_{res}), divided by degrees of freedom to give the MS_W, sometimes symbolized by $s^2_{Y \cdot X}$ or as $s^2_{y|x}$ to show that the variability of Y is dependent on X. Its square root $s_{y|x}$ is the standard deviation from regression.

What does the F ratio indicate? It indicates that the null hypothesis of zero slope can be rejected confidently. Imagine, for example, a population of unrelated X−Y points with no association so that the true population slope $\beta = 0$. Regression analysis on a sample from that population would very likely get a nonzero slope at random. To find out if the null hypothesis (H_0: $\beta = 0$) is true, test the difference between the observed slope b and zero against a measure of variability. As seen from Table 27.5, the less association there is between X and Y, the smaller the model component of regression and the larger the residual SS will be.

Problem 27.1

Nagy et al. (2014) compared the pulmonary capillary wedge and left atrial pressures in patients with mitral stenosis. The table below presents a subset of their results.

x	y
2.098	3.980
6.055	6.964
6.115	7.959
7.134	8.036
9.113	9.031
10.132	10.026
10.132	11.020
11.091	12.015
11.151	13.010
11.271	14.005
13.129	13.852
13.129	15.230
14.029	15.995
14.029	15.077
14.149	13.929
15.048	13.010
15.108	14.923
15.168	16.148
15.108	16.913
15.228	17.985
16.067	15.995
16.067	15.077
16.127	13.852
17.146	15.000
17.086	15.995
17.086	16.990
17.026	18.214
18.106	21.964
18.106	21.046
18.106	19.974
18.106	18.903
18.165	16.990
18.165	15.995
19.065	15.918
19.125	16.990

Draw an XY plot, and calculate the linear regression for these data.

Additional Calculations

These basic calculations are used to compute other useful statistics, such as the significance of the slope and the intercept, the confidence interval of the estimated value of Y_i, and even the confidence interval of the standard deviation from regression.

To test the significance of the slope, calculate the variance of the slope as

$$s_b^2 = \frac{s_{res}^2}{\sum(X_i - \overline{X})^2},$$

and then do a t-test

$$t_{0.05} = \frac{b - \mu}{s_b}. \text{ For the null hypothesis, } \mu = 0.$$

For the example used above in Table 27.6, $s_{res}^2 = 3.1$, $\sum(X_i - \overline{X})^2 = 404.29$ (calculated from the platelet counts above), so that $s_b = \sqrt{\frac{3.1}{404.29}} = 0.088$ and $t_{0.05,N-2} = \frac{2.52-0}{0.088} = 28.64$. Therefore reject the hypothesis that the slope is zero, exactly as shown in Table 24.5. From this it is simple to calculate the 95% confidence limits as $-2.52 \pm t_{0.05,N-2} \times 0.088 = -2.52 \pm 2.004 \times 0.088 = -2.70$ to -2.34.

A slope of zero means that either there is no relationship between X and Y, or else that there is a very nonlinear relationship.

Occasionally the population mean is not zero; for example, if theoretically there should be a 1:1 ratio with a slope of 1. Then the t-test is done with $\mu = 1$.

To determine the 95% confidence interval of the predicted value of Y_i at X_i, first determine the variance of Y_i as

$$s_{res}^2 \left(\frac{1}{N} + \frac{(X_i - \overline{X})^2}{\sum(X_i - \overline{X})^2} \right).$$

To calculate the 95% confidence limits for the intercept, use the same equation but substitute zero for X_i. For the data of Table 27.4, this becomes

$$Variance = 3.1 \left(\frac{1}{52} + \frac{5.633^2}{404.29} \right) = 0.30,$$

so that the standard deviation is $\sqrt{0.30} = 0.55$. Then the 95% confidence limits of c are $29.41 \pm 2.004 \times 0.55 = 28.31$ to 30.51.

Many of these additional statistics can be calculated online at http://home.ubalt.edu/ntsbarsh/Business-stat/otherapplets/Regression.htm and http://www.wessa.net/slr.wasp.

Residuals

Before going further, check linearity and homogeneity of variance. One simple way is to plot the residuals, the values of $Y_i - \widehat{Y}_i$ against the corresponding value of X_i (or $\widehat{Y}_i$ which has an exact correspondence to X_i) (Figure 27.11(a)). If there is reason to suspect an influence of time, the residuals can be plotted against the order or the time at which they were acquired.

Although free online programs for plotting residuals directly are not available, the online programs http://vassarstats.net/corr_stats.html and http://www.xuru.org/rt/LR.

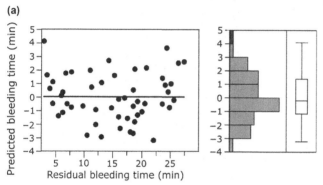

(a)

Figure 27.11 (a) Residual plot. This shows a satisfactory plot with the residuals scattered equally above and below the line. Residual variability does not change materially as Y changes. (b) Normal quantile plot of residuals.

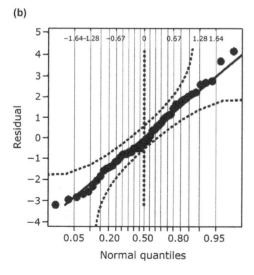

(b)

asp# calculate the residuals (termed "error" in the latter), and these can then be plotted against the original X or Y values. Another useful assessment of residuals is to plot them on normal probability paper to find out if they form a straight line (as they should) (Figure 27.11(b)) or if there are distortions that might indicate some abnormality of their distribution (Montgomery and Peck, 1982).

Figure 27.12 to 27.15 show data from Jamal et al. (2001) who were comparing how changes in dP/dt max affected systolic strain (%).

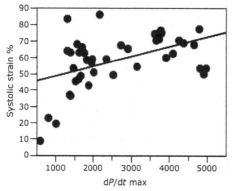

Figure 27.12 Data from Jamal et al. of systolic strain % versus dP/Dt max. The line of best fit by linear regression (which they did **not** use) fits the points poorly, as confirmed by the residual plot (Figure 27.13).

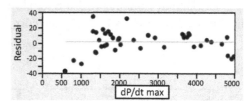

Figure 27.13 Residual plot of linear regression. At each end of the X values the residuals are below the line, and in the center most are above it. This is typical of a curvilinear association. When the data were correctly fitted by a second-order polynomial (as they did correctly), the residuals show more acceptable behavior (Figures 27.14 and 27.15).

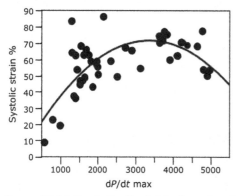

Figure 27.14 Quadratic fit of data from Jamal et al. (2001).

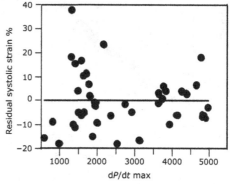

Figure 27.15 Residuals from quadratic fit. The residuals are normally distributed.

Another example of the use of residual plots is shown in Figure 27.16 in which the residuals from the reexpressed curves from Figure 27.4 are shown.

Problem 27.2

Draw the residual plot for the data from Problem 27.1.

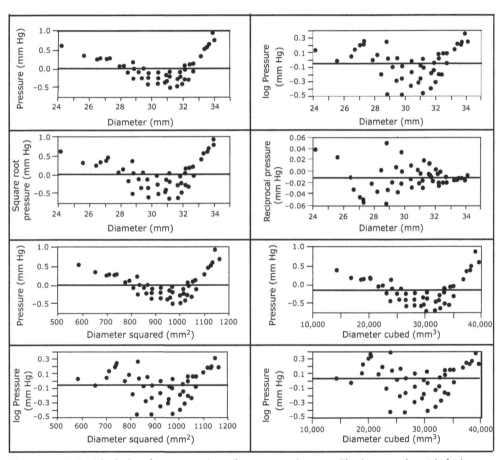

Figure 27.16 Residual plots from a number of reexpressed curves. The best results with fairly even dispersion of the residuals occur with diameter versus reciprocal of pressure and diameter cubed versus logarithm of pressure, confirming the impression of linearity gained from Figure 27.4.

The absolute residual variability varies with the units used and the size of the deviations. To allow for this, standardized residuals are calculated by dividing each absolute residual by the standard deviation from regression. This yields the residuals in standard deviation units, which are dimensionless and scattered above and below a zero line, just as in a univariate distribution the X variate is transformed into standard deviation units above and below zero mean by the z transformation. Then about 95% of the standardized residuals should lie within 2 standard deviations of the zero line.

The effects of a marked increase in variability as X increases can be seen well in a residual plot based on the artificial data of Figure 27.6 (Figure 27.17).

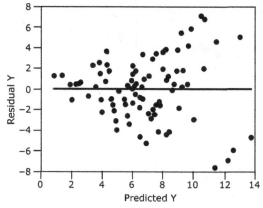

Figure 27.17 Residual plot to show variability increasing greatly as X increases.

Two other residual plots need to be considered. Figure 27.18 shows residuals that are not independent of each other.

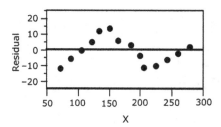

Figure 27.18 Positive autocorrelation of residuals.

The plot shows a tendency for one positive or negative value to be associated with another positive or negative value respectively, suggesting that some factor, frequently time, is influencing these residuals. There are fewer changes in direction than would be expected by chance. Negative autocorrelation is shown if positive and negative residuals alternate, again something unexpected by chance (Figure 27.19). Time-dependent

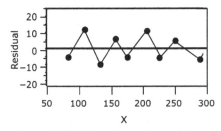

Figure 27.19 Negative autocorrelation.

residuals may be tested specifically by the Wald–Wolfowitz runs test or the Durbin–Watson test (Chapter 31).

Methods of evaluating autocorrelation are described in Chapter 31.

When the results of a linear regression are presented, in addition to the X-Y plot give the equation to the line of best fit, and **always** give the standard deviation from regression. This is the square root of the MS_W (residual or error mean square). In Table 27.5 the MS_W was 5.856, so that the standard deviation from regression was 2.42. (In the computer print out, this value was termed "root mean square error.") In other words, the "average" deviation of data points from the regression line was 2.42. This is the equivalent of the standard deviation of data from a mean in a univariate distribution.

In Chapter 25, ANOVA was used for different dietary additions of vitamin B_{12} to determine the effect in growing pigs (Richardson et al., 1951). The different groups were labeled as A, B, C, and D. If these were different vitamins, then an ANOVA would be the right form of analysis. In fact, the columns represented increasing amounts added to the diet (in µg/lb ration): 0, 5, 10, and 20 µg/lb. This means that there is the possibility of a regression relationship between amount of additive and weight gain, and this is shown in Figure 27.20.

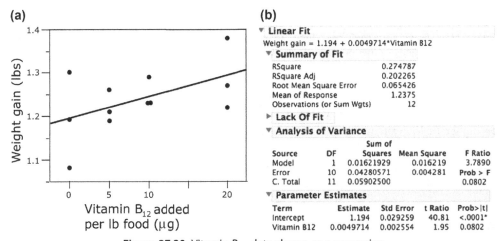

Figure 27.20 Vitamin B_{12} data shown as a regression.

There is a rough linear relationship between the amount of vitamin B_{12} added and the weight gain with a low slope that is not significantly different from zero, with P = 0.0802. This is getting close to significance, and the 95% confidence limits for the slope are $0.0049714 \pm 2.228 \times 0.002554$, or from -0.0007189 to 0.01066. In the direct ANOVA of Chapter 25, the standard deviation of weight was 0.0730, and the F ratio was 1.08, with a P value of 0.4109. Therefore, introducing the regression relationship has reduced the standard deviation of Y to 0.065 when X has been taken into account. If the effect of vitamin B_{12} additive might be important, it would be worth repeating the experiment with more animals.

Confidence Limits

The next order of business is to set confidence limits on the slope, just like confidence limits for the mean of a univariate distribution. It is more complicated for a bivariate distribution because there are two ways in which the slope can vary (Figure 27.21).

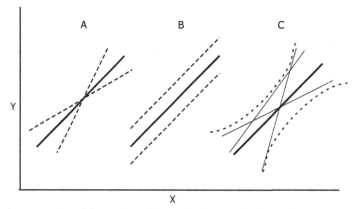

Figure 27.21 Diagram of confidence limits for a line of best fit. Thick solid line—observed sample slope. Thin solid lines—other possible slopes. Dashed lines—possible variations.

Panel A shows that the population slope might be steeper or less steep, pivoting about the same central point. Panel B shows that the population line of best fit might be higher or lower than the sample value, that is, that the intercept may be higher or lower with the same slope. Both of these changes can occur independently; the population slope might be higher and steeper, higher and less steep, lower and steeper, or lower and less steep. When these choices are combined the confidence limits appear as curved biconcave lines around the sample line. Any straight line that can be fitted to lie completely within those boundaries is a possible population slope, as shown by the thin lines in the figure.

An example of 95% limits for the platelet count—bleeding time data shown in Figure 27.10 is given in Figure 27.22.

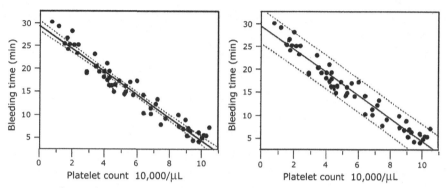

Figure 27.22 Left panel: 95% confidence limits for line of best fit. Right panel: 95% confidence limit for points.

A crucial distinction must be made between confidence limits for the line (which is a mean that changes as X changes) and confidence limits for individual points. (Strictly speaking, the term "confidence limits" should not be applied to a single estimate of Y because Y is not a parameter. The term "prediction interval" might be more accurate.) For example, to use the data shown in Figure 27.10 to determine if an individual value was abnormal and outside expected limits, add another component of variability, as shown in the right-hand panel. The points are the same in both panels.

The outer boundaries for individuals are set so that not more than 5% of individual points lie outside the boundaries. These boundaries are further from the line of best fit than are the inner boundaries because individual values vary more than means do. The computations and the regression line with confidence limits for individual points can be performed online at http://www.xycoon.com/ simple_linear_regression.htm. This requires considerable experience with Excel as well as downloading the free module StatPlus:mac LE. The confidence interval for the intercept can be calculated at http://easycalculation.com/statistics/regression- intercept-interval.php.

To report how much steeper or less steep the slope could be, calculate s_b^2, the variance of the slope, as

$$\frac{MS_W}{\sum(X_i - \overline{X})^2} = \frac{3.1}{404.29} = 0.0077.$$

Then the standard deviation of the slope is $\sqrt{0.0077} = 0.088$. (This is shown in Table 27.6, bottom line.)

Therefore, the 95% confidence limits of the slope are $b \pm t_{0.95,n-2}s_b$, or $-2.52 \pm 0.0088 \times 2.004 = -2.54$ to -2.50.

Sometimes we want to know how much the mean of Y related to X can vary, that is, we calculate the square root of $s_{\hat{Y} \cdot X}^2$. This value is obtained from $s_{Y \cdot X}^2 / N = 3.1/50 = 0.2662$, the square root of which is 0.062. This is comparable to the standard deviation of the mean for a univariate distribution.

It is from these values that the confidence limits for the line of best fit and for individuals are computed. The curved confidence boundaries shown in Figures 27.21 and 27.22, however, cannot be derived from measurements at a single point, but for the reasons given in Figure 27.21 are narrowest at the mean of X and become wider on each side of it. They are a function of $\sum(X_i - \overline{X})^2$, and this means that the boundaries get wider as they move away from the mean of X. This is not unreasonable for values above the mean of X because these larger values should vary more. At the lower end, however, there is a mathematical artifact. Examine the data in Figure 27.23, redrawn from Buckberg et al. (1971).

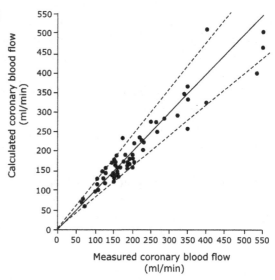

Figure 27.23 Measured versus calculated coronary blood flow in sheep and dogs.

The dashed lines on either side of the solid line of identity indicate 20% above and below the line of identity and thus are one type of boundary. Most measurements fall within the range of +20% to −20%. The smaller values of X and Y show less variation than do the larger values, something expected when the coefficient of variation remains constant. Had confidence limits about the regression line been calculated, as described above, they would have widened out at the lower end (Figure 27.24). The degree to which the lines flare out depends on the correlation between the two variables, being minimal if all the points are near the line, and flaring widely if the points are widely scattered about the line.

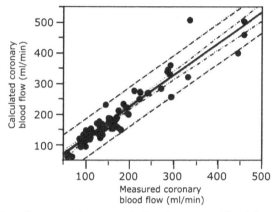

Figure 27.24 Regression of measured versus calculated coronary blood flow, with 95% confidence limits.

In any linear regression, it is important not to extrapolate beyond the observed limits. The relationship might change direction or even curvature if measurements are made outside the observed limits.

Comparison Methods (Basic)

Some comparisons involve two ways of measuring the same thing, for example, comparing a new quicker or cheaper test against an older very reliable but complex method of measuring the concentration of a particular chemical. Because neither value is dependent on the other, but rather both rely on the same underlying phenomenon (the amount of material present), some authorities consider it wrong to designate one as X and the other as Y (Bland and Altman, 1986, 1999; Ludbrook, 1997). They pointed out that in these comparison measurements the slope of the regression line and the correlation between the two methods were not the main objects of the study. Rather, it was to show how much the two methods differed from one another. Bland and Altman (1999) and Ludbrook (1997) argued that the classical Model I regression provides the degree of association between the two variables, merely tests their linear relationship, and may not emphasize important differences between the methods. Furthermore, because both the X and Y variables have error but neither is dependent on the other, there are really two regression lines, one minimizing the vertical Y differences from regression and one minimizing the horizontal X differences from regression.

What such a comparison should show is whether there is a systematic difference between the two measurements, a difference that might be fixed (constant at all values of X) or proportional (increasing as X increases). Frequently these methods obtain some type of average of the slopes of Y on X and X on Y. Bland and Altman recommended plotting the difference between the two measurements on the Y-axis against the mean of the two measurements on the X-axis. This is based on the fact that the X−Y difference is uncorrelated with either X or Y when X and Y are both measurements of the same object (Bland and Altman, 2003). (However, as shown below, when X and Y are completely uncorrelated, the difference Y−X will be negatively correlated with X.) They also calculated what they termed the 95% limits of agreement as mean difference ± standard deviation of the difference, a range expected to include about 95% of the observations. An Excel calculator can be found at http://analyse-it.com/docs/220/standard/bland-altman_agreement.htm

An example is provided in Figure 27.25, using the microsphere data of Buckberg et al. (1971) that were plotted in Figures 24.23 and 24.24.

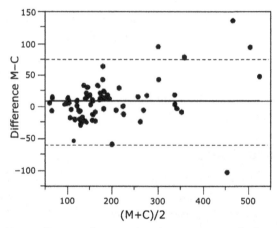

Figure 27.25 Bland–Altman diagram of comparison between a standard method (C) and a microsphere method (M) of calculating coronary blood flow. The mean difference (solid line) is shown, and is close to zero. The two dashed lines show 2 standard deviations above and below the mean, and encompass approximately 95% of the observations. This depiction makes it easier to see differences.

Problem 27.3
Use the data set from Nagy et al. above to construct a Bland–Altman plot.

Bland and Altman were careful to point out that certain requirements were needed, the most important of which were that the differences were constant over the range of measurements and were normally distributed. These can be checked visually on the scattergram, or more formally if needed. If the differences increase as the size of the measurement increases, then the mean might be correct but the limits of agreement would be too wide at small measurements and too narrow at large ones. To deal with this problem they advocated taking the logarithms of the measurements. If this is done, then the limits of agreement refer to proportions of the measurement rather than the original units. Other ways of dealing with this problem as well methods for determining the variability of the deviations are presented below.

Cautionary Tales

1. It is essential to examine the XY scatterplot before assessing regression or correlation. Examine Figure 27.26.

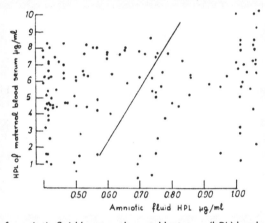

Figure 27.26 Plot of amniotic fluid human placental lactogen (hPL) levels on the X-axis versus maternal serum hPL level on the Y-axis (Lolis et al., 1977). *(Reproduced with permission of the publishers.)*

In the publication, the correlation coefficient was given as 0.21, with P < 0.005. The only way I can interpret this data is to state that the two variables are virtually completely unrelated, no matter what the significance test shows, and what the slope indicates is unclear. Not everything with a high significance value has meaning.

2. All data points must be represented in the figure and the calculations. Mackler et al. (1979) related iron deficiency and plasma phenylalanine concentration in rats. Instead of plotting all the points, they grouped averages for hemoglobin concentrations (g/100 ml blood): 4.5—5, 5—5.5, 5.5—6, 6—6.5, and 6.5—7. Each average had different numbers of measurements. Although the authors did not give a regression equation or a significance value, they did state that the relationship was linear.

(Continued)

Cautionary Tales—cont'd

In a letter to the editor, Bryant (1980) pointed out that pooling different numbers for the means masked the variability. In the original publication the authors presented a table with the individual measurements (a most unusual occurrence), and these are plotted in Figure 27.27.

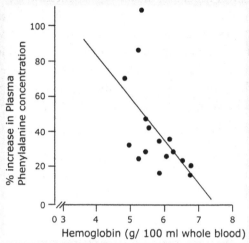

Figure 27.27 XY plot with individual points.

There is an inverse correlation between X and Y, but this is not linear, and perhaps there is a threshold at about 5.5 g/100 ml hemoglobin, or a curved relationship. Taking averages with different sample sizes gave a false impression of linearity.

3. The importance of examining the graphs was stressed in an instructive fictitious example devised by Anscombe (1973). He created four data sets (Table 27.7).

Table 27.7 Anscombe's data sets

Data set	1-3	1	2	3	4	4
Variable	x	y	y	y	x	y
	10.0	8.04	9.14	7.46	8.0	6.58
	8.0	6.95	8.14	6.77	8.0	5.76
	13.0	7.58	8.74	12.74	8.0	7.71
	9.0	8.81	8.77	7.11	8.0	8.84
	11.0	8.33	9.26	7.81	8.0	8.47
	14.0	9.96	8.10	8.84	8.0	6.89
	6.0	7.24	6.13	6.08	8.0	5.25
	4.0	4.26	3.10	5.39	19.0	12.50
	12.0	10.84	9.13	8.15	8.0	5.56
	7.0	4.82	7.26	6.42	8.0	7.91
	5.0	5.68	4.74	5.73	8.0	6.879

Four data sets, each with 11 x,y pairs. Each set yields the same regression statistics
Number of observations 11; mean of x values 9.0; mean of y values 7.5
Slope b=0.5; regression equation y=3+0.5x
Regression sum of squares=27.50(1 df); residual sum of squares=13.75 (9df)
Standard error of b=0.118;
Reproduced with permission of the American Statistical Association

Cautionary Tales—cont'd

Despite the fact that all of these data sets have identical equations and derived values, they are hugely different as shown by their plots (Figure 27.28).

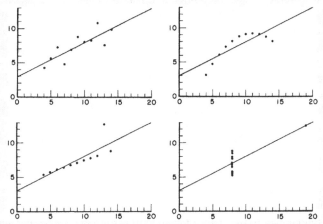

Figure 27.28 Plots of Anscombe's data sets. Despite the identity of the regression equations (indicated by the solid lines), all four sets demonstrate different distributions of the XY values. *(Reproduced with permission from the American Statistical Association.)*

4. It is unwise to rely on a linear regression formula and a significant correlation coefficient to evaluate a relationship. Consider Figure 27.29, a prototype of many in the literature.

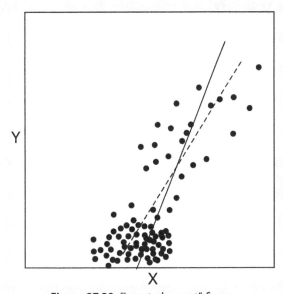

Figure 27.29 "Inverted comet" figure.

(Continued)

Cautionary Tales—cont'd

There is a dense cluster of points at small values of Y, based on the ease of obtaining normal values. These dominate the graph, and may give a slope (solid line) that is unrepresentative of the data; the dashed line might be more representative. Because of a large number of data points the correlation is high, but with the wide scatter the ability to predict Y from X is poor. The graph is not useless, but its use is limited. See Figure 1 in Nakauchi et al. (1981) and Figure 5 in Olivié et al. (1995) as examples.

5. It is unwise to extrapolate a value of Y from a value of X that is much smaller than the lowest or much bigger than the highest X value used in constructing the regression line. Unless there is evidence for extended linearity based on other work, linear extrapolation may lead to incorrect predictions. An obvious example is the asymptotic curvature seen at the top of a dose—response curve (Figure 32.1 et seq). The fact that 10 units of an agonist cause a 15% increase in cardiomyocyte shortening does not mean that 20 units will cause a 30% shortening. In fact, 15% is close to the maximal shortening of a muscle cell. In the platelet bleeding time discussed above, the linear relationship between the variables was absent at very low or very high platelet counts (Figure 27.30).

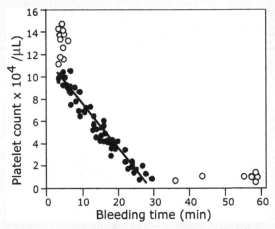

Figure 27.30 Platelet count versus bleeding time, based on data from reference 26. Note departure from linearity at the extremes, shown as open circles. Dark circles and line indicate linear range for the data.

ADVANCED OR ALTERNATIVE CONCEPTS

Heteroscedasticity

If the scattergram suggests heteroscedasticity, it may be worth testing this formally before deciding on the need for transformations. A plot of residuals will confirm the appearance of heteroscedasticity. Many tests of heteroscedasticity have been developed. You do not need them all, but they are frequently mentioned and used so that an understanding of what they are is useful. Two are basically ANOVA tests:

1. The Goldfeld–Quandt test divides the data set into two groups (omitting c measurements—about 20%—in the middle of the distribution), regresses Y on X for each group, calculates the SS_{res} for each group, and does an F test:

$$\frac{SS_{res(larger)}}{SS_{res(smaller)}} = F_{(n_1-c, n_2-c)},$$

where n_1 and n_2 are the numbers in the lower and upper data sets. A high value for F suggests heteroscedasticity.

Example: For the data shown in Figures 27.6 and 27.17, the SS_{res} was 10,636 for the lower 34 X values, and 52,710 for the upper 34 X values. Their ratio of 4.96 is assessed by $F_{(17,17)}$, with P $\approx$ 0.001. Therefore the two error terms are not similar, and the hypothesis of significant heteroscedasticity is supported.

2. The modified Levene test divides the data into halves, regresses Y on X for each half, estimates the median of each residual group, determines for each residual group separately the absolute deviations from the median, calculates the mean absolute deviation in each group, and then compares these two mean deviations by t-test or ANOVA. A significant t or F value indicates that the null hypothesis can be rejected. An advantage of the Levene test is that if the regression appears to be curvilinear as well as heteroscedastic, the data set can be divided into three or more groups, and an ANOVA can be performed on the absolute deviations.

Example: Dividing the data into two groups, the mean absolute deviations of the residuals are 18.9 for lower values of X and 34.6 for the higher X values. By t-test the difference of 15.7 is significant with P $= 0.0003$.

These tests may lose power if the Y distributions are not normal and numbers are small, and cannot readily be extended to more than one X variable, so other tests are often used. Those most often used are tests by Park, Glejser, and Breusch and Pagan (the latter test described independently by Cook and Weisberg). They all have similar forms in that an auxiliary regression is performed between the residuals (ε_i) obtained by regressing Y on X.

1. Park test: $\log \varepsilon_i^2 = c + \beta_1 \log X_1 + v_i$, where v_i is the new error term in the auxiliary regression. This is tested by the Lagrange multiplier (LM) method, in which Nr^2 is approximately equal to chi-square with degrees of freedom equal to the number of

independent variables, here 1. The regression equation was $Y = 3.26 + 0.077X$, and r^2 was 0.168658. Therefore the metric was $85 \times 0.168658 = 14.34$ with 1 df, so that $P = 0.0002$, again attesting to heteroscedasticity.

2. Glejser test: $|\varepsilon_i| = c + \beta_1 X_i + v_i$, where $|\varepsilon_i|$ is the absolute value of the deviation. The resultant linear regression equation was $Y = 1.0057X - 5.85$, with $r^2 = 0.36$. Using the LM method, the chi-square approximation was $85 \times 0.36 = 30.6$, also with 1 df and $P = <0.00001$.

3. Breusch–Pagan test: This test is used more often than the others. The basis of the test is to determine if the squared residuals are constant at each value of X. If the sum of squares due to regression is small relative to the residual (or error) sum of squares, then the null hypothesis cannot be rejected.

To perform the test:

1. Regress Y on X, determine the residuals ε_i, square these residuals, and scale them by dividing each squared residual by the mean of the squared residuals:

$$Scaled\ \varepsilon_i^2 = \frac{\varepsilon_i^2}{\sum \varepsilon_i^2 / N}.$$

This results in a mean squared residual of 1 that is necessary for evaluating the expression.

2. Then perform auxiliary regression (A) of these scaled squared residuals against X_i.

3. Take the resultant auxiliary regression sum of squares (model SS_A or SS_{reg_A}), divide it by 2, and then use that as an approximation to chi-square with 1 df.

4. The same result can be obtained by regressing the unscaled squared residuals against X_i, dividing by 2, and then scaling at the end by dividing by square of the mean squared residual:

$$\frac{SS_{reg_A}}{2\left(\overline{\varepsilon^2}\right)^2}.$$

An alternative expression is

$$\frac{SS_{reg_A}}{2\left(\frac{SS_{res_O}}{N}\right)^2},$$

where SS_{res_O} is the residual sum of squares of the original regression of Y on X. The two expressions in the parentheses are identities. Any of these three forms may appear in the literature.

As an example, consider the scattergram and residual plot shown in Figures 27.6 and 27.17.

The regression equation (numerical data not shown) is $\widehat{Y}_i = 0.31 + 2.40X_i$ with $r^2 = 0.4566$. The mean squared residual was 63,014.23, and the SS_{res} was 74,987.74, with $N = 85$.

Regressing the scaled squared residuals against X_i yields 61.21 for the regression sum of squares. This divided by 2 gives 30.6 as an estimate of chi-square with 1 df, for $P = 3.18e-8$, confirming our belief that variance was not independent of X.

With the unscaled squared residuals the expression in parentheses would be

$$\left(\frac{SS_{res_0}}{N}\right)^2 = \left(\frac{74,987.74}{85}\right)^2 = 778,292.2,$$

and this divided into the regression sum of squares for the unscaled squared residuals of 47,635,724 gives 61.205 as before. This is then divided by 2 to give the metric.

An alternate way to approximate the chi-square value is to use the LM method and multiply the value of r^2 by N.

In this data set, r^2 for regressing the squared residuals (scaled or unscaled) was 0.356746. This multiplied by 85 gives 30.32, close to the estimate for chi-square obtained above.

For this test to be interpreted, the relationship between Y and X must be linear.

The Comparison Problem (Advanced)

Because the limits of agreement shown above for the Bland–Altman plot are point estimates, Bland and Altman (1999, 2009) also advised setting confidence intervals about these limits. They used as an approximation for the standard error of the limits $\sqrt{\frac{3s^2}{N}}$, where s was the standard deviation of the differences, and N the total number of comparisons. Thus if, as in an example that they used, the mean difference of 231 comparisons was 0.2 mm with $s = 3$ mm and the 95% limits of agreement being −5.8 to +6.1 mm, then the standard error would be $\sqrt{\frac{3(3)^2}{231}} = 0.34$, and the 95% confidence interval is $\pm 1.96 \times 0.34 = 0.67$, so that the 95% confidence intervals for the limits will be: lower limit $= -5.8 \pm 0.67 = -5.13$ to -6.47 and for the upper limit $= 6.1 \pm 0.67 = 5.43$ to 6.77. Ludbrook (2010) has taken this further. Instead of the term 95% limits of agreement he prefers to use the concept of 95% tolerance limits with 95% confidence, an approach more in keeping with the well-known tolerance intervals. Ludbrook modified the plot of difference versus mean to show the mean difference (as in the usual Bland–Altman plot) and two pairs of limit lines: the inner pair is the upper and lower 95% confidence limits for the population, and the outer pair is the 95% tolerance limits with 95% confidence. For the inner limits he proposed using a slightly more accurate formula:

$$\overline{X_{diff}} \pm (t_{0.05N-1})s_{diff}\sqrt{1 + \frac{1}{N}}.$$

Therefore for the example used above, the 95% population confidence limits are

$$0.2 \pm 1.96 \times 3\sqrt{1 + \frac{1}{231}} = 0.2 \pm 5.89 = 6.09 \text{ to } -5.69.$$

These are slightly different from those calculated from the simpler formula. For the tolerance limits Ludbrook used mean difference $\pm k s_{diff}$, where k is taken from the tolerance tables referred to in Chapter 7. For $N = 231$, k is ~ 2.131, and the tolerance limits are $0.2 \pm 2.131 \times 3 = 6.56$ to -6.16. If the differences increase in proportion to the size of the measurement, then instead of taking logarithms, Ludbrook recommends carrying out Model I regression of differences versus mean values, and then calculating the hyperbolic 95% limits for points; these are essentially the tolerance limits.

Finally, it is common for the differences to be proportional to the size of the measurement and to be heteroscedastic, that is, for their variability to increase as the measurements increase in size. This can be dealt with by transforming the data: taking logarithms and plotting differences against averages; plotting ratios against averages; or plotting the percent difference against the average (Bland and Altman, 2003; Montgomery and Peck, 1982). Alternatively, a V-shaped confidence interval can be constructed. To do this, Model 1 regression is performed for differences (Y) against averages (X), the residuals are calculated for each value of X, and then the signs are removed to obtain absolute residual values. These absolute residuals are regressed against the averages to obtain the standard regression equation

Absolute residual $= c + b$ (average).

The c and b coefficients are then multiplied by $\sqrt{\frac{\pi}{2}} = 1.2533$ to give the equation

Standard deviation (SD) of difference $= 1.2533c + 1.2553b$ (average). (For derivation, see Bland (2009).)

Then the 95% limits at any average value are predicted difference ± 1.96SD. To be more accurate in allowing for sample size, use $t_{0.05, N-1}$ instead of 1.96.

As an example, a partial list of data adapted from a study of venous versus capillary blood cholesterol (Greenland et al., 1990) is given in Table 27.8. It is set out as recommended by Bland (2009).

These data lead to the regression equation:

Difference $= -0.3759 + 0.0214$*average. From this calculate the predicted difference at each average pressure, and the residuals and absolute residuals, that is, the residuals without minus signs. Then regress the absolute residuals against the average to get

Absolute residual $= 0.3769 + 0.0112$*average, and when the coefficients are multiplied by 1.2533 the equation becomes

SD difference $= 0.4724 + 0.014$*average

Table 27.8 Cholesterol data

Difference	Average	Predicted difference	Residuals	Absolute residuals
4.4	136	3.6364285714	0.7635714286	0.7635714286
4.7	145	3.6364285714	1.0635714286	1.0635714286
3.2	151	3.6364285714	−0.436428571	0.4364285714
4.3	159	3.6364285714	0.6635714286	0.6635714286
3.3	176	3.6364285714	−0.336428571	0.3364285714
0.5	187	3.6364285714	−3.136428571	3.1364285714
5.3	183	3.6364285714	1.6635714286	1.6635714286
5.2	187	3.6364285714	1.5635714286	1.5635714286
6.1	190	3.6364285714	2.4635714286	2.4635714286
4.9	200	3.6364285714	1.2635714286	1.2635714286
3.28	204	3.6364285714	−0.356428571	0.3564285714
2.8	208	3.6364285714	−0.836428571	0.8364285714
2.8	212	3.6364285714	−0.836428571	0.8364285714

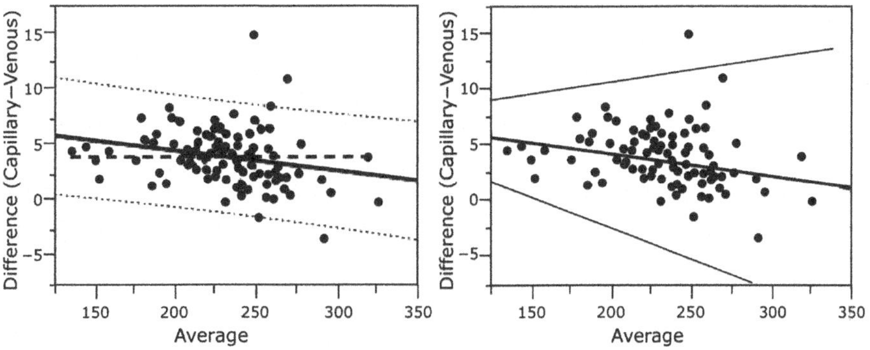

Figure 27.31 Bland—Altman diagram showing 95% confidence limits with progressive increase in differences and heteroscedasticity. Left panel: Conventional diagram with mean (dashed line), line of best fit, and 95% confidence limits. Right panel: Allowance for heteroscedasticity, with better fit to data.

Then the limits are $\pm 1.96 \times$ SD difference on either side of the predicted value. The scatterplot with 95% confidence limits is shown in Figure 27.31 the limits are drawn by calculating the SD difference at two average values, and joining them by a straight line.

The Bland—Altman comparison method starts with the assumption that the two methods are giving approximately the same results for each measured datum. However, it is possible that one method might measure proportionately more or less than the other; for example, the new method might measure twice as much as the standard method. If that occurred, the slope of much greater or less than one would cast doubt on the new method, although possibly the regression could be used as a calibration curve. If a Bland—Altman diagram was made under these circumstances (Figure 27.32), the departure of the

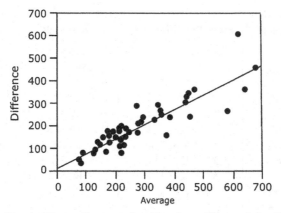

Figure 27.32 Bland–Altman diagram when the slope differs substantially from 45°.

slope from the line of identity will be obvious. This could also be shown simply by a slope significantly more than 45°.

Comparing Two or More Lines

If two sets of linearly related X and Y variables are drawn at random from a population, the two sets will probably have different regression lines of best fit, both in terms of slope and elevation. Did these two lines come from the same population? The method used is termed analysis of covariance or ANCOVA, and it is a two-step process. In the first step, the procedure determines if the slopes are significantly different. If they are different, it may not make sense to continue (Figure 27.33).

If the slopes really are different, then pooling them makes little sense and predicting Y from X will be incorrect everywhere except where the two lines cross. Below the

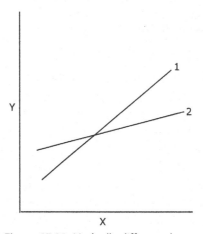

Figure 27.33 Markedly different slopes.

crossing point Y values of group 1 for any X value are lower than those of group 2, but above the crossing point the Y values of group 1 are higher than those of group 2.

To determine if the two slopes are significantly different, the calculations pool the data in a specific way to obtain a mean slope that is the weighted average of the two slopes (Figure 27.34). The test requires normality, independent errors, and homogeneity of variance.

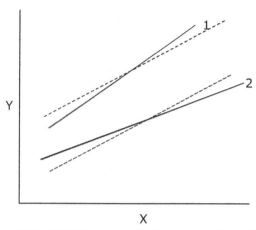

Figure 27.34 ANCOVA stage 1. Pooled slope in dashed lines.

The average slope b_{pooled} is calculated by weighting sums of squares of X by the respective slopes (Maxwell and Delaney, 1990)

$$b_{pooled} = \frac{\sum\left(X_{i1} - \overline{X_1}\right)^2 b_1 + \sum\left(X_{i2} - \overline{X_2}\right)^2 b_2}{\sum\left(X_{i1} - \overline{X_1}\right)^2 + \sum\left(X_{i2} - \overline{X_2}\right)^2}.$$

This can be done simply by pooling the derived data from each group. I prefer to perform these calculations by a program to avoid arithmetic errors, but Table 27.9 shows the steps.

The third line adds the first two lines together, and provides the weighted pooled value for the common slope.

The total sum of squares due to linear regression is

$$\sum\left(\widehat{Y}_i - \overline{Y}\right)^2 = \frac{\sum\left(X_i Y_i - \frac{\sum X_i \sum Y_i}{N}\right)^2}{\sum\left(X_i - \overline{X}\right)^2}.$$

This can be calculated easily from the expression

$$r^2 = \frac{SS_{reg}}{SS_{total}} = \frac{SS_{reg}}{\sum\left(Y_i - \overline{Y}\right)^2}.$$

Table 27.9 The first two lines show the individual group data

Group	N	N − 1	SSx	SSy	SxSy	b	r²	N − 2	SS_reg/Df	SSw/Df	MS_reg	MS_res	F	P
Artery	7	6	2489.71	31.43	−253.95	−0.102	0.8236	5	25.8838/1	5.544/5	25.8831	1.109	23.34	0.0048
Vein	6	5	1566.33	409.33	−725.68	−0.4633	0.8216	4	336.288/1	73.046/4	336.288	18.2	18.42	0.0127
Pooled	13	10	4056.84	440.76	−979.63	−0.2415	0.5367	9	236.556/1	294.204/9				
Total			4135.05	4409.23	1539.55	−0.3723	0.1300		573.221/1	3836.01/11	573.221	348.728	1.644	0.2262

If this is subtracted from SSy (the total sum of squares), the residual, or error term (or SSw), can be derived, and the ANOVA can be calculated.

The effect of this procedure is that the average slope is calculated and substituted for each actual slope, as shown by the dashed lines. Then an ANOVA is done for each line separately. Recall that the line of best fit is by the least squares principle, so that the sum of the squared deviations $\sum(Y_i - \widehat{Y}_i)$ will be less from the observed line than from the recalculated average slope. Is this difference big enough to reject the null hypothesis that $b_1 = b_2$? The difference is compared to the within-group means square to obtain an F ratio (see Table 27.10C).

If the two slopes are not significantly different, then the next step is done. This compares the elevations of the two regression lines. To do this, the original data are pooled, the derived sums of squares are calculated, and the usual regression components are calculated. Once again, an ANOVA is done. If the two regression lines do not have very different elevations that is, the means of Y for each group are not very different, then the total sum of squares will be similar to the sums of squares derived by adding up the groups separately. If the two lines are separated by a long way, then the discrepancy will be marked and can be tested by the F ratio. Online calculations may be done easily at http://vassarstats.net/vsancova.html.

To give a specific example, consider the relationship between blood pressure and the diameter of retina arteries and veins (Leung et al., 2003). The results for each group are shown in Figure 27.35.

The ANOVA for the vein and the artery are shown in Tables 27.10A and 27.10B.

The slopes of these two data sets are different, but are they consistent with random drawing from a population?

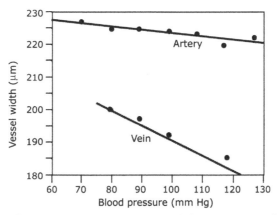

Figure 27.35 Relation of blood pressure to retinal vessel diameter. A significant linear relation is shown for each. The linear equations are: Retinal artery diameter = 233.76 − 0.1020 blood pressure; R square adj = 0.7883; Retinal vein diameter 236.63 − 0.4634 blood pressure; R square adj = 0.7769.

Table 27.10A Vein

Source	Df	Sum of squares	Mean square	F	P
Total	5	409.3333			
Linear regression	1	336.2879	336.2879	18.4153	0.0127
Residual	4	73.0454	18.261		

Table 27.10B Artery

Source	Df	Sum of squares	Mean square	F	P
Total	6	31.4286			
Linear regression	1	25.8839	25.8839	23.3411	0.0048
Residual	5	5.5447	1.1089		

Table 27.10C ANCOVA for slopes

Source	Df	Sum of squares	Mean square	F	P
Total	12	440.76			
Linear regression	1	236.56	236.56	12.74	0.0044
Residual	11	204.20	18.56		

Table 27.10C gives superimposed data from both states.

In this example, the slopes are significantly different, and we would normally stop. For purposes of illustration, however, we will calculate a common slope and test the positions of the two regression lines. In fact, even if the slopes are different, comparing positions of the lines over a restricted range is legitimate.

The second stage is then done with identical slopes, and gives the results shown in Figure 27.36.

The final ANOVA is in Table 27.11.

As is obvious from the combined graph (Figure 27.37) one line is much higher than the other line. Although the lines appear to be far apart, zero is suppressed in the graph and the difference is exaggerated.

A common error is to compare the means of two groups, for example, to determine if cholesterol is higher in one of the groups. Because cholesterol has a relationship to age, the means are of value only if the age distribution is identical in the two groups. If not, the ANCOVA is the best way to make the comparison (Vickers, 2001; Vickers and Altman, 2001).

The same method can be applied to comparing several different slopes, but unless there are specific hypotheses there are the same multiple comparison problems as occur with ANOVA without previous planning.

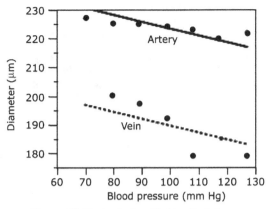

Figure 27.36 Analysis with identical slopes.

Table 27.11 Final ANCOVA for position, R square adj 0.0509

Source	Df	Sum of squares	Mean square	F	P
Total	12	4409.2308			
Linear regression	1	573.2206	573.221	1.64	0.262
Residual	11	3836.0102	348.728		

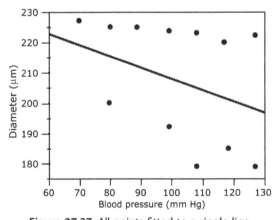

Figure 27.37 All points fitted to a single line.

Outliers

In univariate distributions if a measurement apparently far removed from the remaining measurements is not due to an error, it will produce inefficient estimates of the mean and standard deviation, and thus make it more difficult to show differences between two

Figure 27.38 Outliers. The upper panel shows a data set with little relationship between X and Y. The lower panel shows the same data points with four outliers (open circles) added. The slope of Y on X is now significantly different from 0, due entirely to the influence of a small number of measurements. *(Based on Figure 2.1 in Chatterjee and Price (1977).)*

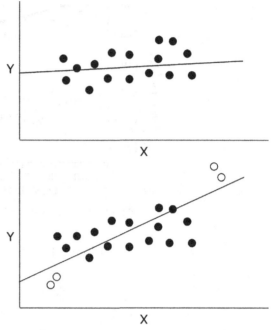

groups. The same problem occurs in bivariate distributions, and is important because un-usual values can greatly alter the calculated regression line and the correlation coefficient (Figure 27.38).

The problem is more complicated for bivariate than for univariate distributions because the point with unusual influence on the calculations is not always the point that appears to be the most different from the rest.

Comparable to the univariate distribution, an outlier in regression can affect the mean and the standard deviation. The mean in a regression equation, however, has two com-ponents: the slope and the mean of the fitted value for Y (or the intercept). Any outlier may have a predominant effect on the slope, the mean of fitted Y, or the standard deviation from regression, or all three.

Leverage
Think back to the description of determining the confidence limits for a slope (Figure 27.20). The reason why the slope is encased by concave lines was as the X value moves farther and farther from the mean of X, the squared deviation gets larger and larger. Therefore points far from the mean have more effect than points near the mean, just as a weight placed on a beam on a fulcrum has more effect when far from the fulcrum than when close to it.

Consider Figure 27.39.

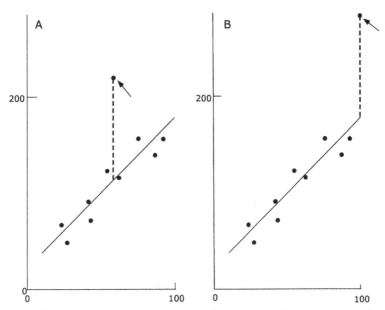

Figure 27.39 Two XY plots identical except for the outliers (marked with an arrow) that have the same deviations from the regression line (dashed line).

The regression results are shown in Table 27.12.

Table 27.12 Regression constants for groups A and B compared with results when the aberrant point is omitted. The aberrant point in B has a much greater effect on the slope and intercept. Both aberrant points increase the residual mean square that is not a method for distinguishing them.

Group	Intercept	Slope	MS residual
A	31.8	1.545	1569.5
B	−7.0	2.181	1178.4
No outlier	21.8	1.525	231.7

The discussion to follow is based on the superb description given by Glantz and Slinker (2001). The effect of the position of an outlier on the regression line is known as leverage. In simple linear regression the leverage is

$$h_{ij} = \frac{1}{N} + \frac{\left(X_i - \overline{X}\right)^2}{\sum \left(X_j - \overline{X}\right)^2},$$

and that is the way in which the standard deviation of $\widehat{Y}$ is calculated for each value of X (see above).

Ideally, all the points should have similar influence on the regression line, with an average value of $(k + 1)/N$, where k represents the number of independent variables (only 1 for a simple linear regression) and N is the sample size. Therefore, the average leverage in the above example is

$$(1 + 1)/9 = 0.22.$$

If any point has a leverage value more than twice the expected value, it should be subjected to further investigation.

There is a more accurate way of assessing leverage, and that is to make use of Studentized residuals. A Studentized residual is defined as

$$r_1 = \frac{e_i}{S_{Y \cdot X} \sqrt{(1 - h_{ii})}}.$$

These are standardized residuals that allow for the effects of the leverage factor h_{ii}. This expression is called the internally Studentized residual because it includes all the data points. There is also an externally Studentized residual in which each point in turn is omitted from the calculation of the residual, a technique known as the jackknife (Chapter 34):

$$r_{-1} = \frac{e_i}{S_{Y \cdot X - 1} \sqrt{(1 - h_{ii})}}.$$

These externally Studentized residuals should have an approximately normal distribution with most of the values within 2 standard deviations of the mean of zero, and these relationships can be shown in box plots or stem-and-leaf diagrams. They can also be tested in a normality plot constructed by plotting the ordered residuals against the cumulative frequencies derived from the equation

$$\frac{i - 3/8}{N + 1/4},$$

where i is the rank of the residual and N is the number of residuals (Chapter 6).

Leverage refers not specifically to unusual deviations from the regression line, but rather concentrates on the disproportionate effect of those deviations if they are far from the mean of X.

Influence

It is possible for a point to have little leverage, but because it is so far removed from the other data points it has a marked effect on the regression line. To deal with this problem there is a statistic called Cook's distance that incorporates all aspects of an excessive deviation. Each data point is removed in turn from the data set, the new regression line is computed, and the intercept is plotted on the X-axis against the slope on the Y-axis. If all the points are reasonably distributed around the line, the relationship of intercept to slope will be similar for each revised data set, and all the points will be near each other.

If removal of one particular point, however, produces a marked difference in location of the intercept–slope plot, then it is likely to warrant examination as an outlier. To judge the significance of such an outlying point, Cook's distance D is calculated as

$$D_i = \frac{r_i^2}{k+1} \times \frac{h_{ii}}{1 - h_{ii}}.$$

D is a function of the internally Studentized residual (a function of the deviation of the point from the line) and the leverage effect. Cook's D has a distribution similar to the F distribution, specifically $F_{k+1,N-k-1}$. In general, a value of $D > 1$ suggests that the point(s) be considered carefully, and a value >4 suggests a potentially serious outlier.

As a specific example, look at Figure 27.40, redrawn from Butter et al. (2001).

There is one outlying value beyond the 95% limits for individual values. The expected value for leverage is $2/24 = 0.083$. There are two points that exceed $0.083 \times 2 = 0.166$. Neither of these is the apparent outlier; they come from the two with the largest values

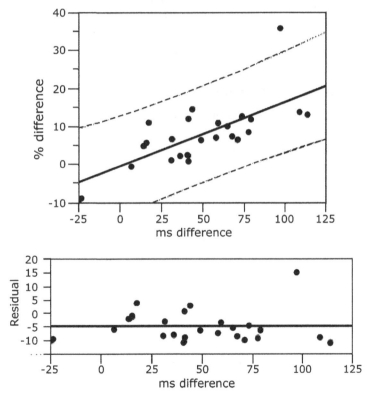

Figure 27.40 Upper panel: Plot of intrinsic conduction delay difference between free wall and anterior wall (ms) versus % dP/dt difference (% difference) with biventricular pacing. The line of best fit and 95% confidence limits for points are shown. Lower panel: Residual plot.

Table 27.13 Three sets of regression results

Group	Intercept	Slope
All values	−0.4765	0.1688
Remove Y 35.7	0.7011	0.1271
Remove X 109, 114	−1.8074	0.2083

of X, even though they do not look very far from the regression line. However, they are pulling the line downward. Cook's D shows that only the distance for the apparently high point warrants examination, with a value of 0.90, the other two having values of 0.15 and 0.06.

If the regression analysis is repeated by removing the apparent high point with a big Cook's distance (97, 35.7) and then again with the full set but removing the two points with high leverage (109.1, 13.7 and 11.2, 13), the changes are shown in Table 27.13.

There are substantial differences depending on which points are omitted. Inasmuch as none of the tests for undue influence showed marked changes, there is no reason to do anything with these data other than to make sure that they are reliable. No matter what statistical tests may show, there is no substitute for common sense. Furthermore, removing data points can, as shown, make big differences to the regression constants, and should never be done without very good cause.

Ratio Measurements and Scaling Factors

Many anatomic or physiologic variables change with age or body size, for example, resting or maximal oxygen consumption or cardiac output, glomerular filtration rate, left ventricular mass, local blood flows, etc. Two approaches are often used to determine if any subject's measurement of one of these variables is abnormal. One is to make a series of normal measurements that cover a range of ages or body sizes. The other is to normalize measurements by taking a ratio to body weight, surface area, or some other base, in order to obtain a single number to use in assessing normality.

If the regression relating the measurement Y to the value of the base X is linear and passes through zero, then we can use simplified arithmetic by using the ratio Y/X as a constant factor (Figure 27.41).

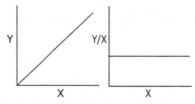

Figure 27.41 If Y and X are linearly related and the regression line passes through zero, then we can use the common ratio of Y/X that is independent of variations in X to determine if a variable Y is normal.

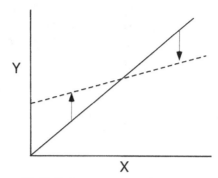

Figure 27.42 Ratio versus nonratio measurements.

Tanner, whose growth charts are well known, analyzed this issue with special reference to calculations of cardiac output (Tanner, 1949a,b). He pointed out that if the regression line between cardiac output and a measure of body size did not go through zero, then errors of judgment would result (Figure 27.42).

The solid line passing through zero implies a constant ratio between Y and X; doubling X will double Y. If, on the other hand, the true (linear) relationship is shown by the dashed line, then at low values of X the constant ratio method underestimates the value of Y (upward arrow), and at high values of X the ratio method overestimates Y (downward arrow). If the two slopes are close the error may be unimportant, and the same conclusion can be made if the working range of X is small on either side of the point at which the two lines cross; the error increases when remote from the crossing point. The ratio method may underestimate cardiac output in infants and overestimate it in very large subjects, although these incorrect estimates probably have little clinical importance except in critical decisions based on pulmonary vascular resistance in infants. In general, incorrect use of a ratio leads to excessive standard deviations from regression and more difficulty comparing groups.

Many studies of oxygen consumption, cardiac output, and glomerular filtration rate, for example, have shown that a simple linear ratio is not accurate. For example, Armstrong and Welsman (1994) studied peak oxygen consumption versus age in boys and girls from 7 to 16 years old. Figure 27.43 (left panel) shows the relationship between peak oxygen consumption on treadmill exercise versus age, and Figure 27.43 (right panel) shows that correcting for body weight does not provide a constant range independent of age. Dallaire et al. (2015) showed recently that predicting z scores for pediatric echocardiography from BMI and age was unsatisfactory, and that polynomial models of the type $y = \sqrt{bx} + c$ or $y = ax^2 + bx + \sqrt{cx} + d$ gave the best predictive values.

Many studies of scaling factors have been done, and most of them have found that linear scaling is almost never satisfactory. On the contrary, allometric scaling (using mass or height or body surface area raised to some fractional power) has provided greater

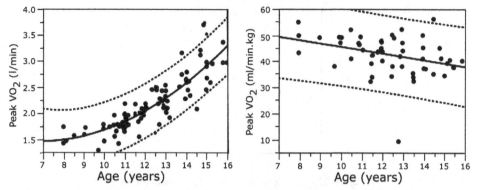

Figure 27.43 Left panel: Relationship of peak oxygen consumption to age. Right panel: Relationship of peak oxygen consumption per unit mass to age. *(Data taken from figures in publication, but only for boys. Data for girls were similar but less markedly curved.)*

constancy for predicting normal values (Chantler et al., 2005; Delanaye et al., 2009; Dewey et al., 2008; Neilan et al., 2009). The base used (weight, height, etc.) varies with the function being studied.

APPENDIX

Derivation of formula for the line of best fit:

The line of best fit is the line that minimizes the sums of squares of deviations of Y_i from the line. That is, minimizes

$$\sum \varepsilon_i = \sum \left(Y_i - \widehat{Y_i}\right)^2 = \sum [Y_i - (c + bX_i)]^2$$
$$= \sum Y_i^2 - 2 \sum Y_i(c + bX_i) + \sum (c + bX_i)^2$$
$$= \sum Y_i^2 - 2c \sum Y_i - 2b \sum X_i Y_i + \sum c^2 + 2bc \sum X_i + b^2 \sum X_i^2$$

Set up partial differentials:

$$\frac{\delta \varepsilon}{\delta c} = -2 \sum Y_i + 2 \sum c + 2 \sum bX_i$$

$$\frac{\delta \varepsilon}{\delta b} = -2 \sum X_i Y_i + 2 \sum cX_i + 2 \sum bX_i^2.$$

For a minimum,

$$-\sum Y_i + \sum c + \sum bX_i = 0$$
$$-\sum X_i Y_i + \sum cX_i + \sum bX_i^2 = 0.$$

Dividing the first expression by N gives

$$c = \overline{Y} - b\overline{X}.$$

Substituting this in the second expression gives

$$\sum X_i Y_i = \left(\overline{Y} - b\overline{X}\right) \sum X_i + b \sum X_i^2,$$

so that

$$\sum X_i Y_i = \left(\frac{\sum Y_i}{N} - b\frac{\sum X_i}{N}\right) \sum X_i + b \sum X_i^2$$

$$= \frac{\sum X_i Y_i}{N} - b\frac{\left(\sum X_i\right)^2}{N} + b \sum X_i^2$$

$$= \frac{\sum X_i Y_i}{N} + b\left(\sum X_i^2 - \frac{\left(\sum X_i\right)^2}{N}\right)$$

$$\therefore b = \frac{\sum X_i Y_i - \dfrac{\sum X_i Y_i}{N}}{\left(\sum X_i^2 - \dfrac{\left(\sum X_i\right)^2}{N}\right)} = \frac{\sum \left(X_i - \overline{X}\right)\left(Y_i - \overline{Y}\right)}{\sum \left(X_i - \overline{X}\right)^2}.$$

REFERENCES

Anscombe, F.J., 1973. Graphs in statistical analysis. Am. Stat. 27, 17–21.

Armstrong, N., Welsman, J.R., 1994. Assessment and interpretation of aerobic fitness in children and adolescents. Exerc. Sport Sci. Rev. 22, 435–476.

Bland, J.M., 2009. How Do I Estimate Limits of Agreement When the Mean and SD of Differences Is Not Constant? (Online). Available: http://www-users.york.ac.uk/~mb55/meas/glucose.htm.

Bland, J.M., Altman, D.G., 1986. Statistical methods for assessing agreement between two methods of clinical measurement. Lancet 8, 307–310.

Bland, J.M., Altman, D.G., 1999. Measuring agreement in method comparison studies. Stat. Methods Med. Res. 8, 135–160.

Bland, J.M., Altman, D.G., 2003. Applying the right statistics: analyses of measurement studies. Ultrasound Obstet. Gynecol. 22, 85–93.

Box, G.E.P., Hunter, W.G., Hunter, J.S., 1978. Statistics for Experimenters. An Introduction to Design, Data Analysis, and Model Building. John Wiley & Sons.

Bryant, R.C., 1980. Masked variability in regression analysis. Pediatr. Res. 14, 352.

Buckberg, G.D., Luck, J.C., Payne, D.B., et al., 1971. Some sources of error in measuring regional blood flow with radioactive microspheres. J. Appl. Physiol. 31, 598–604.

Butter, C., Auricchio, A., Stellbrink, C., et al., 2001. Effect of resynchronization therapy stimulation site on the systolic function of heart failure patients. Circulation 104, 3026–3029.

Chantler, P.D., Clements, R.E., Sharp, L., et al., 2005. The influence of body size on measurements of overall cardiac function. Am. J. Physiol. Heart Circ. Physiol. 289, H2059–H2065.

Chatterjee, S., Price, B., 1977. Regression Analysis by Example. John Wiley & Sons.

Dallaire, F., Bigras, J.L., Prsa, M., Dahdah, N., 2015. Bias related to body mass index in pediatric echocardiographic Z scores. Pediatr. Cardiol. 36, 667–676.

Dallaire, F., Bigras, J.L., Prsa, M., Dahdah, N., 2015. Erratum to: bias related to body mass index in pediatric echocardiographic Z scores. Pediatr. Cardiol. 36, 1316. http://dx.doi.org/10.1007/s00246-015-1212-7.

Delanaye, P., Mariat, C., Cavalier, E., et al., 2009. Errors induced by indexing glomerular filtration rate for body surface area: reductio ad absurdum. Nephrol. Dial. Transplant. 24, 3593–3596.

Dewey, F.E., Rosenthal, D., Murphy Jr., D.J., et al., 2008. Does size matter? Clinical applications of scaling cardiac size and function for body size. Circulation 117, 2279–2287.

Galton, F.I., 1886. Regression towards mediocrity in hereditary stature. J. Anthropol. Inst. 15, 246–263.

Glantz, S.A., Slinker, B.K., 2001. Primer of Applied Regression and Analysis of Variance. McGraw-Hill, Inc.

Greenland, P., Bowley, N.L., Meiklejohn, B., et al., 1990. Blood cholesterol concentration: fingerstick plasma vs venous serum sampling. Clin. Chem. 36, 628–630.

Harker, L.A., Slichter, S.J., 1972. The bleeding time as a screening test for evaluation of platelet function. N. Engl. J. Med. 287, 155–159.

Jamal, F., Strotmann, J., Weidemann, F., et al., 2001. Noninvasive quantification of the contractile reserve of stunned myocardium by ultrasonic strain rate and strain. Circulation 104, 1059–1065.

Leung, H., Wang, J.J., Rochtchina, E., et al., 2003. Relationships between age, blood pressure, and retinal vessel diameters in an older population. Invest. Ophthalmol. Vis. Sci. 44, 2900–2904.

Lolis, D., Konstantinidis, K., Papevangelou, G., et al., 1977. Comparative study of amniotic fluid and maternal blood serum human placental lactogen in normal and prolonged pregnancies. Am. J. Obstet. Gynecol. 128, 724–726.

Ludbrook, J., 1997. Comparing methods of measurement. Clin. Exp. Pharmacol. Physiol. 24, 193–203.

Ludbrook, J., 2010. Confidence in Altman–Bland plots: a critical review of the method of differences. Clin. Exp. Pharmacol. Physiol. 37, 143–149.

Mackler, B., Person, R., Miller, L.R., et al., 1979. Iron deficiency in the rat: effects on phenylalanine metabolism. Pediatr. Res. 13, 1010–1011.

Maxwell, S.E., Delaney, H.D., 1990. Designing Experiments and Analyzing Data. A Model Comparison Perspective. Wadsworth Publishing Company.

Montgomery, D.C., Peck, E.A., 1982. Introduction to Linear Regression Analysis. John Wiley and Sons.

Mosteller, F., Tukey, J.W., 1977. Data Analysis and Regression. A Second Course in Statistics. Addison-Wesley.

Nagy, A.I., Venkateshvaran, A., Dash, P.K., et al., 2014. The pulmonary capillary wedge pressure accurately reflects both normal and elevated left atrial pressure. Am. Heart J. 167, 876–883.

Nakauchi, H., Okumura, K., Tango, T., 1981. Immunoglobulin levels in patients on long-term hemodialysis. N. Engl. J. Med. 305, 172–173.

Neilan, T.G., Pradhan, A.D., King, M.E., et al., 2009. Derivation of a size-independent variable for scaling of cardiac dimensions in a normal paediatric population. Eur. J. Echocardiogr. 10, 50–55.

Olivié, M.A.A., Garcia-Mayor, R.V., Leston, D.G., et al., 1995. Serum insulin-like growth factor (IGF) binding protein-3 and IGF-I levels during childhood and adolescence. A cross-sectional study. Pediatr. Res. 38, 149–155.

Richardson, D., Catron, D.V., Underkofler, L.A., et al., 1951. Vitamin B12 requirement of male weanling pigs. J. Nutr. 44, 371–381.

Senzaki, H., Isoda, T., Paolocci, N., et al., 2000. Improved mechanoenergetics and cardiac rest and reserve function of in vivo failing heart by calcium sensitizer EMD-57033. Circulation 101, 1040–1048.

Tanner, J.M., 1949a. Fallacy of per-weight and per-surface area standards, and their relation to spurious correlation. J. Appl. Physiol. 2, 1–15.

Tanner, J.M., 1949b. The construction of normal standards for cardiac output in man. J. Clin. Invest. 28, 567–582.

Vickers, A.J., 2001. The use of percentage change from baseline as an outcome in a controlled trial is statistically inefficient: a simulation study. BMC Med. Res. Methodol. 1, 6.

Vickers, A.J., Altman, D.G., 2001. Statistics notes: Analysing controlled trials with baseline and follow up measurements. BMJ (Clin. Res. Ed.) 323, 1123–1124.

CHAPTER 28

Variations Based on Linear Regression*

Contents

TRANSFORMING THE Y VARIATE

We may need transformations to stabilize the variance of the Y variate (Natrella, 1963; Schwartz et al., 1988). These transformations have the added advantage that they often restore normality to the distribution of the Y variate. Common transformations are given below:

1. If the Y data are counts and seem to be from a Poisson distribution, $\sqrt{Y}$ or $\sqrt{Y} + \sqrt{Y+1}$ usually works, and has a variance of 0.25.
2. If the data fit a binomial distribution, then $\sin^{-1} \sqrt{Y}$ is effective. Y can be measured in degrees or radians, and if the latter has a constant variance of $0.25/N$.
3. For a continuous distribution, the one most often encountered, because of the likelihood that the coefficient of variation (standard deviation/mean) is constant, then the variance of the residuals is

Var $e_1 = k^2 X_i^2$, where k is the constant of proportionality.

Therefore, divide both sides of the regression equation $(Y_i = c + bX_i + \varepsilon_i)$ by X_i to get

$$\frac{Y_i}{X_i} = \frac{c}{X_i} + b + \frac{\varepsilon_i}{X_i}.$$

---

*For a list of all websites referred to in this chapter, as clickable links, see the book companion website: www.booksite.elsevier.com/9780128023877.

Biostatistics for Medical and Biomedical Practitioners
http://dx.doi.org/10.1016/B978-0-12-802387-7.00028-7

Define the new transformed variables as

$Y_i' = \frac{Y_i}{X_i}$, $X_i' = \frac{1}{X_i}$, $\varepsilon_i' = \frac{\varepsilon_i}{X_i}$ and $c' = \frac{c}{X_i}$ so that the new regression equation in transformed variables is

$$Y_i' = c' + bX_i' + \varepsilon_i'.$$

This new equation will have a constant variance, to be verified by examining residuals (see below).

INVERSE PREDICTION

Regression logic places the independent X value on the horizontal axis and the dependent Y value on the vertical axis, and the least squares principle considers only the vertical deviations of each Y from the regression line. The standard deviation from regression is used to predict the variation of Y at any X value. There are times, however, when we need to do the inverse. In 1975, Hirschfeld et al. (1975) studied the prediction of pulmonary vascular resistance (PVR) from echocardiographically obtained time intervals. Their data are summarized in Figure 28.1, based on a letter to the editor by Silverman and Hoffman (1976).

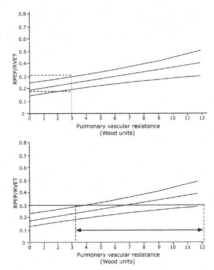

Figure 28.1 Illustration of inverse prediction. RPEP, right ventricular pre-ejection period; RVET, right ventricular ejection time.

The upper panel of Figure 28.1 shows the results obtained when plotting PVR obtained at cardiac catheterization against a simultaneously obtained ratio of right ventricular pre-ejection period (RPEP) to ejection time (RVET). The line of best fit and the 95% confidence limits for individual data are shown, but the individual points are not. To predict the ratio of RPEP to RVET from PVR, draw a vertical line from any value of PVR and predict correctly the range in which 95% of these time ratios would fall by examining the projection of the dashed horizontal lines on the Y-axis. (We could calculate these limits from the basic equations.) That, however, is not what we want. Instead, we want to predict the PVR from the noninvasive echocardiographic method. To do this from the same regression figure shown in the bottom panel, the logic requires drawing a horizontal line from a given ratio, and determining the range within which 95% of the PVR measurements would fall from the projection of the dashed vertical lines on the X-axis. As seen from the figure, this range is so wide as to be of little clinical use. Furthermore, although we could determine the range by eye, the way in which regression calculations are carried out does not permit us to determine the horizontal deviations of the Y values from the regression line. Instead, a special inverse prediction calculation is needed (Zar, 2010). The confidence limits of X for a given value of Y may be determined by:

$$\overline{X} + \frac{b(Y_i - \overline{Y})}{K} \pm \frac{1}{K} \sqrt{\left(S_{Y \cdot X}^2 \left[\frac{(Y_i - \overline{Y})^2}{\sum (X_i - \overline{X})^2} + K\left(1 + \frac{1}{N}\right) \right] \right)}$$

where $K = b^2 - t^2 s_b^2$.

In the lower panel of Figure 28.1, even with correct calculations, the limits of X for a given value of Y are very wide. This per se is not a difficulty due to inverse prediction, but to the lack of precision in the data. Gaddum (1933), working in the field of bioassays, developed an index of precision termed $\lambda = s/b$. To see its effect, consider Figure 28.2.

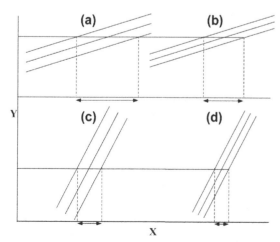

Figure 28.2 Illustration of Gaddum's lambda index. In (a), the slope is not steep and the confidence limits (drawn for simplicity as parallel lines) are quite wide. The confidence limits of X for the given value of Y (shown by the paired vertical dashed lines) are wide, as shown by the double-headed arrow. These confidence limits for X are narrower if the confidence limits are narrower (b), or the slope is steeper (c), and are smallest for the steepest slope and narrowest confidence limits (d).

LINE OF BEST FIT PASSES THROUGH ZERO

It is common in biology and medicine to minimize variation by normalizing a measurement to per kilogram body weight, per square meters body surface area, per unit of blood, and so on. Thus, if we measure in children of different ages absolute cardiac outputs per liter per minute of 1, 3, and 10, and then base these outputs on a body surface area of $1m^2$, the outputs might be 2.9, 3.2, and 4.7 $l.min^{-1}.m^{-2}$, respectively, and are less variable than the original data. Similarly, it may be possible to use a simple surrogate measurement instead of a complicated one provided one can be converted to the other. For example, it is relatively difficult to measure left ventricular volume, but it might be possible to find a power function of a simple linear measurement. For all these normalizing or calibration procedures, we need to know if the relationship is linear and passes through zero, if it is linear but does not pass through zero, or if it is curvilinear. These choices are represented in Figure 28.3.

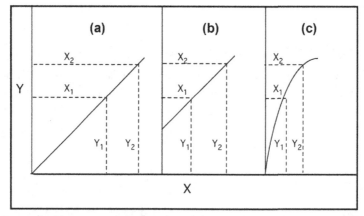

Figure 28.3 Types of calibration or normalizing curves. (a) Straight line through origin. (b) Straight line not through origin. (c) Curved line through origin.

In panel (a), the ratio of Y_i to X_i is constant at any value of X and Y. The constant ratio can be used as a multiplier or divisor, for example, cardiac output is about 3.5 $l.min^{-1}.m^{-2}$ body surface area. For the other panels there is no constant ratio, and the line or curve must be used to determine the X value for any Y value.

For a straight line through the origin, there are three possible scenarios; the variance from regression of Y, $s^2_{Y.X}$, is constant, is proportional to X, or is proportional to X^2. These lead to simplified calculations (Table 28.1).

Table 28.1 Summary of revised formulas

	b	c	SS_{reg}	$s^2_{Y \cdot X}$	s^2_b
Model 1	$\dfrac{\sum(X_i-\overline{X})(Y_i-\overline{Y})}{\sum(X_i-\overline{X})^2}$	$\overline{Y}-b\overline{X}$	$\sum(Y_i-\overline{Y})^2 - \dfrac{[\sum(X_i-\overline{X})(Y_i-\overline{Y})]^2}{\sum(X_i-\overline{X})^2}$	$\dfrac{SS_{reg}}{N-2}$	$\dfrac{s^2_{Y \cdot X}}{\sum(X_i-\overline{X})^2}$
Model 2 $s^2_{Y \cdot X}=k$	$\dfrac{\sum X_i Y_i}{\sum X_i^2}$	0	$\sum(Y_i)^2 - \dfrac{(\sum XY)^2}{\sum X^2}$	$\dfrac{SS_{reg}}{N-1}$	$\dfrac{s^2_{Y \cdot X}}{\sum(X_i)^2}$
Model 2 $s^2_{Y \cdot X} \propto X$	$\dfrac{\sum Y}{\sum X}=\dfrac{\overline{Y}}{\overline{X}}$	0	$\sum\left(\dfrac{Y^2}{X_i}\right) - \dfrac{(\sum Y_i)^2}{\sum X}$	$\dfrac{SS_{reg}}{N-1}$	$\dfrac{s^2_{Y \cdot X}}{\sum(X_i)^2}$
Model 2 $s^2_{Y \cdot X} \propto X^2$	$\dfrac{\sum\left(\frac{Y}{X}\right)}{N}=\dfrac{\sum R}{N}$	0	$\sum(R_i-\overline{R})^2$	$\dfrac{SS_{reg}}{N-1}$	$\dfrac{s^2_{Y \cdot X}}{N}$

Some care is needed in applying the ratio formula of the bottom row. A set of data might provide a regression plot with an intercept that is not zero, but with confidence limits that include zero. Unless the intercept is very small, it is better not to use the ratio formula because then the ratio will not be truly constant. The method is best applied when theoretically the line must go through the origin, as in a chemical reaction in which absence of the input chemicals means absence of the output reaction products.

ERRORS IN THE *X* VARIATE

One of the requirements for regression is that the X variate be measured without error, but that is impossible. Both X and Y must have measurement errors, although it is Y that is our main interest. In reality,

$$\text{Measured Y} = Y^* = \text{true Y} + \varepsilon_Y$$

$$\text{and measured X} = X^* = \text{true X} + \varepsilon_X.$$

The errors in Y and X are each assumed to be normally distributed around zero and to be independent of each other (Altman and Bland, 1983; Strike, 1981).

With measurement errors we actually calculate

$$b = \frac{\sum(X_i^* - \overline{X})(Y_I^* - \overline{Y})}{\sum(X_i^* - \overline{X})^2} = \frac{\text{Covariance } X^* Y^*}{\text{Variance } X^*}.$$

Now because ε_Y and ε_X are independent

$$\text{Covariance } X_i^* Y_i = \text{Covariance } X_i Y \text{ and}$$

$$\text{Variance } X_i^* = \text{Variance } X_i + \text{Variance } \varepsilon_{Xi}.$$

$$b = \frac{\text{Covariance } X_i Y_I}{\text{Variance } X_i + \text{Variance } \varepsilon_X}.$$

Unless X is measured with very little error, we will not calculate the correct slope of the relationship between true X and true Y. This error may be of little importance when, for example, relating height to age, because the error in measuring age can be very small, if necessary not more than 1 day in 365, or 0.27%. If the likely error in X is large, it can materially affect the estimates of slope and correlation.

One of the first procedures to deal with this problem was published in 1949 by Bartlett (1949). (A similar approach had been recommended earlier by Nair and Banerjee (1942), Nair and Shrivastava (1942).) Bartlett divided the data set into three equal-sized groups; if N was not divisible by 3, then the first and third groups were to be of equal size. Then the slope was calculated as

$$b = \frac{\overline{Y_3} - \overline{Y_1}}{\overline{X_3} - \overline{X_1}},$$

where 1 and 3 represent the lowest and highest thirds of X, respectively. The regression equation is as usual: $\widehat{Y_i} = bX_i + (\overline{Y} - b\overline{X})$. If X has minimal error, the slopes calculated by this method and the classical method are the same, but Bartlett's method gives a better estimate of slope if X has large measuring errors. An example of the use of this method can be found in the study by Block et al. (1988) when they compared the arteriovenous differences for oxygen and glucose, arguing that both had similar errors and neither was the independent variable.

More complex ways of handling errors of the X variate are discussed by Ludbrook (2012) but they require specialized programs.

BREAK POINTS

In many chemical or physiological processes, there is a linear relationship between X and Y until a threshold is reached and the slope of the line suddenly changes. Examples of this are the rise in blood lactate when oxygen supply cannot meet oxygen demand (van der Hoeven et al., 1997) or the anaerobic ventilatory threshold is reached (Orr et al., 1982).

Methods for determining the breakpoint, also known as piecewise linear regression (Mendenhall and Sincich, 1986) have been described (Hudson, 1966; Jones and Molitoris, 1984; Mellits, 1968), the easiest description to follow being that of Jones and Molitoris (1984) (Figure 28.4).

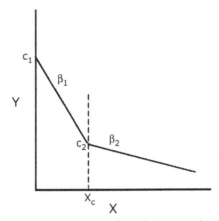

Figure 28.4 Diagram of break point analysis.

They describe two straight lines:

$$\widehat{Y}_i = c_1 + \beta_1 X_c \text{ when } X \leq X_c, \text{ and}$$

$\widehat{Y}_i = c_2 + \beta_2 X_i$ when $X > X_c$. X_c is the critical point at which the two lines meet. Because the lines cross at X_c,

$$c_2 = c_1 + \beta_1 X_c - \beta_2 X_c$$

Therefore there are two new equations:

$$\widehat{Y}_i = c_1 + \beta_1 X_i \quad \text{when } X < X_c,$$
$$\widehat{Y}_i = c_1 + \beta_1 X_c + \beta_2 (X_i - X_c) \text{ when } X \geq X_c.$$

Programs search over different values of X_c so that the residual sum of squares is minimized. (If the break point is known, the two lines can be fitted by multiple regression methods.)

Jones and Molitoris (1984) also gave a method for determining the approximate confidence intervals for the break point, and Graybill and Iyer (1994) described how to determine confidence limits for the slopes and intercepts. An alternative approach to this problem was used by Schwartz et al. (1988) who wanted to determine if there was a threshold value for blood lead concentration below which no nerve damage would occur. In addition to using the above method, they used also logistic regression (see Chapter 29) that gave a similar answer.

RESISTANT LINES

There are ways of determining if one or more points have undue leverage or influence, but how to deal with such aberrant points is not settled. One useful approach is to create a resistant line using median values (Emerson and Hoaglin, 1983; Selvin, 1995; Velleman and Hoaglin, 1981). The breakdown bound, that is, the proportion of data points that can be replaced by arbitrary values without materially changing the slope and the intercept, for the resistant line described below is about 1/6 or 17%.

The basis of the method resembles Bartlett's test (see above) but rather than means uses medians that are less affected by outliers. The X values are divided into three portions with equal numbers of observations ($N/3$) in each: if after dividing by 3 there is one extra number, the middle group has one extra measurement, and if there are two extra numbers they go into the outer groups. Then for each group, determine the median of X and Y. As an example, the data of Butter et al. from Figure 26.42 are presented in Figure 28.5.

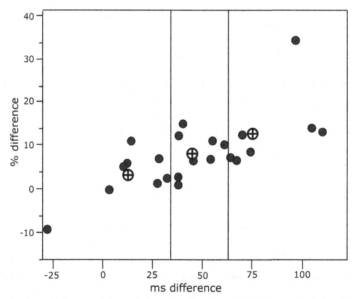

Figure 28.5 Data from Butter et al. (2001) showing X values divided into thirds by the vertical lines, and the median values of X and Y in each third as open circles with an internal cross.

The slope b_1 can be calculated from

$$b = \frac{Y_R - Y_L}{X_R - X_L}$$

where X and Y are the medians for the right (R) and left (L) groups. For the data shown in Figure 25.47, the slope is $b = \frac{12.10 - 3.55}{78.45 - 16.95} = 0.1390$. This is compared to the slope of 0.1688 in the standard regression, and it is likely that the outlier in the upper right part of the graph was responsible for inflating the slope estimate.

The intercept c is determined in standard linear regression as $c = \overline{Y} - b\overline{X}$, but that is not appropriate here. Instead, average c as calculated from each of the three groups:

$$c = \frac{(Y_L - bX_L) + (Y_M - bX_M) + (Y_R - bX_R)}{3}.$$

For this data set, c is calculated as

$$c = \frac{(3.55 - 0.139 \times 16.95) + (8.50 - 0.139 \times 46.55) + (12.1 - 0.139 \times 78.45)}{3}$$

$$= \frac{1.19395 + 2.02955 + 1.19545}{3} = 1.4730$$

c was -0.4765 by the standard regression, again possibly because of the one outlier.

The new equation, $\widehat{Y_i} = c + X_i$, being based on medians, is resistant to outliers, and is often a better estimate of the relationship between X and Y in the population, but it is necessary to examine residuals to determine if they are normally distributed about zero. In standard least squares regression, the sum of the deviations from the regression line is always zero, and a plot of residuals against X has zero slope. This is not necessarily true for the resistant line method, and if the plot of residuals against X has a slope, then the slope of the original regression line must be corrected.

Velleman and Hoaglin (1981) describe an iterative procedure for minimizing the residuals and obtaining the correct slope. The residuals, plotted against X, are divided into the same three groups and the medians taken as before. If the slope is now essentially zero, nothing further is needed. If the slope of the residuals (b') is not zero, it is added to the previous slope, new residuals are calculated, and the process continues until a zero residual slope is obtained. Velleman and Hoaglin (1981) give a way of shortening the iterations by a weighting method.

The final equation becomes

$$\widehat{Y} = 0.1111X_i - 0.2887.$$

The method described above is one of a large class of similar methods (Johnstone and Velleman, 1985). Some are implemented in certain programs, and most do not require complex mathematics. They are not as efficient as the standard linear regression, but like other nonparametric methods gain efficiency when one or more outliers make the standard regression suspect. Confidence limits can also be determined.

APPENDIX

Derivation of Formulas for a Straight Line Passing through Zero

For model 2 with variance constant (second row, Table 28.1), the line of best fit passes through the point 0,0 rather than $\overline{X}, \overline{Y}$. Because the slope is the tangent of the line, this is now $\frac{Y_i - 0}{X_i - 0}$ instead of $\frac{Y_i - \overline{Y}}{X_i - \overline{X}}$. Therefore, whenever there is an expression such as $X_i - \overline{X}$

or $Y_i - \overline{Y}$ in the formula, it is replaced by X_i or Y_i, respectively. As seen from Table 28.1, this applies to the other formulas for lines passing through zero, and simplifies the calculations of the remaining variables. The divisor of $N-1$ for estimating the variance from regression is due to the fact that 0,0 is one fixed point, whereas the point $\overline{X}, \overline{Y}$ uses two degrees of freedom.

For model 2 with constant coefficient of variation (row 4) calculations are even easier. Because s ∞ X, we can use a weighting factor $\omega = 1/X$ and multiply each X by ω. This then gives for the slope

$$b = \frac{\sum \omega X_i Y_i}{\sum \omega X_i^2}$$

But because $\omega = 1/X$, this expression becomes

$$b = \frac{\sum \omega X_i Y_i}{\sum \omega X_i^2} = \frac{\sum \left(\frac{1}{X_i} X_i Y \right)}{\sum \left(\frac{1}{X_i} X_i^2 \right)} = \frac{\sum Y_i}{\sum X_i}.$$

Similarly, the expression for SS_{reg} becomes

$$SS_{reg} = \sum \omega Y_i^2 - \frac{\left(\sum \omega X_i Y_i \right)^2}{\sum \omega X_i^2} = \sum \frac{Y_i^2}{X_i} - \frac{\left(\sum \frac{1}{X_i} X_i Y_i \right)^2}{\sum \frac{1}{X_i} X_i^2} = \sum \frac{Y_i^2}{X_i} - \frac{\left(\sum Y_i \right)^2}{\sum X_i}.$$

As shown in Figure 28.24, panel A, the ratio of Y to X is constant. Therefore, all that is required is to calculate the ratio R for each XY point and average them to get the slope. There is no intercept. The sum of squares of deviations from regression is simply $\sum (R_i - \overline{R})^2$, and the standard deviation of the slope is equivalent to the standard deviation of any mean value.

For model 2 with variance proportional to X, the formulas are derived by weighting each value of Y by multiplying by $\omega = 1/X^2$, with the results shown in row 3.

The slope becomes

$$b = \frac{\sum \omega X_i Y_i}{\sum \omega X_i^2} = \frac{\sum \left(\frac{1}{X_i^2} X_i Y_i \right)}{\sum \left(\frac{1}{X_i^2} X_i^2 \right)} = \frac{\sum \frac{Y_i}{X_i}}{N} = \frac{\sum R}{N}$$

and the SS_{reg} becomes

$$SS_{reg} = \sum \omega Y_i^2 - \frac{\sum (\omega X_i Y_i)^2}{\sum \omega X_i^2} = \sum \frac{1}{X_i^2} Y_i^2 - \frac{\sum \left(\frac{1}{X_i^2} X_i Y_i \right)^2}{\sum \frac{1}{X_i^2} X_i^2}$$

$$= \sum \frac{Y_i^2}{X_i^2} - \frac{\sum \left(\frac{Y_i}{X_i} \right)^2}{N} = \sum (R_i - \overline{R})^2$$

REFERENCES

Altman, D.G., Bland, J.M., 1983. Measurement in medicine: the analysis of method comparison studies. The Statistician 32, 307–317.

Bartlett, M.S., 1949. Fitting a straight line when both variables are subject to error. Biometrics 207–212.

Block, S.M., Johnson, R.L., Sparks, J.W., Battaglia, F.C., 1988. Uterine metabolism of the pregnant guinea pig as a function of gestational age. Pediatr. Res. 23, 45–49.

Butter, C., Auricchio, A., Stellbrink, C., Fleck, E., Ding, J., Yu, Y., Huvelle, E., Spinelli, J., 2001. Effect of resynchronization therapy stimulation on the systolic function of heart failure patients. Circulation 104, 3026–3029.

Emerson, J.D., Hoaglin, D.C., 1983. Resistant lines for y versus x. In: Hoaglin, D.C., Mosteller, F., Tukey, J.W. (Eds.), Understanding Robust and Exploratory Data Analysis. John Wiley & Sons, New York.

Gaddum, J.H., 1933. Methods of biological assay depending on a quantal response. Reports on Biological Standards III Spec. Rep. Ser. Med. Res.Coun. No. 183, 5–46.

Graybill, F.A., Iyer, H.K., 1994. Regression Analysis: Concepts and Applications. Duxbury Press, Belmont, CA.

Hirschfeld, S., Meyer, R., Schwartz, D.C., Kofhagen, J., Kaplan, S., 1975. The echocardiographic assessment of pulmonary artery pressure and pulmonary vascular resistance. Circulation 52, 642–650.

Hudson, D.J., 1966. Fitting segmented curves whose joint points have to be estimated. J. Am. Stat. Assoc. 61, 1097–1129.

Johnstone, I.M., Velleman, P.F., 1985. The resistant line and related regression methods. J. Am. Stat. Assoc. 80, 1041–1054.

Jones, R.H., Molitoris, B.A., 1984. A statistical method for determining the breakpoint of two lines. Anal. Biochem. 141, 287–290.

Ludbrook, J., 2012. A primer for biomedical scientists on how to execute model II linear regression analysis. Clin. Exp. Pharmacol. Physiol. 39, 329–335.

Mellits, E.D., 1968. Statistical methods. In: Cheek, D. (Ed.), Human Growth. Lea & Febiger, Philadelphia.

Mendenhall, W., Sincich, T., 1986. A Second Course in Business Statistics:Regression Analysis. Dellen Publishing Co, San Francisco.

Nair, K.R., Banerjee, K.S., 1942. A note on fitting straight lines if both variables are subject to error. Sankhyā Indian J. Stat. (1933–1960) 6, 331.

Nair, K.R., Shrivastava, M.P., 1942. On a simple method of curve fitting. Sankhyā Indian J. Stat. (1933–1960) 6, 121–132.

Natrella, M.G., 1963. Experimental Statistics. Dover Publications, Inc, Mineola, NY.

Orr, G.W., Green, H.J., Hughson, R.L., Bennett, G.W., 1982. A computer linear regression model to determine ventilatory anaerobic threshold. J. Appl. Physiol. Respir. Environ. Exerc. Physiol. 52, 1349–1352.

Schwartz, J., Landrigan, P.J., Feldman, R.G., Silbergeld, E.K., Baker Jr., E.L., Von Lindern, I.H., 1988. Threshold effect in lead-induced peripheral neuropathy. J. Pediatr. 112, 12–17.

Selvin, S., 1995. Practical Biostatistical Methods. Wadsworth Publishing Company, Belmont CA.

Silverman, N.H., Hoffman, J.I., 1976. Letter: echo assessment of PVR. Circulation 54, 525–526.

Strike, P.W., 1981. Medical Laboratory Statistics. John Wright and Sons, Ltd, Bristol.

Van Der Hoeven, M.A., Maertzdorf, W.J., Blanco, C.E., 1997. Mixed venous oxygen saturation and biochemical parameters of hypoxia during progressive hypoxemia in 10- to 14-day-old piglets. Pediatr. Res. 42, 878–884.

Velleman, P.F., Hoaglin, D.C., 1981. Applications, Basics and Computing of Exploratory Data Analysis. Duxbury Press, Boston, MA.

Zar, J.H., 2010. Biostatistical Analysis. Prentice Hall, Upper Saddle River, NJ.

CHAPTER 29

Correlation

Contents

BASIC CONCEPTS

Introduction

This subject, closely related to the regression concept, asks how closely X and Y are related rather than how much does Y change when X changes. Correlation is calculated so that if all the points lie on the line the value is 1, if X and Y are completely unrelated then the value is 0, and if they are partially related the value is somewhere between 0 and 1. If the slope of the line is negative, so that Y gets smaller as X gets bigger, then the correlation varies between 0 and -1. The sample correlation coefficient (also known as Pearson's product—moment correlation coefficient) has two symbols: r if only two variables are related, and R if more than two variables are involved; the population coefficient is ρ.

The square of the correlation coefficient r^2, termed the coefficient of determination, is defined as $\frac{SS_{reg}}{SS_{total}}$, where SS_{reg} is the sum of squares due to the regression relationship and SS_{total} is the sum of squared deviations from the mean of the Y array. It indicates the

For a list of all websites referred to in this chapter, as clickable links, see the book companion website: www.booksite.elsevier.com/9780128023877.

Biostatistics for Medical and Biomedical Practitioners
http://dx.doi.org/10.1016/B978-0-12-802387-7.00029-9

proportion of the total variability of Y that can be accounted for by the regression relationship. SS_{reg} is

$$\frac{\sum\left[(X_i - \overline{X})(Y_i - \overline{Y})\right]^2}{\sum(X_i - \overline{X})^2}$$

and SS_{total} is $\sum(Y_i - \overline{Y})^2$,

so that $r^2 = \dfrac{SS_{reg}}{SS_{total}} = \dfrac{\sum\left[(X_i - \overline{X})(Y_i - \overline{Y})\right]^2}{\sum(X_i - \overline{X})^2\sum(Y_i - \overline{Y})^2}$

and $r = \dfrac{\sum\left[(X_i - \overline{X})(Y_i - \overline{Y})\right]}{\sqrt{\sum(X_i - \overline{X})^2\sum(Y_i - \overline{Y})^2}}.$

If all the points lie on the line then the total variability of Y is explained by variability of X, so that $SS_{reg} = SS_{total}$, and $r = 1$. If the points are completely unassociated, then SS_{reg} is zero and r is zero.

Rearranging the various components gives other ways of formulating the correlation coefficient. For example,

$$r = \sqrt{1 - \frac{(N-2)s_{Y\cdot X}^2}{(N-1)s_Y^2}}, \quad r = b\frac{s_X}{s_Y}, \quad \text{and } r = \pm\sqrt{b_{X\cdot Y}b_{Y\cdot X}},$$

where r is the bivariate correlation coefficient, b is the slope of the linear regression equation, s_X and s_Y are the standard deviations of the X and Y arrays, respectively, s_Y^2 is the variance of the Y array, $s_{Y\cdot X}^2$ is the variance of the Y deviations from the regression line, and $b_{X\cdot Y}$ and $b_{Y\cdot X}$ are the slopes of the regression of X on Y and Y on X, respectively.

The formulas show that both regression and correlation calculations make use of the same derived values (means, deviations from means) but in different ways.

These considerations can be developed further by a graphic representation (Figure 29.1).

The line of best fit has the same slope for all three panels, but the fit of points about the line is close for the left panel, moderate for the middle panel, and poor for the right panel. As shown by the dashed deviation lines, in the left panel all the points are in the upper right or lower left quadrants, so that the deviations from the means are both positive or both negative and their product is positive. In the middle panel a few points have one positive and one negative deviation, the product of which is negative, so that when all the product deviations from the mean are summed their total is less than the total in the left panel. Finally, in the right panel there are about as many negative as positive product deviations from the mean, and their sum is close to zero.

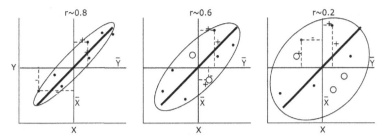

Figure 29.1 Examples of three different correlation coefficients. The line of best fit is the thick solid line that passes through the point where the mean of X and the mean of Y cross. The individual XY points are shown in solid black circles for the upper right and lower left quadrants and in open circles for the other quadrants. The dashed vertical lines show the deviations from the mean of Y, and the dashed horizontal lines show the deviations from the mean of X. Plus and minus signs next to the dashed lines indicate positive or negative deviations respectively. r is the correlation coefficient. The ellipses are drawn by eye to encompass all the data points.

The ellipses each have a long and a short axis. With a high r value the long axis: short axis ratio is high (about 5 here), with a moderate r value the ratio is lower (about 2.2), and with a low r value almost 1. The change in ratio is due to a change in the short axis because the long axis is almost constant.

Online programs for the correlation coefficient are often included in those for linear regression (Chapter 27) but may be calculated separately at http://www.easycalculation. com/statistics/correlation.php, http://easycalculation.com/statistics/r-squared.php, and http://www.alcula.com/calculators/statistics/correlation-coefficient/.

Problem 29.1

Calculate the correlation coefficient for the data in problem 27.1.

Significance and Confidence Limits

The sample correlation coefficient r is an estimate of the population correlation coefficient ρ (rho). If the variables X and Y are normally distributed and ρ is zero, then for $N > 6$, the quantity

$$\frac{r}{\sqrt{\dfrac{1 - r^2}{N - 2}}}$$

is distributed approximately normally like t with $N - 2$ degrees of freedom. Thus for $r = 0.8288$ and $N = 51$, $t = \dfrac{0.8288}{\sqrt{\frac{1 - 0.8288^2}{51 - 2}}} = \dfrac{0.8288}{0.0799} = 10.37$. Therefore $P = {<}0.0001$, allowing us to reject the null hypothesis that $r = 0$. The significance of the correlation coefficient is determined readily from tables or simple interactive online programs, for example, http://vassarstats.net/ and http://www.danielsoper.com/statcalc3/calc. aspx?id=44, and programs such as http://vassarstats.net/rho.html.

To test r against any value for $\rho \neq 0$, the distribution is skewed but can be made approximately normal by a Z (zeta) transformation introduced by Fisher:

$$Z = \frac{1}{2}\ln\left(\frac{1+r}{1-r}\right).$$

(This Z is not to be confused with the z transform for a normal distribution.) Z is normally distributed with a mean of $\frac{1}{2}\ln\left(\frac{1+\rho}{1-\rho}\right)$, and has a standard error of

$$\sigma = \sqrt{\frac{1}{N-3}}$$

for any value of $N > 20$.

To compare any r with $\rho \neq 0$, transform both r and ρ into their respective Z values. Therefore, to test whether $r = 0.8288$ ($N = 51$) is significantly different from $\rho = 0.6075$, the two conversions yield 1.1843 and 0.7049, respectively. Then

$$z = \frac{1.1843 - 0.7049}{0.1443} = 3.3971.$$

$P = 0.000341$, and the observed correlation coefficient of 0.8288 is significantly different from 0.6075.

To compare two observed r values, adapt the above equation by dividing the difference between the two zeta values by the sum of the two standard deviations, calculated by

$$\sqrt{\frac{1}{N_1 - 3} + \frac{1}{N_2 - 3}}.$$

Thus to compare $r_1 = 0.8288$ ($N = 51$) with $r_2 = 0.6075$ ($N = 42$), calculate Z_1 and Z_2 as

$$Z_1 = 0.5\ln\frac{1 + 0.8288}{1 - 0.8288} = 1.1843 \text{ and}$$

$$Z_2 = 0.5\ln\frac{1 + 0.6075}{1 - 0.6075} = 0.7049.$$

The standard deviation of the difference is

$$s_{z_1 - z_2} = \sqrt{\frac{1}{48} + \frac{1}{39}} = 0.2156.$$

Therefore,

$z = \frac{1.1843 - 0.7049}{0.2156} = 2.2236$ g, and so $P = 0.0131$. Although this difference is significant, it is less so than if $r = 0.8288$ is compared with a population value of the same amount (see above). This comparison may be performed online at http://vassarstats.net/index.html, https://www.statstodo.com/HomoCor_Pgm.php.

Fisher's Z transformation is the basis of many other tests of the correlation coefficient (Kleinbaum et al., 1988). For example, to combine several correlation coefficients from a number of small samples, first demonstrate their homogeneity. This can be done readily at http://home.ubalt.edu/ntsbarsh/Business-stat/otherapplets/MultiCorr.htm or http://vassarstats.net/, or to determine if the correlation coefficient is different from some value for ρ that is not zero, or if two experimental correlation coefficients are significantly different from each other. Methods for determining confidence limits and other comparisons are presented by Zar (2010).

The value of r^2 indicates the percentage of change in Y that can be associated with a change in X. Thus if r is 0.8, then 64% of the change in Y is associated with (and possibly caused by) a change in X. If r is 0.5, then only 25% of the change in Y has been explained, and if r is 0.2, then only 4% of the change in Y can be explained by a corresponding change in X. Therefore, the importance (as distinct from the significance) of the correlation coefficient is easy to overestimate. Just as in the t-test the difference (the effect size) may be small, medium, or large, so can the correlation coefficient be small (<0.25), medium ($0.25-0.7$), and large (>0.7) (Cohen, 1988). This is a more important judgment than significance, because any trivial difference may be significant if sample size is large enough.

Finding a significant correlation coefficient is equivalent to finding that the slope b is significantly different from zero. Either test can be used.

Correlation is independent of the units used. On the other hand, the slope of a relationship depends on the units used; the slope of a height–weight relationship is not the same if these are measured in inches and pounds or in centimeters and kilograms.

Sample Size and Power

From the formula for Z above,

$z = \frac{Z_i - Z_\rho}{\sigma_z}$, where z (lower case) is the normal z distribution, Z (upper case) is defined as above, and Z_ρ is a theoretical value from a population with correlation coefficient ρ:

$$Z_\rho = \frac{1}{2}\ln\left(\frac{1 + \rho}{1 - \rho}\right).$$

What is the power of detecting a correlation coefficient of 0.3 with a sample of 20 measurements? Begin with

$$Z_\rho = \frac{1}{2}\ln\left(\frac{1+\rho}{1-\rho}\right) = \frac{1}{2}\ln\left(\frac{1+0.3}{1-0.3}\right) = 0.3095.$$

$$\sigma_z = \sqrt{\frac{1}{20-3}} = 0.2425.$$

Then $z = \frac{0.3095}{0.2425} = 1.2762$ ($P = 0.1009$). This is interpreted as stating that if the true value of the correlation coefficient is 0.0, then 0.1009 of the area under the curve will be as big as 0.3 or more. This is thus not good evidence that the correlation coefficient differs from zero, but what is the power of the test to show a difference of 0.3?

Consider the two normal curves shown in Figure 29.2.

This concept can be simplified to the equation: Power is the area of the standard normal distribution to the right of

$$z_{1-\beta upper} = z_{\alpha/2} - \frac{Z_\rho}{\sqrt{\frac{1}{N-3}}}.$$

For the example given above, then

$1.96 - \frac{0.3095}{0.2425} = 1.96 - 1.28 = 0.68$. The power is the area beyond this value of z.

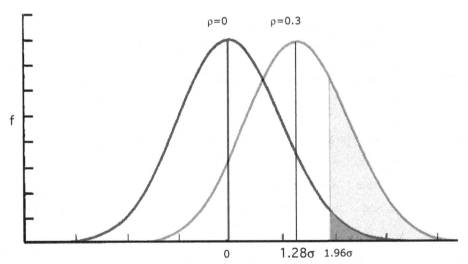

Figure 29.2 Superimposition of two normal curves with the same standard deviation, but one with a mean of $\rho = 0$ and the other with a mean of $r = 0.3$.

To determine the needed sample size for any correlation coefficient, rearrange the above equation to solve for N:

$$N = \left(\frac{z_{\alpha/2} - z_{1-\beta upper}}{Z\rho}\right)^2 + 3$$

(Glantz, 2005).

To compare two observed correlation coefficients, the sample size equation becomes

$$N = 2\left(\frac{Z_\alpha - Z_{\beta(1)}}{z_1 - z_2}\right)^2 + 3.$$

Here α and β are the Type I and Type II errors, respectively.

Sample size or power can be calculated online for a single value of r at http://www.cct.cuhk.edu.hk/stat/other/correlation.htm, or http://www.sample-size.net.

Cautionary Tales

There is nothing wrong with the concept of correlation, but often a great deal wrong with how it is used. Many statisticians disparage the use of correlation coefficients; Winsor and Tukey, for example, belonged to an informal society for the suppression of correlation coefficients!

1. The correlation coefficient is always higher than its square, and thus may confer an impression of greater importance than is justified.
2. In most studies, a low correlation coefficient does not provide much added information for the investigator to use. The one exception is in epidemiology where a disease that has many causes is being studied. Under these circumstances, no one X variable can be expected to have a very high correlation coefficient, and finding a significant correlation coefficient of 0.1 might still indicate the need to consider that variable as one of the underlying causes of the disease.
3. Although the correlation coefficient can be calculated for linear or curvilinear regression, failure to consider linearity may result in incorrect calculations (Figure 29.3).

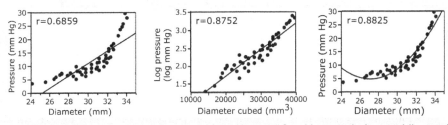

Figure 29.3 Left panel: original data (Senzaki et al., 2000) fitted by straight line. Middle panel: transformed data fitted by a straight line. Right panel: original data fitted by second-order polynomial.

(Continued)

Cautionary Tales—cont'd

Fitting a straight line to a set of XY points with a curved relationship results in an incorrectly low correlation coefficient. Furthermore, although the correlation in the left panel of 0.6854 is quite high, it is no guarantee of linearity.

4. Although no specific criteria have been set for how the X values should be distributed, there are potential problems if the points are bunched at the low end and the high end, with none in the middle (Edwards, 1984). Figure 29.4 shows some data simplified from an actual problem of growth of the right ventricle in fetal sheep.

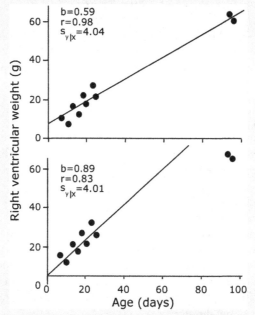

Figure 29.4 Plot of index of age (X: days) versus right ventricular weight (Y: g).

The upper panel shows the effect of fitting a straight line to all the data. The bottom panel shows that if only the initial points are fitted, the slope is steeper and the correlation coefficient is lower. If there are only two bunches of points, then it always possible to join them by a straight line. It is possible that there had been measurements at intervening values of X the relation might have been shown to be curvilinear. See Beer et al. (1982), Lindner et al. (2000), Schwarzacher et al. (2000), and Rim et al. (2001) for similar problems of interpretation. An extreme example of this problem can be shown in the study by Mena et al. (1995) who plotted the relation between two inflammatory mediators and found a correlation of 0.77, even though there were seven points near coordinates of 0, 0, and one point at coordinates 650, 850, with nothing in between them.

Even with intermediate values of X, if there are a disproportionate number of measurements at one end of the curve, these will weight the line and the correlation coefficient in much the same way that an adult at one end of a seesaw outweighs a child at the other end (see Figure 27.28).

Cautionary Tales—cont'd

5. One or a few outlying points can unduly influence not only the slope of the line but also the correlation coefficient that is not a resistant statistic. Consider the uncorrelated XY data of Table 29.1.

Table 29.1 Artificial *XY* data set

X	1	2	3	4	5	6	7	8	9	10	11
Y	4	8	10	1	11	7	2	3	34	6	9

The correlation coefficient is 0.03. After changing the value of Y_1 from 4 to -40 or $+40$, the correlation coefficient becomes 0.46 or -0.52, all because of the influence of a single point. This point was demonstrated nicely by Curran-Everett (2010).

6. There are other concerns with the correlation coefficient. Consider Figure 29.5.

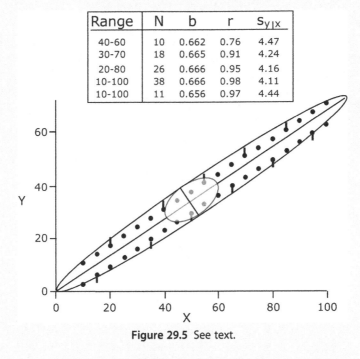

Range	N	b	r	$s_{y|x}$
40-60	10	0.662	0.76	4.47
30-70	18	0.665	0.91	4.24
20-80	26	0.666	0.95	4.16
10-100	38	0.666	0.98	4.11
10-100	11	0.656	0.97	4.44

Figure 29.5 See text.

This is an artificially constructed figure in which each point is exactly four units above or below the line. If all the points from $X = 10$ to $X = 100$ are considered, the slope is 0.666 and the correlation coefficient is 0.98; the standard deviation from regression ($s_{y.x}$) is 4.11, an estimate of the population value of 4. If the range over which X is examined is reduced to 20–80, 30–70, or 40–60, the slope and the standard deviation from regression change little, but the correlation coefficient decreases from 0.98 to 0.95, then 0.91, and then 0.76 respectively. Comparing the two ellipses shows

Cautionary Tales—cont'd

the reason for this. The ellipse that covers the full range of 10—100 has a high long:
short axis ratio, but the ellipse that covers the range 40—60 has a much smaller ratio,
even though its short axis (a function of the standard deviation from regression) has
not changed. To show that the reduced number of points used in the calculation is
not the cause for the change, the final calculation was done with only 11 points (shown
by the short vertical lines attached to some of the points) and it produced almost the
same results as were obtained for the calculation that used all 38 points.

This artifact is one of the reasons why the standard deviation from regression should
always be given, even if the correlation coefficient is given as well.

The mathematical basis of this artifact was discussed by van Belle (2002, page 57).
It is possible to write the formula for the square of the correlation coefficient as

$$r^2 = \cfrac{1}{1 + \cfrac{(n-2)s_{y \cdot x}^2}{b^2 (X_i - \overline{X})^2}}.$$

The bigger the range of the X variate for a given sample size n the closer r is to 1.
Conversely, if measurements are made over a restricted range, the correlation coefficient becomes smaller (Curran-Everett, 2010).

The effect of the range of X can be shown also by Chatillon's balloon trick
(Chatillon, 1984) (Figure 29.6).

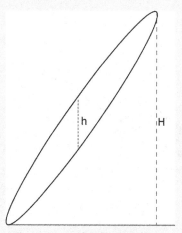

Figure 29.6 Chatillon's balloon.

If an ellipse is drawn around the points (not shown), the length of a vertical through the
center of the ellipse is h, and the total vertical height of the ellipse is H, then
$r \approx \sqrt{1 - \left(\dfrac{h}{H}\right)^2}$. If the range of X is narrowed, then H is reduced relative to h, and
the correlation coefficient becomes smaller.

Cautionary Tales—cont'd

7. Because the correlation coefficient is the square root of the ratio of SS_{reg} to SS_{total}, if SS_{total} decreases with no change in SS_{reg}, the correlation coefficient decreases (Figure 29.7).

	N	b	r	$S_{y|x}$	$\Sigma(Y_i-\bar{Y})^2$	$\dfrac{S(X_i-\bar{X})(Y_i-\bar{Y})}{S(X_i-\bar{X})^2}$
A	11	0.5758	0.9728	4.40	2890.0	2734.9
B	11	0.0812	0.5159	4.33	204.4	54.4

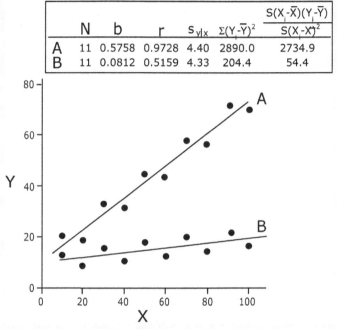

Figure 29.7 Artificial example of effect of change in slope. The points are all exactly four units above or below the lines.

With the steeper slope of 0.5758 (line A) and standard deviation from regression of 4.40, the correlation coefficient is 0.9728. Without any major change in the standard deviation from regression (4.33) but with a slope of 0.0812, the correlation coefficient for line B is 0.5159. As shown in the second last column, this change in r has been due to a marked decrease in the sum of squared deviations from the mean of Y (here shown as $\sum (Y_i - \bar{Y})^2$).

This effect of rotating a set of correlated points has been discussed formally (Loh, 1987). It can also be explained by Chatillon's balloon.

It is therefore imprudent to rely on a number for the correlation coefficient without considering the slope, its linearity, the range of X values, and the distribution of the X values. It is not wrong to mention the correlation coefficient in the publication, but its value is small compared to the vital information provided by the standard deviation from regression.

8. A little recognized requirement for the correlation coefficient is that the X values are normally distributed. We do not often pay attention to this requirement because

(Continued)

Cautionary Tales—cont'd

regression and correlation are quite robust, but the requirement is violated if the X variables are determined in advance (Campbell and Machen, 1993) as, for example, when drug doses are allocated for a dose–response analysis. Even if the dose–response curve is constant, changing the actual doses used may change the correlation coefficient.

Even if the X variables are chosen at random, an abnormal distribution of the X variate can lead to a correlation coefficient that has a large standard error and wide confidence limits, and so makes it harder to compare two or more groups. One way around this problem is to use robust regression lines.

9. Measurement errors reduce the basic correlation between Y and X (Cohen and Cohen, 1975). If Y and X have random errors of ε_Y and ε_X, respectively, each error with a mean of zero, then the correlation coefficient becomes

$$r = \frac{\sum (X_i - \overline{X})(Y_i - \overline{Y})}{\sqrt{\left(\sqrt{\sum (X_i - \overline{X})^2} + \sum \varepsilon_X^2\right)\left(\sum (Y_i - \overline{Y})^2 + \sum \varepsilon_Y^2\right)}}$$

r can only achieve its highest value when $\sum \varepsilon_X^2 = \sum \varepsilon_Y^2 = 0$.

Ordinal Numbers

If the X or Y variables are ordinal numbers, then classical regression cannot be done. For example, an investigator examines aortas at autopsy examination and grades the degree of atherosclerosis as 1+ to 6+, and wants to compare aortic atherosclerosis with a recent serum cholesterol concentration observed in those patients. Because the degree of atheroma (Y variable) is ordinal, it makes no sense to calculate a slope. Instead, calculate a modified correlation coefficient with Spearman's or Kendall's test. Both of these are ranking tests that give a correlation statistic that varies between +1 and −1. They can be used also if the numbers are ratio numbers but the bivariate population is far from normal; like many distribution-free tests, they are relatively insensitive to outliers.

Spearman's Test

For Spearman's rank correlation procedure (Spearman's ρ or r_s), the X and Y variables are each ranked from smallest to largest, the difference in ranks (d) is calculated as $d_i =$ rank of X_i minus rank of Y_i, and then squared to give d^2. (The results will be the same if the data are ranked from largest to smallest.) Then Spearman's rank correlation coefficient (r_s or ρ) is

$$r_s = 1 - \frac{6 \sum d^2}{N(N^2 - 1)}.$$

The significance of r_s can be determined from tables, the computer program, or online programs such as http://www.socscistatistics.com/tests/spearman/Default2.aspx, http://www.fon.hum.uva.nl/Service/Statistics/RankCorrelation_coefficient.html, http://easycalculation.com/statistics/spearman-rank-correlation-calculator.php, http://www.wessa.net/rankcorr.wasp, http://vassarstats.net/corr_rank.html, and https://www.statstodo.com/Contingency_Pgm.php. All allow entry of raw data or ranks.

If there are no tied ranks, the same correlation coefficient can be obtained from the classical formula for Pearson's correlation coefficient. If there are tied ranks, adjustments to the formula are needed, although the differences are minor unless there are very many ties (Zar, 2010).

If this test and classical linear regression are done on the same set of ratio numbers that fit the requirements for regression analysis, the rank correlation test is about 91% as powerful as the parametric test.

As an example, consider the ranking of ice-cream flavors by two judges:

Ice-cream number	Judge A score	Judge A rank	Judge B score	Judge B rank	Rank difference d	d^2
1	5	3.5	7	6	−2.5	6.25
2	8	9	8	7	2	4
3	9	10	5	3	7	49
4	4	2	5	3	−1	1
5	6	5.5	9	8.5	−3	9
6	7	7.5	4	1	6.5	42.25
7	5	3.5	10	10	−6.5	42.25
8	7	7.5	5	3	4.5	20.25
9	3	1	6	5	−4	16
10	6	5.5	9	8.5	−3	9
						$\Sigma d^2 = 199$

For each judge separately, rank the scores from best (score = rank 10) to worst (rank 1). Thus for judge A ice-cream 3 gets a score of 9 and a rank of 10, whereas ice-creams 6 and 8, getting an equal score of 7, share ranks. For these data, Spearman's $\rho = -0.2061$, $P = 0.5097$. The correlation between the two sets of ratings is low. If corrected for ties, $\rho = -0.2360$. Most online calculators correct for ties.

Kendall's τ Test

Kendall's τ test is more tedious to calculate by hand, but can be done by interactive online programs http://www.wessa.net/rwasp_kendall.wasp#output or standard statistical programs. The X data are arrayed and ranked in order from lowest to highest value. Then the corresponding ranked Y data (raw data, or ranked, usually the latter) are examined to determine if they are concordant (arranged in the same order) or discordant (arranged in the opposite order). For example, consider the set in Table 29.2.

Table 29.2 X and Y ranks, based loosely on Table 1.26 in Bland (1995)

Number	X	Y	Y rank	Discordant	Concordant
1	1	4.0	2	1	8
2	2	2.6	1	0	8
3	3	9.2	4	1	6
4	4	7.5	3	0	6
5	5	11.4	5	0	5
6	6	13.0	7	1	3
7	7	14.7	8	1	2
8	8	12.9	6	0	2
9	9	15	9	0	1
10	10	17.2	10	0	0
Total				4	41

Nc, total concordant; Nd, total discordant.

In the Y column, for each row count the number of X ranks that are smaller (=discordant). Thus for Y_1 there is 1; for Y_2 there are none, for Y_7 there is 1 for a total of 2. These discordant ranks sum to 4. Now count the number of ranks that are higher. For Y_1 there are 8, for Y_2 there are 8, etc. and sum these. The sum of concordant ranks is 41. Then calculate, $\tau = \frac{Nc - Nd}{Nc + Nd} = \frac{Nc - Nd}{\frac{1}{2}k(k-1)}$ where $k =$ number of pairs. In the above example this gives $\tau = \frac{41-4}{41+4} = 0.8222$.

There are different formulas with identical results. Corrections for multiple ties may be needed. The total sum of ranks can also be calculated from $\binom{k}{2} = \frac{k!}{2!(k-2)!}$. If $k = 10$, $\binom{k}{2} = \frac{10!}{2!8!} = \frac{3628800}{2 \times 40320} = 45$.

Spearman's and Kendall's tests cannot be converted into each other. For a given set of data, Spearman's ρ tends to be bigger than Kendall's τ.

Problem 29.2

The table presents data on marks for English and Mathematics for each of 11 students. Perform Spearman's r_s and Kendall's τ tests.

English	Mathematics
56	64
77	68
54	43
75	67
60	61
60	55
54	57
78	78
72	63
59	67
44	71

ADVANCED AND ALTERNATIVE CONCEPTS

Partial Correlation

If there are bivariate correlations between age (A), blood pressure (B), and serum choles-terol (C), what is the relationship of blood pressure to cholesterol if age is constant? One way to test this would be to measure blood pressure and serum cholesterol in a narrow age range, but this would require a much bigger sample size to cover several age ranges. Instead calculate the partial correlation coefficient between blood pressure and serum cholesterol independent of age from:

$$r_{BCA} = \frac{r_{BC} - r_{BA}r_{AC}}{\sqrt{\left(1 - r_{BA}^2\right)\left(1 - r_{AC}^2\right)}}.$$

The numerator is the difference between the bivariate correlation coefficient be-tween the two variables under consideration and the product of the remaining two bivar-iate correlation coefficients. The denominator is the square root of the product of 1 minus the first of the remaining correlation coefficients and 1 minus the second of the remaining correlation coefficients.

Swanson et al. (1955) found bivariate coefficients for these three variables of $r_{AB} = 0.3332$, $r_{AC} = 0.5029$, and $r_{BC} = 0.2495$. What is the relationship of blood pressure and serum cholesterol independent of age? Calculate the partial correlation coefficient between blood pressure and serum cholesterol as $r_{BC \cdot A} = \frac{0.2495 - (0.3332 \times 0.5029)}{\sqrt{(1 - 0.3332^2)(1 - 0.5029^2)}} = 0.1005$. Therefore, the correlation between blood pressure and serum cholesterol of 0.2495 was in part because both of these variables increased with age, and removing the effect of age reduced the correlation. We have to be careful that the effect of age is directionally the same at different ages. If the bivariate correlation was negative in younger subjects and the opposite way in older subject, partial correlation would be difficult to interpret. These calculations can be done online at http://vassarstats. net/par.html and http://www.wessa.net/partcorr.wasp.

With four variables A, B, C, and D, it is possible examine the correlation coefficient between any two variables if the other two are held constant by extending the above equation. Individual partial correlation coefficients between sets of three variables are calculated, and then the four-part partial correlation coefficient is

$$r_{AB \cdot CD} = \frac{r_{AB \cdot D} - r_{AC \cdot D}r_{BC \cdot D}}{\sqrt{\left(1 - r_{AC \cdot D}^2\right)\left(1 - r_{BC \cdot D}^2\right)}}.$$

These calculations can be done with the free online program http://vassarstats.net/ index.html.

The confidence limits can be determined (Snedecor and Cochran, 1989). In addition, partial correlations can be determined using Kendall's τ, and Conover (1980) also asserts that partial correlations can be determined using Spearman's ρ coefficient.

There are complexities involved in evaluating multiple and partial correlation coefficients. An excellent discussion of these issues of particular relevance to the social sciences is given by Cohen and Cohen (1975) in their Chapter 3. As an example, consider the relationship between Y and two explanatory variables X_1 and X_2. The multiple correlation coefficient $R_{Y \cdot X_1 X_2}$ is

$$R_{Y \cdot X_1 X_2} = \sqrt{\frac{r_{YX_1}^2 + r_{YX_2}^2 - 2r_{YX_1} r_{YX_2} r_{X_1 X_2}}{1 - r_{X_1 X_2}^2}}.$$

Assume that there is no correlation between Y and X_2, so that $r_{YX_2} = 0$, but there is positive correlation between Y and X_1 as well as between X_1 and X_2. Substitute $r_{YX_2} = 0$ into Eqn (25.11) to get

$$R_{Y \cdot X_1 X_2}^2 = \frac{r_{YX_1}^2}{1 - r_{X_1 X_2}^2}.$$

The denominator is <1, so that

$$R_{Y \cdot X_1 X_2}^2 > r_{YX_1}^2.$$

This produces a paradoxical result. Despite no correlation between Y and X_2, the inclusion of X_2 in the multiple regression increases the correlation between Y and X_1.

Spurious Correlation

This is a subtler trap than any of the issues described above, and was elegantly discussed by Archie (1981) under the heading of Mathematical Coupling of Data. Coupling occurs when two variables are related when they have a common component, when one variable is contained in the other, or a third dependent variable is common to both variables.

Tanner was one of the first to examine this problem (Tanner, 1949) that was discussed in more detail by Oldham (1962). Figure 29.8 shows the results of plotting a random

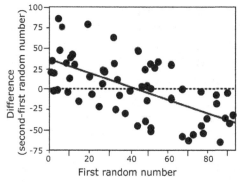

Figure 29.8 A random number on the X-axis is plotted against the difference between a second random number and the first one on the Y-axis.

number (obtained from http://www.random.org/) against the difference between the second and the previous random number.

By choosing at random numbers for X_1 and X_2, and then plotting X_1 against $(X_2 - X_1)$, Oldham showed that there would necessarily be a regression line with a slope of -1 and a correlation coefficient of -0.707, despite the fact that the numbers were chosen at random. This leads to serious errors of interpretation. As one way to escape from this dilemma, Oldham recommended comparing Y_1 and Y_2 where $Y_1 = \frac{X_1 + X_2}{2}$ and, $Y_2 = X_1 - X_2$, instead of comparing X_1 with $X_2 - X_1$, which will produce a spurious correlation. This method avoids spurious correlations between X_1 and X_2, because the sums and differences are not correlated. Other possible combinations are described in his publication. It is permissible to plot X_1 against X_2 and avoid this particular problem.

The theoretical basis for Oldham's results can be seen by considering the relation between total X and its components. Thus if $X_{iT} = X_{iA} + X_{iB}$, where X_{iT} is the total and is correlated with one of its components, say X_{iA}, then the partial correlation r_{TA} between these two variates is

$$r_{TA} = \frac{S_A + r_{AB}S_b}{\sqrt{S_B^2 + 2r_{AB}S_BS_A + S_A^2}}.$$

If r_{AB} is really zero, this expression simplifies to $r_{TA} = \dfrac{1}{\sqrt{1 + \frac{S_B^2}{S_A^2}}}$, and if in addition the

variances of X_A and X_B are the same, as they were in Oldham's random selection, this becomes $\frac{1}{\sqrt{2}} = 0.707$.

Archie discussed in detail different types of coupling. In one of his examples, he derived a plot of cardiac output against oxygen consumption, for example, and even though he used random numbers for the arteriovenous oxygen difference, he obtained a linear relationship between the two variables with a correlation coefficient of 0.75. Oxygen consumption is the product of the arteriovenous oxygen difference and the cardiac output, so that in effect cardiac output appeared on both axes. Similarly, cardiac output and heart rate are highly correlated because heart rate is a major determinant of cardiac output (cardiac output = heart rate × stroke volume).

As another of his examples, a linear relationship was found in a study of the effect of hepatectomy on the relation between hepatic delivery of insulin and glucagon and the hepatic uptake of these substances (Caruana and Gage, 1980). However, hepatic uptake is defined as the flux of the substance in the portal vein plus the flux in the hepatic artery, minus flux in the hepatic vein, all divided by the hepatic weight, and hepatic delivery is defined as flux of the substance in the portal vein plus the flux in the hepatic artery divided by total body weight. Therefore, hepatectomy that changes liver weight automatically changes the calculated uptake, and the linear relationship between hepatic delivery and uptake is mainly due to the relationship between body and hepatic weight and unrelated to metabolism. Statistical analyses of these types of relationships in the literature produce faulty conclusions, not because of incorrect statistics but because they have been applied incorrectly to mathematically coupled variables. Everyone involved in scientific research should study Archie's publication and its examples. Moreno et al. (1986) presented an approach to correct this problem.

A recent survey of dental research has emphasized the erroneous deductions drawn by ignoring these problems (Tu et al., 2004a,b).

Cautionary Tales

The problems of comparing a change in some measurement due to an intervention with the first measurement are ubiquitous and serious. An example is a study of the relationship between pre- and postdialysis concentrations of norepinephrine in uremic patients (Musso et al., 1989). The slope obtained by plotting the difference in concentrations against the initial concentration was close to -1, the theoretical value if there was in reality no correlation (Figure 29.9, left panel). In a subsequent letter, Boer (1990) showed that if pre- and postdialysis values were plotted against each other, the slope of the relationship was close to zero (Figure 29.9, right panel). (The investigators actually plotted the difference on the X-axis against the initial value, but this had almost no effect on the results.)

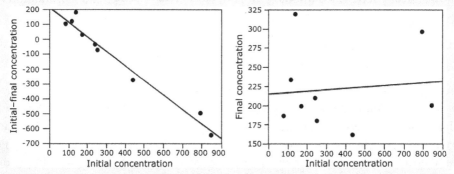

Figure 29.9 Left panel: initial values plotted against difference between initial and final concentrations. Right panel: initial values plotted against final concentrations.

The slope of almost -1 is similar to that obtained by Oldham who used random numbers. In Figure 29.9 (left panel), the slope was -0.9811 and r^2 was 0.961 ($P < 0.0001$), and in the right panel the slope was 0.0189, with r^2 of 0.1308 ($P = 0.79$). What did the experiment show? It seems simplest to regard the right panel as indicating no relationship between initial and final values. Another example is a study of carbamazepine dosage purporting to show a high correlation between the metabolite–drug ratio and the drug dose–concentration ratio (van Belle and Friel, 1986). The previous finding of a high correlation (0.89–0.94) that would allow accurate estimates of patient compliance was shown to be spurious, and corrected analyses were given.

Cautionary Tales—cont'd

The fallacy in many of these studies comes from ignoring the pervasive phenomenon of regression to the mean. Any subject's measurements vary from time to time. For example, systolic blood pressure is not constant. If subject A has a high pressure at time t_0, it is likely that it will be lower at time t_1. Conversely, a subject whose initial pressure is low is likely to have a later pressure that is higher. This phenomenon is shown by the data of Musso et al. in Table 29.3.

Table 29.3 Norepinephrine concentrations before and after dialysis

Initial value	Final value	Initial − Final value
81	186	105
119	233	114
140	319	179
174	199	95
245	209	−36
254	180	−74
439	162	−277
794	296	−498
847	200	−647

The high values decreased and the low values increased, and this is more in keeping with regression to the mean than an effect of dialysis. The right panel in Figure 29.9, showing no relation between the initial and final norepinephrine concentrations, suggests that this conclusion is correct.

Ratios and Scaling Factors

When the independent, dependent, or both variables are made into ratios, the possibility of spurious association looms large. Think about the innumerable measurements taken as a ratio to body surface area (cardiac output, glomerular filtration rate, oxygen uptake), or the incidence per million population, to realize that regressions using ratios are common. One of the earliest warnings about this practice was made by Tanner (1949) and was reinforced by many other studies. Although some disagree with the criticisms (Firebaugh and Gibbs, 1985), it would be wise to proceed very cautiously. Positive, negative, or zero correlations may all be incorrectly attained.

Kronmal (1993) recommended using multiple regression equations to avoid the ratio problem, for example, rather than relating FEV1/height^2 to age, as done in some studies (for example, in men FEV1/height^2 = 1.42 − 0.008Age), it would be better to calculate the multiple regression equation (Chapter 30).

$$FEV1 = 1.61 - 0.023 \text{ Age} + 0.899 \text{ height}^2 \text{ (for men).}$$

Others have recommended this approach, or else use analysis of covariance to avoid these problems (Vickers, 2001; Williams et al., 1984; Vickers and Altman, 2001), Nevill et al. advised using logarithmic functions. For example, they showed that when relating running speed (Y) to oxygen uptake (X) and body weight (Z), spurious correlation was avoided by calculating

$$Z = 84.3 Y^{1.01} X^{1.03}$$

Kronmal (1993) summed up the field by quoting Neyman: "Spurious correlations have been ruining empirical statistical research from times immemorial."

Intraclass Correlation

In Chapter 25, Table 25.2 gave weight gains of piglets with different added amounts of Vitamin B_{12}, and the question about whether the amount of vitamin added affected weight gain was answered by a one-way analysis of variance (ANOVA). We could also ask about the correlation between the different groups, something known as the intraclass correlation coefficient (ICC). There is variability between doses, estimated as S_B^2, the between group mean square. There is also a common within group mean square, estimated by S_W^2. Then the ICC (Snedecor and Cochran, 1989; Uebersax, 2008; Everitt, 1989) is

$$ICC = \frac{S_B^2}{S_B^2 + S_W^2}.$$

If there were no variability within each dose, then all the variability would be between the groups (classes), and ICC would be 1. In practice ICC is never 1, but the higher it is, the more the variability is due to intraclass variability than to intersubject variability.

In Chapter 15, the kappa statistic was used to examine the correlation between two raters. To examine the correlation between more than two raters, a modified intraclass correlation can be used. The model is based on the relationship X = true value + rater effect + error. Each of these components has variability. The variability of the true value is S_B^2, the variability due to error is S_W^2, and the variability due to rater differences is s_r^2. These variances are assumed to be independent, and the rater and error terms are assumed to each have a mean of zero. Then the variance of X is estimated by $S_B^2 + S_W^2 - S_r^2$, and the ICC is

$$ICC = \frac{S_B^2}{S_B^2 + S_W^2 - S_r^2}.$$

Assume that the data shown previously in Table 25.1 from a two-way ANOVA, with the different doses of vitamin being replaced by four raters, the replicates by three different subjects, and the data being some form of clinical score (Table 29.4).

Table 29.4 Hypothetical clinical scores

	Rater A	Rater B	Rater C	Rater D
Subject 1	1.30	1.26	1.29	1.38
Subject 2	1.19	1.21	1.23	1.27
Subject 3	1.08	1.19	1.23	1.22

These produce the ANOVA table in Table 29.5.

Table 29.5 ANOVA table for hypothetical rater data. In this table, r is the number of raters, and n is the number of subjects per group. E(MS) indicates what the mean square estimates

Source of variation	SS	DF	MS	E(MS)
Total	0.059025	11		
Between raters	0.016425	3	0.005475	$\sigma_W^2 - n\sigma_b^2$
Between subjects	0.03345	2	0.01672	$\sigma_W^2 + r\sigma_b^2$
Within	0.00915	6	0.001525	σ_W^2

These formulas allow estimation of the individual variances:

$$S_r^2 = \frac{MS_r - MS_W}{N} = \frac{0.005475 - 0.001525}{3} = 0.001317,$$

$$\text{and } S_B^2 = \frac{MS_B - MS_W}{r} = \frac{0.01672 - 0.001525}{4} = 0.003799.$$

Therefore, $ICC = \frac{0.003799}{0.003799 + 0.001317 + 0.001525} = 0.5721$. In this example interrater variability is fairly large; if it had been small, the ICC would have been closer to 1.

Some variations on this theme are presented by Uebersax (2008) depending on how the raters are selected. Fleiss (1986) also describes various methods of handling discrepancies among raters.

Another way of looking at the intraclass correlation is to assess reliability (Fleiss, 1986). Consider measuring some variable (e.g., blood pressure, attitude to some social issue), and repeating the measurement several times. Then the measured value X_i may be thought of as having two components: a "true" or "error-free" value T_i and a random error ε_i. Thus, $X_i = T_i + \varepsilon_i$. Assume that a variable such as blood pressure or attitude may vary from moment to moment around some "true" value μ, with variance σ_T^2, and that the random error is unrelated to the value of T, and has a mean of zero and a variance of σ_ε^2. Then the variance of X will be $\sigma_X^2 = \sigma_T^2 + \sigma_\varepsilon^2$. The relative magnitude of these two components of variability is $R = \frac{\sigma_T^2}{\sigma_T^2 + \sigma_\varepsilon^2}$. R is another form of intraclass correlation, but in view of its components is termed the coefficient of reliability. R varies between 0 and 1, and can be interpreted directly as a proportion of variance due to random error, unlike the usual interpretation in which r^2 expresses the proportion of variance explained by the regression relationship.

One consequence of unreliability is that it lowers the calculated correlation between two variables. In estimating the correlation between two variables T and U, what is actually measured are $X_i = T_i + \varepsilon_i$, and $Y_j = U_j + \varepsilon_j$, where ε_i and ε_j are unrelated, and the true correlation between T and U is ρ_{TU}. The correlation between the measured values X and Y is

$$\rho_{XY} = \rho_{TU}\sqrt{R_X R_Y},$$

where R_X and R_Y are the reliabilities of the two measured variables. Thus, if the reliability of each measurement is 0.7 and 0.8, respectively,

$$\rho_{XY} = \rho_{TU}\sqrt{0.7 \times 0.8} = 0.75\rho_{TU}$$

so that the true correlation has been reduced by 25%.

This relationship can be used also to determine the sample sizes needed to determine significance of a given mean difference (Everitt, 1989), and the required number is always bigger than the error-free number (N_f) by a factor of N_f/R.

As expected, replication improves reliability. If m replicate measurements are made, then

$$R_m = \frac{mR}{1 + (m-1)R},$$

where R is the reliability of a single measurement (Everitt, 1989).

APPENDIX

1. Spearman's rank correlation coefficient is merely the Pearson correlation coefficient with ranks replacing the numerical values:

$$r_s = \frac{\sum\left[Xrank - \left(\frac{N+1}{2}\right)\right]\left[Yrank - \left(\frac{N+1}{2}\right)\right]}{\dfrac{N(N-1)(N-2)}{12}}.$$

2. Related expressions

   The equations for slope (b) and correlation coefficient (r) can be displayed in several equivalent forms. It may be useful to know some of these if you want to recalculate results from a report that does not give the original data:

$$r = \frac{S_x}{S_y}b \text{ and } b = \frac{S_y}{S_x}r.$$

REFERENCES

Archie Jr., J.P., 1981. Mathematic coupling of data: a common source of error. Ann. Surg. 193, 296—303.

Beer, D.J., Osband, M.E., McCaffrey, R.P., Soter, N.A., Rocklin, R.E., 1982. Abnormal histamine-induced suppressor-cell function in atopic subjects. N. Engl. J. Med. 306, 454—458.

Bland, M., 1995. An Introduction to Medical Statistics. Oxford University Press, Oxford.

Boer, P., 1990. Misleading statistics: predialysis norepinephrine and its change after hemodialysis. Nephron 55, 78—80.

Campbell, M.J., Machen, D., 1993. Medical Statistics. A Commonsense Approach. John Wiley & Sons, Chichester.

Caruana Jr., J.A., Gage, A.A., 1980. Increased uptake of insulin and glucagon by the liver as a signal for regeneration. Surg. Gynecol. Obstet. 150, 390—394.

Chatillon, G., 1984. The balloon rules for a rough estimate of the correlation coefficient. Am. Stat. 1.

Cohen, J., 1988. Statistical Power Analysis for Behavioral Sciences. Lawrence Erlbaum Associates, Hillsdale, NJ.

Cohen, J., Cohen, P., 1975. Applied Multiple Regression/Correlation Analysis in the Social Sciences. John Wiley& Sons, New York.

Conover, W.J., 1980. Practical Nonparametric Statistics. John Wiley & Sons, New York.

Curran-Everett, D., 2010. Explorations in statistics: correlation. Adv. Physiol. Educ. 34, 186—191.

Edwards, A.L., 1984. An Introduction to Linear Regression and Correlation. W.H.Freeman and Co, New York.

Everitt, B.S., 1989. Statistical Methods for Medical Investigations. Oxford University Press, New York.

Firebaugh, G., Gibbs, J.P., 1985. User's guide to ratio variables. Am. Sociol. Rev. 50, 713—722.

Fleiss, J.L., 1986. The Design and Analysis of Clinical Experiments. John Wiley & Sons, New York.

Glantz, S.A., 2005. Primer of Biostatistics. McGraw-Hill, New York.

Kleinbaum, D.G., Kupper, L.L., Muller, K.E., 1988. Applied Regression Analysis and Other Multivariable Methods. PWS-KENT Publishing Company, Boston.

Kronmal, R.A., 1993. Spurious correlation and the fallacy of the ratio standard revisited. J. R. Stat. Soc. Ser. A Stat. Soc. 3, 379—392.

Lindner, J.R., Coggins, M.P., Kaul, S., Klibanov, A.L., Brandenburger, G.H., Ley, K., 2000. Microbubble persistence in the microcirculation during ischemia/reperfusion and inflammation is caused by integrin- and complement-mediated adherence to activated leukocytes. Circulation 101, 668—675.

Loh, W.-Y., 1987. Does the correlation coefficient really measure the degree of clustering around a line? J. Educ. Stat. 12, 235—239.

Mena, E.A., Kossovsky, N., Chu, C., Hu, C., 1995. Inflammatory intermediates produced by tissues encasing silicone breast prostheses. J. Invest. Surg. 8, 31—42.

Moreno, L.F., Stratton, H.H., Newell, J.C., Feustel, P.J., 1986. Mathematical coupling of data: correction of a common error for linear calculations. J. Appl. Physiol. (1985) 60, 335—343.

Musso, N.R., Deferrari, G., Pende, A., Vergassola, C., Saffioti, S., Gurreri, G., Lotti, G., 1989. Free and sulfoconjugated catecholamines in normotensive uremic patients: effects of hemodialysis. Nephron 51, 344—349.

Nevill, A.M., Holder, R.L., Mcshane, P., Kronmal, R.A., Letters to the Editor. Spurious correlations and the fallacy of the ratio standard revisited. J. R. Stat. Soc. Ser. A Stat. Soc. 158, 619—625.

Oldham, P.D., 1962. A note on the analysis of repeated measurements on the same subjects. J. Chronic Dis. 15, 969—977.

Rim, S.J., Leong-Poi, H., Lindner, J.R., Wei, K., Fisher, N.G., Kaul, S., 2001. Decrease in coronary blood flow reserve during hyperlipidemia is secondary to an increase in blood viscosity. Circulation 104, 2704—2709.

Schwarzacher, S.P., Uren, N.G., Ward, M.R., Schwarzkopf, A., Giannetti, N., Hunt, S., Fitzgerald, P.J., Oesterle, S.N., Yeung, A.C., 2000. Determinants of coronary remodeling in transplant coronary disease: a simultaneous intravascular ultrasound and Doppler flow study. Circulation 101, 1384—1389.

Senzaki, H., Isoda, T., Paolocci, N., Ekelund, U., Hare, J.M., Kass, D.A., 2000. Improved mechanoenergetics and cardiac rest and reserve function of in vivo failing heart by calcium sensitizer EMD-57033. Circulation 101, 1040—1048.

Snedecor, G.W., Cochran, W.G., 1989. Statistical Methods. Iowa State University Press, Ames, Iowa.

Swanson, P., Leverton, R., Gram, M.R., Roberts, H., Pesek, I., 1955. Blood values of women: cholesterol. J. Gerontol. 10, 41–47.

Tanner, J.M., 1949. Fallacy of per-weight and per-surface area standards, and their relation to spurious correlation. J. Appl. Physiol. 2, 1–15.

Tu, Y.K., Clerehugh, V., Gilthorpe, M.S., 2004a. Ratio variables in regression analysis can give rise to spurious results: illustration from two studies in periodontology. J. Dent. 32, 143–151.

Tu, Y.K., Maddick, I.H., Griffiths, G.S., Gilthorpe, M.S., 2004b. Mathematical coupling can undermine the statistical assessment of clinical research: illustration from the treatment of guided tissue regeneration. J. Dent. 32, 133–142.

Uebersax, J., 2008. Statistical Methods for Rater Agreement [Online]. Available: http://john-uebersax.com/stat/agree.htm.

van Belle, G., 2002. Statistical Rules of Thumb. Wiley Interscience, New York.

van Belle, G., Friel, P.N., 1986. Problem of spurious correlation in the evaluation of steady-state carbamazepine levels using metabolite data. Ther. Drug Monit. 8, 177–183.

Vickers, A.J., 2001. The use of percentage change from baseline as an outcome in a controlled trial is statistically inefficient: a simulation study. BMC Med. Res. Methodol. 1, 6.

Vickers, A.J., Altman, D.G., 2001. Statistics notes: analysing controlled trials with baseline and follow up measurements. BMJ 323, 1123–1124.

Williams, G.W., Forsythe, S.B., Textor, S.C., Tarazi, R.C., 1984. Analysis of relative change and initial value in biological studies. Am. J. Physiol. 246, R122–R126.

Zar, J.H., 2010. Biostatistical Analysis. Prentice Hall, Upper Saddle River, NJ.

CHAPTER 30

Multiple Regression

Contents

BASIC CONCEPTS

Introduction

This chapter is advanced, and inexperienced statisticians should not perform these analyses on their own. Nevertheless all investigators and even most readers should be aware of the issues. Few dependent variables are related to only one independent variable, and nonlinear relationships are common. The intent of this chapter is to provide

For a list of all websites referred to in this chapter, as clickable links, see the book companion website: www.booksite.elsevier.com/9780128023877.

Biostatistics for Medical and Biomedical Practitioners
http://dx.doi.org/10.1016/B978-0-12-802387-7.00030-5

basic understanding of when and how to proceed with these analyses and what difficulties to take into account.

Frequently, a dependent variable Y is a function of more than one explanatory variable, so that the general equation is $\widehat{Y}_i = c + b_1 X_1 + b_2 X_2 + ... b_k X_k$ or $Y_i = c + b_1 X_1 + b_2 X_2 + ... b_k X_k + \varepsilon_i$ for the dependence of Y on k different X variables. In principle the same procedure is used as for simple bivariate regression. An equation is sought that minimizes the sum of the squared deviations from regression $\sum \varepsilon_i^2$ and maximizes the (multiple) correlation coefficient, here termed R.

To minimize $\sum \varepsilon_i^2$, the coefficients are calculated by formulas similar to those used for bivariate regression (Edwards, 1984; Glantz and Slinker, 2001). The computations should be done with computer programs. Despite the complexity, there are several freeware online programs. One of them named AutoFit at http://www.eskimo.com/~brainy/ allows you to run the regression, or send the data to the Web site for free analysis. The site at http://home.ubalt.edu/ntsbarsh/Business-stat/otherapplets/MultRgression.htm allows 4 X variables but only 16 samples. The sites at http://www.xuru.org/rt/MLR.asp and http://vassarstats.net/ allow many more samples and dependent variables. Many of these programs allow you to copy and paste from your data sheet. These free programs will usually not perform the subsidiary analyses discussed below.

Multiple Linear Regression with Two X Variables

This is the simplest form of multiple regression and illustrates the main features. The basic regression equation is

$$\widehat{Y}_i = c + b_1 X_1 + b_2 X_2, \quad \text{or} \quad Y_i = c + b_1 X_1 + b_2 X_2 + \varepsilon_i.$$

The equation of best fit (it is no longer a line) has an intercept that represents the value of Y when all the X values are zero. This intercept is

$$c = \overline{Y} - \left(b_1 \overline{X_1} + b_2 \overline{X_2} \right).$$

For two independent X variables the equation defines a plane or surface. Imagine this as a set of bivariate relations relating Y to X_1 with X_2 held constant, and Y to X_2 holding X_1 constant. The requirements for multiple regression are similar to those for bivariate regression—ratio numbers, independence, normal distributions, equal variances—but these are more difficult to evaluate with several independent variables.

Once the regression equation has been obtained, the question is if each of the two coefficients is significantly different from zero. Even though two independent variables have been measured, one of them might not offer any predictive information. To test the individual coefficients, use the formula

$$S_{b_1} = \sqrt{\frac{s_{Y \cdot X}^2 (or\ MS_{res})}{\sum \left(X_i - \overline{X_1} \right)^2 \left(1 - r_{X_1 X_2}^2 \right)}}$$

for b_1, and a corresponding formula for b_2

$$S_{b_2} = \sqrt{\frac{s_{Y \cdot X}^2 (or\ MS_{res})}{\sum (X_i - \overline{X_2})^2 (1 - r_{X_1 X_2}^2)}}.$$

This formula uses the squared correlation between X_1 and X_2, $r_{X_1 X_2}^2$. If X_1 and X_2 are completely uncorrelated so that $r^2 = 0$, the expression for the standard deviation of b becomes the same as that for a bivariate linear relationship. If X_1 and X_2 are highly correlated, for example, $r = 0.9$, then the variance of b_1 or b_2 becomes 10 times larger, making it much more difficult to reject the null hypothesis that $b_i = 0$. The variance of b_i is also large if $s_{Y \cdot X}^2$ is big or $\sum (X_i - \overline{X_i})^2$ is small, so that the correlation between explanatory variables is not the only factor to be considered.

Perform a t-test on each coefficient. Then

$$t_1 = \frac{b_1}{s_{b_1}} \quad or \quad t_2 = \frac{b_2}{s_{b_2}}.$$

t is evaluated with $n - 3$ degrees of freedom—one for each variable.

In the multiple regression equation, the coefficient c is the intercept, and just as in simple linear regression it represents the value of $\overline{Y}$ when all the X variables are zero. Each coefficient (b_1 or b_2), shows how much $\overline{Y}$ changes for a one unit change in one variable when the other is kept constant, and is termed a partial regression coefficient.

The above example with two independent variables can be extended to more independent variables. In a study relating systolic blood pressure to age, weight, height, subcutaneous fat thickness, and arm size, Whyte (1959) observed

Systolic pressure (mm Hg) $= 165 + 0.35$ weight (lbs) $- 0.01$ age (years) $- 1.55$ height (in) $- 0.09$ fat (mm) $+ 0.81$ arm size (cm).

It is also possible to calculate standardized coefficients, represented by $b*$, as

$$b^* = b_1 \frac{s_{X_i}}{s_Y},$$

where b_i is the regression coefficient in question, s_{X_i} is the standard deviation of variate X_i, and s_Y is the standard deviation of variate Y. This is interpreted as the change in standard deviation of predicted Y for a 1 standard deviation change in X_i if the remaining X variates remain constant. The value for $b*$ ranges from $+1$ to -1, and indicates the strength of the association between Y and X_i without the need to consider units. The regression equation obtained by Whyte (above) can be changed into standardized units to give.

Systolic pressure (mm Hg) $= 0.513$ weight (lbs) $- 0.004$ age (years) $- 0.272$ height (in) $- 0.086$ fat (mm) $+ 0.133$ arm size (cm). (The coefficients for fat and arm thickness were not significant.)

In this form the coefficients indicate the relative importance of the X variables. Weight is therefore the single most important variable because it has the highest standardized coefficient of 0.513. Neither equation tells us how good the prediction equation is. This has to be determined by the multiple correlation coefficient that, at 0.24, was small.

Multiple Collinearity

This is an important complicating factor. The expression for the standard deviation from regression shows that s_b is smallest when $r^2_{X_1 X_2}$ is smallest. The more closely X_1 and X_2 are correlated with each other the higher their correlation is, the smaller the component $1 - r^2_{X_1 X_2}$ will be, so that the denominator of the expression for s_b becomes smaller, and s_b becomes bigger.

High degrees of correlation are common. When they occur, the resulting analyses become erratic, with unpredictable consequences. The R^2 in predicting Y is still accurate, with perhaps a low P value, but the contributions of individual predictors may be incompatible with a high predictive value. In addition, the confidence limits will be very wide, and adding or subtracting a single value can materially alter the regression equation.

A different random sample from the populations of Y, X_1, and X_2 should give similar even if not identical coefficients, and we can envisage a stack of planes that are close to each other and approximately parallel. If X_1 and X_2 are highly correlated, however, other samples could have wildly different coefficients and planes. This is the serious consequence of multicollinearity. Glantz and Slinker (Glantz and Slinker, 2001; Slinker and Glantz, 1985) give examples of this problem and explain it well. Other helpful descriptions of multicollinearity appear in the books by Kleinbaum et al. (1988) and Neter et al. (1996).

The multiple regression technique used above can be extended to many X variates.

Prerequisites

These are ratio numbers, normality of distribution, independence of measurements, linearity, and homoscedasticity, as well as absence of multicollinearity. The requirements may be more difficult to determine by casual inspection than in simple bivariate regression because a single scattergram may not suffice to show problems. Normality can be tested but is not important if sample size is large. Independence of observations is often obvious, but if, for example, a time-dependent relationship is present, a test such as the Durbin–Watson test (Chapter 31) can be done. Of more importance are linearity and homoscedasticity, because in their absence the tests of hypotheses may be erroneous. Linearity and homoscedasticity can be examined by plotting residuals of predicted against observed dependent variables for the whole data set.

This global test, however, does not mean that all individual relationships are linear. One way to test this is to do residual analyses for the bivariate relationship of the dependent variable to each of the independent variables. Examples are shown in the advanced section below.

Determining the "Best" Regression

After determining the regression equation relating Y to several X variates, decide which of the X variates adds significantly to the prediction of Y. Ideally, the model should include all the relevant X variates that determine Y. If these are all present there is a *correctly specified* model, one in which the various components are estimated without bias. If some important determinants are left out, the model is *underspecified*, leading to incorrect and biased coefficients and increased variability, as shown by comparing linear with quadratic regression described in the previous chapter. If there are *extraneous* factors unrelated to the Y or any of the other X variates, they do not affect the results except that it takes more work to collect and analyze the data. Finally, if redundant factors are present, the model is *overspecified* and risks multicollinearity problems.

With many X variables, there are several ways of proceeding. One is to examine all possible combinations of the X variables, known as all subsets regression. The program determines R^2 and residual sums of squares (SS_{res}) for all possible combinations of the X variates. If there are many variables, and especially if powers of the variables and cross products of the variables are included, not only may this overwhelm the computer but it provides so many results that selecting the best one is difficult. Some criterion is needed to indicate which of the many equations gives a useful relationship. One of the ways of doing this is to examine the multiple correlation coefficient R^2, and especially the adjusted R^2. One way of telling if additional X variates contribute to the regression is to calculate R^2 that increases as more variates are introduced. In applying this technique to a regression with many independent X variates, R^2 always increases with each added factor, even if in the population no change in correlation has occurred. R^2 has a slight positive bias that is particularly likely to occur if the number of variates (k) is large relative to sample size, N (Lucke and Whitely, 1984); the expected value of R^2 by chance is $k/(N-1)$. To allow for this source of error most programs calculate an adjusted R^2:

Adjusted $R^2 = 1 - (1 - R^2)\frac{N-1}{N-k-1}$, where N is the sample size and k is the number of regressors. If k is small relative to N then the adjusted R^2 and R^2 will be similar, but if k is large relative to N the two forms of R^2 will differ. There is a convenient online calculator for this adjustment at http://danielsoper.com/statcalc3/calc.aspx?id=25.

The better the equation fits the data the higher the value for R^2 and the lower the SS_{res} will be.

Another method for assessing the number of variables needed to avoid underspecification (see below) is the C_p statistic developed by Mallows in 1964 (Mallows, 1973). In essence, C_p is the ratio between the residual mean square (MS_{res}) calculated from a subset of the variates to the total MS_{res} with a correction. Formally, it is

$$C_p = \frac{MS_{res \cdot p}}{MS_{res \cdot k}} - (N - 2p).$$

N is the total sample size, k is the total number of variates, and p is the reduced number of X variates being examined. Because the model includes the intercept, p is one more than the number of variates included. The closer C_p is to p, the better specified is the equation. The statistic should not be used to choose one "best" model, but rather to choose models to exclude because their values of C_p are much greater than p. Small differences for C_p should not be used to decide which models to include.

Some programs include the Akaike "an information criterion (AIC)" based on maximal likelihood principles. $\text{AIC} = 2k + N \ln\left(\frac{2\pi SS_{res}}{N}\right) + 1$, where k is the number of parameters (here X variates plus the equation constant). Because the AIC is a ranking rather than an absolute index, the constant 2π and $+1$ values can be removed, leaving

$$\text{AIC} = 2k + N \ln\left(\frac{SS_{res}}{N}\right).$$

The AIC attempts to find the minimum number of free parameters that explains the data, so that the lower the value of AIC, the more likely is it that superfluous parameters are excluded. As for C_p, the AIC should be used to select the few regressions with the lowest values to concentrate on, rather than being used to select the best single combination of parameters.

Other criteria have been proposed, one of which is Schwarz's Bayesian information criterion (BIC) (Schwarz, 1979). This may be written as

$\text{BIC} = N \ln\left(\frac{SS_{res}}{N}\right) + k \ln N$, where N is the number of data points, and k is the number of X variates. It is similar to the AIC except for the logarithm of N in the second term. This expression penalizes excess parameters more heavily than does the AIC, and it also penalizes larger sample sizes that have the disadvantage of making even small differences significant (Ramsey and Schafer, 2002). Like the AIC, the smaller the value for BIC, the more useful the model is likely to be.

There is no perfect way of selecting the best regression. Probably the combination of good fit and biological sense allows for effective data fitting.

If there are too many variables for all subsets regression, some alternatives are forward stepwise regression, backward stepwise regression, and mixed regression. Forward stepwise regression starts with the highest bivariate correlation, say between Y and X_3. Then it adds another variable, perhaps one with the next highest bivariate correlation, and tests by analysis of variance (ANOVA) to determine if there has been a significant reduction in the SS_{res} and thus a significant increase in adjusted R^2. The process continues until no further significant change in adjusted R^2 occurs. Backward stepwise regression begins with all the variables included, and then recalculates the adjusted R^2 after omitting the X variate with the lowest bivariate correlation with Y. If the change is not significant, the inference is that the deleted X variate was not a factor. Then the next X variate is deleted, and the process continues until deleting an X variate produces a significant change in adjusted R^2, so then that variate is retained and the final equation is determined. If there are many X variates these two stepwise regression techniques may reach different conclusions, and sometimes the order in which variates are included or excluded makes a difference. As an alternative, the mixed (sometimes called stepwise) regression technique is used. The procedure begins like the forward regression method, but after each addition of a variable a backward elimination is done to see if any of the variables previously included have become redundant. It is possible for variables to be added, removed, added in again, and so on as the regression equation changes. In fact, different results can occur if variables are entered in a different order, or if variables are entered in sets. It is also possible for the forward, backward, and stepwise regression methods to end up with different sets of variables. The more variables there are in the full regression equation the more the potentiality for error. If the different regression methods selected a common set of variables, then these could very well be the important ones to consider. If they selected different sets of variables, then it is for the investigator to evaluate the usefulness of each variable as a predictor, based on prior knowledge, or even to select a likely subset of variables and repeat the experiment or observational study.

Which Is the Best Regression?

Numerous methods have been proposed to determine the "best" regression model, but the notion of "best" is not well defined (Hocking, 1976). The investigator has to use common sense and not rely too much on complex and often poorly understood statistical techniques. An excellent discussion of the advantages and disadvantages of each selection method is presented by Katz (2006). He recommends the forward selection method for relatively small sample sizes or if there is concern about multicollinearity, the backward selection method if there are likely to be suppressor variables, and the best subset regression if the number of explanatory variables is small. Katz comments too that elimination of regressor variables is usually better justified by biological insights than statistical techniques.

One difficulty with all of these complex regressions is that they are designed to minimize the errors for that particular set of data. Despite achieving significant coefficients, there is no guarantee that another data set will find the same coefficients or even the same set of variables. To guard against this contingency, use a criterion sample. If the sample is big enough, divide it into two portions at random. Then determine the regression equation for the first portion of the data, sometimes referred to as the training portion. If the regression based on the second portion, sometimes referred to as the validation portion, matches that of the first half, it gives reassurance that the selected variables are important contributors to the regression. In one such study (Thursz et al., 1995), the effect of various MHC class I and class II antigens in the clearance of hepatitis B virus (HBV) was examined in 1344 children, about one-third of whom were positive for HBV core antibody. Many apparent associations were detected. When these associations were assessed in 235 adults exposed to HBV, only a few of these associations were confirmed. Other examples of this validation procedure are readily found (Haricharan et al., 2009; Richardson et al., 2001).

Residual analysis is important, especially if sample size is <100. One approach is to plot the residuals (predicted − observed values) for the full model against the dependent variable and each independent variable. As with any other regression residuals, linearity, normality, and homoscedasticity can be tested (Glantz and Slinker, 2001; Mendenhall and Sincich, 1986). If any residual plots seem to depart substantially from the ideal, it may be worth transforming one of the variables.

Nonlinear Regression: Polynomial Regression

If in a bivariate regression the relationship is clearly alinear, then linear regression is inefficient. If there is a known mechanism, for example, a logarithmic or exponential relationship, then either the Y or the X variate can be transformed, and a linear regression can be done on the transformed variables. If logarithmic transformations are to be performed, some practical issues are described clearly by Motulsky (2009). If no suitable transformation is known, then fitting a power function, a specific form of multiple regression, may be valuable. These functions are of the form

$$\widehat{Y}_i = c + b_1 X_1 + b_2 X_i^2 + b_3 X_i^3 + ...b_k X_i^k.$$

A function including X^2 is a quadratic, X^3 is cubic, X^4 is quartic, X^5 is quintic, and so on. A quadratic expression produces a parabola, and because parabolas have different curvature in different portions and because curvature varies with the parabola's focal length, this is often the most general form of curved regression used. These computations are computer intensive, and can be done online at http://www.xuru.org/rt/PR.asp and http://polynomialregression.drque.net/online.php.

Although in theory any number of powers can be used, it seldom makes sense to go beyond a cubic form. This point was emphasized by Montgomery and Peck (1982) who wrote:

> It is important to keep the order of the model as low as possible. When the response function appears to be curvilinear, transformations should be tried to keep the model first-order...If this fails, a second-order polynomial should be tried. As a general rule the use of high-order polynomials ($k > 2$) should be avoided unless they can be justified for reasons outside the data. A low-order model in a transformed variable is almost always preferable to a high-order model in the original metric. Arbitrary fitting of high-order polynomials is a serious abuse of regression analysis.

Conclusions about Regression Methods in General

The key to effective multiple regression methods is to design the study correctly. Apart from asking significant questions and making the required measurements accurately, care must be taken to have an adequate sample size. Unlike the usual power calculations, what is at stake here is the number of variables examined relative to the total number of subjects. Altman (1992) recommends no more than $N/10$ variables, where N is the total sample size. Katz (14) recommends determining the power of the various bivariate relationships; if any of these have inadequate power then the multiple regression is also likely to be underpowered. Commercial programs such as Power and Precision or PASS are available. Discussions of these issues are presented in a number of studies (Concato et al., 1995; Harrell et al., 1985; Peduzzi et al., 1995).

Fitting the data by a regression equation should be regarded as the beginning of the analysis and not an end in itself. After checking for outliers and errors, the resulting equation has to be useful. The purpose of the modeling is not merely to produce an equation that fits the data, but to be able to predict future values of the dependent Y variable and to assess the relative importance of the explanatory factors.

As summarized by Chatfield (1988), the objectives in model building include:

1. To provide a parsimonious summary or description of one or more sets of data.

2. To provide a basis for comparing several sets of data.

3. To confirm or refute a theoretical relationship suggested a priori.

4. To describe the properties of the random or residual variation…to assess the uncertainty in any conclusion.

5. To provide predictions which act as a "yardstick" or norm, even when the model is known not to hold for some reason.

6. To provide physical insight into the underlying physical process….

Chatfield does not consider "trying lots of different models until a good-looking fit is obtained" to be one of the purposes of model building, and points out further that the "choice between models which fit data approximately equally well should be made on grounds external to the data." The more complex the statistical analysis, for example, multiple regression, the more his advice should be taken to heart.

There are several ways of validating these models after their construction.

One is to evaluate the coefficients to see if they make sense from a physical or biological point of view. Test the model by inserting reasonable values for the independent variable(s) to make sure that the predicted value of Y appears to be reasonable, and that, for example, an impossible negative value is not calculated.

A second is to add new data and then make sure that the revised prediction equation is little altered from the original equation. This is essential, because any form of regression modeling is designed to optimize the prediction for that data set, and it is important to know if it remains stable and predictive when more data are added.

A third approach is to split the existing data set into two portions, sometimes called the training and holdout (or validation) portions, and compare the resulting equations. There are several ways of doing this (Chatfield, 1989; Garfinkel and Fegley, 1984; Jamal et al., 2001; Ramsey and Schafer 2002). One simple approach is to compute the predicted values in the training and holdout groups separately, and then for each group calculate r^2 between observed and predicted Y values. The difference r^2(training) $- r^2$ (holdout) is called shrinkage and is usually positive. If it is small (e.g., about 0.10), then the fitting process was probably reliable and it is reasonable to pool the two data sets and determine a final regression equation. Greater shrinkage suggests unreliability and suggests caution.

ADVANCED CONCEPTS AND EXAMPLES

For those who want to see the principles mentioned above in practice, detailed examples are presented below.

Multiple Regression with Many Independent *X* Variates

Table 30.1 features a number of variables in patients with cystic fibrosis (O'Neill et al., 1983). These variables were considered those most likely to predict maximal static expiratory pressure (*PEmax*), a measure of malnutrition, and can be tested to determine the most useful explanatory or predictive model.

   PEmax is the dependent variable.

   Linearity and homoscedasticity can be examined by plotting residuals of predicted against observed *PEmax* for the whole data set (Figure 30.1).

Table 30.1 Cystic fibrosis data

Subject	Age	Gender	Height	Weight	BMP	FEV1	RV	FRC	TLC	PEmax
1	7	0	109	13.1	68	32	258	183	137	95
2	7	1	112	12.9	65	19	449	285	134	85
3	8	0	124	14.1	64	22	441	268	147	100
4	8	1	125	16.2	67	41	234	146	124	85
5	8	0	127	21.5	93	52	202	131	104	95
6	9	0	130	17.5	68	44	308	155	118	80
7	11	1	139	30.7	89	28	305	179	119	65
8	12	1	150	28.4	69	18	369	198	103	110
9	12	0	146	25.1	67	24	312	194	128	70
10	13	1	155	31.5	68	23	413	225	136	95
11	13	0	156	39.9	89	39	206	142	95	110
12	14	1	153	42.1	90	26	253	191	121	90
13	14	0	160	45.6	93	45	174	139	108	100
14	15	1	158	51.2	93	45	158	124	90	80
15	16	1	160	35.9	66	31	302	133	101	134
16	17	1	153	34.8	70	29	204	118	120	134
17	17	0	174	44.7	70	49	187	104	103	165
18	17	1	176	60.1	92	29	188	129	130	120
19	17	0	171	42.6	69	38	172	130	103	130
20	19	1	156	37.2	72	21	216	119	81	85
21	19	0	174	54.6	86	37	184	118	101	85
22	20	0	178	64	86	34	225	148	135	160
23	23	0	180	73.8	97	57	171	108	98	165
24	23	0	175	51.1	71	33	224	131	113	95
25	23	0	179	71.5	95	52	225	127	101	195

Gender 0 male, 1 female; BMP—body mass index as a percentage of age-specific normal median value; FEV1—forced expiratory volume in 1 s; RV—residual volume; FRC—functional residual capacity; TLC—total lung capacity; *PEmax*—maximal static expiratory pressure (cm H_2O).

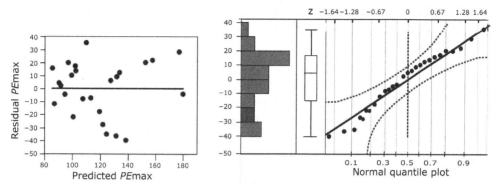

Figure 30.1 Left panel: Residual plot with all variables. Right panel: Quantile plot for Residual *PE*max. The plots do not show any marked alinearity or heteroscedasticity.

This global test, however, does not mean that all individual relationships are linear. One way to test this is to do residual analyses for the bivariate relationship of the dependent variable to each of the independent variables (Figure 30.2).

Although none of these individual bivariate regressions appear to be grossly alinear, there is an advantage to testing the linearity of all of the independent variates simultaneously. Some programs offer tests such as Ramsey's RESET test, also referred to as the

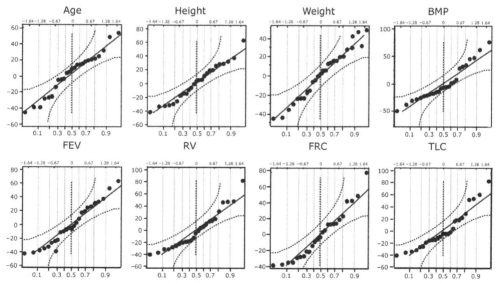

Figure 30.2 Residual distributions of *PE*max for different variables, and normal quantile plots for bivariate regressions.

Powers of Y (POY) test or a misspecification test (Ramsey, 1969). If the original equation can be summarized as $Y_{ii} = c + \sum b_i X_i + \varepsilon_i$, where $b_i X_i$ represents all the possible explanatory variables, then Ramsey's auxiliary equation is $Y_i = c + \sum b_i X_i + b_{i+1} \widehat{Y}^2 + b_{i+2} \widehat{Y}^3 \ldots + \varepsilon_i$; power >4 is seldom justified. The power functions are applied to the predicted values of Y. The null hypothesis is that the coefficients of the extra terms are all zero. If the hypothesis is rejected, then nonlinear terms must be included in the final analysis. To test the null hypothesis, the multiple correlation coefficients for the original data set R_O^2 and the auxiliary data set R_A^2 are compared by

$$\frac{\frac{R_A^2 - R_O^2}{k-1}}{\frac{1-R_A^2}{N-k}} \sim F_{(k-1, N-1)},$$ where N is the sample size and k is the number of auxiliary

parameters.

When this equation was calculated for the cystic fibrosis data,

$$\widehat{Y}_i = -437.31 + 4.93 Age - 7.19 Gender + 3.33 Height - 12.17 Weight + 6.03 BMP$$
$$- 4.79 FEV1 - 0.086 RV + 0.96 FRC - 0.040 TLC + 0.017 PEmax^2$$
$$+ 0.000023 PEmax^3$$

and $R_A^2 = 0.7591$. The adjusted R_O^2 without the power functions was 0.6349. Then the formula above gives

$\frac{\frac{0.7591 - 0.6349}{10}}{\frac{1 - 0.7591}{14}} = 0.72$. This value for F is too low to reject the null hypothesis, so there is

no evidence that alinearity is a problem; this confirms what is in Figure 30.2. Thursby and Schmidt (1977) suggested that a similar test based on powers of the explanatory variables might be better. This test can be performed online at http://www.wessa.net/esteq.wasp.

Other programs provide tests for heteroscedasticity, such as the tests by White, Glejser, or Breusch—Pagan—Godfrey (Chapter 27). These tests involve regressing the residuals or their logarithms against the independent variables, and some of the tests include power functions of the variables and their cross products.

White's test is important for assessing heteroscedasticity. It uses an auxiliary regression of the form

$$\widehat{\varepsilon_i}^2 = c + \beta_1 X_1 + \beta_2 X_2 + \ldots \beta_k X_k$$
$$+ \beta_{k+1} X_1^2 + \beta_{k+2} X_2^2 + \ldots \beta_{2k-1} X_k^2$$
$$+ \beta_{2k} X_1 X_2 + \beta_{2k+1} X_1 X_3 + \ldots \beta_{\frac{k(k-1)}{2}+1} X_{k-1} X_k + v_i,$$

where v_i is a normally distributed error term independent of ε. In other words, regress the square of the residuals against a constant, the original explanatory variables, the squares of the original explanatory variables, and the cross products of the explanatory variables.

As an example, consider the regression of *PE*max against weight, *FEV*1, and *BMP*. This results in the equation

$$\widehat{Y}_i = 126.01 + 1.53\,Weight + 1.11FEV1 - 1.46BMP.$$

From this, obtain the residuals and derive the auxiliary equation

$$\widehat{\varepsilon_i}^2 = -27295 - 6.42\,Weight + 644.01BMO + 166.02FEV1 + 0.21\,Weight^2$$
$$- 2.18FEV1^2 - 4.13BMP^2 + 0.11\,Weight \times BMP + 0.20\,Weight \times FEV1$$
$$+ 2.69BMP \times FEV1.$$

This equation has $R_A^2 = 0.355858$. To evaluate this, multiply it by N to get $24 \times 0.355858 = 8.54$. This is evaluated like chi-square with degrees of freedom equal to the number of coefficients excluding the constant. There are 9 such coefficients, and a chi-square of 8.54 with 9 degrees of freedom, so that P = 0.4807. There is thus no reason to consider heteroscedasticity, again confirming the results in Figure 30.2.

Analysis of Cystic Fibrosis Example

Begin by examining the regressions between *PE*max and each of the other (explanatory) variables (Table 30.2).

Table 30.2 Bivariate regression between *PE*max and the remaining variables

Variable	b	R^2	Adj R^2	RMSres	se	t	P
Age	4.0547	0.3764	0.3492	26.9736	1.0884	3.73	0.0011
Gender	−19.045				13.176	−1.45	0.16
Height	0.9319	0.3591	0.3312	27.3448	0.2596	3.59	0.0015
Weight	1.1867	0.4035	0.3776	26.3794	0.3009	3.94	0.0006
BMP	0.6392	0.0527	0.01149	33.2443	0.5652	1.13	0.2698
FEV1	1.3539	0.2056	0.1710	30.4440	0.5550	2.44	0.0228
RV	−0.1227	0.0996	0.0604	32.110	0.769	−1.59	0.1244
FRC	−0.2859	0.1662	0.1300	31.1883	0.1335	−2.14	0.0431
TLC	−0.3579	0.0330	−0.0091	33.5880	0.4041	−0.89	0.3849

Returning to Table 30.2, as R^2 gets smaller, the residual root mean square (RMSres) becomes bigger, because it is derived from the SS_{res} that is closer to the total sum of squares (SS_{total}) of the dependent variable that was 26,832.640. For the dichotomous variable gender, the coefficient −19.045 is the difference between the mean values for males and females, with females having a lower value than males.

The bivariate correlations in Table 30.2 are useful only to determine the best single explanatory variable, but give no information about combining explanatory variables. The next step is to examine the bivariate correlations between each of the explanatory

X variables to get more information about the model, and in particular determine the possibility of multicollinearity (Table 30.3).

Table 30.3 Bivariate correlation coefficients

	PEmax	Age	Gender	Height	Weight	BMP	FEV1	RV	FRC
Age	0.6135								
Gender	−0.289	−0.167							
Height	0.5992	**0.9261**	−0.1680						
Weight	0.6352	**0.9059**	−0.1990	**0.9207**					
BMP	0.2295	0.3778	−0.138	0.4413	0.6725				
FEV1	0.4534	0.2945	−0.528	0.3167	0.4483	0.5455			
RV	0.3156	0.5519	0.271	0.5695	0.6215	0.5824	0.6659		
FRC	0.4077	0.6378	0.184	0.6387	0.6157	0.4369	0.6588	**0.9136**	
TLC	0.1816	0.4694	0.024	0.4571	0.4185	0.3649	0.4430	0.5891	0.6870

R values >0.9 shown in bold type.

An extension of this matrix, suggested by Weisberg (1985) (see his Figure 6.2), is the matrix plot developed by Chambers et al. (1983). The correlation matrix shown in Table 30.3 is supplemented by a grid of bivariate plots, one for each pair of variates. This shows more clearly the form of the relationship and whether there are any obvious outliers.

Detecting Multicollinearity

Multicollinearity should be suspected if R^2 is high but the individual coefficients have unexpected values or unusually high standard errors. If any two variables, X_j and X_k, have a correlation coefficient above 0.8 you should be suspicious, and multiple collinearity is almost certain to be a problem if the correlation coefficient is over 0.95. This check is less useful if there are more than two X variables, because it is possible for redundancy to be present by virtue of the combination of several variables, not just two.

As an example, examine the regression between PEmax and both age and height. This yields the equation.

$\widehat{PE}\text{max} = 17.8600 + 2.7278Age + 0.3397Height$, with adjusted R^2 of 0.3271. The standard errors or the coefficients of age and height are respectively 2.9326 and 0.6900, both large.

Now regress PEmax on age, height, and weight to get

$$\widehat{PE}\text{max} = 64.3793 + 1.5553Age - 0.0728Height + 0.8689Weight.$$

The adjusted R^2 has increased slightly to 0.3277, and the standard errors of the coefficients are respectively 3.1489, 0.8016, and 0.8601. Thus although we have gained little predictive ability by adding in weight (and did not expect to because weight and height are highly correlated), there have been big changes in the standard errors and big changes in the coefficients; for example, the coefficient for height has changed from 0.3397 to -0.0728, and for age from 2.7278 to 1.5553. Similarly, if another highly correlated variate, *BMP*, is added, the coefficients and standard errors change unpredictably (Table 30.4). Such changes suggest that multicollinearity is involved.

Table 30.4 Effect of multicollinearity

	Intercept	Age	Height	Weight	BMP	RV	FEV1	FRC
Coefficient	17.8600	2.7178	0.3397					
se		2.9326	0.6900					
Coefficient	64.6550	1.5765	−0.0761	0.8695				
se		3.1436	0.8028	0.8592				
Coefficient	274.63	−3.0832	−0.6985	3.6338	−1.9621			
se		3.6566	0.8008	1.5354	0.9318			
Coefficient	45.3677	4.1756				0.01289		
se		0.3337				0.0784		
Coefficient	−52.4425	4.5416				0.1621	1.5742	
se		1.1944				0.0900	0.6032	
Coefficient	−51.9147	4.5314				0.1633	1.5716	−0.0053
se		1.3052				0.1501	0.6356	0.2958

If this is true then regression involving less highly correlated variables should be more stable. Thus regressing *PE*max on age and RV, and then with age, RV, and *FEV1*, gives
$$\widehat{PE}\text{max} = 45.3677 + 4.1756Age + 0.01289RV,$$ with adjusted R^2 being 0.3205, and the coefficient standard errors being respectively 1.3337 and 0.0784, and
$$\widehat{PE}\text{max} = -52.4425 + 4.5416Age + 0.1612RV + 1.5742FEV1,$$ with adjusted R^2 of 0.4625, and standard errors of 1.1944, 0.0900, and 0.6032 respectively. The coefficients remain stable when *FRC* is included, because it is not as highly correlated with the other variates.

The coefficients and standard errors in the two examples are compared in Table 30.4.

In the upper part of the table, the coefficients for weight and height all alter unpredictably as new variates are added to age, whereas in the lower part of the table the coefficients are stable.

To detect this type of multicollinearity without having to calculate all these combinations, consider the expression for the standard error of a coefficient of X_j when there are more than two X variables:

$$s_{\beta_j}^2 = \frac{s^2}{n-1} \times \frac{1}{s_{X_j}^2} \times \frac{1}{1 - R_j^2} \sqrt{\frac{MS_{res}}{\sum(X_j - \overline{X}_j)\left(1 - R_j^2\right)}}$$

This shows that the variability of the coefficient β_j will be bigger if there is more variability of the Y values from the response surface $\left(\frac{s^2}{n-1} = MS_{res}\right)$, if the variability of $X_j \left(\frac{1}{s_{X_j}^2}\right)$ is smaller, that is, X_j has a small range, or if the multiple correlation coefficient among the X variables $\left(R_j^2\right)$ is very large.

The equation above resembles the expression for the standard error if there are only two X variables except that R_j^2 is the multiple correlation coefficient between all the X variables. The expression $(1 - R_j^2)$ is referred to as tolerance. If R_j^2 is high then the tolerance is low, and values below 0.1 demand close inspection of the data to avoid problems due to multicollinearity. If R_j^2 is zero, then the standard error s_{bjmin} is

$$s_{bjmin} = \sqrt{\frac{MS_{res}}{\sum(X_j - \overline{X}_j)}}.$$

When there is no redundant information

$$s_{bj} = \frac{1}{1 - R_j^2} s_{bjmin}.$$

The term $\frac{1}{1-R_j^2}$ is known as the variance inflation factor (VIF) and is the reciprocal of tolerance as defined above. With no redundant information the VIF is 1. The more redundant information there is the higher the value of VIF. If it is >10 there are almost certain to be problems due to multicollinearity, and any VIF > 4 requires serious consideration. VIF must be calculated for each independent (X) variable, and is done automatically by most programs.

A high VIF indicates redundant information. It would be reasonable to remove variables with VIF > 10 and then repeat the regression on the reduced set of variables. This approach, however, does not allow for possible interaction between the explanatory variables, and another way to identify these redundant variables is by *auxiliary regression*. One at a time each X variate is regressed against the remaining $k - 1$ X variates to produce an expression

$$\widehat{X_j} = c + b_1 X_1 + b_2 X_2 + \ldots b_{j-1} X_{j-1} + b_{j+1} X_{j+1} + \ldots b_k X_k.$$

If none of the variables are correlated with X_j, then none of the coefficients will be significantly different from zero. Any that are correlated will have coefficients that are significantly different from zero. Furthermore, if the multiple correlation coefficient for any of the auxiliary regressions exceeds that for the primary regression (involving Y), multicollinearity should be suspected (Kleinbaum and Klein, 2010).

If in the example used above we regress any X variate against the remaining X variates, the R^2 and the coefficients (unadjusted) are shown in Table 30.5.

Most of the coefficients are not significantly different from zero, those that are significant at P < 0.05 are in bold type, and those that are significant at P < 0.00625 (using a Bonferroni correction) are shown in bold italic type. For the prediction equation of *PEmax* using all the X variables, the multiple correlation coefficient was 0.6349, much less than some of the results from auxiliary regression. Multicollinearity is therefore a problem with this data set.

Table 30.5 Auxiliary regression. The empty squares show the variates used as the dependent variable

R^2	c	Age	Gender	Height	Weight	BMP	FEV1	RV	FRC	TLC	VIF
0.9557	31.90		0.5565	−0.0496	**0.3578**	**−0.1533**	**−0.1113**	0.0107	−0.0392	−0.0384	22.6
0.5710	−101.43	2.1501		0.2495	−0.7814	0.0740	0.7887	−0.0866	0.2463	0.1146	2.3
0.9378	202.45	−1.2572	2.4411		**1.5868**	−0.5526	−0.5097	0.0496	−0.1836	−0.1364	16.1
0.9816	−99.97	**1.8638**	−1.3051	**0.3258**		**0.4265**	**0.2736**	−0.0249	0.0895	0.0981	61.0
0.8753	155.35	**−2.7796**	0.6548	−0.3949	**1.4846**		−0.1638	−0.0183	−0.0170	−0.1800	8.0
0.8118	141.30	**−2.3150**	**4.7810**	−0.4181	**1.0930**	−0.1880		0.0586	**−0.2748**	−0.1154	5.3
0.9034	−220.23	6.7744	−13.5236	1.2325	−3.0183	−0.6373	1.7758		**1.9248**	−0.0650	10.4
0.9393	229.65	−4.7719	7.5830	−0.8812	2.0917	−0.1142	**−1.4465**	**0.3718**		0.1241	16.5
0.6024	264.05	−3.8785	4.0312	−0.5430	1.9002	−1.0020	−0.5597	−0.0104	0.1028		2.5

All the regressions with coefficients significantly different from zero are associated with VIF values ≥ 8. There are two clusters of redundant variables. *Age, height, weight,* and *BMP* are highly interrelated, and so are *RV* and *FRC*. These interrelationships make good physiological sense, and suggest that it would be advantageous to eliminate some of the redundant variables before carrying out the final multiple regression analysis.

Determining the Correct Model

Testing the significance of the individual coefficients gives some guidance, as shown in the last two columns of Table 30.2. Unfortunately these tests do not tell us whether retaining those variates with significant coefficients is the best choice. The question is to how to tell when an increase in adjusted R^2 is significant and denotes that the factor should be retained in the final model. Several methods have been suggested (see Glantz and Slinker, 2001).

All Subsets Regression

In the cystic fibrosis example, the regression program starts with the 9 X variables. Then it examines the regression for the 9 combinations with one of the X variates removed, then the regression for all the 36 combinations of 7 variables, 84 combinations of 6 variables, and so on. The procedure is computer intensive, and with more variates, including power functions and interaction terms, may tax the computer. More importantly, the investigator faces the decision about which of the many hundreds of regression equations to select. The program used here, JMP, highlights the best fit for each set of variables—9, 8, 7, and so on (Table 30.6).

In addition, the program plots out the MS_{res} for each combination, as shown in Figure 30.3.

The investigator is not required to pick the lowest of these values, and a decision about which is the best should not be made from this test. What it does do is to provide a short list of acceptable candidates for the investigator to decide which combinations make the best sense.

To shorten the calculations, certain sequential techniques have been developed. These techniques have in common successive addition or removal of variates until some specified criterion is met. In statistical programs, the final results are usually given immediately, but it is possible to follow step-by-step, thus gaining insight into the process.

Forward Selection

The forward selection method begins with the variate with the largest bivariate regression sum of squares (SS_{reg}) between Y and X. Then the X variate with the next largest SS_{reg} is added. This addition almost always increases R^2, increases regression mean square (MS_{reg}) and decreases MS_{res}. Then test the incremental effect. Some programs will do calculations for each of the possible second variates, add the variate that achieves the highest F ratio,

Table 30.6 Small section of results of all subsets analysis. The highlighted sets give the best predictions for the respective numbers of variables

Model	Number	RSquare	RMSE	AICc	BIC
Age,Gender{1–0},Height,Weight,BMP,FEV1,RV,FRC,TLC	9	0.6349	25.5545	262.525	255.625
Age,Height,Weight,BMP,FEV1,RV,FRC,TLC	8	0.6339	24.7794	256.005	252.479
Age,Gender{1–0},Height,Weight,BMP,FEV1,RV,FRC	8	0.6330	24.8093	256.065	252.539
Gender{1–0},Height,Weight,BMP,FEV1,RV,FRC,TLC	8	0.6282	24.9702	256.388	252.863
Age,Gender{1–0},Weight,BMP,FEV1,RV,FRC,TLC	8	0.6270	25.0121	256.472	252.947
Age,Gender{1–0},Height,Weight,BMP,FEV1,RV,TLC	8	0.6259	25.0491	256.546	253.020
Age,Gender{1–0},Height,Weight,BMP,FEV1,FRC,TLC	8	0.6109	25.5451	257.526	254.001
Age,Gender{1–0},Height,Weight,BMP,RV,FRC,TLC	8	0.6098	25.5798	257.594	254.069
Age,Gender{1–0},Height,BMP,FEV1,RV,FRC,TLC	8	0.5825	26.4615	259.289	255.763
Age,Gender{1–0},Height,Weight,FEV1,RV,FRC,TLC	8	0.5727	26.7685	259.865	256.340
Age,Height,Weight,BMP,FEV1,RV,FRC	7	0.6308	24.1394	250.498	249.467
Height,Weight,BMP,FEV1,RV,FRC,TLC	7	0.6282	24.2248	250.674	249.644
Age,Weight,BMP,FEV1,RV,FRC,TLC	7	0.6269	24.2658	250.759	249.729

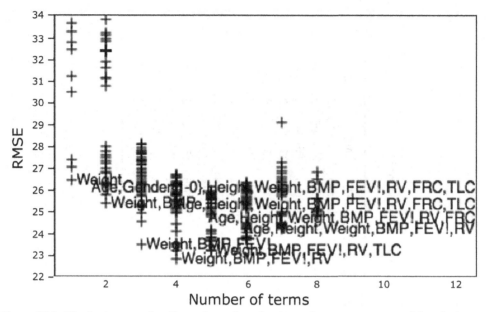

Figure 30.3 All subsets regression. For each number of variates, the components providing the lowest RMSE are listed.

then evaluate the effect of adding in each of the remaining variates as the third variate, put in the variate with the highest F ratio, and so on until the addition of the next variate produces an F ratio below some critical value, often termed F enter or F*in*. Frequently F*in* is set at 4, but this is not a universal default and must be checked for in any given program. Other programs may examine the effect of adding the first of the remaining variates, and if this achieves an F*in* above the critical value leave that variate in and proceed to the next.

As an example, look at the successive steps applied to the cystic fibrosis data.

After the first step (Table 30.7, page 557).

Because the bivariate F ratio is high, weight has been selected and is associated with the highest SS_{reg}—10827.95. Then the program adds in *BMP* that has the next highest SS_{reg} to give Table 30.8, page 558.

The adjusted R^2 has increased, and C_p, *AIC*, and *BIC* are lower. The F ratio is borderline, but *BMP* has increased adjusted R^2 and is retained.

To see what effect *BMP* has made, perform an ANOVA (Table 30.9a, page 559).

Comparing the models with one and two independent variables (left vs right panels), including two independent variables increases the model SS from 10827.947 to 12723.139, and reduces the SS_{res} (labeled Error) from 16004.693 to 14109.501. To determine if the reduction in error SS is significant, perform a one-way ANOVA, and test the reduction in the SS_{res} by relating it to the smaller of the two MS_{res} (Table 30.9b, page 559).

Table 30.7 First forward step

SSE	DFE	RMSE	RSquare	RSquare Adj	Cp	p	AICc	BIC
16004.693	23	26.379087	0.4035	0.3776	3.5083272	2	239.6338	242.1476

Current Estimates

Lock	Entered	Parameter	Estimate	nDF	SS	"F Ratio"	"Prob>F"
☑	☑	Intercept	63.568172	1	0	0.000	1
☐	☐	Age	0	1	213.7819	0.298	0.59073
☐	☐	Gender{1-0}	0	1	788.7532	1.140	0.29714
☐	☐	Height	0	1	36.62306	0.050	0.82434
☐	☑	Weight	1.18686368	1	10827.95	15.561	0.00065
☐	☐	BMP	0	1	1895.191	2.955	0.09965
☐	☐	FEV1	0	1	954.2458	1.395	0.2502
☐	☐	RV	0	1	270.9908	0.379	0.5445
☐	☐	FRC	0	1	12.22795	0.017	0.89798
☐	☐	TLC	0	1	225.0707	0.314	0.58102

Step History

Step	Parameter	Action	"Sig Prob"	Seq SS	RSquare	Cp	p	AICc	BIC
1	Weight	Entered	0.0006	10827.95	0.4035	3.5083	2	239.634	242.148

Table 30.8 Second step

SSE	DFE	RMSE	RSquare	RSquare Adj	Cp	p	AICc	BIC
14109.501	22	25.324711	0.4742	0.4264	2.6061802	3	239.3401	242.2156

Current Estimates

Lock	Entered	Parameter	Estimate	nDF	SS	"F Ratio"	"Prob>F"
☑	☑	Intercept	124.486719			0.000	1
☐	☐	Age	0	1	666.7947	1.042	0.31905
☐	☐	Gender{1-0}	0	1	824.6327	1.304	0.26642
☐	☐	Height	0	1	679.7208	1.063	0.31429
☐	☑	Weight	1.63666146	1	11309.67	17.634	0.00037
☐	☑	BMP	-0.9987454	1	1895.191	2.955	0.09965
☐	☐	FEV1	0	1	2552.977	4.639	0.04302
☐	☐	RV	0	1	17.88261	0.027	0.87188
☐	☐	FRC	0	1	27.82682	0.041	0.84054
☐	☐	TLC	0	1	91.90814	0.138	0.71431

Step History

Step	Parameter	Action	"Sig Prob"	Seq SS	RSquare	Cp	p	AICc	BIC
1	Weight	Entered	0.0006	10827.95	0.4035	3.5083	2	239.634	242.148
2	BMP	Entered	0.0997	1895.191	0.4742	2.6062	3	239.34	242.216

Table 30.9a Left panel, only weight included. Right panel, both weight and BMP included

▶ Summary of Fit

R.Square	0.403536
R.Square Adj	0.377603
Root Mean Square Error	26.37909
Mean of Response	109.12
Observations (or Sum Wgts)	25

▶ Analysis of Variance

Source	DF	Sum of Squares	Mean Square	F Ratio
Model	1	10827.947	10827.9	15.5606
Error	23	16004.693	695.9	**Prob > F**
C. Total	24	26832.640		0.0006*

▶ Parameter Estimates

Term	Estimate	Std Error	t Ratio	Prob>|t|
Intercept	63.568172	12.69574	5.01	<.0001*
Weight	1.1868637	0.300876	3.94	0.0006*

▶ Summary of Fit

R.Square	0.474166
R.Square Adj	0.426363
Root Mean Square Error	25.32471
Mean of Response	109.12
Observations (or Sum Wgts)	25

▶ Analysis of Variance

Source	DF	Sum of Squares	Mean Square	F Ratio
Model	2	12723.139	6361.57	9.9192
Error	22	14109.501	641.34	**Prob > F**
C. Total	24	26832.640		0.0008*

▶ Parameter Estimates

Term	Estimate	Std Error	t Ratio	Prob>|t|
Intercept	124.48672	37.47528	3.32	0.0031*
Weight	1.6366615	0.389743	4.20	0.0004*
BMP	−0.998745	0.580995	−1.72	0.0997

Table 30.9b ANOVA after second step

Source of variation	Sum of squares	Degrees of freedom	Mean square	F
With weight and BMP	12723.14	2		
Weight alone	10827.95	1		
Difference	1895.19	1	1895.19	2.96
SS_{res} due to W, BMP	14109.50	22	641.34	

The reduction in SS_{res} is not significant because $F < 4$, but nevertheless the program retains BMP because of substantial decreases of C_p, AIC, and BIC. It is also too soon to stop the process. The difference of 1895.19 is the same as the SS due to BMP in Table 30.8.

Next $FEV1$ is added, with a further increase in adjusted R^2 and decrease of C_p (Table 30.10, page 561).

The F ratio is adequate, being >4. An ANOVA gives Table 30.11, page 561.

The decrease in SS_{res} is now significant because the $F > Fin$.

The variate with the next highest SS_{reg} is RV, and including this gives Table 30.12, page 562.

The reduction in SS_{res} after adding TLC is not significant, and no advantage is gained by adding other variates, so the process terminates (Table 30.13, page 563).

The full model is

$$\widehat{PE}\text{max} = 63.8243 + 1.7438\,Weight + 1.5461\,FEV1 + 0.1252\,RV - 1.3702\,BMP,$$

with an adjusted R^2 of 0.5357. This is the same set as all subsets analysis selected as having the lowest RMSE (Figure 30.1). These are not the same variates that would have been selected by inspecting the individual coefficients in isolation in Table 30.2. Testing the residuals showed satisfactory distribution.

Backward Elimination

The backward selection program starts with all the variates included in the regression. Then the effect of removing a variable on MS_{res} is assessed for each variable, and the variable with the least effect on increasing MS_{res} is removed if it does not increase the F ratio for removal, $Fout$. As for the forward selection process, $Fout$ is often but not always set at 4. The process continues until removal causes a significant change in MS_{res}, when that variate is left in and no further removals are done. Eventually the reduced model that provides the regression equation is

$$\widehat{PE}\text{max} = 126.3336 + 1.5365\,Weight + 1.10863\,FEV1 - 1.4653\,BMP.$$

The adjusted R^2 was 0.5086.

Comparing the forward and backward selection methods, RV was selected only in the forward method, and as a result there are some differences in the coefficients of the variates. Which of these procedures should we accept? That answer depends on the purpose of the study. If the objective was to obtain the best possible prediction of PEmax, then choose the model with the higher adjusted R^2, namely the model that includes RV (Adjusted R^2 0.5369 vs 0.5086). Remember, though, that another random sample from the same population might give a slightly different prediction. If the objective is to understand what factors are important in predicting PEmax, then statistics will not answer the question. For that, you need physiological and experimental insights. If the inclusion or exclusion of RV is potentially important for understanding the process, further experiments will be needed.

Table 30.10 Third step

SSE	DFE	RMSE	RSquare	RSquare Adj	Cp	p	AICc	BIC
11556.524	21	23.458702	0.5693	0.5078	0.6967521	4	237.5081	240.4445

▶ Current Estimates

Lock	Entered	Parameter	Estimate	nDF	SS	"F Ratio"	"Prob>F"
✓	✓	Intercept	126.007181			0.000	1
☐	☐	Age	0	1	570.6859	1.039	0.32024
☐	☐	Gender{1-0}	0	1	3.329585	0.006	0.94024
☐	☐	Height	0	1	517.2305	0.937	0.34459
☐	✓	Weight	1.53296348	1	9748.56	17.715	0.00039
☐	✓	BMP	-1.4591073	1	3493.923	6.349	0.01991
☐	✓	FEV1	1.10877314	1	2552.977	4.639	0.04302
☐	☐	RV	0	1	1174.58	2.263	0.14815
☐	☐	FRC	0	1	815.3789	1.518	0.23218
☐	☐	TLC	0	1	645.6409	1.183	0.28959

▶ Step History

Step	Parameter	Action	"Sig Prob"	Seq SS	RSquare	Cp	p	AICc	BIC
1	Weight	Entered	0.0006	10827.95	0.4035	3.5083	2	239.634	242.148
2	BMP	Entered	0.0997	1895.191	0.4742	2.6062	3	239.34	242.216
3	FEV1	Entered	0.0430	2552.977	0.5693	0.6968	4	237.508	240.445

Table 30.11 ANOVA after third step

Source of variation	Sum of squares	Degrees of freedom	Mean square	F
With weight, BMP, and FEV1	15276.12	3		
Weight and BMP alone	12723.14	2		
Difference	2552.98	1	2552.98	4.64
SS_{res} due to W, BMP	11556.52	21	550.31	

Table 30.12 Fourth step

▶ Current Estimates

Lock	Entered	Parameter	Estimate	nDF	SS	"F Ratio"	"Prob>F"
☑	☑	Intercept	63.8242644	1	0	0.000	1
☐	☐	Age	0	1	169.2978	0.315	0.58121
☐	☐	Gender{1-0}	0	1	1.665115	0.003	0.95655
☐	☐	Heigh	0	1	173.641	0.323	0.57636
☐	☑	Weight	1.74379041	1	10902.83	21.003	0.00018
☐	☑	BMP	-1.3702183	1	3047.545	5.871	0.02501
☐	☑	FEV1	1.54608863	1	3709.674	7.146	0.01461
☐	☑	RV	0.12519417	1	1174.58	2.263	0.14815
☐	☐	FRC	0	1	0.483083	0.001	0.97659
☐	☐	TLC	0	1	190.5608	0.355	0.55818

▶ Step History

Step	Parameter	Action	"Sig Prob"	Seq SS	RSquare	Cp	p	AICc	BIC
1	Weight	Entered	0.0006	10827.95	0.4035	3.5083	2	239.634	242.148
2	BMP	Entered	0.0997	1895.191	0.4742	2.6062	3	239.34	242.216
3	FEV1	Entered	0.0430	2552.977	0.5693	0.6968	4	237.508	240.445
4	RV	Entered	0.1481	1174.58	0.6131	0.8981	5	238.337	240.984

Table 30.13 After entering *TLC*, there is an increase in C_p, *AIC*, and *BIC*, so that no advantage had been obtained. This is confirmed in the ANOVA in Table 30.14a and 30.14b

SSE	DFE	RMSE	RSquare	RSquare Adj	Cp	p	AICc	BIC
10191.384	19	23.160065	0.6202	0.5202	2.6062834	6	241.7957	243.7396

▶ Current Estimates

Lock	Entered	Parameter	Estimate	nDF	SS	"F Ratio"	"Prob>F"
☑	☑	Intercept	44.3404922	1	0	0.000	1
☐	☐	Age	0	1	56.05601	0.100	0.75599
☐	☐	Gender{1-0}	0	1	25.36652	0.045	0.83454
☐	☐	Heigh	0	1	84.01574	0.150	0.70343
☐	☑	Weight	1.7624741	1	11065.04	20.629	0.00022
☐	☑	BMP	-1.3802475	1	3089.674	5.760	0.0268
☐	☑	FEV1	1.57582816	1	3826.201	7.133	0.051511
☐	☑	RV	0.10532008	1	719.4996	1.341	0.26114
☐	☐	FRC	0	1	72.63393	0.129	0.72344
☐	☑	TLC	0.20693936	1	190.5608	0.355	0.55818

▶ Step History

Step	Parameter	Action	"Sig Prob"	Seq SS	RSquare	Cp	p	AICc	BIC
1	Weight	Entered	0.0006	10827.95	0.4035	3.5083	2	239.634	242.148
2	BMP	Entered	0.0997	1895.191	0.4742	2.6062	3	239.34	242.216
3	FEV1	Entered	0.0430	2552.977	0.5693	0.6968	4	237.508	240.445
4	RV	Entered	0.1481	1174.58	0.6131	0.8981	5	238.337	240.984
5	TLC	Entered	0.5582	190.5608	0.6202	2.6063	6	241.796	243.74

Table 30.14a Left panel, excluding *TLC*. Right panel, including *TLC*

▶ **Summary of Fit**

RSquare	0.613085
RSquare Adj	0.535702
Root Mean Square Error	22.78371
Mean of Response	109.12
Observations (or Sum Wgts)	25

▶ **Analysis of Variance**

Source	DF	Sum of Squares	Mean Square	F Ratio
Model	4	16450.695	4112.67	7.9227
Error	20	10381.945	519.10	Prob > F
C. Total	24	26832.640		0.0005*

▶ **Parameter Estimates**

Term	Estimate	Std Error	t Ratio	Prob>|t|
Intercept	63.824264	53.34835	1.20	0.2455
Weight	1.7437904	0.380495	4.58	0.0002*
BMP	-1.370218	0.565508	-2.42	0.0250*
FEV1	1.5460886	0.57835	2.67	0.0146*
RV	0.1251942	0.083228	1.50	0.1481

▶ **Summary of Fit**

RSquare	0.620187
RSquare Adj	0.520236
Root Mean Square Error	23.16007
Mean of Response	109.12
Observations (or Sum Wgts)	25

▶ **Analysis of Variance**

Source	DF	Sum of Squares	Mean Square	F Ratio
Model	5	16641.256	3328.25	6.2049
Error	19	10191.384	536.39	**Prob > F**
C. Total	24	26832.640		0.0014*

▶ **Parameter Estimates**

Term	Estimate	Std Error	t Ratio	Prob>|t|
Intercept	44.340492	63.31977	0.70	0.4922
Weight	1.7624741	0.388049	4.54	0.0002*
BMP	-1.380247	0.575096	-2.40	0.0268*
FEV1	1.5758282	0.590017	2.67	0.0151*
RV	0.1053201	0.090936	1.16	0.2611
TLC	0.2069394	0.347189	0.60	0.5582

Table 30.14b ANOVA

Source of variation	Sum of squares	Degrees of freedom	Mean square	F
With weight, BMP, and FEV1, RV, and TLC	16641.26	5		
Weight, BMP, FEV1, and RV	16450.70	4		
Difference	190.56	1	190.56	0.37
SS$_{res}$ due to W, BMP, FEV1, RV	10381.95	20	519.10	

Both of these techniques work reasonably well but have a tendency to stop too soon. Neither of them guards against revealing redundancy when a subsequent variable is added or subtracted.

Nonlinear Regression: Polynomial Regression

In Chapter 27, Figures 27.12–27.15, some data from a study by Jamal et al. (2001) were used to show the difference between a linear and a quadratic fit. The curved regression line seems to be a better fit with more evenly scattered residuals, but the question is if this could have occurred by chance or whether the curvilinear relationship is better. We also need to ask if higher powers would produce better fits. Figure 30.4 shows fitting up to five power functions, and Table 30.15 presents some of the regression results for the different power functions.

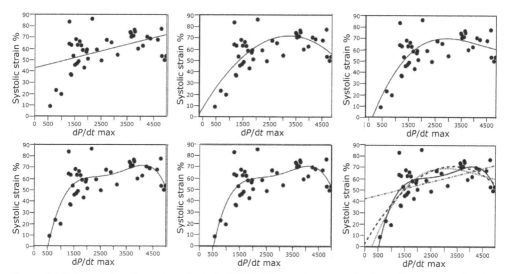

Figure 30.4 Data taken from Jamal et al. (2001). Upper three panels show linear, second-order (quadratic), and third-order (cubic) fits. Lower three panels show fourth-order (quartic) and fifth-order (quintic) fits, and finally all power functions superimposed. In this last panel the second-order fit is the dashed curve, third-order fit is the dotted curve, and the fourth- and fifth-order fits are superimposed.

The results of analyzing the different functions are shown in Table 30.15.

Before analyzing these data in detail, examine the general effects of increasing power functions on the results.

1. There are changes in the intercept c and the linear coefficient b_1.
2. The second-order coefficients are all 1000-fold smaller than the first-order coefficients, and the third-, fourth-, and fifth-order coefficients are smaller still. This does not mean that they can be neglected; these coefficients are multiplied by large numbers.

Table 30.15 Power fits to data

	Power				
	1	2	3	4	5
c	42.37	2.01	−18.79	−85.40	−91.16
b_1X	0.005945	0.04097	0.06970	0.21089	0.22706
b_2X^2		$-6.0479e^{-6}$	−0.0000174	−0.0001134	−0.000129
b_3X^3			$+1.3236e^{-9}$	$+2.6682e^{-9}$	$+3.3393e^{-8}$
b_4X^4				$-2.268e^{-12}$	$-3.3578e^{-12}$
b_5X^5					$+9.841e^{-17}$
R^2	0.2264	0.4783	0.4994	0.5657	0.5658
$s_{Y \cdot X}$	14.4559	12.0182	11.9231	11.2511	11.4005
SS_{reg}	2506.92	5297.30	5530.49	6264.47	6265.90
Df	1	2	3	4	5
MS_{reg}	2506.92	2648.65	1843.50	1566.12	1253.18
SS_{res}	8567.88	5777.50	5544.31	4810	4808.90
Df	41	40	39	38	37
MS_{res}	208.97	144.44	142.16	126.59	129.97
SS_{total}	11,074.80	11,074.80	11,074.80	11,074.80	11,074.80

3. R^2, a measure of fit, increased substantially from linear to quartic, and then did not improve with the quintic fit. This change went hand in hand with an increase in SS_{reg} (sum of squares due to regression) because $R^2 = SS_{reg}/SS_{total}$.
4. Increasing the power function reduced the standard deviation from regression and is to be expected because the standard deviation from regression is what is left over when the variability due to regression is accounted for. The standard deviation from regression did not improve with the quintic fit.

Determine if the changes are consistent with the null hypothesis by ANOVA. First determine if the improved results obtained by a quadratic fit over a linear fit are significant (Table 30.16).

Table 30.16 ANOVA for quadratic versus linear fit

Source of variation	Sum of squares	Degrees of freedom	Mean square	F
Quadratic	5297.30	2		
Linear regression	2506.92	1		
Quadratic after linear	5297.3 − 2506.92 = 2790.38	1	2790.38	19.31 P < 0.0001
$SS_{res}(X^2)$	5777.50	40	144.44	

The change in SS_{reg} due to the higher power gives one mean square, and that is compared with the minimal SS_{res} that comes from the higher power fit. The F ratio is very high, so reject the null hypothesis that these data fit a linear model. Then perform the next ANOVA to compare the quadratic with the cubic fits (Table 30.17).

Table 30.17 ANOVA to compare cubic with quartic

Source of variation	Sum of squares	Degrees of freedom	Mean square	F
Cubic	5530.49	3		
Quadratic	5297.30	2		
Cubic after quadratic	233.19	1	233.19	1.64 P = 0.2079
$SS_{res}(X^3)$	5544.31	39	142.16	

The improvement is not significant, so that a cubic fit does not improve on a quadratic fit. Nevertheless proceed with the quartic comparison (Table 30.18).

Table 30.18 Comparison of quartic and cubic functions

Source of variation	Sum of squares	Degrees of freedom	Mean square	F
Quartic	6264.47	4		
Cubic	5530.49	3		
Quartic after cubic	733.57	1	733.57	5.80 P = 0.021
$SS_{res}(X^4)$	4810.0	38	126.58	

The quartic is significantly better than the cubic.

If the purpose of the regression analysis was to determine the best fit, then a quartic regression is the best choice. As a model for understanding the subject, however, quartic regression may make less physiological sense than quadratic regression.

More information about curvilinear regression can be found in the book by Hamilton (1992).

If the data appear to fit an exponential model,

$$\widehat{Y} = \alpha \beta^X e,$$

deal with this by realizing that this is an intrinsically linear model because taking logarithms of both sides gives

$$\log \widehat{Y} = \log \alpha + X \log \beta + \log e.$$

Logarithms to base 10 or base e are equally effective.

Splines

Some data cannot be fitted by any simple power function. Interpolating splines, in particular, cubic splines, can fit a smoothed curve connecting each data point. A cubic spline is a piecewise cubic polynomial whose coefficients change in different portions of the data set according to certain rules. As a result a complex smooth curve (a Bezier curve) can be fitted to the points. The procedure is best implemented by a computer program, but understandable online tutorials are available (Lancaster; McKinley and Levine). Online programs for creating these splines are found at http://www. solvemymath.com/online_math_calculator/interpolation.php and http://www.akiti. ca/CubicSpline.html. A simple applet for demonstrating interpolating splines can be found at http://www.math.ucla.edu/~baker/java/hoefer/Spline.htm. If the data consist of a cloud of points and what is needed is a curve with varying shapes that produces a moving average, then smoothing basis splines (B-splines) can be constructed.

Correcting for Multicollinearity

If it is apparent that two variables are virtually measuring the same thing, one of them should be eliminated. If, for example, cardiac output is measured after infusing different volumes of blood, there is little to be gained by regressing cardiac output against total blood volume and infused volume because these volumes will be highly correlated. If the variables cannot be eliminated, a procedure known as centering is used. To do this, the mean of each X variate is subtracted from its components to give $X_i - \overline{X}_i$, and the regression is calculated with these transformed variates. Sometimes this deviation is divided by the standard deviation to give a z score. Both of these transformations give a mean of zero that helps to avoid multicollinearity problems. A particularly clear explanation of why this is useful is presented by Glantz and Slinker (2001). In addition, the transformation may be done in such a way as to simplify the numbers, and this helps the computation because even high-powered computers may have difficulties with matrix inversion (used in the computation) of large numbers.

Multicollinearity is very likely to be present in polynomial regression of the form $\widehat{Y}_i = c + b_1 X_1 + b_2 X_i^2 + b_3 X_i^3 + \dots b_k X_i^k$, and also when interactions are present as in

$$\widehat{Y}_i = c + b_1 X_1 + b_2 X_2 + b_3 X_1 X_2.$$

With centered values for the calculations presented in relation to Figure 30.1 there is no change to the fitted curve, the residuals and the correlation coefficient, but there are

Polynomial Fit Degree=3

systolic strain % = 68.374061 + 0.0054525*Centered dtmax − 6.8901e−6*Centered dp/dtmax^2 + 1.3236e−9*Centered dp/dtmax^3

Summary of Fit

RSquare	0.499376
RSquare Adj	0.460866
Root Mean Square Error	11.92316
Mean of Response	58.1
Observations (or Sum Wgts)	43

▶ Lack of Fit

Analysis of Variance

Source	DF	Sum of Squares	Mean Square
Model	3	5530.488	1843.50
Error	39	5544.312	142.16
C. Total	42	11074.800	

Parameter Estimates

Term	Estimate	Std Error
Intercept	68.374061	2.903608
Centered dp/dt max	0.0054525	0.003164
Centered dp/dt max^2	−6.89e−6	1.515e−6
Centered dp/dt max^3	1.3236e−9	1.033e−9

Polynomial Fit Degree=3

systolic strain % = −18.79141 + 0.0697042*dP/dt max − 0.0000174*dP/dt max^2 + 1.3236e−9*dP/dt max^3

Summary of Fit

RSquare	0.499376
RSquare Adj	0.460866
Root Mean Square Error	11.92316
Mean of Response	58.1
Observations (or Sum Wgts)	43

▶ Lack of Fit

Analysis of Variance

Source	DF	Sum of Squares	Mean Square	F Ratio
Model	3	5530.488	1843.50	12.9676
Error	39	5544.312	142.16	Prob > F
C. Total	42	11074.800		<.0001*

Parameter Estimates

Term	Estimate	Std Error	t Ratio	Prob>|t|
Intercept	−18.79141	19.08381	−0.98	0.3309
dP/dt max	0.0697042	0.023829	2.93	0.0057*
dP/dt max^2	−1.74e−5	8.965e−6	−1.94	0.0596
dP/dt max^3	−1.3236e−9	1.033e−9	1.28	0.2079

differences of the X coefficients. This can be seen by comparing the cubic polynomial with and without centering (Figure 30.5).

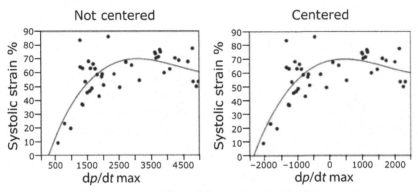

Figure 30.5 Cubic regression without (left panel) and with (right panel) centering.

The accompanying table (on previous page) gives the basic data for these curves.

The fitted curves are identical as are the values for R^2, MS_{res}, mean response, and the ANOVA. Differences are noted in the intercepts and coefficients, and particularly in the much wider standard errors of the coefficients without centering. (The intercept occurs when X is zero, and so is not at the left vertical axis line for the centered graph.) Centering also emphasizes the central part of the distribution where the greatest accuracy occurs (Glantz and Slinker, 2001). When uncentered, low, middle and high values of X are associated respectively with low, middle and high values of X^2, their relationship is monotonic, and their correlation is high. When centered, low values of X and X^2 become larger numbers, middle values are low and larger values are high. There is no longer a monotonic relationship and the correlation is lower.

Other ways of avoiding multicollinearity are described by Katz (2006) whose book on multivariate analysis is easy to read and instructive. It is wise to omit a variable if it seems to have no plausible biological function (unless it is being tested for this specifically), or if it is an intermediate explanatory variable. For example, in a study of explanatory variables for essential hypertension, it is unnecessary to include prorenin, renin, and angiotensin. Angiotensin alone is a useful predictor of response. A second technique is to use a categorical scale with an "and/or" response. Thus rather than include renin and angiotensin as ratio numbers, specify that a renin concentration in excess of X_1 units or an angiotensin concentration in excess of Y units counts as a positive response. A third technique is to construct a multivariable scale in which closely related questions are coded to fit $1 - N$ groups (the same for each variable). For example, if in predicting a coronary artery calcium score by using *BMI*, insulin resistance, and fasting blood glucose, all of which are related, assign each factor a score of $1-5$ (e.g., *BMI* <20, 20−25, 26−30, 31−35, >35), and then use the cumulative score as a single explanatory factor. Finally, if the variables are unrelated, it is still possible to define a combined score; as example, see Apgar score in Table 3.3, or create a score for degree of exercise, weight, use of beta blockers, and a measure of psychological stress as a combined predictor of myocardial infarction.

Principles of Nonlinear Regression

Nonlinear fits are frequently used in biochemical and pharmacological systems that examine rate constants, feedback controls, cooperativity, and other complex interactions. They may be simple exponential curves, or else equations such as those defining Michaelis–Menten kinetics:

$v = \frac{V_{max}S}{K_m+S}$. Sometimes complex equations with partial derivatives are involved.

Some simple curved XY relationships can be transformed to make them linear. A polynomial smoothing spline was used by Sherrill et al. (1989) to model pulmonary and somatic growth functions.

The principle of least squares is used for these nonlinear fits, and the procedure requires several iterations. At first, guesses are made about the values of the different parameters. The program then adjusts these estimates, and if the SS_{res} is diminished then a second iteration with new values is done. The procedure continues until negligible improvement occurs in the SS_{res}. There are a variety of considerations and techniques used in the fitting process, and many of these are described by Hamilton (9), Motulsky and Ransnas (1987) (Motulsky was the originator of the statistics program Prism that is particularly well adapted to nonlinear solutions), and by Garfinkel and Fegley (1984). Online programs can be found at http://statpages.org/nonlin.html, http://www.colby.edu/chemistry/PChem/scripts/lsfitpl.html, and http://www.xuru.org/rt/NLR.asp. Although these programs perform complex calculations, they should be used with care. An excellent online tutorial is provided at http://graphpad.com/curvefit/.

Dummy or Indicator Variables

It is possible to introduce a qualitative (nominal or ordinal) factor into regression. In Chapter 27, an example of the relationship between blood pressure and diameter in retinal arteries and veins was used to illustrate ANCOVA. A different analysis could be done using an indicator (or dummy) variable and multiple regression. This variable allows us to identify different categories of a qualitative variable. For k categories of the qualitative variable, there are $k - 1$ dummy variables. (The reason for using $k - 1$ variables instead of k variables 1,2,3,…k is to avoid implications of ordering of variables (Gunst and Mason, 1980).)

Coding with dummy variables can be performed by reference cell coding (more common) or by effect cell coding. In reference cell coding, commonly used for comparisons with a designated control group, assign 0s to the control group and combinations of 0 and 1 to the other groups. With effect cell coding, the various groups are compared with their average. Thus if there are two categories, designate one of the states (which one is immaterial) as 1, and the other as −1 for effect coding, or as 0 (basal state) and 1 for reference coding, and then perform multiple regression:

$\widehat{Y}_i = c + b_1X_{1i} + b_2X_{2i}$, where X_1 is the independent variable and X_2 is the indicator variable. (Different programs have different defaults, JMP being one of the few that uses effect coding as the default. Therefore, JMP treats 1 and 0 as if they were 1 and −1.)

Thus when comparing diameters of retinal arteries and veins at different blood pressures (Leung et al., 2003), set out the data as shown in Table 30.19.

Table 30.19 In this data set, the retinal artery is coded 1, and the vein 0

Retinal vessel	Diameter (micron)	Systolic blood pressure (mm Hg)
1	227	70
1	225	80
1	225	89
1	224	99
1	223	108
1	220	117
1	222	127
0	200	79.8
0	197	89.3
0	192	99
0	179	108
0	185	118
0	179	127

Multiple regression produces two parallel regression lines (See Figure 27.39). The results by effect coding are shown in Table 30.20.

Table 30.20 Effect coding of retinal vessel data

Source of variation	Sum of squares	Degrees of freedom	Mean square	F
Total	4409.2308	12		
Linear regression	4205.0696	2	2102.53	102.9841
Residual	204.1611	10	20.42	P < 0.0001

Rsquare adj 0.6389.

The regression equation is

Diameter = 230.5948 − 0.2415 × Blood Pressure − 16.9266 if vein, or +16.9266 if artery. The two parallel lines in Figure 27.39 show the effect, the intercepts differing by 2 × 16.9266 = 33.85.

Analyzing this data by reference coding (by changing the modeling type in the JMP program) gives the same data as in Table 30.20 but the prediction equation is now

Diameter = 213.6682 − 0.2415 × Blood Pressure + 0 if vein, or 33.8532 if artery

Thus for the vein, diameter = 213.6682 × Blood Pressure, and for the artery it is

Diameter = 213.67682 × Blood Pressure + 33.8532.

The difference between the two intercepts is the same for the two types of coding, and the ANOVA and lack of fit statistics are the same for both methods, as are the t-tests for the parameters. The parameters themselves and the intercepts are different because they measure different things.

The models imply that the slope of the relationship is the same in both groups that differ only in their mean value or intercept, but the two data sets might also differ by mean and slope, that is, that there is interaction. This is handled by using as a model

$$\widehat{Y}_i = c + b_1 X_1 + b_2 X_2 + b_3 X_1 X_2.$$

Considering variable X_1, for which $X_2 = 0$,

$$\widehat{Y}_i = c + b_1 X_1.$$

Considering variable X_2,

$$\widehat{Y}_i = c + b_1 X_1 + b_2(1) + b_3 X_1(1) = (c + b_2) + (b_1 + b_3)X_1.$$

This shows that the change from group 1 to group 2 in intercept is reflected by the parameter b_2, and in slope by the parameter b_3.

There is no reason to restrict the number of groups to 2. For example, compare the relationship between age and cholesterol in four states by setting up three more variables (Table 30.21).

Table 30.21 Indicator variables for four states

State	X_2	X_3	X_4
Iowa (*I*)	0	0	0
Nebraska (*N*)	1	0	0
California (*C*)	0	1	0
Texas (*T*)	0	0	1

Then the prediction equation is

$$\widehat{Y}_i = c + b_1 Age + b_2 X_2 + b_3 X_3 + b_4 X_4 + \varepsilon_i.$$

For Iowa, the equation becomes
$\widehat{Y}_i = c + b_1 Age + \varepsilon_i$, and for California it becomes

$$\widehat{Y}_i = c + b_1 Age + b_3 X_3 + \varepsilon_i.$$

As another example, relate blood pressure to the dose of norepinephrine in control patients, diabetic patients, and patients who have had a myocardial infarct. Then code the control group as (0,0), the diabetic group as (1,0), and the infarct group as (0,1). The equation is then

$$\widehat{Y}_i = c + b_1 Dose + b_2 Diabetic + b_3 Infarct.$$

The intercept alone, c, represents the blood pressure in the absence of agonist, diabetes, and infarction.

If the agonist is infused, then if the subject is a control, the relationship is $\widehat{Y}_i = c + b_1 Dose$, because both diabetics and infarct patients are coded zero.

If the patient is a diabetic, the equation is $\widehat{Y}_i = c + b_1 Dose + b_2 Diabetic$ and the difference between control and diabetic subjects at any dose is b_2.

If the patient has had an infarct, the equation is $\widehat{Y}_i = c + b_1 Dose + b_3 Infarct$, and the difference between control and infarct subjects at any dose is b_3.

Effect cell coding, on the other hand, allows comparison of the mean of a group from the overall mean of all the groups. To achieve this, code as shown in Table 30.22.

Table 30.22 Effect cell coding model

Group code	Group 2	Group 3	Group 4
Iowa (1)	−1	−1	−1
Nebraska (2)	1	0	0
California (3)	0	1	0
Texas (4)	0	0	1

When this is done, the regression equation is $\widehat{Y}_i = c + b_1 I + b_2 N + b_3 C + b_4 T$. Because of effect coding, the intercept c is the overall mean value of the measured variable. The coefficient b_1 shows the difference between the mean for Iowa and the overall mean, coefficient b_2 shows the difference between the mean for Nebraska and the overall mean, and so on.

An excellent discussion of dummy (categorical) variables is presented by Katz (2006).

Repeated Measures Regression

The examples discussed above all had a single observation of the dependent variable for each subject, and are referred to as *between-subjects* designs. It is, however, common to use a number of subjects and then make a series of measurements on each of them; this is referred to as a *within-subjects* design. The repeated measurements may be for example, measurement of left ventricular volume (1) Before anesthesia, (2) After anesthesia with closed chest, (3) Open chest, closed pericardium, and (4) Open chest, open pericardium. Alternatively the repeated measurements may be serial times, doses, pressures, and so on. If repeated measurements are done, it would be a mistake to pool them all without considering how homogeneous they are. For example, examine Figure 30.6.

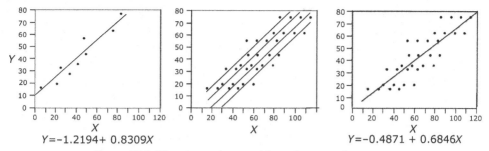

$$Y=-1.2194+ 0.8309X \qquad\qquad\qquad\qquad Y=-0.4871 + 0.6846X$$

Figure 30.6 Diagram to show problem of repeated measures.

The left panel shows a linear artificial XY relationship in a single subject with eight measurements. (It resembles the regression obtained when relating arterial oxygen tension measured directly in blood to arterial oxygen tension measured with a skin electrode.) The center panel shows three other subjects with identical slopes but different intercepts. If differences among subjects were ignored and all 32 measurements were pooled (right panel), the pooled regression line could have a substantially different slope, as shown by the regression equations.

Therefore the analysis must allow for differences among subjects. Glantz and Slinker (10) recommend dummy variables to account for differences among the subjects. This can be done by defining two dummy variables:

$$D_1 \begin{cases} 1 \text{ if subject } 1 \\ 0 \text{ if subject } 2 \\ -1 \text{ if subject } 3 \end{cases} \text{ and } D_2 \begin{cases} 0 \text{ if subject } 1 \\ 1 \text{ if subject } 2 \\ -1 \text{ if subject } 3 \end{cases}.$$

The regression model then becomes

$$\widehat{Y}_i = c + b_1 X_1 + b_2 D_1 + b_3 D_3.$$

Then the regression equations are respectively

$$\widehat{Y}_i = c + b_1 X_1 + b_2 \cdot 1 + b_3 \cdot 0, \text{ (subject 1)}$$
$$\widehat{Y}_i = c + b_1 X_1 + b_2 \cdot 0 + b_3 \cdot 1, \text{ (subject 2) and}$$
$$\widehat{Y}_i = c + b_1 X_1 + b_2 \cdot -1 + b_3 \cdot -1 \text{ (subject 3)}.$$

For each subject designated by the dummy variable, the appropriate number is inserted into the regression formula. With this procedure, the slope for each subject is shown to be zero, and there are differences only in the intercepts.

Multivariate Analysis

This is not the same as multiple regression, in which a single dependent variable is related to a set of independent explanatory variables. In contrast, multivariate analysis, also termed MANOVA, has two or more dependent variables that may not themselves be independent of each other. "Multivariate data are data for which each observation consists of values for more than one random variable on each experimental unit" (Fisher and van Belle, 1993).

As an example, consider a study, described by Everitt and Hay (1992), to determine whether postpartum depression is associated with delayed intellectual development of the infants. Two groups are examined: mothers without postpartum depression and mothers with depression, and at several months of age a variety of psychological tests are performed. As part of the study, comparisons are made between three components of IQ scores: perceptual, verbal, and quantitative. It certainly would be possible to perform separate t-tests on each of these components, but not only does this raise problems due to multiplicity but it also loses some information because these components are interrelated. In addition, doing single variable comparisons results in a loss of power. A simple ANOVA is not appropriate, because the components of a factor may be correlated.

Another example might be testing the effect of several drugs on systolic and diastolic blood pressures.

The correct analysis is to use Hotelling's T^2 test. This test requires calculation of a variance—covariance matrix and is implemented in most standard statistics programs. It can also be performed by the free program BrightStats http://www.brightstat.com/.

Multivariate methods are used in discriminant analysis and in logistic regression.

Longitudinal Regression

Regression studies in which several members of a group are each followed for many time periods are considered as longitudinal studies. Unlike the repeated measures described above in which the variability among subjects is allowed for in examining the relationship of the dependent to the independent variables, in longitudinal studies the whole set of outcome variables is of interest; an example is the assessment of growth curves or glucose tolerance curves in two or more experimental groups. Frequently the mean values at each time period these data are joined to form average curves, and multiple t-tests are calculated at each time point. Not only must these tests be corrected for multiplicity, but also in fact the curve may be misleading because the average curve may not reflect any individual curve; see Figures 2 and 3 in Matthews et al. (1990). These studies pose several problems (Matthews et al., 1990). Ideally they are balanced, that is, each subject has the same number of measurements made at the exact same times. In practice, there are often missing values, or else values are obtained opportunistically at different times for each subject. In addition, successive measurements in each subject are likely to be highly correlated, some being hypo- and others hyperresponders. As a consequence, the successive t-tests are not independent, and these time-varying covariances involving the individuals' responses make the usual multivariate methods unsuitable (Schwartz et al., 1988; Ware, 1985).

Instead of rushing into complex calculations, it is often simpler to select summary measures to be analyzed before the experiment is started. Examples might be the peak glucose concentrations, time to peak concentration, duration for concentration to exceed some specified value, total area under the curve, rate of rise of concentration in the first 30 min, or any other relevant measure. These can be analyzed simply by standard tests. Accompanying the analyses by a graph to show each individual set of responses may be helpful.

If more formal and complex analyses are indicated, there are many proposed solutions, one of the most general being that is developed by Zeger and Liang (1986). Their method is based on estimating a common correlation between all repeated measurements on each subject. Assume that the response over time is linear. In principle, determine a common intercept β_0, and a common slope β_1. Any one subject may have a response Y_i with a different intercept and slope, so characterize that subject's response as $Y_i = (\beta_0 - b_0) + (\beta_1 - b_1) + \varepsilon_i$, where b_0 and b_1 are the individual differences from the common values. Dummy variables to indicate a specific group or treatment can be incorporated. The method is robust, can accommodate linear or curvilinear relations, but requires specialized general estimating equations.

REFERENCES

Altman, D.G., 1992. Practical Statistics for Medical Research. Chapman and Hall.

Chambers, J.M., Cleveland, W.S., Kleiner, B., et al., 1983. Graphical Methods for Data Analysis. Wadsworth.

Chatfield, C., 1988. Problem Solving. A Statistician's Guide. Chapman & Hall.

Concato, J., Peduzzi, P., Holford, T.R., et al., 1995. Importance of events per independent variable in proportional hazards analysis. I. Background, goals, and general strategy. J. Clin. Epidemiol. 48, 1495–1501.

Edwards, A.L., 1984. An Introduction to Linear Regression and Correlation. W.H. Freeman and Co.

Everitt, B.S., Hay, D., 1992. Talking about Statistics. A Psychologist's Guide to Design & Analysis. Edward Arnold.

Fisher, L.D., van Belle, G., 1993. Biostatistics. A Methodology for the Health Sciences. John Wiley and Sons.

Garfinkel, D., Fegley, K.A., 1984. Fitting physiological models to data. Am. J. Physiol. 246, R641–R650.

Glantz, S.A., Slinker, B.K., 2001. Primer of Applied Regression and Analysis of Variance. McGraw-Hill, Inc.

Gunst, R.F., Mason, R.L., 1980. Regression Analysis and Its Applications. Marcel Dekker.

Hamilton, L.C., 1992. Regression with Graphics. A Second Course in Applied Statistics. Duxbury Press.

Haricharan, R.N., Barnhart, D.C., Cheng, H., et al., 2009. Identifying neonates at a very high risk for mortality among children with congenital diaphragmatic hernia managed with extracorporeal membrane oxygenation. J. Pediatr. Surg. 44, 87–93.

Harrell Jr., F.E., Lee, K.L., Matchar, D.B., et al., 1985. Regression models for prognostic prediction: advantages, problems, and suggested solutions. Cancer Treat. Rep. 69, 1071–1077.

Hocking, R.R., 1976. The analysis and selection of variables in linear regression. Biometrics 32, 1–49.

Jamal, F., Strotmann, J., Weidemann, F., et al., 2001. Noninvasive quantification of the contractile reserve of stunned myocardium by ultrasonic strain rate and strain. Circulation 104, 1059–1065.

Katz, M.H., 2006. Multivariate Analysis. A Practical Guide for Clinicians. Cambridge University Press.

Kleinbaum, D.G., Kupper, L.L., Muller, K.E., 1988. Applied Regression Analysis and Other Multivariable Methods. PWS-KENT Publishing Company.

Kleinbaum, D.G., Klein, M., 2010. Logistic Regression. A Self-learning Test. Springer.

Lancaster, D. The Math behind Bezier Cubic Splines (Online). Available: http://www.tinaja.com/glib/cubemath.pdf.

Leung, H., Wang, J.J., Rochtchina, E., et al., 2003. Relationships between age, blood pressure, and retinal vessel diameters in an older population. Invest. Ophthalmol. Vis. Sci. 44, 290.

Lucke, J.F., Whitely, S.E., 1984. The biases and mean squared errors of estimators of multinomial squared multiple correlation. J. Educ. Stat. 9, 183–192.

Mallows, C.L., 1973. Some comments on Cp. Technometrics 15, 661–675.

Matthews, J.N., Altman, D.G., Campbell, M.J., et al., 1990. Analysis of serial measurements in medical research. BMJ (Clin. Res. Ed.) 300, 230–235.

McKinley, S. Levine, M. Cubic Spline Interpolation (Online). Available: http://www.academia.edu/8488245/Cubic_Spline_Interpolation.

Mendenhall, W., Sincich, T., 1986. A Second Course in Business Statistics: Regression Analysis. Dellen Publishing Co.

Montgomery, D.C., Peck, E.A., 1982. Introduction to Linear Regression Analysis. John Wiley and Sons.

Motulsky, H.J., 2009. Statistical Principles: The Use and Abuse of Logarithmic Axes (Online). Available: http://www.graphpad.com/faq/file/1487logaxes.pdf.

Motulsky, H.J., Ransnas, L.A., 1987. Fitting curves to data using nonlinear regression: a practical and nonmathematical review. FASEB 1, 365–374.

Neter, J., Kutner, M.H., Nachtsheim, C.J., et al., 1996. Applied Linear Statistical Models. Irwin.

O'Neill, S., Leahy, F., Pasterkamp, H., et al., 1983. The effects of chronic hyperinflation, nutritional status, and posture on respiratory muscle strength in cystic fibrosis. Am. Rev. Respir. Dis. 128, 1051–1054.

Peduzzi, P., Concato, J., Feinstein, A.R., et al., 1995. Importance of events per independent variable in proportional hazards regression analysis. II. Accuracy and precision of regression estimates. J. Clin. Epidemiol. 48, 1503–1510.

Ramsey, J.B., 1969. Tests for specification errors in classical least squares regression analysis. J. R. Stat. Soc. Ser. B 31, 350–371.

Ramsey, F.L., Schafer, D.W., 2002. The Statistical Sleuth. A Course in Methods of Data Analysis. Duxbury.

Richardson, D.K., Corcoran, J.D., Escobar, G.J., et al., 2001. SNAP-II and SNAPPE-II: simplified newborn illness severity and mortality risk scores. J. Pediatr. 138, 92–100.

Schwartz, J., Landrigan, P.J., Feldman, R.G., et al., 1988. Threshold effect in lead-induced peripheral neuropathy. J. Pediatr. 112, 12–17.

Schwarz, G.E., 1979. Estimating the dimension of a model. Ann. Stat. 6, 461–464.

Sherrill, D.L., Morgan, W.J., Taussig, L.M., et al., 1989. A mathematical procedure for estimating the spatial relationships between lung function, somatic growth, and maturation. Pediatr. Res. 25, 316–321.

Slinker, B.K., Glantz, S.A., 1985. Multiple regression for physiological data analysis: the problem of multicollinearity. Am. J. Physiol. 249, R1–R12.

Thursby, J.G., Schmidt, P., 1977. Some properties of tests for specification error in a linear regression model. J. Am. Stat. Assoc. 72, 635–641.

Thursz, M.R., Kwiatkowski, D., Allsopp, C.E., et al., 1995. Association between an MHC class II allele and clearance of hepatitis B virus in the Gambia. N. Engl. J. Med. 332, 1065–1069.

Ware, J.H., 1985. Linear models for the analysis of longitudinal studies. Am. Stat. 2, 95–101.

Weisberg, S., 1985. Applied Linear Regression. John Wiley & Sons.

Whyte, H.M., 1959. Blood pressure and obesity. Circulation 19, 511–516.

Zeger, S.L., Liang, K.-Y., 1986. Longitudinal data analysis for discrete and continuous outcomes. Biometrics 42, 121–130.

CHAPTER 31

Serial Measurements: Time Series, Control Charts, Cusums

Contents

INTRODUCTION

Frequently observations are obtained serially over time: hourly or daily body temperatures, daily blood creatinine concentrations, weekly hemoglobin concentrations, weekly check of a standard sodium salt concentration in a laboratory, annual birth rates in a country, weekly rainfall, or the Dow-Jones index. Figure 31.1 shows the weekly incidence over several years of influenza-associated illness in children.

The mean value and variability of such serial measurements are of interest, and so is the trend toward increasing and decreasing. Analysis of time series is important in engineering, and many textbooks deal with the subject. Various methods of smoothing the graphs and exposing underlying regularities in the apparently erratic data are used (Brown and Rothery, 1993; Chatfield, 1980; Diggle, 1990; Hamilton, 1992). Oscillatory behavior is common in biological studies, ranging from electroencephalograms to calcium cycling in cells to pulsatile secretion of gonadotrophic hormones. An easy introduction to the subject is provided by Everitt (1989), Mendenhall and Sincich (1986), Neter et al. (1978), Pollard (1977), and by Wonnacott and Wonnacott (1981). Biological oscillations may be less regular than those occurring in engineering studies, and are correspondingly difficult to analyze (Filicori et al., 1984; Merriam and Wachter, 1982; Veldhuis et al., 1986; Velduis et al., 1986). It is even possible to

For a list of all websites referred to in this chapter, as clickable links, see the book companion website: www.booksite.elsevier.com/9780128023877.

Biostatistics for Medical and Biomedical Practitioners
http://dx.doi.org/10.1016/B978-0-12-802387-7.00031-7

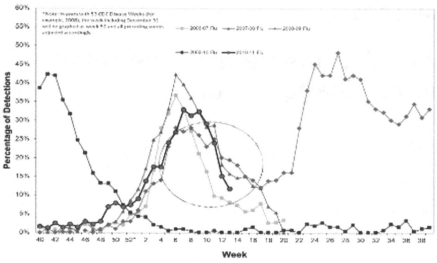

Figure 31.1 Influenza detections in Respiratory Laboratory Network and Sentinel Laboratories, 2006–2011.

find artifactual oscillations that are induced by the mathematical process used, as discussed in an article entitled "Biological clock in the unicorn" (Cole, 1957).

SERIAL CORRELATION

A question about any data collected serially over time is whether consecutive measurements are correlated with each other. Serial correlation may seriously underestimate the standard deviation from regression and all the assessments of variability derived from it, leading to a false estimate of accuracy.

Wald–Wolfowitz Runs Test

There are several ways of determining serial correlation. A simple method for nominal scale data is the Wald–Wolfowitz runs test. Consider a study in which 20 men (M) and 20 women (F) are enrolled. To evaluate randomness, define a run as a series of one kind without interruption. Thus if the order of entry into the study was *MMFFFMFFFMMMMFMMFFMFFMMMFFMMMFFMMMFFMF*, there are 17 runs: 2M, 3F, 1M, 3F etc. (even a single member constitutes a run). A table of probabilities for this test gives P > 0.20, so that there is no evidence against randomness. The test can be done online at http://www.quantitativeskills.com/sisa/statistics/ordinal.htm, If selection is randomized, it is unlikely that the first 20 subjects will be of one gender, and the next 20 the other gender; this sequence has only 2 runs, and P < 0.001.

An exact alternation of men and women is also unlikely; a set with 40 runs also has $P < 0.001$.

With ≥ 20 members of each group, use the normal approximation.

The expected mean μ if the null hypothesis is true is

$$\mu = \frac{2n_1 n_2}{N} + 1,$$

where n_1 and n_2 are the numbers in each group, and $N = n_1 + n_2$.

The variance σ^2 is calculated from

$$\sigma^2 = \frac{2n_1 n_2 (2n_1 n_2 - N)}{N^2(N - 1)}.$$

Therefore the value for W, the standardized estimate of the difference between the number of runs observed R and the number expected from the null hypothesis, is estimated as

$$W = \frac{R - \frac{2n_1 n_2}{N} - 1}{\sqrt{\frac{2n_1 n_2 (2n_1 n_2 - N)}{N^2(N-1)}}}.$$

The value for W is obtained from the z tables.

Some authorities recommend a correction for continuity in the numerator.

$$W = \frac{\left| R - \frac{2n_1 n_2}{N} - 1 \right|}{\sqrt{\frac{2n_1 n_2 (2n_1 n_2 - N)}{N^2(N-1)}}}$$

where the demarcating lines $\|$ indicate the absolute value of the argument. An extension to more than two groups is described by Zar (2010).

Up-and-Down Runs Test

A slightly different procedure, the up-and-down procedure, is used to determine if the alternation is between measurements on a ratio, interval, or ordinal scale. If a series of temperatures are taken successively, it would be suspicious if the temperatures alternated regularly or if a steady rise occurred for half the temperatures followed by a consistent fall. This is not quite the same as the runs method described above, although it would be if temperatures were classified as high or low. To examine the up-and-down problem, the method of first differences has been used (Edgington, 1961). Determine if the difference between X_n and X_{n+1} is positive or negative, and then determine the number of runs. For total number <50, there are tables of critical values (Durbin and Watson, 1950;

Madansky, 1988; Zar, 2010), and for larger numbers there is a normal approximation. The expected mean value of the number of runs R if the numbers are random is

$$\mu_R = \frac{2N-1}{3},$$

and the standard deviation σ_R is

$$\sigma_R = \sqrt{\frac{16N-29}{90}}.$$

Therefore

$$z = \frac{R - \frac{2N-1}{3}}{\sqrt{\frac{16N-29}{90}}}.$$

Table 31.1 shows a set of daily temperatures.

The number of runs is 8 ($2+, 1-, 2+, 1-, 2+, 2-, 2+, 2-$). From the runs table, the probability of ≤ 8 runs in 15 consecutive observations is 0.2216. Therefore there is no reason to reject the null hypothesis that the temperatures were random. The relevant table may be found online at http://www.scribd.com/doc/53565230/100/Table-E-Runs-Up-and-Down-Distribution or as Table 1 at http://www.iasri.res.in/ebook/EB_SMAR/e-book_pdf%20files/Manual%20II/4-Non-Parametric_test.pdf. The test can be done with Excel—see http://www.youtube.com/watch?v=YWlod6Jdu-k, but is easier to do by hand.

Rank von Neumann Ratio

A more powerful test than the up-and-down test just described is to associate the measured values of X_i with ranks r_i (from lowest to highest), and then calculate the rank von Neumann ratio v as

$$v = \frac{\sum\limits_{i=2}^{N} (r_i - r_{i-1})^2}{\frac{N(N^2-1)}{12}}.$$

The critical values for v are given by Bartels (1982) or online by Table S, p607 at http://www.scribd.com/doc/53565230/14/A-TEST-BASED-ON-RANKS. Just as the Durbin–Watson test (below) the ratio varies from 0 to 4.

Applying this method to the data of Table 31.1 gives Table 31.2.

Then the rank ratio is

$$v = \frac{(7-8)^2 + (1-7)^2 + (14-1)^2 \ldots + (5.5-5.5)^2}{\frac{15(15^2-1)}{12}} = \frac{540.25}{280} = 1.93.$$

Table 31.1 Daily temperatures

Day	1	2	3	4	5	6	7	8	9	10	11	12	13	14	15
T	37.6	37.8	37.9	36.5	37.3	37.7	36.6	36.9	37.6	36.9	36.2	36.8	37.4	37.1	36.8
Sign Δ		+	+	−	+	+	−	+	+	−	−	+	+	−	−

Table 31.2 Daily temperatures

Day	1	2	3	4	5	6	7	8	9	10	11	12	13	14	15
T	37.6	37.8	37.9	36.5	37.3	37.7	36.6	36.9	37.6	36.9	36.2	36.8	37.4	37.1	36.8
ΔT		0.2	0.1	−1.4	0.8	0.4	−0.9	0.3	0.7	−0.6	−0.7	0.5	0.6	−0.3	−0.3
Rank		8	7	1	14	10	2	9	13	4	3	11	12	5.5	5.5

This value yields $P > 0.10$, so that the null hypothesis of randomness cannot be rejected. Tied ranks are averaged, and the formula is unreliable with many ties.

These tests can be used for more than time series. For example, they are recommended for assessing the independence of residuals in a regression equation or an analysis of variance (Kennedy and Neville, 1986).

Ratio Measurements

If the data consist of ratio measurements, one of the tests commonly used is the Durbin–Watson test for first-order autocorrelation (Durbin and Watson, 1950, 1951). For example, if blood pressures are measured serially throughout the day, there would be positive autocorrelation because of lower pressures at night than in the daytime. The coefficient of autocorrelation is termed ρ, and the null hypothesis is that $\rho = 0$.

Autocorrelation affects the ability to estimate accurately the standard deviation from regression. The requirements for linear regression assume that the residuals (error terms) have zero mean constant variance, and are uncorrelated, as well as being normally distributed. If these requirements are not met and there is positive autocorrelation, then the standard errors of the regression coefficient tend to be too small.

To assess autocorrelation, the Durbin–Watson test examines successive residuals about the regression line. The test statistic d is given by

$$ d = \frac{\sum_{i=2}^{N} (e_i - e_{i-1})^2}{\sum_{i=1}^{N} e_i^2}. $$

where e_i represents the residuals. The statistic can be calculated online at http://www.wessa.net/slr.wasp and http://home.ubalt.edu/ntsbarsh/Business-stat/otherapplets/Trend.htm and tables of critical values at http://eclectic.ss.uci.edu/~drwhite/courses/Durbin-Watson.htm.

Autocorrelation, if present, is usually positive (Figure 27.18), and then the differences between any two consecutive residuals will be small, and the sum of the squared differences will be small relative to the sum of the squared residuals. d has a maximal value of 4 (Montgomery and Peck, 1982). The tables have both upper and lower critical values that need to be judged. The usual null hypothesis H_0 is that the coefficient of autocorrelation $\rho = 0$, and the usual alternative (for positive autocorrelation) is that $\rho > 0$. Then if $d < d_L$ (the lower of the two tabulated values), conclude that d is significant, and reject the null hypothesis at level α; if $d > d_U$ d is not significant and do not reject H_0; and if $d_L < d < d_U$, the test is inconclusive.

In general, $d = 2$ means no autocorrelation, $d < 1$ suggests marked positive autocorrelation, and $d > 3$ suggest marked negative autocorrelation, although the latter is rare (Figure 27.19). To test the alternative hypothesis $\rho < 0$, repeat the above tests but use $4-d$ instead of d.

CONTROL CHARTS

Quality control refers to determining the limits within which a process functions. A *process* is a series of operations that produces an outcome, such as an accurate measurement of a blood constituent. In measuring a blood constituent, for example, the process includes pipetting out the correct initial amount of blood, adding an exact amount of a diluent with precisely known property, perhaps adding an accurately measured amount of a chemical reagent with precisely known composition and concentration, and estimating the absorption of the resulting solution in an accurately calibrated spectrophotometer. A process is regarded as being in statistical control if repeated samples act like random samples from a stable probability distribution (Natrella, 1963). Ideally, repeating a measurement of a standard sodium concentration of 140 mMol should give the same value. However, repeated measurements of the same standard sodium solution will vary. The problem then is to determine stability of the signal in the face of noise, that is, natural variability. When is variability excessive and when does it indicate bias? If the samples are shown to be out of statistical control, then the source must be determined so that corrective action can be taken.

Early in the twentieth century Shewhart, working at the Bell Telephone Laboratories, introduced the notion of control charts. These in general take the form of a chart in which the value of the measurement is plotted against time, usually in regular increments.

A typical control chart is given in Figure 31.2.

Each point is a measurement made at successive times. The thick center line is the mean value, determined by theory or prior observation. The lines above and below the center line are drawn at values corresponding to 1, 2, and 3 standard deviations above the mean, based on prior observations. The values of 17.7–18.3 are artificial values used here for illustration. In an actual control chart they are determined by the subject being measured: for example, the mean might be 140 mMol for a normal

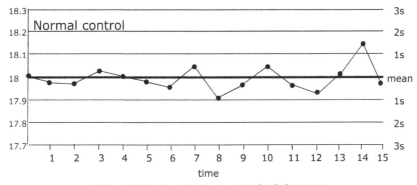

Figure 31.2 Control chart. s-standard deviation.

serum sodium concentration, and the standard deviation is determined by observation of repeated measurements.

Determining the correct standard deviation depends in part on the number of "control" measurements used in its calculation. Although a large sample size yields a sample standard deviation closer to the population value, it is the short-term variation that we want. One recommendation is that the control period is divided into successive subgroups (natural or artificially determined), the range of each subgroup is calculated, then the mean range is determined, and a working standard deviation is derived by dividing the mean range by Hartley's constant that depends on the number of subgroups and their sample size (Caulcutt, 2004). The constants are found at http://dfx.nl/userfiles/file/pdf/Control%20Chart%20Constants%20and%20Formulas.pdf. Other tables at or Figure 4.17 give constants for multiplying the mean range to get the upper and lower control limits directly. Frequently a range of 2 is chosen. Then consecutive ranges $|Y_1 - Y_2|, |Y_2 - Y_3|...$ are averaged and divided by the constant 1.28 to provide an estimated standard deviation (Caulcutt, 2004).

The control chart in Figure 31.2 shows the accuracy and precision of a process. For it to be more useful, a series of rules have been created. These specify sets of one or more unusual events that help in deciding when a process is out of control enough to warrant further investigation. The Western Electric Company (1956) defined some of these events, and a fuller set was defined by Nelson's rules (Nelson). Nelson's rules are:

1. One point is >3 standard deviations from the mean.
2. 9 or more consecutive points are on the same side of the mean.
3. 6 or more consecutive points are increasing or decreasing.
4. 14 or more points in a row alternately increase and decrease.
5. 2 or 3 out of 3 consecutive points are >2 standard deviations of the mean on the same side of the mean.
6. 4 or 5 out of 5 consecutive points are >1 standard deviation of the mean on the same side of the mean.
7. 15 points in a row are all within 1 standard deviation on either side of the mean.
8. 8 consecutive points are all >1 standard deviation on either side of the mean.
   Each of these rules is illustrated in Figure 31.3.

In some publications the lines 3 standard deviations above and below the mean are termed respectively the upper control limit (UCL) and the lower control limit (LCR). Companies and laboratories are free to determine their own rules, and sometimes the control limits are determined not by standard deviation units but by practical considerations of what tolerance should be allowed.

It is also possible to have control charts for the means, ranges, or standard deviations of small groups. Each of these has use in a particular field. Many other types of control charts

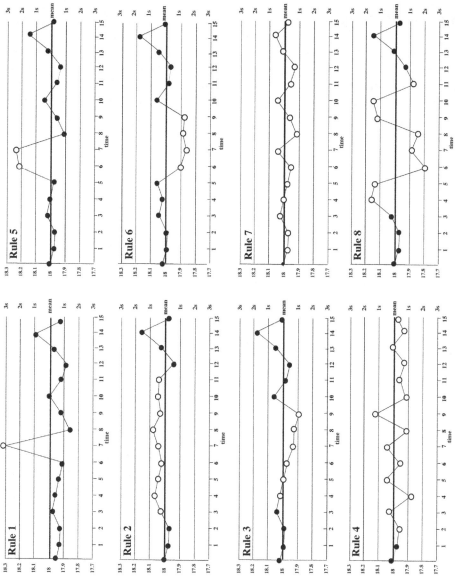

Figure 31.3 Nelson's rules. The open circles indicate the abnormal points that fit each rule.

are described by Hogg and Ledolter (1987), Roberts (1966), Betteley et al. (1994), Kennedy and Neville (1986), and Oakland (2003) Control charts can be created in Excel at (http://www.vertex42.com/ExcelTemplates/control-chart.html)

CUMULATIVE SUM TECHNIQUES (CUSUMS)

In medical practice, as well as laboratory control, there may be a quicker way to determine when a process is changing. This is a particularly challenging problem because often the signal is almost undetectable in the noise level. Consider Figure 31.4, taken from an article entitled "Why don't doctors use Cusums?" by Chaput de Saintonge and Vere (1974).

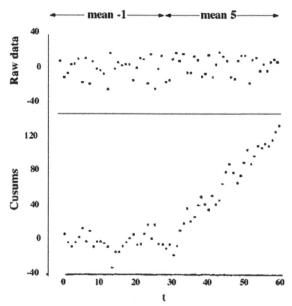

Figure 31.4 Upper panel: Artificial example of a low signal:noise ratio. The first portion shows randomly scattered values about a mean of −1. The second portion shows similar random variation after the mean has been altered to 5. The change is undetectable by eye. Lower panel: Cusums of the raw data.

The cumulative sum technique could not be simpler. By eye, a mean value is selected for the first few points; the exact value chosen is not important. The difference between the next point (X_1) and the mean is d_1. Then the difference $d_2 = X_2 - X_1$ is added to d_1 to obtain $\sum d_i$.

Then $d_3, d_4, \ldots d_n$ are added sequentially, and $\sum d_i$ is plotted against sample number. If the values of X continue to scatter above and below the mean, some of the deviations will be positive, some will be negative and the cumulative sum (Cusum) of the deviations tends to remain near zero. If, on the other hand, the values of X tend to increase or decrease consistently, even though the trend is hidden by the scatter, the Cusum of the deviations becomes increasingly positive or negative respectively. The results of the procedure on the data shown in Figure 31.4 are given in the lower panel (Chaput de Saintonge and Vere, 1974).

Another example is from a study by Davey et al. (1986) of the discharge rate of a single gamma motor neurone in the cat hind limb before and after facilitation by episodic stretch (Figure 31.5).

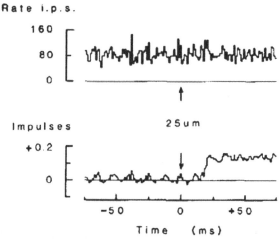

Figure 31.5 Discharge rate of motor neurone after facilitation. Basic record of rate in impulses per second above, Cusums below. It is doubtful that any change could have been detected by eye.

Instructions and sample charts can be found at https://www.statstodo.com/CUSUM_Exp.php, http://www.ehow.com/how_5305567_calculate-cusum.html, with instructions for using Excel at http://webbut.unitbv.ro/bu2009/BULETIN2009/Series%20I/BULETIN%20I%20PDF/Industrial%20Enginering/Eftimie%20N_09.pdf and at http://analysisjoe.blogspot.com/2007/03/applying-cusum-to-your-spreadsheet-data.html.

Problem 31.1

The following gives daily white cell counts (1000/c.mm) in a patient. Can you tell when the white count has begun to increase?

Day	1	2	3	4	5	6	7	8	9	10	11	12	13	14	15
WBC	9.4	8	9.3	11.7	12.2	10.2	8.1	11.5	9.2	10.4	9	11.5	10.5	9.4	10.1

Day	16	17	18	19	20	21	22	23	24	25	26	27	28	29	30
WBC	9.4	10.6	10.3	8.5	10.8	10.9	9.3	12.3	11.5	10.6	11.1	10.4	11.6	11.3	10.5

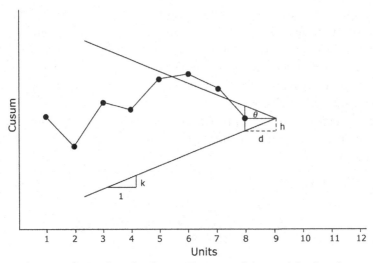

Figure 31.6 Application of V mask to the Cusum. The apex of the mask is placed one or more units ahead of the last measurement. The appearance of Cusum values that cross the upper line shows an upward slope that warrants investigation.

How can we tell when a deviation from zero slope is significant enough to warrant further investigation? The most commonly used method is to use a V mask, illustrated in Figure 31.6.

The V mask is based on the desired average run length (ARL), that is, the average length of the Cusum while the failure or deviation rate is acceptable. The ARL equals the number of patients or measurements seen before the Cusum exceeds the control limit. A wide mask angle reduces the number of false alarms, whereas a narrow angle allows early detection of a change that could lead to corrective action. The angle of the V depends on how many units ahead of the last Cusum point the apex is placed, how many standard deviations from the mean are acceptable, and how many units of divergence from the mean can be tolerated before some action is taken (Barnard, 1959; Woodward and Goldsmith, 1964). Some of these issues are more important in industry than medicine. For example, in Medicine, we often need to take action early, for example, to stabilize blood pressure or control ventilation, so that a one-unit lead and a short run time in which the Cusum departs from the mean are preferred.

V masks are implemented in most statistical programs.

To calculate the V mask, determine a deviation δ in standard deviation units that should be detected. The V mask has a half angle θ that the slope of the upper or the lower arm makes, as defined by the rise or fall of the slope (k) for a 1 unit change. This is the same as the vertical height h divided by the distance d (that is the number of units the apex is ahead of the last point) so that $d = h/k$. Then specifying the type I error α and the type II error β, calculate

$$\theta = \frac{2}{\delta} \frac{\log n(1 - \beta)}{\alpha} \text{ and } k = \frac{\delta}{2}.$$

In terms of type I (α) and type II (β) errors, write (Montgomery, 2000)

$$d = \frac{2}{\delta^2} \ln \left(\frac{1 - \beta}{\alpha} \right)$$

As a rule of thumb, if k is half of δ, h should be about 4 or 5. If a high sensitivity to small changes or slow trends is wanted, $h = 8$ and $k = 0.25$ are appropriate, and if large changes or rapid shifts need to be detected, then $h = 2.5$ and $k = 1$ are appropriate. As an example, if $d = 8$ and $\tan \theta = 0.25$, a change of 2σ in performance will be detected on the average after 4 measurements, a 1σ change after 8 measurements, and a 0.5σ change after 18 measurements (Marshall, 1979). The selection of a suitable V mask depends on what the investigator wants to do with the data. Alternative ways of assessing changes from the process mean have been described (Everitt, 1989).

Although some investigators have not found Cusums to be useful in biomedical studies (Mitchell et al., 1980), this is not the predominant view (Barnard, 1959; Chang and McLean, 2006; Chaput de Saintonge and Vere, 1974; Chatfield, 1980; Diggle, 1990; Draper and Smith, 1981; Grunkemeier et al., 2003; O'Brien and Christie, 1997; Rowlands et al., 1980; Westgard et al., 1977) and these methods may be particularly useful in infectious diseases with erratic swinging fevers (Kinsey et al., 1989; Walters and Griffin, 1986). Cusums are used extensively in industry. A clear description of their use and evaluation is given by Chatfield (1995) and Woodward and Goldsmith (1964).

Various extensions of the Cusum method have been used to follow surgical complications (death, excessive blood transfusion, etc.) so as to detect a change in their incidence. One variation is the exponential weighted moving average that resembles the Cusum method except that for each sum the previous observations are given exponentially decreasing weights (Smith et al., 2013). The second variation allows for the possibility that successive patients may have very different associated problems by creating a risk-adjusted Cusum (Steiner et al., 2000). Consultation with a statistician is recommended in deciding which variation to use.

SERIAL MEASUREMENTS

It is common for a group of animals or patients to be given a stimulus, and then to have serial observations made at successive time intervals of some response, for example, glucose or catecholamine concentrations, blood pressures, tumor size. Chapter 26 discussed repeated measures analysis, and this certainly enters into analyses of the results of such experiments. There are, however, other problems to deal with. The most important is that the successive measurements are not independent of each other, but are serially correlated.

As pointed out by Matthews et al. (1990) two types of responses are typically seen. One is the peaked response, where the response rises above control values to a maximum (or falls below them to a minimum), and then falls back to baseline. In the other there is a monotonic rise or fall over the duration of the study. Frequently several subjects are in each group. An example of the peaked response can be seen in Figure 31.1.

The first comment about such a figure is that joining the means of the results at different time periods gives a curve that may conceal the individual responses (Figure 31.7).

It is possible to construct a mean curve, but instead of conveying useful information it conceals information. This same problem may make it difficult to compare two groups. Many statisticians have recommended measuring the area under the curve for each subject. Then each subject's responses are summarized by a single number, and the sets of areas under the curves can be compared by a standard two-sample test.

On the other hand, the question of interest may be the time to reach the maximum in the two groups, and once again the mean curves may be misleading. Matthews et al. (1990) recommend plotting the maximal value against the mean time for each group, and then either compare the mean times to maximum or perhaps the slopes of the resulting plots. Alternatively, the question might be what the maxima or the minima are, and these are again easy to compare as sets of summary figures.

For monotonic curves, the analysis also depends upon the question being asked. This might be the rate of change, estimated by (linear) regression lines, the maximal values at a given time after the stimulus, or the time taken to reach a given change from the baseline. Whatever the question, it is best approached by summarizing each subject's response in a single measurement, rather than blending all the subjects in a group into one curve that might not be representative of the variability of the subjects.

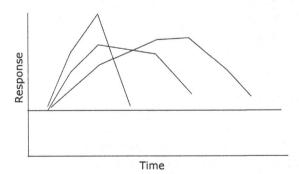

Figure 31.7 Serial responses. Hypothetical results of three patients.

REFERENCES

Barnard, G.A., 1959. Control charts and stochastic processes. J. R. Stat. Soc. Ser. B 21, 239–271.

Bartels, R., 1982. The rank version of von Neumann's ratio test for randomness. J. Am. Stat. Assoc. 77, 40–46.

Betteley, G., Mettrick, N., Sweeney, E., et al., 1994. Using Statistics in Industry. Prentice Hall.

Brown, D., Rothery, P., 1993. Models in Biology: Mathematics, Statistics and Computing. John Wiley & Sons, Inc.

Chatfield, C., 1980. The Analysis of Time Series. An Introduction. Chapman & Hall.

Chatfield, C., 1995. Statistics for Technology. A Course in Applied Statistics. Chapman & Hall.

Caulcutt, R., 2004. Control charts in practice. Significance 1, 81–84.

Chang, W.R., McLean, I.P., 2006. CUSUM: a tool for early feedback about performance? BMC Med. Res. Methodol. 6, 8.

Chaput de Saintonge, D.M., Vere, D.W., 1974. Why don't doctors use cusums? Lancet 1, 120–121.

Cole, L.C., 1957. Biological clock in the unicorn. Science 125, 874–876.

Davey, N.J., Ellaway, P.H., Stein, R.B., 1986. Statistical limits for detecting change in the cumulative sum derivative of the peristimulus time histogram. J. Neurosci. Methods 17, 153–166.

Diggle, P.J., 1990. Time Series. A Biostatistical Introduction. Clarendon Press.

Draper, N., Smith, H., 1981. Applied Regression Analysis. John Wiley & Sons.

Durbin, J., Watson, G.S., 1950. Testing for serial correlation in Least Squares Regression, I. Biometrika 37, 409–428.

Durbin, J., Watson, G.S., 1951. Testing for serial correlation in Least Squares Regression, II. Biometrika 38, 159–179.

Edgington, E.S., 1961. Probability table for number of runs of signs of first differences in ordered series. J. Am. Stat. Assoc. 56, 156–159.

Everitt, B.S., 1989. Statistical Methods for Medical Investigations. Oxford University Press.

Filicori, M., Butler, J.P., Crowley Jr., W.F., 1984. Neuroendocrine regulation of the corpus luteum in the human. Evidence for pulsatile progesterone secretion. J. Clin. Invest. 73, 1638–1647.

Grunkemeier, G.L., Wu, Y.X., Furnary, A.P., 2003. Cumulative sum techniques for assessing surgical results. Ann. Thorac. Surg. 76, 663–667.

Hamilton, L.C., 1992. Regression with Graphics. A Second Course in Applied Statistics. Duxbury Press.

Hogg, R.V., Ledolter, J., 1987. Applied Statistics for Engineers and Physical Scientists. Macmillan Publishing Company.

Kennedy, J.B., Neville, A.M., 1986. Basic Statistical Methods for Engineers and Scientists. Harper and Row.

Kinsey, S.E., Giles, F.J., Holton, J., 1989. Cusum plotting of temperature charts for assessing antimicrobial treatment in neutropenic patients. BMJ (Clin. Res. Ed.) 299, 775–776.

Madansky, A., 1988. Prescriptions for Working Statisticians. Springer-Verlag.

Marshall, R.A.G., 1979. The analysis of counter performance by cusum techniques. J. Radioanal. Chem. 54, 87–94.

Matthews, J.N., Altman, D.G., Campbell, M.J., et al., 1990. Analysis of serial measurements in medical research. BMJ (Clin. Res. Ed.) 300, 230–235.

Mendenhall, W., Sincich, T., 1986. A Second Course in Business Statistics: Regression Analysis. Dellen Publishing Co.

Merriam, G.R., Wachter, K.W., 1982. Algorithms for the study of episodic hormone secretion. Am. J. Physiol. 243, E310–E318.

Mitchell, D.M., Collins, J.V., Morley, J., 1980. An evaluation of cusum analysis in asthma. Br. J. Dis. Chest 74, 169–174.

Montgomery, D.C., Peck, E.A., 1982. Introduction to Linear Regression Analysis. John Wiley and Sons.

Montgomery, D.C., 2000. Introduction to Statistical Quality Control. Wiley.

Natrella, M.G., 1963. Experimental Statistics. Dover Publications, Inc.

Nelson, L.S., 1984. Technical Aids. J. Qual. Technol. 16, 238–239.

Neter, J., Wasserman, W., Whitmore, G.A., 1978. Applied Statistics. Allyn and Bacon, Inc.

Oakland, J.S., 2003. Statistical Process Control. Butterworth-Heinemann.

O'Brien, S.J., Christie, P., 1997. Do CuSums have a role in routine communicable disease surveillance? Public Health 111, 255–258.

Pollard, J.H., 1977. A Handbook of Statistical and Numerical Techniques. Cambridge University Press.

Roberts, S.W., 1966. A comparison of some control chart procedures. Technometrics 8, 411–430.

Rowlands, R.J., Wilson, D.W., Nix, A.B., et al., 1980. Advantages of CUSUM techniques for quality control in clinical chemistry. Clin. Chim. Acta 108, 393–397.

Smith, I.R., Garlick, B., Gardner, M.A., et al., 2013. Use of graphical statistical process control tools to monitor and improve outcomes in cardiac surgery. Heart Lung Circ. 22, 92–99.

Steiner, S.H., Cook, R.J., Farewell, V.T., et al., 2000. Monitoring surgical performance using risk-adjusted cumulative sum charts. Biostatistics 1, 441–452.

Veldhuis, J.D., Rogol, A.D., Evans, W.S., et al., 1986. Spectrum of the pulsatile characteristics of LH release in normal men. J. Androl. 7, 83–92.

Velduis, J.D., Weiss, J., Mauras, N., et al., 1986. Appraising endocrine pulse signals at low circulating hormone concentrations: use of regional coefficients of variation in the experimental series to analyze pulsatile luteinizing hormone release. Pediatr. Res. 20, 632–637.

Walters, S., Griffin, G.E., 1986. Resolution of fever in Staphylococcus aureus septicaemia—retrospective analysis by means of Cusum plot. J. Infect. 12, 57–63.

Western Electric Company, 1956. Statistical Quality Control Handbook. Western Electric Co.

Westgard, J.O., Groth, T., Aronsson, T., et al., 1977. Combined Shewhart-cusum control chart for improved quality control in clinical chemistry. Clin. Chem. 23, 1881–1887.

Wonnacott, T.H., Wonnacott, R.J., 1981. Regression: A Second Course in Statistics. John Wiley & Sons.

Woodward, R.H., Goldsmith, P.L., 1964. Cumulative Sum Techniques. Oliver and Boyd.

Zar, J.H., 2010. Biostatistical Analysis. Prentice Hall.

CHAPTER 32

Dose—Response Analysis

Contents

GENERAL PRINCIPLES

An increasing stimulus (dose or concentration of an agent, rate of nerve stimulation, degree of stretch, etc.) is given to a responding system that may be a bacterial culture, insect larvae, lymphocytes in culture, a muscle strip, a blood vessel, or even a whole organism in which the response or effect may be blood pressure, temperature, white cell count, percentage of organisms killed, amount of cytokine released, and so on. At extremely low stimuli, there may be no response. Then, as the stimulus increases, a response occurs and usually increases monotonically to reach some maximum value, after which increasing stimuli might have no further effect. (It is possible for the response to decrease after some maximal stimulus has been given.) The basic response curve is usually tripartite—a horizontal portion of no response at low stimuli, a rising response at higher stimuli, and then another horizontal maximal response at the highest stimuli. This gives an S-shaped or sigmoid curve (Figure 32.1).

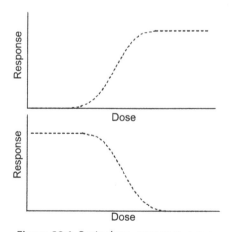

Figure 32.1 Basic dose—response curve.

For a list of all websites referred to in this chapter, as clickable links, see the book companion website: www.booksite.elsevier.com/9780128023877.

Biostatistics for Medical and Biomedical Practitioners
http://dx.doi.org/10.1016/B978-0-12-802387-7.00032-9

In the top panel, the dose increases from left to right, and the response increases from bottom to top. In the bottom panel, the response decreases as dose increases because of inhibition. Frequently, using a logarithmic scale for doses produces an approximately linear intermediate (nonhorizontal) phase that may be easier for analysis. In addition, the logarithmic scale expands the regions of low dosage where rapid changes are occurring and compresses the scale at higher doses where the response is changing more slowly. The response may be continuous, such as a gradual increase in muscle tension as the agonist concentration increases, or may be quantal, as when a particular effect is or is not reached. The quantal response is an ungraded response; it may be a fixed effect such as reduction of coughing below x times per hour, or may be an all-or-none response such as living or dying.

The typical dose—response curve is a plot of the logarithm of the dose on the X axis and the response on the Y axis. Frequently, the responses and/or the doses are transformed into response or dose metameters. Judicious selection of transformation for the dose can be selected so that the dose metameters are simple numbers such as -1 and $+1$ for two dose levels, -1, 0, and $+1$ for three dose levels, and so on (Colquhoun, 1971; Finney, 1952, 1964). The response is obtained by direct measurement in whatever units are appropriate to the subject, but then is converted into percentages based on no effect as 0% and full effect as 100%. Almost all responses are the result of binding of an agonist to a receptor, and the degree of binding is known as the affinity, that is, how chemical interactions result in occupancy of the receptors. This is not the same as efficacy, which refers to the response induced by that binding. This in turn is distinguished from potency that refers to the amount of agonist required to produce a given effect and is a function of affinity and efficacy; potency is often defined as the effect of 1 unit of a standard preparation. The concentration of agonist required to produce 50% of the maximal effect is known as the ED50, and in some experiments, the concentration of agonist required to kill 50% of the animals or cells is termed the LD50. If an agonist shifts the curve to the left (curve B in Figure 32.2), it has increased potency because the

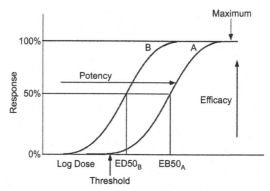

Figure 32.2 Some typical features in a dose—response curve.

ED50 is seen at a lower concentration; the maximal response and thus the maximal efficacy may not change. Some of these features are shown in Figure 32.2.

The slope of the middle portion of the curve often supplies information. The concentrations at which the response first begins (threshold) and first reaches maximum are also of interest, but may be difficult to define accurately. Sigmoid dose—response curves are of major importance in analyzing receptor-binding information. Analysis of sigmoid curves is mathematically complex, and requires good programs to achieve it. The analysis has to handle a complex equation:

$$Y_i = \frac{a - d}{1 + \left(\frac{X_i}{c}\right)^b},$$

where Y is the response, X is the dose, a is the response when $X = 0$, d is the maximal response, c is the ED50, and b is a steepness factor. Another more general formulation for the sigmoid dose—response curve is:

$$\widehat{Y} = \text{Bottom} + \frac{\text{Top} - \text{Bottom}}{1 + 10^{\text{LogEC50} - X}}.$$

See excellent online discussion by Motulsky at http://www.graphpad.com/manuals/prism4/RegressionBook.pdf

Multiple nonlinear regression techniques are needed to solve these problems.

One general statistical program that features these analyses prominently is Prism, but all large programs allow dose—response analysis, and there are a host of specialized programs for this purpose, one of the best known being Ligand (Curran-Everett, 2005; DeLean et al., 1978; Munson and Rodbard, 1980).

QUANTAL DOSE—RESPONSE CURVES

Some responses are all-or-none, and are termed quantal. Examples are whether an insect does or does not survive a given dose of insecticide, or whether a patient does or does not respond to a painful stimulus when given a particular concentration or amount of an anesthetic. Analysis of such responses differs from other forms of dose—response analysis, because the investigator does not give increasing doses of the agonist and measure a corresponding response in any subject. Instead, a specific dose of agonist is given to a number of subjects (insects, patients) and how many do or do not react (survive for insects, move with patients) are recorded. Then a higher dose is given to a new set of subjects, and so on. How any given individual responds to a particular dose is unknown, but the percentage responding at that dose can be determined. In general, the percentage responding plotted against the dose, or the log of the dose, produces an S-shaped curve (Figure 32.2).

It is possible to straighten out the cumulative normal sigmoid curve by plotting the X variate against the normal equivalent distribution (NED) (Chapter 6). By converting a normal Gaussian curve into standard form, $z = \frac{X_i - \mu}{\sigma}$, any given area under the curve can be specified in z units. Thus, the lowest 2.5% under the curve occurs at -2 units (2σ below the mean), the lowest 15.87% at -1 units, 50% at 0 units, 84.2% at 1 unit, and so on. This scale is symmetrical about zero, and although in theory it extends to infinity above and below the mean, in practice only 0.0000002867 of the area is more than 5 units below or above the mean, so that virtually all the area lies between 5 units below and 5 units above the mean of 0. To avoid negative numbers 5 is added to the scale, and the new transformed NED numbers are termed probits. Therefore, if the quantal dose—(log)response curve is approximately symmetrical and normal, a plot of the dose against the percent response transformed into probits (derived from tables) gives a straight line (Figure 32.3).

$$\text{Probit} = 5 + \frac{X_i - \mu}{\sigma} = \left(5 - \frac{\mu}{\sigma}\right) + \left(\frac{1}{\sigma}\right)X_i$$

and this is the equation to a straight line with intercept $\left(5 - \frac{\mu}{\sigma}\right)$ and slope $\left(\frac{1}{\sigma}\right)$.

A simple explanation of probits and accompanying tables can be found online at http://www.ncbi.nlm.nih.gov/pmc/articles/PMC1624212/. A nice explanation of probit analysis and the tables are given at http://userwww.sfsu.edu/efc/classes/biol710/probit/ProbitAnalysis.pdf.

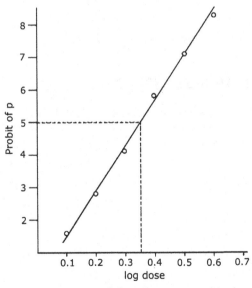

Figure 32.3 Quantal dose—response probit plot.

If the points can be fitted reasonably well by a straight line, then the value of X corresponding to a probit of 5 (shown by the dotted lines) is the median log dose required for a 50% response. The reciprocal of the slope is the standard deviation, and this can be used to set confidence limits (in log units).

Precise fitting of the line is complex, because the binomial response results in larger variability for high proportions than for low proportions (heteroscedasticity). Fitting is done by weighted least squares methods, and usually has several iterations.

Precision of estimate is greatest for the ED50 (median), but often a lower value is required. There is not much interest in knowing how much radiation is needed to kill or cause cancer in 50% of people, but much importance in knowing at what lower limit of radiation exposure the risk is very low. This means working at the low extreme of the curve, but here data are more difficult to assess and the number required to reach a firm conclusion may be very large. This is why we are still arguing about whether there is or is not a threshold for radiation damage.

REFERENCES

Colquhoun, D., 1971. Lectures on Biostatistics. Clarendon Press.

Curran-Everett, D., 2005. Estimation of dose-response curves and identification of peaks in hormone pulsations: classic marriages of statistics to science. Am. J. Physiol. Endocrinol. Metab. 289, E363—E365.

DeLean, A., Munson, P.J., Rodbard, D., 1978. Simultaneous analysis of families of sigmoidal curves: application to bioassay, radioligand assay, and physiological dose-response curves. Am. J. Physiol. 235, E97—E102.

Finney, D.J., 1952. Probit Analysis. Cambridge University Press.

Finney, D.J., 1964. Statistical Method in Bioassay. Hafner Publishing Co.

Munson, P.J., Rodbard, D., 1980. Ligand: a versatile computerized approach for characterization of ligand-binding systems. Anal. Biochem. 107, 220—239.

CHAPTER 33

Logistic Regression

Contents

INTRODUCTION

Until now, the regression discussion has involved a continuous Y variate. Sometimes, however, the Y variate is discontinuous, and in particular has a dichotomous value: an outcome either happens or does not happen. Examples are the response of an organism (say, an insect) to a toxin—it either lives or dies; survival of a premature infant related to birth weight; the presence or absence of a disease related to certain clinical or laboratory findings. Therefore, Y can take on only one of two values—no or yes. If many subjects are studied at different doses of a drug or different birth weights, then at each dose or weight a probability (P) of an event such as death or a disease can be assigned.

If in a typical regression equation $\hat{Y}_1 = c + b_1X_1$ P is replaced by Y, then

$$P = c + bX_1.$$

This is unsuitable because P can vary only from 0 to 1, whereas Y can be any value, including values above 1 or being negative. To avoid a negative result, the equation might be written as $P = e^{c+bX}$, but this, although always positive, can be greater than 1. The desired criterion can be met by an expression of the form $P = \frac{1}{1+e^{-(c+bX)}}$ that can never exceed 1.

This is termed the logistic function that has an S shape (Figure 33.1).

When the coefficient b in the equation is $-\infty$, the value of the function is 0, and when it is $+\infty$, the value is 1.

In normal regression c represents the intercept on the Y-axis when $X = 0$, but in logistic regression it has a slightly different interpretation (see below), and β_0 is used in its place. Then the logistic function becomes

For a list of all websites referred to in this chapter, as clickable links, see the book companion website: www.booksite.elsevier.com/9780128023877.

Biostatistics for Medical and Biomedical Practitioners
http://dx.doi.org/10.1016/B978-0-12-802387-7.00033-0

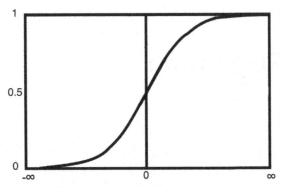

Figure 33.1 Logistic function curve.

$$P = \frac{1}{1 + e^{-(\beta_0 + \beta_1 X)}}.$$

β_0 takes the place of c in the usual regression equation, and β_1 is the coefficient of the X variate.

P is the probability of success and $1 - P$ is the probability of failure.

Then,

$$1 - P = 1 - \frac{1}{1 + e^{-(\beta_0 + \beta_1 X)}} = \frac{1 + e^{-(\beta_0 + \beta_1 X)} - 1}{1 + e^{-(\beta_0 + \beta_1 X)}} = \frac{e^{-(\beta_0 + \beta_1 X)}}{1 + e^{-(\beta_0 + \beta_1 X)}}.$$

The odds of success are defined as $\frac{P}{1-P}$, and this is therefore

$$\frac{P}{1 - P} = \frac{\frac{1}{1+e^{-(\beta_0 + \beta_1 X)}}}{\frac{e^{-(\beta_0 + \beta_1 X)}}{1+e^{-(\beta_0 + \beta_1 X)}}} = \frac{1}{e^{-(\beta_0 + \beta_1 X)}} = e^{(\beta_0 + \beta_1 X)}.$$

Taking natural logarithms gives

$$\log n \frac{P}{1 - P} = \log n e^{(\beta_0 + \beta_1 X)} = \beta_0 + \beta_1 X.$$

This is the equation of a linear regression between X and $\log n \frac{P}{1-P}$.

The expression $\log n \frac{P}{1-P}$ is the logit transformation.

After deriving the linear equation, convert the log of the odds of success to the probability P of success, even though this latter relationship is alinear. These calculations can be performed online at http://statpages.org/logistic.html, http://vassarstats.net/logreg1.html#down, http://www.wessa.net/rwasp_logisticregression.wasp, but only for simple problems.

What meaning is attached to the different coefficients? If the X variate is 0, then $P = \frac{1}{e^{-\beta_0}}$ or logit $P = \beta_0$. This is true, whether or not X can physically be 0. Thus, in the examples used below for artificial ventilation in neonates, it is impossible to have a neonate with zero gestational weight. In this instance, β_0 is the background risk of artificial ventilation in the absence of any explanatory factors; that is, it is the average risk for the whole studied population.

The β_1 coefficient also has a meaning. It is the change in logit P for a one-unit change in the X variable. If there are multiple explanatory factors (X_1, X_2, X_3, etc.), β_i is the change in logit P for a one-unit change in the X_i variable when the other variables are constant.

Logit transformation can be used also with odds ratios. If there are logits P_1 for one group and P_2 for another, for example, the probability of having a myocardial infarction related to age in subjects who do or do not smoke, then

$$\text{logit } P_1 - \text{logit } P_2 = \log\frac{P_1}{1-P_1} - \log\frac{P_2}{1-P_2} = \log\left[\frac{\log\frac{P_1}{1-P_1}}{\log\frac{P_2}{1-P_2}}\right]$$

$$= \log\left[\frac{P_1(1-P_2)}{P_2(1-P_1)}\right].$$

This is the logarithm of the odds ratio (Chapter 20), and it can also be written as

$$\log n \ OR = \frac{e^{(\beta_0+\beta_1 X_1)}}{e^{(\beta_0+\beta_1 X_2)}} = e^{(\beta_0+\beta_1 X_1)} - e^{(\beta_0+\beta_1 X_2)} = e^{\beta_1(X_1-X_2)}.$$

SINGLE EXPLANATORY VARIABLE

In a newborn nursery, the risk of dying or of needing artificial ventilation is known to be a function of birth weight or gestational age. From a data set of 315 newborn infants, kindly supplied by Dr Terri Slagle of the California Pacific Medical Center in San Francisco, examine these relationships by logistic regression. Figure 33.2 shows the results for the probability of needing ventilation, based on birth weight.

At very low birth weights almost 100% of the neonates needed artificial ventilation, a percentage that decreased to very low values at high birth weights.

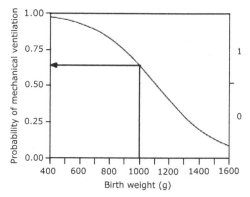

Figure 33.2 Birth weight versus probability of artificial ventilation.

The results of the calculations are in Table 33.1.

Table 33.1 Logistic regression analysis of birth weight and need for ventilation.

Model	−Log-Likelihood		DF	Chi-Square	Prob > ChiSq
Difference	54.14953		1	108.2991	<0.0001
Full	163.92351				
Reduced	218.07303				
RSquare (U)		0.2483			
Observations (or sum weights) converged by gradient		315			

Whole model test

Parameter estimates

Term	Estimate	Std error	Chi-Square	Prob > ChiSq
Intercept	5.50796392	0.6521633	71.33	<0.0001
Birth weight in grams for log odds of 0/1	−0.0049233	0.0005675	75.27	<0.0001

The programs use the method of maximum likelihood estimation to fit the curve. Under the heading, Whole Model Test is what resembles an Analysis of variance (ANOVA) table. "Full" refers to a measure with no explanatory variables, (here there is only one—birth weight) and "Reduced" refers to the measure after addition of the explanatory variable. The "Difference" is analogous to the between group sum of squares in an ANOVA, and is tested by the negative log-likelihood to give a chi-square value. As in any chi-square, the higher the value for given degrees of freedom the more likely is the result to be significant, that is, to reject the null hypothesis that birth weight did not affect the need for artificial ventilation. The RSquare of 0.2483 shows that the explanatory variable can account for no more than 24.83% of the variability.

In each panel, the negative log-likelihood is calculated for all the data points without regard to any explanatory factors (full) and this is compared with the negative log-likelihood calculated when the factor is included (reduced). The difference resembles the within groups mean square in ANOVA, and is tested for significance. There is a significant reduction in variability due to the explanatory factor.

The parameter estimates provides the prediction equation as

$$P = \frac{1}{1 + e^{-(5.5080 - 0.004923BW)}},$$

and this can be used to calculate probabilities at any desired birth weight. For example, a neonate weighing 1000 g at birth has a probability of needing artificial ventilation of $P = \frac{1}{1 + e^{-(5.5080 - 0.004923 \times 1000)}} = 0.6422$, as in Figure 33.1 (arrow).

If the birth weight is 2000 g, then the probability is $P = \frac{1}{1+e^{-(5.5080-0.004923\times1600)}}, = 0.0856$.

Repeat the above calculations using gestational age as the explanatory variable (Figure 33.3; Table 33.2).

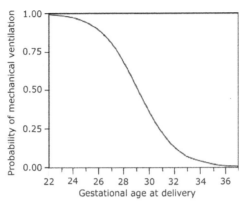

Figure 33.3 Gestational age versus probability of artificial ventilation. The analytic data are in Table 33.2.

Table 33.2

Whole model test

Model	−Log-Likelihood	DF	Chi-Square	Prob > ChiSq
Difference	76.10544	1	152.2109	<0.0001
Full	141.96759			
Reduced	218.07303			
RSquare (U)	0.3490			
Observations (or sum weights) converged by gradient	315			

Parameter estimates

Term	Estimate	Std error	Chi-Square	Prob > ChiSq
Intercept	19.4010702	2.1349654	82.58	<0.0001
Gestational age at delivery for log odds of 0/1	−0.6662323	0.07313	83.00	<0.0001

The fit is better as shown by an RSquare of 0.3490. The prediction equation is $P = \frac{1}{1+e^{-(19.4011-0.6662GA)}}$. The probability of ventilation at a gestational age of 30 weeks is

$$\text{logit } P = 19.4011 - 0.6662 \times 30 = -0.5849.$$

Then taking antilogs of both sides gives $\frac{P}{1-P} = e^{-0.5849} = 0.5572$.

Solving for P gives $P = 0.3578$ which fits nicely with the graph above.

MULTIPLE EXPLANATORY VARIABLES

An advantage of logistic regression is that it allows the evaluation of multiple explanatory variables by extension of the basic principles. The general equation is

$$P = \frac{1}{1 + e^{-(\beta_0 + \beta_1 X_1 + \beta_2 X_2 + \ldots \beta_n X_n)}} = \frac{1}{1 + e^{-(\beta_0 + \sum \beta_i X_i)}}.$$

For example, consider predicting the probability of artificial ventilation from birth weight, gestational age, and maternal age, first separately (Figure 33.4).

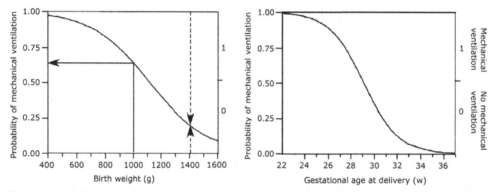

Figure 33.4 Individual probability curves for birth weight and age. The curve for maternal age was almost flat and is not shown.

The probability of artificial ventilation is almost 1 for the smallest and youngest neonates. It is possible to interpret each curve as splitting the area into a portion with risk of ventilation and a portion with no risk of ventilation; the two vertical dashed lines show that at a birth weight of 1400 g, the odds of artificial ventilation are about one-quarter the odds of no artificial ventilation.

The statistics of these curves are shown in Table 33.3.

Table 33.3 Probability of artificial ventilation

		Whole model test			
Model	−Log-Likelihood		DF	Chi-Square	Prob > ChiSq
Difference	54.14953		1	108.2991	<0.0001
Full	163.92351				
Reduced	218.07303			**Birth weight**	
RSquare (U)		0.2483			
Observations		315			
(or sum weights)					

Table 33.3 Probability of artificial ventilation—cont'd

Whole model test

Model	−Log-Likelihood		DF	Chi-Square	Prob > ChiSq
Difference	76.10544		1	152.2109	<0.0001
Full	141.96759				
Reduced	218.07303			**Gestational age**	
RSquare (U)		0.3490			
Observations (or sum weights)		315			

Whole model test

Model	−Log-Likelihood		DF	Chi-Square	Prob > ChiSq
Difference	4.89681		1	9.793625	<0.0018
Full	213.17622				
Reduced	218.07303			**Maternal age**	
RSquare (U)		0.0225			
Observations (or sum weights)		315			

All three explanatory factors are significant on their own, with the best single predictor being gestational age. Although maternal age as a predictor is significant, with $P = 0.0018$, the RSquare value of 0.0225 shows that maternal age by itself can explain only 2.25% of the variability.

The question is what happens if all the three explanatory factors are included in a single equation. Will it provide more information than any of the single regressions? Will it show if any of the variables are redundant? The results are shown in Table 33.4.

The RSquare has increased slightly to 0.3662 from the highest single value of 0.3490 for gestational age alone. Birth weight is no longer a predictor; it has an insignificant chi-square ($P = 0.3062$) and the confidence limits for its coefficient range from positive to negative. Therefore omit birth weight and produce a final regression with two variables (Table 33.5).

The final equation is

$$P = \frac{1}{1 + e^{-(21.5626 - 0.6704\,GA - 0.0604\,MA)}},$$

where GA is gestational age and MA is maternal age.

For gestational ages of 25, 30, and 35 weeks, and maternal ages of 20 and 40 years, the probabilities of needing artificial ventilation calculated from the formula are given in Table 33.6.

Table 33.4 Regression with three variables

Whole model test

Model	−Log-Likelihood	DF	Chi-Square	Prob > ChiSq
Difference	79.86792	3	159.7358	<0.0001
Full	138.20511			
Reduced	218.07303			
RSquare (U)	0.3662			
Observations (or sum weights)	315			
converged by gradient				

Lack of fit

Parameter estimates

Term	Estimate	Std error	Chi-Square	Prob > ChiSq	Lower 95%	Upper
Intercept	20.4402255	2.622536	60.75	<0.0001	15.5825235	25.9006
Birth weight in grams	−0.0008706	0.0008508	1.05	0.3062	−0.0025389	0.00080
Gestational age at delivery	−0.5993864	0.100158	35.81	<0.0001	−0.8054551	−0.411
Maternal age at delivery. For log odds of 0/1	−0.0591915	0.0244469	5.86	0.0155	−0.1085991	−0.0123

Table 33.5 Two variable regression

Whole model test

Model	–Log-Likelihood	DF	Chi-Square	Prob > ChiSq
Difference	79.34711	2	158.6942	<0.0001
Full	138.72592			
Reduced	218.07303			
RSquare (U)	0.3639			
Observations (or sum weights)	315			

Lack of fit

Source	DF	–Log-Likelihood	Chi-Square	Prob > ChiSq
Lack of fit	258	117.22481	234.4496	0.8509
Saturated	260	21.50111		
Fitted	2	138.72592		

Parameter estimates

Term	Estimate	Std error	Chi-Square	Prob > ChiSq
Intercept	21.5626217	2.4170882	79.58	<0.0001
Gestational age at delivery	–0.6703814	0.0744915	80.99	<0.0001
Maternal age at delivery. For log odds of 0/1	–0.0603604	0.0244109	6.11	0.0134

Table 33.6 Selected probabilities

Gestational age (weeks)	Maternal age (years)	Probability of artificial ventilation
25	20	0.9732
25	40	0.9158
30	20	0.5603
30	40	0.2758
35	20	0.0427
35	40	0.0139

In keeping with the coefficients that were determined, maternal age plays a small role in determining the need for artificial ventilation.

Alternatively, write $\ln\frac{P}{1-P} = 21.5626 - 0.6704GA - 0.0604MA$. The value for β_0 of 21.5626 is the average risk of artificial ventilation independent of any explanatory variables. β_1, the coefficient for gestational age, is 0.6704. Therefore, the logit decreases by 0.6704 units for each week increase in gestational age if maternal age is constant.

APPROPRIATENESS OF MODEL

Is the statistical model, appropriate for the data? Other possible models, such as discriminant analysis and Hotelling's T^2, test have been used (Cupples et al., 1984). The logistic regression model has advantages over the other two in not needing normally distributed variables. Many different approaches have been used (Glantz and Slinker, 2001; Lemeshow and Hosmer, 1982), and different programs implement these in different ways. In Table 33.3 above the lack of fit is tested and the fit was found to be acceptable.

In previous chapters on regression, several tests were discussed: plotting residuals or studentized residuals, leverage, Cook's distance, and others. Some of these tests can be applied to examining the results from logistic regression models (Glantz and Slinker, 2001). Furthermore, the model may contain interaction terms that also need to be evaluated.

Sample size and power calculations are as important here as in other statistical tests. The recommendation of Altman (1992) that the sample size should be at least 10 times the number of variables holds here as it does for multiple regression, with the exception that the sample size refers to the number of positive events. If examining the outcome (death or survival) of premature infants is related to six possible explanatory variables, then at least 60 deaths are needed for an adequate sample size with enough power.

Then, just like multiple regression methods, multicollinearity is a concern. For example, birth weight and gestational age are correlated. Will this interfere with the estimates? To check this to determine what the correlation is (Figure 33.5).

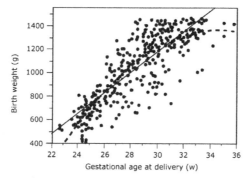

Figure 33.5 Relationship between birth weight and gestational age.

For linear regression R^2 was 0.6632, and for quadratic regression it was 0.7034, and neither of these is high enough to suggest that multicollinearity will cause problems. If there is concern, then better estimates can be obtained by centering the data.

Because this is a form of multiple regression there is the choice of forward, backward, or step-wise regressions, with the same potential problems as discussed in Chapter 30.

REFERENCES

Altman, D.G., 1992. Practical Statistics for Medical Research, Chapman & Hall, London, p. 611.

Cupples, L.A., Heeren, T., Schatzkin, A., et al., 1984. Multiple testing of hypotheses in comparing two groups. Ann. Intern. Med. 100, 122–129.

Glantz, S.A., Slinker, B.K., 2001. Primer of Applied Regression and Analysis of Variance. McGraw-Hill, Inc.

Lemeshow, S., Hosmer Jr., D.W., 1982. A review of goodness of fit statistics for use in the development of logistic regression models. Am. J. Epidemiol. 115, 92–106.

CHAPTER 34

Poisson Regression

Contents

INTRODUCTION

Poisson regression requires advanced statistical programs and is complex so that it is not featured in most basic textbooks. Nevertheless, it is often used in epidemiology, sociology, and psychology. In 2004—2008, 1568 articles using Poisson regression had appeared in the medical literature (Kleinman and Norton, 2009), so that investigators need to know when it is appropriate, how to interpret the results, and what precautions should be taken before using it.

Standard regression, linear, or multiple, is used to predict a dependent variable that may be of any size and could be positive or negative from one or more explanatory variables that may be continuous ratio numbers or dummy variables. Logistic regression is used to predict a dichotomous variable, for example, survival or dying, from similar explanatory variables. What can be used for counted data that probably fit a Poisson distribution? Neither of the previous methods will be useful. The results are not dichotomous, and counts violate the requirements for standard regression in at least three ways (Coxe et al., 2009):

1. Poisson data are skewed, whereas standard regression requires a symmetric distribution of errors.
2. Standard regression can sometimes produce negative values that cannot occur in a Poisson distribution.
3. Whereas in standard regression the variance should be (reasonably) constant, in a Poisson distribution the variance increases in proportion to the mean.

Poisson regression overcomes these three problems by a logarithmic transformation that compensates for skewness, prevents a negative predicted value, and also includes the proportionality between variance and the mean.

For a list of all websites referred to in this chapter, as clickable links, see the book companion website: www.booksite.elsevier.com/9780128023877.

Biostatistics for Medical and Biomedical Practitioners
http://dx.doi.org/10.1016/B978-0-12-802387-7.00034-2
613

If Y has a Poisson distribution, then a log-linear model can be constructed as $\ln \hat{Y} = a + \beta X$, and can be extended to several explanatory variables

$$\ln \hat{Y} = \alpha + \beta_1 X_1 + \beta_2 X_2 + ... \beta_k X_k.$$

The difficulty is that the prediction is in terms of log counts, whereas in practice actual counts are needed. This can be handled by exponiating both sides

$$e^{\ln \hat{Y}} = e^{(\alpha + \beta_1 X_1 + \beta_2 X_2 + ... \beta_k X_k)}.$$

Because $e^{\ln \hat{Y}} = \hat{Y}$, rewrite the equation as

$$\hat{Y} = e^{(\alpha + \beta_1 X_1 + \beta_2 X_2 + ... \beta_k X_k)}.$$

Now the predicted value of Y is in counts. This equation can be manipulated further to give

$$\hat{Y} = e^{\alpha} e^{\beta_1 X_1} e^{\beta_2 X_2} ..... e^{\beta_k X_k}.$$

Therefore, if all the variables except X_i are held constant, a one-unit change in X_i causes a change in predicted Y of $\hat{Y} e^{\beta_i}$.

Fitting the Poisson regression is done by maximum likelihood methods that are beyond the scope of this book. Examples of the use of these principles in epidemiological investigations, for example, of the risk of cancer and radiation exposure, are given by Selvin (1995).

In standard regression, the departure from perfect prediction is assessed by the value of $1 - R^2$, but this cannot be calculated for Poisson regression. In its place, the maximum likelihood method calculates a *deviance* that represents variability. Deviance is a relative and not an absolute metric. A large deviance indicates a poor fit, whereas a small deviance indicates a better fit. The deviance is used to calculate a pseudo R^2 from Coxe et al. (2009).

$$R^2_{\text{deviance}} = 1 - \frac{\text{deviance(fitted model)}}{\text{deviance(intercept alone)}}.$$

This pseudo R^2 varies from 0 to 1, and gets bigger as more explanatory variables are included. Variations on estimates of pseudo R^2 are also used (Coxe et al., 2009). The significance of the difference between two deviances obtained by adding in more explanatory variables is tested by chi-square, with degrees of freedom equal to the difference in the number of parameters tested (Coxe et al., 2009). More complex programs for assessing model adequacy, leverage, and outliers are available (Coxe et al., 2009).

SUITABILITY OF POISSON REGRESSION

Sometimes Poisson regression is inappropriate, for example, when the observed variance is much greater than the mean. This is termed overdispersion, and is usually due to failure to include all the explanatory variables or to nonindependence between events, a condition referred to as a contagious distribution (Chapter 19). Poisson regression may be inefficient if there are too many zeros, something that is quite frequent. Both of these factors may be present. For example, Table 34.1 shows the frequency of 12-year-old children with decayed, missing, or filled teeth (DMFT) in an Iranian study (Moghinbeigi et al., 2008).

Table 34.1 Distribution of DMFT in 12-year-old Iranian children

DMFT	Frequency
0	652
1	55
2	69
3	56
4	75
5	36
6	29
7	22
8	22
9	11
10	6
11	2
12	2
13	1
14	4
15	1
16	0
17	1
18	0
19	1

There were 1045 children, the mean number of DMF teeth was 1.598, and the standard deviation was 2.706. If this were a Poisson distribution, the number of children with different numbers of DMF teeth are shown in Table 34.2 and compared with the observed numbers.

Table 34.2 Observed and expected numbers, based on Poisson distribution

Number of DMFT	Proportion from Poisson	Expected number from Poisson (E)	Observed number (O)	O − E	$(O - E)^2/E = \chi^2$
0	0.202	211.09	652	440.91	920.94
1	0.323	337.54	55	−282.54	236.50
2	0.258	269.61	69	−200.61	149.27
3	0.138	144.21	56	−88.21	53.96
4	0.055	57.47	75	17.53	5.35
5	0.018	18.81	36	17.19	15.71
6	0.005	5.22	29	23.78	108.33
>6	0.001	1.05	73	71.95	4930.29
Total	1.000	1045	1045	0.0	$\chi^2_T = 6420.35$

With the discrepancy shown, there is hardly any need to do a chi-square test to show that the two sets of numbers do not fit. This distribution of DMF teeth differs from a Poisson distribution in two respects: there is an excess of zeros, and the standard deviation exceeds the mean.

DETECTING OVERDISPERSION

Because overdispersion causes the standard deviation to exceed the mean, it needs to be tested for. Some statistics programs report in addition to the deviance the Pearson statistic (total chi-square) (Dallal, 2008). If the total chi-square is divided by the corresponding degrees of freedom, it provides an index of dispersion; if there is no overdispersion the ratio should be 1. (Remember that the 0.50 value is about the same as the degrees of freedom for any chi-square with more than 4 degrees of freedom.) Furthermore, the ratio mean to standard deviation should also be 1. Unfortunately, these two indexes do not necessarily agree (Dallal, 2008).

Because the programs performing Poisson regression are complex and have to be selected with care, it is important to consider the advice given by Dallal (2008), "...virtually any sin that can be committed with least squares regression can be committed with Poisson and negative binomial regression. These include stepwise procedures and arriving at a final model by looking at the data."

CORRECTING FOR OVERDISPERSION

This is done most simply by using a scaling factor

$$\phi = \frac{\text{chi-square}}{df}.$$

The model then becomes a Poisson regression with mean μ and variance $\phi(\mu)$, and the standard deviation becomes $\sqrt{\phi(\mu)}$. The deviance of the new model becomes deviance$/\phi$, and being smaller, indicates a better fit.

In the example shown in Table 34.2,

$\phi = \frac{6420.35}{6} = 1070.06$, so that the standard deviation becomes 32.72.

As an alternative, a negative binomial regression can be done (Coxe et al., 2009).

It may also be necessary to correct for excess numbers of zeros.

There are many possible variations for testing the assumptions and performing the analyses, and several different types of analysis that can be done. Apart from variants of the zero-inflated Poisson, there are models for zero-inflated negative binomial regression that, in addition to the excess zeroes, can also take heterogeneity into account (Rose et al., 2006). In some data sets the events are very sparse, for example, the admission of children with Kawasaki syndrome to hospital may occur on the average once in

10–12 days, and then a variation known as gamma regression has advantages (Bateson, 2009; Checkley et al., 2009; Keenan et al., 2007). Consultation with a statistician is essential.

REFERENCES

Bateson, T.F., 2009. Gamma regression of interevent waiting times versus Poisson regression of daily event counts: inside the epidemiologist's toolbox-selecting the best modeling tools for the job. Epidemiology 20, 202–204.

Checkley, W., Guzman-Cottrill, J., Epstein, L., et al., 2009. Short-term weather variability in Chicago and hospitalizations for Kawasaki disease. Epidemiology 20, 194–201.

Coxe, S., West, S.G., Aiken, L.S., 2009. The analysis of count data: a gentle introduction to Poisson regression and its alternatives. J. Pers. Assess. 91, 121–136.

Dallal, G.E., 2008. Poisson Regression [Online]. Available: http://www.jerrydallal.com/LHSP/Poisson.htm.

Keenan, S.P., Dodek, P., Martin, C., et al., 2007. Variation in length of intensive care unit stay after cardiac arrest: where you are is as important as who you are. Crit. Care Med. 35, 836–841.

Kleinman, L.C., Norton, E.C., 2009. What's the risk? A simple approach for estimating adjusted risk measures from nonlinear models including logistic regression. Health Serv. Res. 44, 288–302.

Moghinbeigi, A., Eshragian, M.R., Mohammad, K., et al., 2008. Multilevel zero-inflated negative binomial regression modelling for over-dispersed count data with extra zeros. J. Appl. Stat. 25, 1193–1202.

Rose, C.E., Martin, S.W., Wannemuehler, K.A., et al., 2006. On the use of zero-inflated and hurdle models for modeling vaccine adverse event count data. J. Biopharm. Stat. 16, 463–481.

Selvin, S., 1995. Practical Biostatistical Methods. Wadsworth Publishing Company.

## PART 8

Miscellaneous Topics

CHAPTER 35

Survival Analysis

Contents

BASIC CONCEPTS

Introduction

Statistical methods are used extensively to determine time-to-failure in industry and have been adapted to medical purposes; the techniques are known as survival analysis. Survival may be defined as "the absence of a specific event after prolonged surveillance" (Muenz, 1983). An event has been defined as "a transition from one discrete stage to another" (Allison, 1995). Death is the prime example of an event, but other end points can be used: recurrence of a supraventricular arrhythmia after ablation, pacemaker failure, relapse after leukemia treatment, or readmission for congestive heart failure are all events. Survival analysis in these events shows the rate at which failure or the event occurs. It might take many years before the arrhythmia returns, the pacemaker fails, or the leukemia returns. The question then becomes how to determine survival rates in a timely fashion? In two or more different techniques of ablation, we would not want to wait for 50 years before deciding on the best technique. This problem is of particular interest in comparing different forms of treatment for cancer.

The techniques used in medicine are based on the life table (survivorship) method. A life table may be defined as "...a graph or table giving an estimate of the proportion of a

For a list of all websites referred to in this chapter, as clickable links, see the book companion website: www.booksite.elsevier.com/9780128023877.

Biostatistics for Medical and Biomedical Practitioners
http://dx.doi.org/10.1016/B978-0-12-802387-7.00035-4

group of patients that will still be alive at different times after randomization, calculated with due allowance for incomplete follow-up" (Peto et al., 1977). In general, the table or graph starts with the time of entry, t_0, and 100% survival, and survival decreases with time. Occasionally, the plot shows failures (deaths, events), and then the table starts at time t_0 and events 0%, and events increase with time.

The life table method has been developed over the last several hundred years, perhaps starting with the *Observations on the Bills of Mortality* published in 1662 by John Graunt (1620−1674), and an article about life tables and annuities published in 1693 by the astronomer Edmund Halley (1656−1742) (Dick, 1949). Details of the method can be found in textbooks of Epidemiology or Public Health, and from many books (Allison, 1995; Armitage et al., 2002; Kalbfleisch and Prentice, 1980; Kaplan and Meier, 1958; Mantel, 1966; Selvin, 1991). Survival analysis is a major tool used in clinical trials, and all the precautions needed for a successful trial need to be followed or else the statistical analysis will be fruitless. Perhaps the most easily understood reference sources for understanding such trials are the two articles by Peto et al. entitled "Design and analysis of randomized clinical trials requiring prolonged observation of each patient" (Peto et al., 1976, 1977).

An early influential medical publication was the study of survival in systemic lupus erythematosus by Merrell and Shulman (1955). They emphasized the need to define the starting point from which the disease is followed and also observed that the accrual of patients over time meant that at any time point patients still alive would have been followed for different time periods, and that during the follow-up some patients would have become lost from the study without any information about their survival. A typical data set is shown in Figure 35.1.

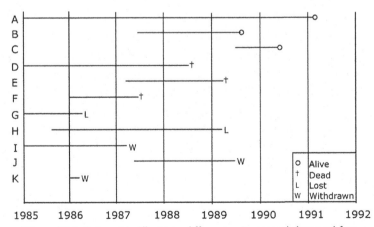

Figure 35.1 Data set to illustrate differences in accrual data and fate.

Patients A, B, and C were all alive in 1989, 1990, and 1991, respectively, but A has been followed for 6 years, B for 2 years, and C for less than 1 year. Patients D, E, and F have all died, but at different times after entry into the study. Patients G and H were lost to the study, and could not be found, either because they had moved and left no new address or because they did not want to cooperate. Patients I, J, and K were all withdrawn at different times after entry because of death due to an unrelated disease, transfer to another treatment, or failure to maintain the treatment.

Merrell and Shulman developed a method of dealing with these problems, and Cutler and Ederer (Cutler and Ederer, 1958) in 1958 extended the procedure to handle patients with different periods of follow-up (Figure 35.2).

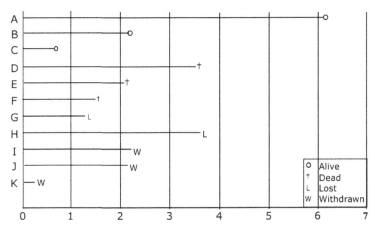

Figure 35.2 Same data set arranged so that all patients start at a common time, t_0.

Kaplan and Meier (1958) published a rigorous version of this method and termed it the product-limit method. The publications in 1974 (Anderson et al., 1974) and 1977 (Grunkemeier and Starr, 1977) by Grunkemeier, Starr, and colleagues introduced these methods into surgical practice and revolutionized the way in which surgeons analyzed their results.

Basic Method

The basis of the actuarial method (Berkson and Gage, 1950) is to follow patients for a period, for example 1 year, determine how many die in that year, and calculate the proportion p_1 who survive as

$$p_1 = 1 - \frac{\text{\# of deaths in period}}{\text{\# alive at beginning of period}}.$$

Then take those alive at the start of the second time period, determine how many die in this period, and calculate the probability p_2 of surviving the second period. Then the cumulative probability of surviving both periods is $p_1 \times p_2$, and so on. This is a conditional probability, because it concerns the survival during the second period conditional on having survived the first period. This method allows for subjects who have not yet completed the second period so that the base number for p_1 can be greater than the base number for p_2.

Table 35.1 shows how the data are presented.

Table 35.1 Basic life table. The symbols for the various columns vary in different texts

Start of period t_k	# Alive at start of period l_k	# Deaths in period d_k	# Alive < full period w_k	# Lost or withdrawn u_k	Adjusted number alive at start of period l'_k	Probability of dying in period q_k	Probability of surviving period p_k	Cumulative survival Π_{pk}
0–1	309	27	0	0	309	27/309 = 0.0874	0.9126	0.9126
1–2	282	14	6	2	278	14/278 = 0.0504	0.9496	0.8667
2–3	260	9	15	11	247	9/247 = 0.0364	0.9636	0.8352
3–4	225	5	13	6	215.5	5/215.5 = 0.0232	0.9768	0.8158

The first column shows the period (t_k). The second column shows how many patients entered the trial at the beginning of each period (l_k). The third column shows how many patients died in that period (d_k). When calculating the probability of dying, there are patients who did not complete a given period, either because they had been followed for less than a full period (w_k), or were lost to the study or withdrawn from it (u_k). The conventional approach is to assume that patients in columns w_k and u_k are evenly distributed across the period and so the average contribute one half of their number to be deducted from the total entering that period alive; the results would be biased if patients in columns D and E were treated as if all were alive or if all were dead. Therefore

$$l'_k = l_k - 0.5(w_k + u_k).$$

Then the probability of dying (q_k) is

$$q_k = \frac{d_k}{l'_k}.$$

The next column shows the probability of surviving that period as $p_k = 1 - q_k$. This is then multiplied by the cumulative probability up to that period (Π_{pk}) to give the probability of surviving period t_k given that the patient has already survived periods 1, 2, 3,...,t_{k-1}, and this is shown in the final column. Clear descriptions of this procedure are provided by Anderson et al. (1974) and Kleinbaum (1966).

The reasons for loss or withdrawal must be independent from the disease being studied. For example, in a study of breast cancer, a patient dying from a myocardial infarction is classified as withdrawn, not as death due to cancer. On the other hand, if the patient died from a hemorrhage probably caused by one of the treatments for cancer, this is not an independent event.

In the actuarial method the periods are usually years, but could be months, weeks, 5-year groups, or any other appropriate period. The Kaplan–Meier method is identical to the actuarial method except that the cumulative probability is recalculated whenever a failure occurs. Therefore, graphs drawn by the actuarial method show evenly spaced probabilities as against irregularly spaced values with the Kaplan—Meier method.

Figure 35.3 shows a survival plot for the persistence of sinus rhythm in children with episodes of supraventricular tachycardia after ablation of pathways by two different-sized cooling tips; they were followed for the duration of the study (Courtesy of Dr F. Collins and Dr N. Chanani).

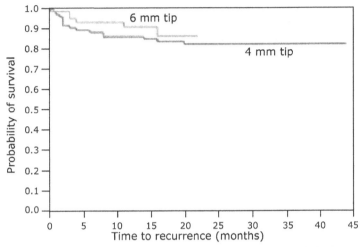

Figure 35.3 Kaplan—Meier plot comparing small 4 mm tip (lower line) with larger 6 mm tip (upper line). It cannot be an actuarial plot because the intervals at which the lines change are irregular.

Patients entered the study at different times, and thus were followed for different periods. A partial data set is shown in Table 35.2.

Table 35.2 Partial data set for ablation study

▼	ID	Date of study	Group (tip size)	Censored	Time to recurrence (months)
1	1	10/27/05	0	1	23
2	2	6/16/05	0	0	3
3	3	5/16/05	0	1	28
4	4	6/15/04	1	1	39
5	5	8/1/05	1	0	16
6	6	6/6/05	0	1	28
7	7	4/20/06	0	1	17
8	8	2/13/06	1	1	19
9	9	10/17/05	1	1	23
10	10	5/23/06	1	0	0.75
11	11	8/16/05	0	1	25
12	12	12/9/04	1	1	34

Column 1 is the identifier (nominal variable), which could be an admission hospital number or an arbitrary number or letter. Column 2 is the date of study. Column 3 is tip size (nominal variable) with 0 being 4 mm and 1 being 6 mm diameter. Column 4 indicates censoring, with 0 being recurrence and 1 being no recurrence. (The choice of 0 or 1 for censored data is arbitrary. Programs allow for either.) Column 5 is the time to recurrence (continuous variable). (Other columns of data in the study are not reproduced here.) If the patient had a recurrence, indicated by a 0 in the censor column, then the time shows when recurrence occurred. If the patient had not yet had a recurrence when the data were analyzed, as indicated by a 1 in the censor column, the time shows the length of follow-up to that date. Some of these patients may develop recurrences in the future, and because they have not been followed until failure has occurred, they are described as right censored. They contribute information about how long patients can be followed without failure, but there is no way to know how much longer this state will continue. The censor variable 0 or 1 tells the program which patients have and have not had an event.

Some investigators provide details of the numbers of successes and failures at each time point. Figure 35.4 gives a hypothetical example.

Occasionally, these figures display smoothed curves, but these should be considered approximations to the actual data.

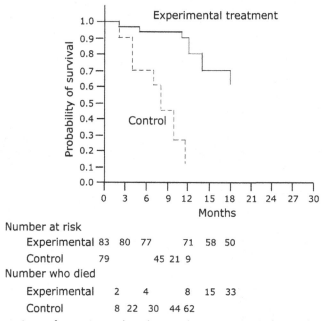

Figure 35.4 Comparison of experimental and control treatments, with supplementary numbers provided.

Online programs for these plots have two formats. One requires entry for each subject line by line, as in Table 35.2, and these can be found at http://biostat.hitchcock.org/BSR/Analytics/CompareTwoSurvivalDistributions.asp, which is best done via an Excel file, http://in-silico.net/statistics/survivor, http://www.ehow.com/how_8369388_make-survivorship-curve-chart-excel.html, with instructions for performing the test, https://www.statstodo.com/Survival_Pgm.php (but this needs membership for large data sets), and http://in-silico.net/statistics/survivor. The other allows entry of the life table, as in Table 35.1, and can be found at http://vassarstats.net/survival.html and https://statcom.dk/K-M_plot.php, the latter allowing easy importation of data and drawing the graph. Files must be set up as text files. None of these are easy to use.

Problem 35.1

Two groups of patients are randomized to receive either conventional therapy (C) or a new experimental therapy (E) for breast cancer. Use the Kaplan–Meier method to decide if the new treatment is better.

Experimental treatment			Conventional treatment		
Time of event t (months)	# At start of the month	# Who died at time t	Time of event t (months)	# At start of the month	# Who died at time t
1	25	0	1	49	0
5	24	0	3	48	0
6	23	2	5	47	0
9	21	0	6	46	8
10	20	2	8	38	2
12	17	4	9	36	0
13	12	1	10	36	2
15	11	0	12	34	6
16	10	0	13	28	0
20	9	0	15	25	0
24	8	1	16	22	0
27	7	0	18	21	1
32	5	1	20	18	1
44	5	0	22	17	0
			24	16	2
			27	13	0
			28	12	0
			30	9	1
			32	7	1
			33	6	0
			34	5	0
			36	4	0
			42	2	1
			44	2	0

Confidence Limits

As in any sample from a larger population, the survival curve is a point estimate at each time period, and similar samples would have slightly different data. The confidence limits at each point can be calculated from (Berkson and Gage, 1950)

$$Var\widehat{\Pi_{pk}} = \Pi_{pk}^2 \sum_{k=0}^{k-1} \frac{q_k}{l_k' p_k}$$

$$= \Pi_{pk}^2 \sum_{k=0}^{k-1} \frac{d_k}{l_k'(l_k' - d_k)}$$

$$= \Pi_{pk}^2 \sum_{k=0}^{k-1} \frac{d_k}{l_k' l_{k+1}'}.$$

The three expressions are the same because $q_k = \frac{d_k}{l_k'}$, and whichever is easier can be used.

The results of these calculations are shown as SE_{exact} in Table 35.3. As an example, for time period 3 (Table 35.1), the calculation is

$$Var\widehat{\Pi_{p3}} = 0.8352^2 \left[\frac{0.0874}{309 \times 0.9126} + \frac{0.0504}{278 \times 0.9496} + \frac{0.0364}{247 \times 0.0636} \right] = 0.000456056$$

so that $SE\widehat{\Pi_{p3}} = \sqrt{Var\widehat{\Pi_{p3}}} = 0.0214$. Then calculate 95% confidence limits as

$$0.8352 \pm 1.96SE = 0.8352 \times 1.96(0.0214) = 0.7933 \text{ to } 0.8771$$

Table 35.3 Calculations of standard error

Period	SE(exact)	Peto
0–1	0.0161	0.0156
1–2	0.0194	0.0196
2–3	0.0214	0.0226
3–4	0.0225	0.0247

In statistical programs such as JMP, the standard errors are printed out for each group. A partial printout is given for the 4 mm tip in the ablation example (Table 35.4). Standard errors may be calculated online at http://iscc-serv2.imm. dtu.dk/%7Emerser/K-M_plot.php, http://www.hutchon.net/Kaplan–Meier.htm, and http://vassarstats.net/survival01.html#next.

Table 35.4 Partial printout of data for the 4 mm tip used for ablation. The standard error increases progressively

Time to recurrence (months)	Survival	Failure	SurvStdErr	Number failed	Number censored	At risk
0.0000	1.0000	0.0000	0.0000	0	0	91
0.0000	1.0000	0.0000	0.0000	0	1	91
0.5000	0.9889	0.0111	0.0110	1	0	90
0.7500	0.9778	0.0222	0.0155	1	0	89
1.0000	0.9667	0.0333	0.0189	1	0	88
1.5000	0.9556	0.0444	0.0217	1	0	87
2.0000	0.9111	0.0889	0.0300	4	0	86
3.0000	0.9000	0.1000	0.0316	1	0	82
4.0000	0.8889	0.1111	0.0331	1	0	81
6.0000	0.8778	0.1222	0.0345	1	0	80
7.0000	0.8778	0.1222	0.0345	0	1	79
8.0000	0.8553	0.1447	0.0371	2	0	78
9.0000	0.8553	0.1447	0.0371	0	1	76
10.0000	0.8553	0.1447	0.0371	0	1	75

The final column in Table 35.3 headed "Peto" gives a simple approximation described by Peto et al. (1977). For any value of the computed probability of survival Π_{pk} (final column of Table 35.1), the standard error is approximately

$$SE\widehat{\Pi_{pk}} = \pi p_k \sqrt{\frac{1 - \pi p_k}{N}},$$

where N is the number of patients alive at the end of the year in question. The approximation is close to the exact value.

Some programs allow confidence limits to be plotted on the graph.

Comparison of Different Survival Curves

This is most often done by the log-rank test of Mantel (1966), although similar methods based on a modified Wilcoxon test can also be performed (Gehan, 1965; Kalbfleisch and Prentice, 1980; Peto and Peto, 1972; Tarone and Ware, 1977). The log-rank test examines the 2×2 table consisting of observed versus expected failures in each group whenever a failure occurs, and tests significance across all the tables with a Mantel–Haenszel test. The test can be extended to more than two groups.

The test statistic can be formalized as $\chi^2_{\log\text{ rank}} = \sum_g \frac{(O_g - E_g)^2}{E_g}$, where O and E are the observed and expected events in group g, calculated each time an event occurs. Various weighting systems can be used. In the Gehan test, the statistic is $\chi^2_{\text{Gehan}} = \sum_g \frac{R_t(O_{gt} - E_{gt})^2}{R_t^2 E_{gt}}$, where R is the number of patients at risk in each group at each time point.

The log-rank test places more weight on longer survival times, and the Wilcoxon tests place more weight on early survival times because they obtain a weighted average of each $O-E$ deviation by using the number of survivors in the group at each time. Different investigators have recommended different weighting systems; Gehan (1965) used weights $\omega_i = l_i$, Tarone and Ware (1977) used $\omega_i = \sqrt{l_i}$, and the Peto test (Peto and Peto, 1972; Prentice and Marek, 1979) gives more weight to the higher numbers at the beginning of the curve and much less weight to the smaller numbers near its end. There is another Gehan test based on ranks, as in the basic Wilcoxon test, and this gives results almost identical to Gehan's chi-square test (Selvin, 1991). If the publication does not mention which form of Wilcoxon's test was used, it matters very little because they all give similar results. Furthermore, it would be folly to reject the null hypothesis at $p = 0.045$ with one test but not reject it if another test had $P = 0.067$.

In the ablation study described above (Table 35.5), there was no significant difference between the groups.

Table 35.5 Comparison between groups. In this example, neither test shows significant differences between the two tip sizes

Tests between groups

Test	Chi-square	DF	Prob > chi-square
Log-rank	0.6330	1	0.4262
Wilcoxon	0.8421	1	0.3588

Caveats: If patients are accrued over several years, there must be stationarity, that is, all features of the patients and any other treatments must remain constant. Then it is unwise to extrapolate beyond the observed curves. It is possible for curve A to show better survival than curve B for 10 years, but then for survival to deteriorate in later years in group A and by 20 years be worse than the final survival for group B. Finally, because there will be smaller numbers of patients followed for the longest times, a single failure might have a large effect; for example, if at 5 years there are 100 patients, 1 failure changes the probability of survival little, but 1 failure out of 3 survivors at 10 years produces a large decrease in survival. Although this is obvious and would be made more obvious by examining the confidence limits, many reports do not include these limits.

Creating survival curves that describe the time course of events in one or more groups is simple, and provides useful information about whether treatment A or B prolongs life more, or keeps patients out of hospital longer. The description, however, is not an end in itself, but often the prelude to determining underlying mechanisms by defining a function that fits the curve, for example, log-normal, Weibull, or other type of curve. This requires more extensive examination and consultation with a statistician.

Sample Size

Before beginning the study, an attempt should be made to estimate the likely sample size needed. This can be done online at http://www.quesgen.com/SSSurvival.php, https://www.statstodo.com/SSizSurvival_Pgm.php, http://www.sealedenvelope.com, http://www.cct.cuhk.edu.hk/stat/survival/Rubinstein1981.htm and http://www.sample-size.net. As for other sample size estimates, some guesses or provisional data must be obtained for the likely event rate and the proportion in each group.

ADVANCED CONCEPTS

Calculating the Log-Rank Test

The test involves pooling the two groups and arranging the survival times in rank order. Then a series of 2 × 2 tables is constructed each time when there is a failure (Table 35.6).

Table 35.6 Components of 2 × 2 table

Group	Failure	No failure	Total exposed
A	O_A	$l'_A - O_A$	l'_A
B	O_B	$l'_B - O_B$	l'_B
Total	O_T	$l'_T - O_T$	l'_T

As in any chi-square table, the expected value for failure in group A (E_A) is

$$E_A = \frac{O_T l'_A}{l'_T}.$$

As a rule, because a new table is set up each time an event occurs, O_T is usually 1, and O_A and O_B are either 0 or 1. Therefore, $E_A = \frac{l'_A}{l'_T} = p_A$.

The calculations are shown in the hypothetical example (Table 35.7).

Table 35.7 Data set for Mantel–Haenszel log-rank test. l'_A, l'_B, and l'_T are the number of subjects in group A, group B, and the total, respectively; O_A, O_B, and O_T are the number of failures (deaths or other events) in group A, group B, and the total, respectively; $\frac{E_A = O_T l'_A}{l'_T}$

Time	l'_A	l'_B	l'_T	O_A	O_B	O_T	E_A	$O_A - E_A$	V
3	35	45	80	0	1	1	$\frac{35 \times 1}{80} = 0.4375$	−0.4375	0.2461
7	35	44	79	0	1	1	$\frac{35 \times 1}{79} = 0.4430$	−0.4430	0.2468
8	35	43	78	0	2	2	$\frac{35 \times 2}{78} = 0.8974$	−0.8974	0.2442
1	35	41	76	1	0	1	$\frac{35 \times 1}{76} = 0.4605$	0.5395	0.2484
29	34	41	75	0	1	1	$\frac{34 \times 1}{75} = 0.4533$	−0.4533	0.2478
54	34	40	74	1	2	3	$\frac{35 \times 3}{74} = 1.4189$	−0.4189	0.2416
Σ				2	7	9	4.1106	−2.1106	1.4749

The variance V of the difference $O_A - E_A$ is calculated as $V = \frac{l'_A l'_B (l'_T - O_T)}{l'^2_T (l'_T - 1)}$ (Altman, 1992). When a single event occurs, this reduces to

$$V_{O_A} = \frac{(l'_T - 1) l'_A l'_B}{(l'_T)^2 (l'_T - 1)} = \frac{l'_A l'_B}{(l'_T)^2} = \frac{l'_A}{l'_T} \times \frac{l'_B}{l'_T} = p_A p_B = p_A (1 - p_A).$$

Then calculate chi-square as $\chi^2 = \frac{\left[\sum (O_A - E_A)\right]^2}{V} = \frac{-2.1106}{1.4749} - 1.4310$. In this example, the critical 0.05 value of chi-square of 3.84 has not been reached, although the trend seems to be for more events to occur in group B. The log-rank test examines cumulative $O - E$ differences for one group. If the two groups are not significantly different, then sometimes the $O - E$ differences will be positive (an event occurs in group A) or sometimes negative (an event occurs in group B). If these are random occurrences, then the sum will be small and indicate no significant differences.

An alternative calculation that does not involve V is

$$\chi^2 = \frac{\left(\sum O_A - \sum E_A\right)^2}{\sum E_A} + \frac{\left(\sum O_B - \sum E_B\right)^2}{\sum E_B},$$

where $\sum E_B = \sum O_T - \sum E_A$.

This formula gives a slightly different answer

$$\chi^2 = \frac{-2.1106^2}{4.1106} + \frac{-2.1106^2}{9 - 4.1106} = 1.9948.$$

This variant is regarded as more conservative than the previous one (Armitage et al., 2002).

Examples of the calculations are given by Armitage et al. (2002) and by Altman (1992). The log-rank test can be done with more than two data sets, and on data sets stratified into subgroups. The test can be performed online at http://iscc-serv2.imm.dtu.dk/%7 Emerser/K-M_plot.php that also draws the survival curves and provides confidence limits.

The Hazard Function

The survival function $S(t)$ is

$$S(t) = \frac{\text{number of patients surviving more than time } t}{\text{total number of patients in study}}.$$

This is also termed the cumulative survival function because it gives the probability of surviving all time intervals from the start to the selected time point.

When following a group of patients over time, some patients die between times t_x and t_{x+1}. The instantaneous hazard function $h(t)$ is the risk of dying (or failure in general) in a very small time period Δt, if the patient has survived to time t_x. It represents the risk of dying in subjects who have survived up to that time. It can be symbolized formally by

$$\widehat{h(t)} = \lim_{\Delta t \to \infty} \frac{P(t_x \leq T \leq t_x + \Delta t | T \geq t_x)}{\Delta t}.$$

This is the conditional probability that a person who has survived for t_x periods $(T \geq t_x)$ will die between the short period t_x and $t_x + \Delta t$. It is the slope of the survival curve at any given time t, and can also be written as

$$\widehat{h(t)} = -\left[\frac{dS(t)/dt}{S(t)}\right].$$

The hazard function is a probability per unit time, and is thus a rate.

There is also a cumulative hazard function that adds up all the instantaneous hazard functions to a given point. It can be calculated as $\Delta t = -\log_e S(t)$, and produces a curve that is almost a mirror image of the cumulative survival curve. See Figure 35.5.

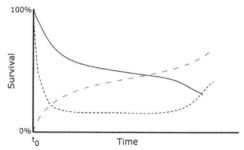

Figure 35.5 Survival $S(t)$ (solid line), instantaneous hazard $h(t)$ (short dashed line), and cumulative hazard $\Delta(t)$ (long dashed line) curves. Immediately after surgery there is a rapid decrease in survival, confirmed by the steep initial hazard curve. After that there is a period of very slow decrease in survival where the hazard function is low and steady, and then the hazard function increases as late complications become manifest. The instantaneous hazard function in the middle of the figure is low, but the cumulative hazard function continues to rise because patients die from time to time.

As an example, if in the month after a coronary bypass operation the hazard rate is calculated as 0.015, then on average 0.015 patients are expected to die in the first month. In a database of 1000 patients, 15 will die in the first month. This figure does not apply to subsequent months that might have different hazard functions.

Typically in examining the results after cardiac surgery, curves as in Figure 35.5 are shown.

These hazard functions can be fitted to different distributions that might throw some light on the underlying processes (Altman, 1992).

If the survival curve is approximately exponential, as it often is, then the hazard rate H is estimated from

$$H = \frac{d}{\sum f + \sum c}$$

where d is the number of failures, $\sum f$ is the sum of the failure times, and $\sum c$ is the sum of the times of the censored individuals. The reciprocal of H is the estimate of mean survival time

$$\bar{t} = \frac{1}{H}.$$

These two formulas can be used to set approximate confidence limits. The 95% confidence limits for mean survival time are $\bar{t} \pm 1.96 \times SE_x$, and the standard error can be approximated by

$$\sqrt{\frac{X^2}{d}}.$$

Hazard Ratio

The log-rank test, like any other test of significance, indicates whether survival between two groups is significantly different, but does not indicate how different they are. One way to show the difference is to state the survival in each group at comparable times, for example, 56% at 10 years in group A as against 32% at 10 years in group B. Another way is to compare observed and expected numbers in each group. If the survival is the same in the two groups, then the number of observed events will be proportional to the expected numbers, and will be the same in each group. To examine this, the hazard ratio is computed. This ratio R is

$$R = \frac{\sum O_A / \sum E_A}{\sum O_B / \sum E_B},$$

where O and E are the observed and expected numbers of events, and A and B indicate the groups being compared. For the example in Table 35.6, the hazard ratio is $R = \frac{2/4.1106}{7/3.2974} = 0.2292$. If the hazard ratio is >1, it indicates that the treatment group has a shorter survival than the control referenced group, and if it is <1, it indicates that the group of interest is less likely to have a shorter time to the event than the reference group. The ratio does not quantify the magnitude of the difference.

It is possible to determine approximate confidence limits for the logarithm of the hazard ratio (Simon, 1986). Calculate

$$K = \frac{\sum O_A - \sum E_A}{\sum V}$$

an estimate of the logarithm of the hazard ratio with an approximate standard error of $\frac{1}{\sqrt{\sum V}}$.

Thus for the data in Table 35.7,

$$K = \frac{2 - 4.096}{1.4749} = -1.4310 \quad \text{and} \quad \frac{1}{\sqrt{\sum V}} = \frac{1}{\sqrt{1.4749}} = 0.8234.$$

Then the 95% confidence limits of K are $K \pm 1.96 \times 0.8234 = -1.4749 \pm 1.6139 = -3.0888$ to 0.139. Therefore the 95% confidence limits for the hazard ratio are $e^{-3.0888}$ to $e^{0.139}$, or 0.0456 to 1.1491. These limits are wide, include 1, and confirm the findings that the two groups are not significantly different.

Spruance et al. (2004) emphasized that the hazard ratio quantifies the degree of difference between the groups, but does not indicate what the absolute difference in duration of the illness is. (In a race, for example, the hazard ratio gives the probability that A will win, but does not tell us by how much.) They wrote: "The hazard ratio is equivalent to the odds that an individual in the group with the higher hazard reaches the endpoint first." In a trial of treatment to shorten the duration of symptoms in herpes zoster, for example, the hazard ratio represents the odds that the time to remission of symptoms is less in a patient from the treated group than from the control group. The probability of getting better first is the odds of healing first divided by the probability of not healing first. Therefore, in this setting,
Odds of healing first $(HR) = \frac{\text{Probability of healing first}}{\text{Probability of not healing first}} = \frac{P}{1-P}.$ This can be rearranged to give Probability of healing first $= \frac{HR}{1+HR}.$

Thus a hazard ratio of 2 matches a 67% chance that the treated patient will heal first, and a ratio of 3 corresponds to a 75% chance of healing first. The actual difference in time to healing requires absolute numbers, such as the median ratio that may give values that are not the same as the hazard ratio. It is possible for a hazard ratio to be greater or less than the median ratio.

Hernan (2010) pointed out that in epidemiologic studies, mean hazard ratios are usually cited, but this practice ignores the possibility that the hazard ratios change with time. In the Women's Health Initiative, for example, in which hormone therapy was compared with a placebo, the successive annual hazard ratios for coronary heart disease were 1.81, 1.34, 1.27, 1.25, 1.45, and 0.70. Therefore depending on how long the study continues and thus how many hazard ratios are averaged will yield different averages. Examining year-specific hazard ratios overcomes this problem but leads to another one related to selection bias. Some people are more prone to develop heart disease than are others. These may be detected early, leaving a pool of slightly less susceptible people to enter the next period. After several years the control and treated groups are no longer comparable and the hazard ratio may decrease to 1 or below 1.

Cox Proportional Hazards Regression

What factors influence the survival curves? In assessing survival after a myocardial infarction, how important are covariates such as the age at time of infarction, body mass index, diabetes, serum LDL concentration, and blood pressure; in assessing survival with cirrhosis of the liver, how important are serum albumin, alkaline phosphatase, alcohol intake; in assessing survival with kidney disease, how important are age, gender, creatinine concentration, hemoglobin concentration, serum albumin? One way of assessing these variables is to realize that the survival function $S(t)$ has values between 0 and 1, and thus might be suitable for logistic multiple regression analysis.

However, logistic regression does not take survival times or censoring into account, and is replaced by the Cox regression model (Cox, 1972). (Sir David Cox, b. 1924, an eminent British statistician.) This is a robust nonparametric model. Cox's publication is the most highly cited reference in the entire literature of statistics and ranks among the top 100 publications in all of science (Altman, 1992). If a trial of a large number of patients with coronary artery disease is done to compare medical and surgical treatment, there will inevitably be differences in the proportions of potentially important cofactors such as diabetes, gender, LDL concentration, hypertension, smoking history, and body mass index. Do one or more of these had undue influence on the survival in each group? It would be difficult to interpret the results of comparing two treatments for coronary artery disease if one group had severe renal involvement and the other did not. Cox regression helps to adjust the imbalance between the two groups.

One way of analyzing the data is to assume that the hazard functions related to the two survival curves are proportional to each other, that is, if the hazard function for curve A is 20% less than that for curve B at a given time, it is approximately 20% less at other times too. More generally, $h_A(t) = k h_B(t)$ where k is a constant. The survival curves for these two groups can be related to the equation $S_B(t) = [S_A(t)]^k$ (Glantz and Slinker, 2001; Selvin, 1991).

If the proportional hazards requirement is met, then Cox regression is applicable. Cox regression is semiparametric, applies to many different survival functions, and its requirements are quite robust, but would certainly not apply if the two curves crossed.

Cox regression assumes that the ratio of the two hazard functions R is logistic, so that $R = h_0(t)e^{\beta_1 X_1 + \beta_2 X_2 + \cdots + \beta_K X_K}$. The proportionality constant k can therefore be written as

$$k = \left(e^{\beta_1 X_1}\right)\left(e^{\beta_2 X_2}\right)\cdots\left(e^{\beta_j X_j}\right).$$

When all the β coefficients are zero, $e^0 = 1$, and $h_0(t)$ is the baseline, time-dependent hazard function. Furthermore, if all the β coefficients except one $\left(e^{\beta_i X_i}\right)$ are set to zero, the value of $e^{\beta_i X_i}$ represents the hazard function for that variable alone. The exponential components that are the potential explanatory variables are subject, but not time dependent. (Although weight, age, serum lipoprotein concentrations do change with time, in this type of study each contributes only one fixed value.)

Taking logarithms of both sides gives

$$\log R = \log\frac{h_A(t)}{h_B(t)} = h_0(t) + \beta_1 X_1 + \beta_2 X_2 + \cdots + \beta_k X_k$$

Once the data are fitted to the model, the calculations estimate the coefficients β_1, β_2, etc., together with their standard errors so that the significance of each coefficient can be tested. (Precautions for dealing with multiple regression and multicollinearity are involved in these calculations.) Then the contributions of each variable can be assessed for the change in hazard. A positive coefficient for any variable, for example, 2, means that the variable makes survival worse relative to the reference group, and a negative coefficient, for example, -0.35, means that the factor improves survival.

An alternative formulation mentioned by Selvin (1991) is

$$\log\left(\frac{\lambda_j(t)}{\lambda_0(t)}\right) = \sum_{t-1}^{k} b_i\left(X_{ij} - \overline{X_i}\right),$$

or

$$\log\left[\lambda_j(t)\right] = \log[\lambda_c(t)] - \sum_{t-1}^{k} b_i\left(X_{ij} - \overline{X_i}\right).$$

These formulas show clearly that as in a multiple regression model, there are two terms: a first term that is time dependent and equivalent to the intercept, and a second term that is a weighted sum of explanatory variables independent of time.

As an example, consider the arrhythmia ablation data presented above, and add in age and number of cryoablation lesions as possible explanatory variables (data not shown). The analysis is given in Table 35.8.

The upper panel (Table 35.8) shows the results for survival time in the two tip sizes with no other explanatory variables added. As shown by the chi-square and probability for the model, the differences are not significant. The parameter estimates indicate that arrhythmias in the new group (6 mm tip) are 19% less likely to recur than in the old group (4 mm tip), but with a wide standard error this is not significant. The risk ratio was 0.8265 with wide confidence limits.

In the lower panel (Table 35.8), age and number of attempts at ablation (# cryo lesions) have been added. As shown under Model, chi-square has increased and is almost significant. Tip size has a larger effect (27% difference) though this is still not significant, age has no effect (small estimate, large standard error), but lesion number increases

Table 35.8 Cox regression for ablation data

A. Whole model

Number of events		22
Number of censorings		124
Total number		144

Model	-LogLikelihood	Chi-square	DF	Prob>Chi-square
Difference	0.3260	0.6521	1	0.4194
Full	106.0179			
Reduced	106.3439			

Parameter estimates

Term	Estimate	Std error	Lower 95%	Upper 95%
Group	0.1905	0.2419	−0.7068	0.2600

Effect Likelihood Ratio Tests

Source	DF	Chi-square	Prob>Chi-square
Group	1	0.6521	0.4914

B. Whole model

Number of events		18
Number of censorings		102
Total number		120

Model	-LogLikelihood	Chi-square	DF	Prob>Chi-square
Difference	3.3948	6.78971	3	0.0789
Full	80.3836			
Reduced	83.7765			

Parameter estimates

Term	Estimate	Std error	Lower 95%	Upper 95%
Group	−0.2716	0.3974	−1.2208	0.4192
# cryo lesions	0.1227	0.0489	0.0143	0.2101
Age	0.0253	0.0551	−0.0828	0.1340

Effect Likelihood Ratio Tests

Source	DF	Chi-square	Prob>Chi-square
Group	1	0.5185	0.4715
# cryo lesions	1	4.7764	0.0289*
Age	1	0.2105	0.6464

Unit Risk Ratios (per unit change in regressor)

Term	Risk ratio	Lower 95%	Upper 95%	Reciprocal
Group	0.7622	0.2950	1.5208	1.3120
# cryo lesions	1.1306	1.0144	1.2338	0.8845
Age	1.0256	0.9205	1.1434	0.9750

*P<0.05

failure rate by 13% per unit increase, and this is significant (see lowest panel). As shown in the lowest section, a 1-unit increase in lesion number increases the hazard function by 13% (but with 95% confidence limits of 1—23%). Because age is not an explanatory variable, delete it and leave in only tip size and lesion number (Table 35.9).

Table 35.9 Only two explanatory variables used from ablation data

Whole model

Total number				120

Model	-LogLikelihood	Chi-square	DF	Prob>Chi-square
Difference	3.2896	6.5792	2	0.0373*
Full	80.4889			
Reduced	83.7785			

Parameter estimates

Term	Estimate	Std error	Lower 95%	Upper 95%
New Group	−0.2454	0.3937	−1.1901	0.4357
# cryo lesions	0.1198	0.0482	0.0123	0.2051

Effect Likelihood Ratio Tests

Source	DF	Chi-square	Prob>Chi-square
Group	1	0.4289	0.5125
# cryo lesions	1	4.6431	0.0312*

Unit Risk Ratios (per unit change in regressor)

Term	Risk ratio	Lower 95%	Upper 95%	Reciprocal
Group	0.7824	0.3042	1.5460	1.2781
# cryo lesions	1.1272	1.0124	1.2277	0.8871

*P<0.05

As the model shows, adding in lesion number has made a significant improvement as shown by the significant chi-square. The 6 mm tip size now has a 22% lower failure rate as compared with the reference group with 4 mm tip size, and the lesion number increases failure rate by 12%. $e^{-0.2453694} = 0.782415$, and $e^{0.11975937} = 1.127226$, that is, e to the coefficient gives the hazard ratio for that variable.

Knowing that the number of lesions affects the survival curves, keep that data in the final model and have a more accurate hazard ratio for tip size that is now not influenced by any effect that the number of lesions has on the outcome. If hypothetically there were data with the same numbers of lesions in the two groups, then lesion number would no longer be an influencing or confounding factor and no allowance for it would be needed. More complex analyses involving interactions among the explanatory factors can also be performed.

Online calculations can be done at http://statpages.org/prophaz.html, but this is not very flexible. There are good descriptions of Cox regression in nephrology and hepatology (Christensen, 1987; Elashoff, 1983; Schlichting et al., 1983; van Dijk et al., 2008).

Competing Risks Analysis

If a group of elderly patients having replacement of the aortic valve with a mechanical prosthetic valve are followed, the survival curve drops off quite rapidly, but not all the deaths are due to complications or aortic valve surgery. Older people have a higher incidence of cancer or renal disease that may cause death. Therefore the survival curve is due to all causes of death, not just postsurgical causes. Epidemiologists define two probabilities of dying: crude probability refers to death of an individual in the presence of multiple causes of death, whereas net probability refers to death from a particular cause when other causes of death are not present. Survival after aortic valve surgery would differ if some people did not die from cancer or accidents.

Two approaches are used to evaluate competing risks (Selvin, 1991). One approach assumes that the net probabilities can be described by exponential functions with hazard rates of λ_1 and λ_2, net probability rates of $Q_1 = 1 - e^{-\lambda 1}$ and $Q_2 = 1 - e^{-\lambda 2}$, and that the probability of surviving an interval $= P_1 P_2 = (1 - Q_1)(1 - Q_2) = e^{-(\lambda 1 + \lambda 2)}$.

This implies that causes 1 and 2 are independent, an assumption probably true for aortic valve surgery and cancer, but perhaps not true for aortic valve surgery and renal failure.

Crude probability of death from either cause is $q = 1 - P_1 P_2 = 1 - e^{-(\lambda 1 + \lambda 2)}$.
Because $P_i = 1 - Q_i$,

$$Q_i = 1 - P_i = 1 - (1 - q)\frac{\lambda_i}{\lambda_1 + \lambda_2}.$$

The ratio of the two hazard rates $\frac{\lambda_i}{\lambda_1 + \lambda_2}$ is estimated by $\frac{d_i}{d_1 + d_2}$, where d_i is the number of deaths from cause 1 and $d_1 + d_2$ is the total number of deaths from all causes. This estimate is used to determine the net probability of death from cause 1 as

$$Q_i = 1 - \left(1 - \frac{d}{l}\right)^{\frac{d_i}{d_1 + d_2}}$$

where l is the number of individuals at risk at the beginning of the interval. This is less than the crude rate based on d by virtue of the quantity in parentheses. For example, if $l = 150$, $d_1 = 5$, and $d_2 = 7$, the net death rate will be $\widehat{Q_i} = 1 - \left(1 - \frac{12}{150}\right)^{\frac{5}{12}} = 0.0341$. This is less than the crude death rate, that is, $12/150 = 0.08$.

An alternative that does not involve the exponential assumptions is to regard individuals at risk as dying from cause 1, dying from cause 2, or living through the interval.

Considering those who die from cause 2 as being lost to follow-up, then deaths from cause 1 are underestimated because if subjects had not died from cause 2 they would be exposed to the risk of dying from cause 1. On the usual assumption that the lost individuals are exposed to risk for half the interval, the number exposed to risk of dying from cause 2 had been decreased by $0.5d_2$. Therefore corrected net probability of death from cause 1 is

$$\widehat{Q_i} = \frac{d_1}{l - 0.5d_2}.$$

Using the numbers from the previous example, $\widehat{Q_i} = \frac{5}{150 - 0.5 \times 12} = 0.0347$, similar to the value obtained by the previous formula.

The problem of competing risks is prominent in evaluating the results of heart valve replacement surgery. Younger patients who do not have many competing causes of death may have a valid postoperative survival curve. Investigators have then used the same life table methods to assess valve failure that did not result in death. Unfortunately, if patients have died it is not possible to tell if they would have had valve failure at a later stage, so that estimates of valve failure will be incorrect (Blackstone, 1999; Blackstone and Lytle, 2000; Grunkemeier et al., 1977; Grunkemeier and Wu, 2001; Grunkemeier et al., 2007). The issue of competing risks is important also in oncology. An excellent discussion by Kim stresses that many competing risks are not independent; for example, relapse after allogeneic stem cell transplantation and transplant-related mortality are both associated with immunologic effector mechanisms and so not suitable for the usual life table calculations that assume independent events.

There is much discussion in the medical literature about how to deal with competing risks (Blackstone, 1999; Blackstone and Lytle, 2000; Bodnar and Blackstone, 2005; Grunkemeier et al., 1997, 2001, 2007; Kaempchen et al., 2003). Consider a simple example of 200 patients followed after aortic valve replacement. If 50 of them die early from noncardiac causes before any valve failure, then there are only 150 patients who remain at risk for valve failure. If after 20 years 15 patients have needed valve replacement, then the risk of valve failure is 10% after 20 years. On the other hand, if none had died of noncardiac causes, we would have followed 200 patients and might (who knows?) have observed 25 valve (12.5%) failures. On the other hand, there might still have been 15 failures for a final percentage of 7.5 after 20 years. Both values are correct, but are based on different considerations. Kim recommends solutions for these problems, although they require commercial programs.

Grunkemeier and colleagues (Grunkemeier and Starr, 1977; Grunkemeier et al., 1977, 1997, 2001, 2007; Grunkemeier and Wu, 2001) have argued in favor of determining cumulative incidences of each of the competing events, something that can be done simply from the primary data. This results in a set of cumulative curves (Figure 35.6).

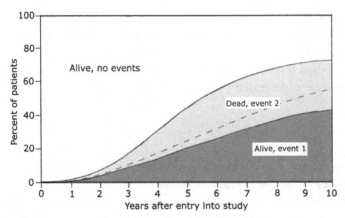

Figure 35.6 Cumulative curves to show competing risks effect. These are the observed data. If the Kaplan–Meier method had been used with event 1 as the event of interest, then both those with event 2 (died) and those alive with no events are regarded as censored, and the dashed line shows that the incidence of event 1 is exaggerated.

REFERENCES

Allison, P.D., 1995. Survival Analysis Using SAS. A Practical Guide.

Altman, D.G., 1992. Practical Statistics for Medical Research, 611 p.

Anderson, R.P., Bonchek, L.I., Grunkemeier, G.L., et al., 1974. The analysis and presentation of surgical results by actuarial methods. J. Surg. Res. 16, 224–230.

Armitage, P., Berry, G., Matthews, J.N.S., 2002. Statistical Methods in Medical Research. Blackwell.

Berkson, J., Gage, R.P., 1950. Calculation of survival rates for cancer. Proc. Staff Meet. Mayo Clin. 25, 270–286.

Blackstone, E.H., 1999. Actuarial and Kaplan-Meier survival analysis: there is a difference. J. Thorac. Cardiovasc. Surg. 118, 973–975.

Blackstone, E.H., Lytle, B.W., 2000. Competing risks after coronary bypass surgery: the influence of death on reintervention. J. Thorac. Cardiovasc. Surg. 119, 1221–1230.

Bodnar, E., Blackstone, E.H., 2005. Editorial: an 'actual' problem: another issue of apples and oranges. J. Heart Valve Dis. 14, 706–708.

Christensen, E., 1987. Multivariate survival analysis using Cox's regression model. Hepatology 7, 1346–1358.

Cox, D.R., 1972. Regression models and life tables. J. R. Stat. Soc. Ser. B 34, 187–220.

Cutler, S.J., Ederer, F., 1958. Maximum utilization of the life table method in analyzing survival. J. Chronic Dis. 8, 699–712.

Dick, O.L., 1949. Aubrey's Brief Lives. Secker and Warburg.

van Dijk, P.C., Jager, K.J., Zwinderman, A.H., et al., 2008. The analysis of survival data in nephrology: basic concepts and methods of Cox regression. Kidney Int. 74, 705–709.

Elashoff, J.D., 1983. Surviving proportional hazards. Hepatology 3, 1031–1035.

Gehan, E.A., 1965. A generalized Wilcoxon test for comparing arbitrarily singly-censored samples. Biometrika 52, 203–223.

Glantz, S.A., Slinker, B.K., 2001. Primer of Applied Regression and Analysis of Variance. McGraw-Hill, Inc.

Grunkemeier, G.L., Starr, A., 1977. Actuarial analysis of surgical results: rationale and method. Ann. Thorac. Surg. 24, 404–408.

Grunkemeier, G.L., Thomas, D.R., Starr, A., 1977. Statistical considerations in the analysis and reporting of time-related events. Application to analysis of prosthetic valve-related thromboembolism and pacemaker failure. Am. J. Cardiol. 39, 257–258.

Grunkemeier, G.L., Anderson, R.P., Miller, D.C., et al., 1997. Time-related analysis of nonfatal heart valve complications: cumulative incidence (actual) versus Kaplan-Meier (actuarial). Circulation 96, II-70–II-74.

Grunkemeier, G.L., Anderson, R.P., Starr, A., 2001. Actuarial and actual analysis of surgical results: empirical validation. Ann. Thorac. Surg. 71, 1885–1887.

Grunkemeier, G.L., Wu, Y., 2001. Actual versus actuarial event-free percentages. Ann. Thorac. Surg. 72, 677–678.

Grunkemeier, G.L., Jin, R., Eijkemans, M.J., et al., 2007. Actual and actuarial probabilities of competing risks: apples and lemons. Ann. Thorac. Surg. 83, 1586–1592.

Hernan, M.A., 2010. The hazards of hazard ratios. Epidemiology 21, 13–15.

Kaempchen, S., Guenther, T., Toschke, M., et al., 2003. Assessing the benefit of biological valve prostheses: cumulative incidence (actual) vs. Kaplan-Meier (actuarial) analysis. Eur. J. Cardiothorac. Surg. 23, 710–734.

Kalbfleisch, J.D., Prentice, R.L., 1980. Statistical Analysis of Failure Time Data. Wiley.

Kaplan, E.L., Meier, P., 1958. Nonparametric estimation from incomplete observations. J. Am. Stat. Assoc. 53, 457–481.

Kleinbaum, D.G., 1966. Survival Analysis. A Self-learning Text. Springer Verlag.

Mantel, N., 1966. Evaluation of survival data and two new rank order statistics arising in its consideration. Cancer Chemother. Rep. 50, 163–170.

Merrell, M., Shulman, L.E., 1955. Determination of prognosis in chronic disease, illustrated by systemic lupus erythematosus. J. Chronic Dis. 1, 12–32.

Muenz, L.R., 1983. Comparing survival distributions: a review for nonstatisticians. Cancer Invest. 1, 455–466.

Peto, R., Peto, J., 1972. Asymptotically efficient rank invariant test procedures. J. R. Stat. Soc. Ser. A 135, 185–207.

Peto, R., Pike, M.C., Armitage, P., et al., 1976. Design and analysis of randomized clinical trials requiring prolonged observation of each patient. I. Introduction and design. Br. J. Cancer 34, 585–612.

Peto, R., Pike, M.C., Armitage, P., et al., 1977. Design and analysis of randomized clinical trials requiring prolonged observation of each patient. II. Analysis and examples. Br. J. Cancer 35, 1–39.

Prentice, R.L., Marek, P., 1979. A qualitative discrepancy between censored rank tests. Biometrics 35, 861–867.

Schlichting, P., Christensen, E., Andersen, P.K., et al., 1983. Prognostic factors in cirrhosis identified by Cox's regression model. Hepatology 3, 889–895.

Selvin, S., 1991. Statistical Analysis of Epidemiologic Data. Oxford University Press.

Simon, R., 1986. Confidence intervals for reporting results of clinical trials. Ann. Intern. Med. 105, 429–435.

Spruance, S.L., Reid, J.E., Grace, M., et al., 2004. Hazard ratio in clinical trials. Antimicrob. Agents Chemother. 48, 2787–2792.

Tarone, R.E., Ware, J., 1977. On distribution-free tests for equality of survival distribution. Biometrika 64, 156–160.

CHAPTER 36

Meta-analysis

Contents

INTRODUCTION

Meta-analysis is a set of techniques used "to combine the results of a number of different reports into one report to create a single, more precise estimate of an effect" (Ferrer, 1998). The aims of meta-analysis are "to increase statistical power; to deal with controversy when individual studies disagree; to improve estimates of size of effect, and to answer new questions not previously posed in component studies" (Hunter and Schmidt, 1990). All definitions stress that there must be a valid reason to combine the studies. Egger et al. (2002) wrote "Indeed, it is our impression that reviewers often find it hard to resist the temptation of combining studies when such meta-analysis is questionable or clearly inappropriate." Although the frequency at which meta-analysis is used is increasing (Egger and Smith, 1997), meta-analysis has its detractors. In reality, if carefully performed, it yields useful information, but a meta-analysis of badly designed studies produces erroneous statistics and may be misleading. Ignoring heterogeneity and combining apples and oranges is a pervasive error in meta-analysis (Eysenck, 1995) and techniques exist to assess it (Ferrer, 1998; Tang and Liu, 2000). Other forms of bias also interfere with effective meta-analysis (Egger and Smith, 1998).

There are several advantages to meta-analysis. It allows investigators to pool data from many trials that are too small by themselves to allow for secure conclusions. Although ideally any clinical trial should plan an adequate sample size, historically most trials have been underpowered. In 2002, a study of 5503 clinical trials (McDonald et al., 2002) identified 69% as having fewer than 100 subjects. Small trials make it more difficult to reject the null hypothesis because they lead to larger standard deviations and standard errors. There is also a risk of bias. A small trial that does not show a significant effect might

For a list of all websites referred to in this chapter, as clickable links, see the book companion website: www.booksite.elsevier.com/9780128023877.

Biostatistics for Medical and Biomedical Practitioners
http://dx.doi.org/10.1016/B978-0-12-802387-7.00036-6

not be submitted for publication, whereas the same sized trial that reached significance (whether warranted or not) will probably be published (Stern and Simes, 1997). Egger et al. (2002) concluded that on average unpublished trials underestimate treatment effects by 10%. Furthermore, Stanbrook et al. (2006) found that clinical trials named with an acronym were more likely to be published in a major journal or to be cited than trials not named, independent of whether the results were positive or negative.

FOREST GRAPHS

The results of the meta-analysis are presented in tables and graphs (Bax et al., 2009). A common variety of graph, sometimes called a forest graph, is shown in Figure 36.1.

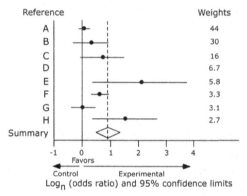

Figure 36.1 Typical figure of response to some new treatment. The dots are the mean log odds ratio, and the horizontal lines indicate 95% confidence limits. Figures in the right-hand column are the weights assigned to each study; the studies are often arranged in descending weights. The solid vertical line at 0 indicates no difference between the groups, and the dashed vertical line indicates the pooled average. Some figures include the numbers of subjects in each group.

As often happens, the largest studies show the least effects.

The weights are usually calculated from $1/(standard error)^2$, and these weights are then used to determine the final mean value and confidence limits. The calculations depend upon whether a fixed or a random effects model is used. The former implies that all the studies estimate the same population mean, whereas the latter implies that there may be variability between the means as well as within each separate study (Borenstein et al., 2010). For example, if the effect of a beta-adrenergic blocker after myocardial infarction is tested on several small groups of identical composition, it is reasonable to consider that they all come from the same population and estimate the same population mean. If, on the other hand, the samples have different compositions (age groups, associated diseases, etc.), although the medication may be useful in all groups, it may affect each subpopulation differently. Therefore, not only the variability within a sample, but also the difference between the various population means need consideration. This additional source of variability changes the weighting factors and makes the confidence intervals wider.

Therefore meta-analysis programs take account of heterogeneity as well, and if necessary, correct for it. Excellent articles featuring these issues are presented by Hulley et al. (Hulley et al., 2007) and Higgins et al. (2003), and the principles and practice of meta-analysis can be found in the book by Borenstein et al. (2009).

Higgins et al. (2003) recommended an index of heterogeneity called I^2, calculated as $I^2 = \frac{100\% \times (Q - df)}{Q}$, where Q is Cochran's heterogeneity calculated by summing each study's weighted squared deviations from the average of the meta-analysis estimate.

In addition to the line indicating no difference, another line indicating the mean change in all the studies combined is good practice (Cuzick, 2005), and allows better assessment of individual samples with confidence limits that include the null hypothesis but also include the average change.

In forest plots, the sample size is sometimes indicated by the size of the symbol for the mean (Lewis and Clarke, 2001). One potential weakness is that the smaller samples with wider confidence limits feature more prominently than those with smaller limits. Forest plots and the relevant calculations may be produced online at http://www.healthstrategy.com/meta/metainput.htm, http://www.singlecaseresearch.org/idea-center/forest-plot-in-excel, and http://commfaculty.fullerton.edu/jreinard/meta-analysis_programs.htm. The last of these gives references to several free meta-analysis programs, mostly for PCs. There is also a complete and well-documented commercial program called Comprehensive Meta-Analysis at http://www.meta-analysis.com/pages/comparisons.html. It comes with an excellent tutorial.

FUNNEL PLOTS

In the funnel plot, the X-axis represents the mean result (that may be an odds or risk ratio, or a percent difference) and the Y-axis shows the sample size or an index of precision (Egger et al., 1997). Sterne and Egger (2001) recommended the inverse standard error for the Y-axis and the log of the odds ratio for the X-axis. The symmetry of the plot may vary depending on whether sample size or inverse standard error is used as an index of precision (Tang and Liu, 2000).

Because there are usually more small than large samples, the points that represent each mean value are widely spread at the base and narrow as they move to the top, thus resembling an inverted funnel or a fir tree (Figure 36.2).

The funnel plot is often used to assess bias (Ferrer, 1998; Song et al., 2002; Souza et al., 2007; Tang and Liu, 2000). Prominent causes of bias are publication bias, with studies giving positive results more frequently submitted for publication and more likely to be published (Roehr, 2012); English language bias—negative studies are less likely to be published in English journals, although this has not always been observed (Juni et al., 2002; Moher et al., 2000; Song et al., 2002); and citation bias—studies with positive conclusions are cited more frequently and thus are more easily identified and incorporated in the

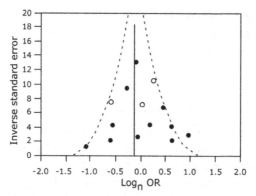

Figure 36.2 Funnel plot. The dashed lines indicate the funnel. Solid and open circles can be used to differentiate subgroups.

database. The basis of assessing bias is that if all the studies give random assessments of the same unbiased mean value, the plot should be symmetrical. If the studies are biased, for example, by having too few small studies with positive results and large effect sizes, then the funnel plot becomes asymmetrical with a deficit near the bottom (Figure 36.3).

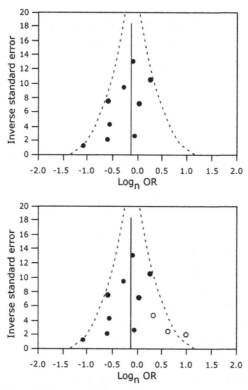

Figure 36.3 Top panel: Deficit of points with large effect and small sample size. Bottom panel: Restoration of symmetrical funnel (added open circles).

The asymmetry may be judged by eye, but can also be tested mathematically. One approach (Egger et al., 1997) is to fit the points by linear regression. In a symmetrical funnel plot, the intercept on the X-axis should be close to zero, whereas with asymmetry it may deviate considerably from zero. Egger et al. (1997) analyzed 37 meta-analyses published between 1993 and 1996 in the Annals of Internal Medicine, BMJ, JAMA, and Lancet. Most intercepts were well below zero, showing a deficiency in the lower right-hand corner of the funnel.

Other statistical tests for asymmetry can be done (Begg and Mazumdar, 1994).

A technique called "trim and fill" has been developed to deal with serious asymmetry by modeling the data as if they were symmetrically distributed, as they should be, if all the samples are unbiased estimators of the same mean value (Duval and Tweedie, 2000a,b). An iterative method using rank correlation is used in which some of the extreme values remaining are removed, and a new mean is calculated. If the distribution remains asymmetrical, another iteration is performed. After 2—4 cycles, when the distribution is symmetrical, the trimmed data are replaced and their theoretical counterparts on the other side of the axis of symmetry are inserted.

This technique may improve estimates when there are deficits due to publication bias, but deficits may be due to other factors, and different corrections may be required (Peters et al., 2007; Terrin et al., 2003).

Funnel plots can be drawn by online programs at http://www.kurtosis.co.uk/technique/funnel/index.htm. They can also be drawn with standard XY plot software.

RADIAL PLOTS

To evaluate heterogeneity among the samples, Galbraith (1988) recommended a radial plot in which one axis plotted the z score (log odds ratio/standard error of log odds ratio) and the other axis plotted the log odds ratio on a curved line resembling a speedometer.

The advantages of this graphic display are (after Galbraith) as follows:

1. Each estimate has a unit standard error in the X direction.
2. The numerical value of an odds ratio can be read off by extrapolating a line from $(\mathbf{0}, 0)$ through $(\mathbf{x}, y)$ to the circular scale drawn.
3. Points with a large standard error drop near the origin, whereas points with a small standard error, that is, the more informative estimates, drop well away from the origin.

The Galbraith scale is more often represented as a classical XY plot, with the z score on the Y-axis, the inverse standard error on the X-axis, and two parallel lines indicating ± 2 standard errors (Figure 36.4).

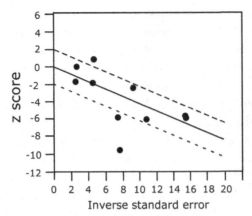

Figure 36.4 Modified Galbraith plot. If the studies all estimate one fixed parameter, then the dots should fall between the two outer lines.

L'ABBÉ PLOTS

In the L'Abbé plot, control versus treated outcome for each study is plotted on a graph that shows the line; of identity (Solid line Figure 36.5).

In some studies, the dots in the L'Abbé plot are circles of different sizes that represent the weights (size) of the samples. The circles may be colored to indicate subgroups.

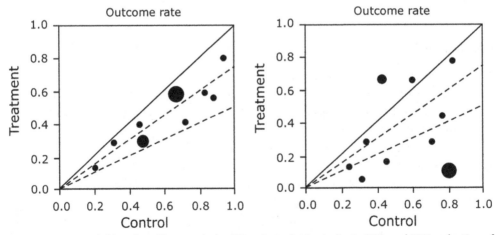

Figure 36.5 Two L'Abbe plots. The two dashed lines in each plot indicate 25% and 50% reduction of effect. The left-hand plot shows homogeneity, but the right-hand plot shows excessive dispersion, casts doubt upon the homogeneity of the samples, and suggests that the studies may be measuring different things.

Bax et al. (2009) also describe box plots, quantile plots, and standard residual histograms. They compared the different plots and concluded that heterogeneity was shown best by the forest plot and the standard residual histogram, that the funnel plot might be best for assessing publication bias, but finally that many problems remained to be solved. They urged caution in interpreting any of these graphic displays.

When used carefully, meta-analysis is a useful technique for many purposes. A useful summary is provided by Anzures-Cabrera and Higgins (2010), and a useful online tutorial together with some online calculations and calculators is provided by Basu.

CRITICISMS OF META-ANALYSIS

Few meta-analyses meet all the criteria for a good study, so that their conclusions are often suspect (Sacks et al., 1987; Chan and Altman, 2005).

One of the severest critics is Ioannidis, whose nontechnical Presidential lecture to the Society for Research Synthesis Methodology should be read by everyone who performs or reads about meta-analysis (Ioannidis, 2010). He analyzed critically several meta-analyses performed to determine if steroids were helpful in bacterial meningitis. The earliest studies concluded that they were very beneficial, but as later studies were analyzed, the conclusions became less certain, and the most recent analysis in 2010 showed no benefit at all. As the author pointed out, historically, there has been a tendency for treatment effects to become smaller with repeated studies. This by itself is not a cause for alarm, because in science, new data always have the ability to correct previous errors or misinterpretations. What was alarming is that the four most cited articles in the meningitis field were two early trials that found an implausibly large treatment effect, one that found an effect only in adults, and one a nonsystematic "expert" review. As Ioannidis wrote "I suspect that the scientific literature is much littered with such wreckages that have not been removed from view."

Even more serious criticisms were offered in a recent publication by Shibata (2013). He pointed out that about 30—50% of large randomized clinical trials failed to confirm the results of previous meta-analyses. The probable reasons for the failure included small trial sizes used in the meta-analyses and, more importantly, clinical heterogeneity.

REFERENCES

Anzures-Cabrera, J., Higgins, J.P.T., 2010. Graphical displays for meta-analysis: an overview with suggestions for practice. Res. Synth. Methods 1, 66—80.

Basu, A. How to Conduct a Meta-analysis (Online). Available from: http://www.pitt.edu/~super1/lecture/lec1171/001.htm.

Bax, L., Ikeda, N., Fukui, N., Yaju, Y., Tsuruta, H., Moons, K.G., 2009. More than numbers: the power of graphs in meta-analysis. Am. J. Epidemiol. 169, 249—255.

Begg, C.B., Mazumdar, M., 1994. Operating characteristics of a rank correlation test for publication bias. Biometrics 50, 1088—1101.

Borenstein, M., Hedges, L.V., Higgins, J.P.T., Rothstein, H.R., 2010. A basic introduction to fixed-effect and random-effects models for meta-analysis. Res. Synth. Methods 1, 97—111.

Borenstein, M., Hedges, L.V., Higins, J.P.T., Rothstein, H.R., 2009. Introduction to Meta-analysis. John Wiley & Sons, Chichester, England.

Chan, A.W., Altman, D.G., 2005. Identifying outcome reporting bias in randomised trials on PubMed: review of publications and survey of authors. BMJ 330, 753.

Cuzick, J., 2005. Forest plots and the interpretation of subgroups. Lancet 365, 1308.

Duval, S., Tweedie, R., 2000a. A nonparametric "Trim and Fill" method of accounting for publication bias in meta-analysis. J. Am. Stat. Assoc. 95, 89—98.

Duval, S., Tweedie, R., 2000b. Trim and fill: a simple funnel-plot-based method of testing and adjusting for publication bias in meta-analysis. Biometrics 56, 455—463.

Egger, M., Davey Smith, G., Schneider, M., Minder, C., 1997. Bias in meta-analysis detected by a simple, graphical test. BMJ 315, 629—634.

Egger, M., Ebrahim, S., Smith, G.D., 2002. Where now for meta-analysis? Int. J. Epidemiol. 31, 1—5.

Egger, M., Smith, G.D., 1997. Meta-analysis. Potentials and promise. BMJ 315, 1371—1374.

Egger, M., Smith, G.D., 1998. Bias in location and selection of studies. BMJ (Clin. Res. Ed.) 316, 61—66.

Eysenck, H.J., 1995. Meta-analysis of best-evidence synthesis? J. Eval. Clin. Pract. 1, 29—36.

Ferrer, R.L., 1998. Graphical methods for detecting bias in meta-analysis. Fam. Med. 30, 579—583.

Galbraith, R.F., 1988. A note on graphical presentation of estimated odds ratios from several clinical trials. Stat. Med. 7, 889—894.

Higgins, J.P., Thompson, S.G., Deeks, J.J., Altman, D.G., 2003. Measuring inconsistency in meta-analyses. BMJ 327, 557—560.

Hulley, S.B., Cummings, S.R., Browner, W.S., Grady, D.G., Newman, T.B., 2007. Designing Clinical Research. Williams & Wilkins, Philadelphia, Lippincott.

Hunter, J.E., Schmidt, F., 1990. Methods of Meta-analysis. Sage, Newbury Park.

Ioannidis, J.P.A., 2010. Meta-research: the art of getting it wrong. Res. Synth. Methods 1, 169—184.

Juni, P., Holenstein, F., Sterne, J., Bartlett, C., Egger, M., 2002. Direction and impact of language bias in meta-analyses of controlled trials: empirical study. Int. J. Epidemiol. 31, 115—123.

Lewis, S., Clarke, M., 2001. Forest plots: trying to see the wood and the trees. BMJ 322, 1479—1480.

McDonald, S., Westby, M., Clarke, M., Lefebvre, C., 2002. Number and size of randomized trials reported in general health care journals from 1948 to 1997. Int. J. Epidemiol. 31, 125—127.

Moher, D., Pham, B., Klassen, T.P., Schulz, K.F., Berlin, J.A., Jadad, A.R., Liberati, A., 2000. What contributions do languages other than English make on the results of meta-analyses? J. Clin. Epidemiol. 53, 964—972.

Peters, J.L., Sutton, A.J., Jones, D.R., Abrams, K.R., Rushton, L., 2007. Performance of the trim and fill method in the presence of publication bias and between-study heterogeneity. Stat. Med. 26, 4544—4562.

Roehr, B., 2012. Routine screening for ovarian cancer harms more than it helps, says US authority. BMJ 345, e6203.

Sacks, H.S., Berrier, J., Reitman, D., Ancona-Berk, V.A., Chalmers, T.C., 1987. Meta-analyses of randomized controlled trials. N. Engl. J. Med. 316, 450—455.

Shibata, M.C., 2013. What is wrong with meta-analysis? The importance of clinical heterogeneity in myocardial regeneration research. Int. J. Clin. Pract. 67, 1081—1085.

Song, F., Khan, K.S., Dinnes, J., Sutton, A.J., 2002. Asymmetric funnel plots and publication bias in meta-analyses of diagnostic accuracy. Int. J. Epidemiol. 31, 88—95.

Souza, J.P., Pileggi, C., Cecatti, J.G., 2007. Assessment of funnel plot asymmetry and publication bias in reproductive health meta-analyses: an analytic survey. Reprod. Health 4, 3.

Stanbrook, M.B., Austin, P.C., Redelmeier, D.A., 2006. Acronym-named randomized trials in medicine—the ART in medicine study. N. Engl. J. Med. 355, 101—102.

Stern, J.M., Simes, R.J., 1997. Publication bias: evidence of delayed publication in a cohort study of clinical research projects. BMJ 315, 640—645.

Sterne, J.A., Egger, M., 2001. Funnel plots for detecting bias in meta-analysis: guidelines on choice of axis. J. Clin. Epidemiol. 54, 1046–1055.

Tang, J.L., Liu, J.L., 2000. Misleading funnel plot for detection of bias in meta-analysis. J. Clin. Epidemiol. 53, 477–484.

Terrin, N., Schmid, C.H., Lau, J., Olkin, I., 2003. Adjusting for publication bias in the presence of heterogeneity. Stat. Med. 22, 2113–2126.

CHAPTER 37

Resampling Statistics

Contents

INTRODUCTION

Resampling occurs when observed data and a data generating mechanism such as a die or a computer is used to produce new samples unrelated to a hypothetical distribution. These techniques are therefore used when the form of the distribution is unknown or the samples are too small for standard methods to be used, for example, determining the interquartile interval for a very small data set.

The techniques are computer intensive. Because the calculations require special programs, resampling is usually out of reach for the average nonstatistician, but investigators will see the methods referred to in publications and need to understand the principles of resampling, and the strengths and weaknesses of the methods. For relatively understandable explanations of resampling methods, see the articles by Bergendahl and Veldhuis (1995), Boos and Stefanski (2010), Stark et al. (2007), Diaconis and Efron (1983), Ludbrook (1994), and Curran-Everett (2009, 2012) and the books by Efron (1994), Manly (1997), and Mosteller and Tukey (1977).

The major techniques include the bootstrap and the jackknife, Monte Carlo methods of random sampling, and permutation (Diaconis and Efron, 1983; Efron, 1979; Efron and Tibshirani, 1986; Ludbrook, 1994, 1995a,b, 2002; Ludbrook and Dudley, 1994; Manly, 1997; Curran-Everett, 2009, 2012). With these techniques computers can produce rapidly thousands of samples from a data set.

BOOTSTRAP

Samples are taken repeatedly, analyzed, and replaced many times, with no limit to the number of resampling runs done. The analyses produce robust estimates of point variables

For a list of all websites referred to in this chapter, as clickable links, see the book companion website: www.booksite.elsevier.com/9780128023877.

Biostatistics for Medical and Biomedical Practitioners
http://dx.doi.org/10.1016/B978-0-12-802387-7.00037-8

(mean, proportion, odds ratio, regression coefficient, etc.) with their standard errors and confidence limits.

Simon, one of the early developers of these methods (Simon, 1997) gives a simple example. Consider 20 people working in an office, and assume that on the average one of them becomes ill on any day and stays at home. How often will three people be away on any given day? This estimate can be made by assuming that the data fit a Poisson process. An alternative estimate is to resample. Generate a batch of 20 random numbers between 1 and 20, and arbitrarily assign one number, say 9, to represent an ill worker. Count how many 9s are present in the batch of 20. Repeat the sampling 1000 times, and determine how often three 9s appear in the sample. This number as a percentage of the total number of samples gives the required answer.

What is the variability of an estimate? Consider a set of experimental weight gains of 10 infant animals fed a particular formula: 50, 54, 46, 42, 51, 56, 61, 54, 48, 47 g/day. The mean value is 50.9 g/day. The usual method for calculating standard deviation gives s = 5.53, se = 1.74, 95% confidence limits 46.94−54.85 g/day. Similar estimates can be obtained by carrying out a bootstrap. Program the computer to select at random 10 numbers from a data set including thousands of each of these 10 numbers. Any one selection may include any of these 10 numbers in any pattern, for example, one of each, or any 10 even numbers, or occasionally 10 of the same number. Determine the mean for each set of 10 numbers and find the 95% confidence limits. In this example, they would be very similar to those calculated above; when I ran 5000 resamplings, the mean was also 50.9 and the standard error was 1.66. This was close to the previous value. The difference is that resampling does not involve any assumptions about the population from which those numbers came.

Sometimes it is difficult or impossible to know what the population distribution is, and therefore resampling the one data set provides data that are independent of any statistical theory. For example, determining the interquartile distance from a set of 10 numbers would be inexact with such a small set. Resampling allows the determination of thousands of interquartile distances, and averages them. An excellent online tutorial is provided by Teknomo (2006). There is one caveat, and that is, that if the sample is very unrepresentative of the population, a biased result may be obtained.

Other examples of calculations that would be difficult to achieve by standard statistical methods are determining the median difference between two independent samples (Efron and Gong, 1983) or the mean and confidence limits for the product or ratio of the means of two data sets (Ludbrook, 1995a). Bootstrapping can be used also to determine regression coefficients when the data do not conform to the usual requirements for parametric regression analysis. The null hypothesis is that there is no correlation between the X and Y variates, so that in theory any X_i could be associated with any Y_i. Therefore, the program draws at random all possible combinations of X and Y, calculates the resulting regression coefficient, and determines the probability that the observed regression coefficient could come from a set in which the regression coefficient is zero. These methods can be used to solve problems for which no parametric solutions apply (Manly, 1997).

There are free online calculators available at http://www.wessa.net/rwasp_bootstrapplot1.wasp, and there is an add-on for Excel at http://www3.wabash.edu/econometrics/EconometricsBook/Basic%20Tools/ExcelAddIns/bootstrap.htm.

As an example, consider the set of differences in weight growth in the peanut problem (Table 20.1). Repeated sampling (bootstrapping) for 1000 simulations gives the results in Figure 37.1.

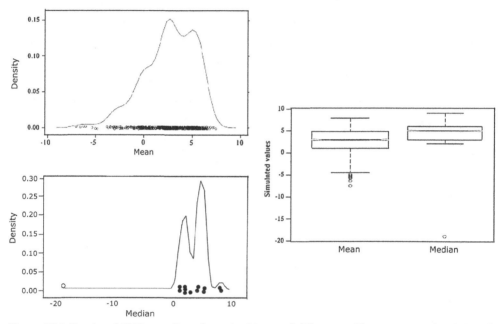

Figure 37.1 Results of 1000 samplings from the 10 sets of differences. The upper panel and the left box plot (third panel) show that the means of these 1000 samples are above zero more than 5% of the time, and confirm the conclusion from the t-test, but without regard to any of the requirements of the t-test. On the other hand, the median, being less sensitive to outliers, suggests that the roasted peanuts cause a consistent although small increase in growth.

PERMUTATIONS

Permutations share features with the bootstrap, but each data set is sampled until all the permutations are acquired; duplicate permutations are not allowed. If the data set is very large, the number of permutations becomes so big that even large computers take excessive time to cover them all, and then random sampling by the Monte

Carlo method can be done to derive a reasonable set of permutations. This is the basis of the Wilcoxon tests, but these had to be done on ranks because of limited computer power. Today the same tests can be done using the individual values in the data set. For example, to assess the difference between the means of two samples, examine all possible permutations, calculate the difference between the means, and do this for every possible permutation. Then the probability of rejecting the null hypothesis is

$$p = \frac{\text{Number of permutations with mean difference} \geq \text{observed difference}}{\text{Total number of possible permutations}}$$

As an example, consider group A with values 20, 11, 8, 7, 6 and group B with values 14, 8, 6, 5, 3. On the null hypothesis, these all come from the same population. Therefore, take successive permutations of the 10 numbers, split them into two groups of 5 and examine the difference between the means. The sampling is repeated for each of the 252 possible permutations (Table 37.1).

Table 37.1 Three of the possible sets of permutations

Group A	Group B	Mean A − Mean B
20, 11, 8, 7, 6	14, 8, 6, 5, 3	3.2
20, 14, 8, 7, 3	11, 8, 8, 7, 5	2.6
11, 6, 6, 5, 3	20, 11, 8, 8, 7	−4.6

When all the permutations are done, the results are shown in Figure 37.2.

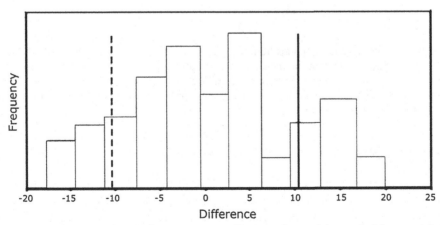

Figure 37.2 Random permutations from two groups. The areas beyond the vertical lines each include 17% of the results.

From these data, confidence limits can be determined without having to postulate any underlying distribution.

Simple instructive examples of permutations are given by Mosteller and Rourke (1973) and Curran-Everett (2012).

JACKKNIFE

This was one of the earliest resampling methods proposed. A sample is drawn and the statistics are recalculated after removing one data value at a time, starting with X_1 and ending with X_n; the number of resamplings is finite. These repeated samples give independent estimates from which parameters, variances and confidence limits may be derived. The procedure has the ability to remove bias.

The jackknife is a limited version of the bootstrap. Both methods can be used to determine confidence limits, but these are often wider than their parametric equivalents, and the best method of calculating them is still disputed. Outliers may affect the results. Nevertheless, for certain problems no other ways of determining confidence limits exist.

MONTE CARLO METHODS

Monte Carlo methods make random selections from the samples, based on an assumed model. Bootstrapping and permutation methods are specific types of more general Monte Carlo methods that can be applied to many types of data sets for which bootstrapping is inappropriate (Manly, 1997). A simple example, based on a problem illustrated by Bevington and Robinson (1992) is given below.

Consider determining the area of an irregular plane figure (Figure 37.3).

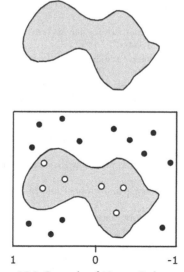

Figure 37.3 Example of Monte Carlo method.

In a relatively simple figure the area could be measured by planimetry or the trapezoid rule, but random sampling gives the same results. Place the figure inside a square with the base of two units, and arrange to plot on the figure, a series of points determined by random sampling from a set of numbers ranging from −1 to +1. After many samples, say 1000, there will be a distribution of points resembling the few shown in the figure. Because the distribution is random, the ratio of the number of points in the irregular figure to the total number of points will be the same as the ratio of the two areas. Because the area of the square is known, it is possible to determine the area of the irregular figure.

Many problems pertaining to these resampling methods are unsolved, and not every bootstrapped derived value is automatically correct. Outliers and severe heteroscedasticity may distort results (Stine, 1990). It is a field in which considerable experience is needed to avoid errors.

REFERENCES

Bergendahl, M., Veldhuis, J.D., 1995. Altered pulsatile gonadotropin signaling in nutritional deficiency in the male. Trends Endocrinol. Metab. 6, 145–159.

Bevington, P.R., Robinson, D.K., 1992. Data Reduction and Error Analysis for the Physical Sciences. McGraw-Hill, Inc., New York.

Boos, D., Stefanski, L., 2010. Efron's bootstrap. Significance 7, 186–188.

Curran-Everett, D., 2009. Explorations in statistics: the bootstrap. Adv. Physiol. Educ. 33, 286–292.

Curran-Everett, D., 2012. Explorations in statistics: permutation methods. Adv. Physiol. Educ. 36, 181–187.

Diaconis, P., Efron, B., 1983. Computer-intensive methods in statistics. Sci. Am. 248, 116–130.

Efron, B., 1979. Bootstrap methods; another look at the jackknife. Ann. Stat. 7, 1–26.

Efron, B., 1994. The Jackknife, the Bootstrap, and Other Resampling Plans. Capital City Press, Montpelier, VT.

Efron, B., Gong, G., 1983. A leisurely look at the bootstrap, the jackknife, and cross-validation. Am. Stat. 37, 36–48.

Efron, B., Tibshirani, R.J., 1986. Bootstrap methods for standard errors, confidence intervals and other measures of statistical accuracy. Stat. Sci. 1, 54–77.

Ludbrook, J., 1994. Advantages of permutation (randomization) tests in clinical and experimental pharmacology and physiology. Clin. Exp. Pharmacol. Physiol. 21, 673–686.

Ludbrook, J., 1995a. Issues in biomedical statistics: comparing means by computer-intensive tests. Aust. N. Z. J. Surg. 65, 812–819.

Ludbrook, J., 1995b. Issues in biomedical statistics: comparing means under normal distribution theory. Aust. N. Z. J. Surg. 65, 267–272.

Ludbrook, J., 2002. Statistical techniques for comparing measurers and methods of measurement: a critical review. Clin. Exp. Pharmacol. Physiol. 29, 527–536.

Ludbrook, J., Dudley, H., 1994. Issues in biomedical statistics: statistical inference. Aust. N. Z. J. Surg. 64, 630–636.

Manly, B.F.J., 1997. Randomization, Bootstrap and Monte Carlo Methods in Biology. Chapman and Hall, London.

Mosteller, F., Rourke, R.E.K., 1973. Sturdy Statistics. Nonparametrics and Order Statistics. Addison-Wesley Publishing Company, London.

Mosteller, F., Tukey, J.W., 1977. Data Analysis and Regression. A Second Course in Statistics. Addison-Wesley, Reading, CA.

Simon, J.L., 1997. Resampling: The New Statistics. Wadsworth, Boston.

Stark, J., Chan, C., George, A.J., 2007. Oscillations in the immune system. Immunol. Rev. 216, 213–231.

Stine, R., 1990. An introduction to bootstrap methods. In: Fox, J., Long, J.S. (Eds.), Modern Methods of Data Analysis. Sage Publications, Inc., Newbury Park, CA.

Teknomo, K., 2006. Bootstrap Sampling Tutorial [Online]. Available from: http://people.revoledu.com/kardi/tutorial/Bootstrap/examples.htm.

CHAPTER 38

Study Design: Sampling, Clinical Trials

Contents

SAMPLING PROBLEMS

We can put our knowledge to use to show how to design studies efficiently. It is essential to start by asking important questions, identifying the likely important relationships, and using effective methods of assessing them. This is what training programs are for. *In addition, whatever the question and the study design it is essential know ahead of time how to analyze the results.* Without this knowledge, the designs may inefficient or even produce unanalyzable results (Hulley et al., 2007). The two main types of study are observational and experimental; the former observes what happens in a sample, the latter perturbs the sample for specific purposes. To determine if smoking cigarettes caused bladder cancer, it would be unethical to take two groups of people, make one group smoke cigarettes, and then after 40 years find out if there was more bladder cancer in the smoking than the nonsmoking group. The best alternative is to follow two groups, one consisting of cigarette smokers and one of nonsmokers, and find out if they developed different incidences of bladder cancer.

If the cigarette smokers did indeed have more bladder cancer, what more needs to be done? The first consideration is to decide what population was being investigated. Is it a target or a convenience population? The target population is the theoretical population desired. The target might be a group of men and women with a racial mixture and range of socioeconomic classes equivalent those in the US population, all of whom began smoking cigarettes in their teens and continued to smoke cigarettes throughout the period of study. What we might get is a convenience sample, a selection of people

For a list of all websites referred to in this chapter, as clickable links, see the book companion website: www.booksite.elsevier.com/9780128023877.

Biostatistics for Medical and Biomedical Practitioners
http://dx.doi.org/10.1016/B978-0-12-802387-7.00038-X

with the time or inclination to join the study, and if a financial reward was offered for joining the study then we might get an excess of poorer people. The results would apply only to the observed sample and hence could be cautiously extended only to the base population from which the sample came. This might not be the same as the target population. A second major problem concerns confounders, that is, hidden differences that might be the true explanation for the observations. For example, could smoking be innocuous, but could smokers be more likely to take a medication or food that is excreted in urine and will eventually cause bladder cancer? How are we going to find out the true cause of bladder cancer?

The history of observational studies is rich with misleading results. One of the most famous is the Literary Digest survey in 1936 of the likely outcome of the presidential election between Franklin Roosevelt and Alf Landon. The Literary Digest (Poll), having correctly predicted the outcome of the five preceding Presidential elections, mailed 10,000,000 questionnaires (each ballot contained the annual subscription card), and over 2,300,000 responses showed an overwhelming response of 57% to 43% in favor of the Republican candidate Alf Landon. Even the chairman of the National Democratic party, James Farley, was impressed enough to state:

> *Any sane person cannot escape the implication of such a gigantic sampling of popular opinion as is embraced in The Literary Digest straw vote. I consider this conclusive evidence as to the desire of the people of this country for a change in the National Government. The Literary Digest poll is an achievement of no little magnitude. It is a Poll fairly and correctly conducted.*
>
> *Poll.*

Yet in the actual election, it was Roosevelt who won with 62% to 38%, one of the largest majorities in electoral history. A similar poll conducted at the same time with only 50,000 people by George Gallup, a journalist who specialized in assessing public opinion, correctly predicted the Roosevelt victory. Why was there such a discrepancy?

The Literary Digest sent its questionnaire to people whose names were drawn from lists of its subscribers, as well as from lists of automobile and telephone owners, but this was a time when telephones were scarce, cars were relatively expensive, and magazine subscribers were among the minority with money to spare; the United States was just emerging from the Great Depression. Consequently, the people polled were among the more affluent members of society, most of whom detested Roosevelt's policies. Furthermore, even among the affluent, a response to the questionnaire was more likely among those against Roosevelt than in favor of his policies; people who feel strongly about an issue are more likely to respond. Therefore, despite the huge sample, the Literary Digest made two fatal errors. They did not sample the target population that should have been all the potential US voters, and they did not allow for the fact that responders and nonresponders may be different. A 5% failure to respond might not have been important, but when 77% do not respond, the chances of a biased sample are very high. The convenience sample, even one as large as this one was, was totally unrepresentative of the target population. There may indeed be safety in numbers, but only if they represent the desired sample.

How did Gallup with smaller numbers of people polled produce an accurate estimate of the final results? He used a method called quota sampling, in which he attempted to sample representative proportions of all the voters. This has now been replaced by a more accurate method based on randomization. As a footnote to history, the Gallup Organization made a serious error when in 1948 they predicted that Dewey would defeat Truman in the presidential election. Their error was in stopping polling 3 weeks before the election, thereby missing the big late swing of independent voters to Truman.

Under some circumstances, an observational group may be large enough to be more like a target than a convenience population. In the Framingham Heart Study, in 1948 the National Heart Institute (subsequently the National Heart, Lung, and Blood Institute) enlisted the city of Framingham in Massachusetts to help them follow several thousand of its inhabitants by a series of clinical and laboratory tests to find out what factors might lead to cardiovascular disease and stroke. The investigators chose a random selection of 2/3 of the households, and then the occupants were invited to participate. The majority of subjects approached enrolled. Initially, they recruited 5209 people aged 30−62 years, and have followed them and two cohorts of their children since then. By maintaining good relations with the community, there have been few subjects defecting from the study, and almost all of them return every 2 years for testing and examination. Nevertheless, despite what was close to a random sample for the Framingham population, this was far from being representative of all adults of that age. There are vast cultural and socioeconomic differences between the population of Framingham and comparably sized cities in Louisiana or Bulgaria, and what is true of one city might not be true of another. One study in Great Britain (Brindle et al., 2003) showed that the criteria established in Framingham for several cardiovascular risk factors overestimated the risk in Great Britain.

Another prominent study of this type is the Nurses' Health Study (NHS), started in 1976 with the primary objective of evaluating the long-term consequences of oral contraceptives. Subsequently, other factors such as diet were also investigated. Nurses were selected because they had a high educational standard so that they could respond accurately to questionnaires and also be motivated to join the study. Invitations were sent out to the population of 170,000 nurses aged 30−55 years in the 11 most populous states, and 122,000 responded and have been followed since then.

One important component of the NHS was evaluating the effects of hormone replacement therapy in healthy postmenopausal women with respect to deaths from cardiovascular disease. A major finding was that over 20 years there was about a 50% reduction in deaths from cardiovascular disease among those who took hormone replacement (Manson and Martin, 2001).

The NHS sample was large, with a widely based selection. It is likely but not certain that the 122,000 responders and the 48,000 (28%) nonresponders were similar. On the other hand, this is not the same as a universal target for women because it was restricted to subjects with a specific educational and perhaps socioeconomic criterion. Whether they respond in the same way to diet and contraceptives as do, say, women who are poor, uneducated, and belong to underprivileged minorities is uncertain. In fact, when the results of this study on deaths from cardiovascular disease were tested formally by randomized clinical trials (Grady et al., 2002; Grodstein et al., 2000), hormone replacement therapy was shown to *increase* the risk of death from cardiovascular disease. One possible explanation of the discrepancy between the observational and randomized studies was that in the NHS, hormone replacement therapy was started at an average age of 51 years, whereas in the randomized trials, the average age at starting therapy was 63–67 years (Coulter, 2011). Once again the target population must match the wider population if the results are to be applicable.

The Royal Society of General Practitioners in the United Kingdom (Hannaford et al., 2007; Hannaford, 2010) carried out another large study of contraceptives in relation to cancer incidence. They recruited 23,777 women using oral contraceptives and 23,796 women who did not use them; the two groups were comparable in important variables such as age, number of pregnancies, social class, smoking habits, and other medical problems. After 48 years, there was a reduction in the incidence of all cancers of about 12% in those who used contraceptives. Although many participants left the study and were lost to follow up, subgroup examination suggested that these losses were unlikely to have affected the conclusions. On the other hand, with an observational study of this type, it was not possible to exclude the effects of confounders. Furthermore, although one of the strengths of this trial was its long duration, this was also its weakness because over 48 years, there were several changes in the chemical composition of contraceptive pills that could not be allowed for in the conclusions.

HISTORICAL CONTROLS

In some studies, instead of performing a randomized clinical trial, a group of subjects exposed to some potential disease-causing factor is compared to historical controls. Historical controls are not randomized, have many drawbacks, and should be avoided if possible. Diseases change over time, especially infectious diseases where severity waxes and wanes during an epidemic. Furthermore, patient selection changes over time. Current patients are often diagnosed earlier than they used to be, so that the average severity of the disease is less. Specific advances in treatment, on the other hand, may attract the more severe forms of disease disproportionately. Nonspecific therapeutic advances have altered outcomes. For example, Harrison et al. (1978, 1986) assessed the natural history of fetuses diagnosed in utero with congenital diaphragmatic hernia born in Norway between 1969 and 1975 and in California between 1980 and 1982; in both groups about 60—75% of the patients died. This observation was the basis for carrying out a clinical trial of surgical correction of the hernia in the fetuses between 1999 and 2001 (Harrison et al., 2003). By the time of the trial, the medical care of these infants had improved survival so much that it was not possible to show any improvement from the surgery. Many more differences are listed in the comprehensive book by Schwartz et al. (1980).

Historical controls may, however, lead to useful hypotheses. In the 1940s, the development of incubators for warming and providing high oxygen concentrations to premature infants increased their survival, but an increasing incidence of retrolental fibroplasia began to be reported (Humes, 2000; Wheatley et al., 2002). In 1951, in Australia Campbell (1951) suggested that high oxygen concentrations could be the cause of the retinopathy, basing this hypothesis on the high incidence of this retinopathy in Australia compared with the low incidence in Great Britain where incubators and high oxygen concentrations were used far less frequently (Silverman, 1980). Nevertheless, it was not until Patz and colleagues (Patz, 1957) carried out a randomized clinical trial that the hypothesis was established.

RANDOMIZATION

An early example of randomization was the Medical Research Council (MRC) trials of the treatment of tuberculosis. In the first trial, they allocated patients at random to receive either streptomycin or the symptomatic therapy in use at the time, and found a marked benefit from streptomycin (Anonymous, 1948). The groups were comparable in all important criteria. They then conducted later trials with patients randomized to receive streptomycin (now the new standard of treatment) or streptomycin and para-amino-salicylic acid (PAS); the combination proved to be superior (Anonymous, 1950). Once again, the groups were comparable in all important respects. In 1952, the MRC conducted another trial in which patients were allocated at random to receive either streptomycin plus PAS or isoniazid (Anonymous, 1952). This time when they compared the degree of lung cavitation, one of the markers of severity, they noted that the isoniazid group had 55% of the patients with bilateral cavitation but only 40% of those with unilateral cavitation. This discrepancy per se biased the results against isoniazid. Furthermore, when they graded the degree of cavitation from nil to 3+, the isoniazid group had 20% with no cavitation as against 7% in the other group, and had 69% with grades 1+ and 2+ as against 84% with these grades in the streptomycin PAS group. This degree of imbalance, not seen in the prior trials, occurred despite a formal randomization procedure. As another example, in the VA Cooperative Study of the treatment of chronic angina pectoris by surgery or medical treatment, patients were randomized based on age (<50, >50) and degree of coronary arterial involvement on angiography. When the investigators examined several other factors, such as blood pressure, previous myocardial infarction, history of smoking, diabetes, and blood cholesterol, all of these were equally distributed in both groups except for cholesterol, with significantly more with high blood cholesterol in the medically treated group. Therefore, randomization, although eliminating conscious bias, does not necessarily eliminate all bias.

Randomization may also be important when studying the potential advantages of a screening test. Chapter 21 described issues associated with selection of an appropriate screening test, but did not address whether the screening test was effective in reducing morbidity and mortality. To study this, there should be two comparable groups, applying the screening test to one and not the other, and determining if indeed screening is beneficial. Randomization and equalization of the groups is essential. If the screened group had more patients with mild disease and the control group had more with severe disease, the screened group would show the better outcomes, but it would be impossible to tell if the better outcome was due to screening or patient selection. The number of possible errors in selecting groups to compare is large, and described in detail by Feinstein (Feinstein et al., 1984).

One particularly subtle type of error, that of *stage migration*, was discussed in 1985 by Feinstein et al. (1985) in an article entitled "The Will Rogers phenomenon. Stage migration and new diagnostic techniques as a source of misleading statistics for survival in cancer." This was based on the quip by the humorist Will Rogers: "When the Okies left Oklahoma and moved to California, they raised the average intelligence level in both states." In one report, the authors observed that cancers treated in 1977 appeared to have higher survival rates compared with those treated between 1953 and 1964. This seemed to be due to the use of newer imaging techniques, because when survival based on initial symptoms was studied, there was no difference between the two time periods.

A modern example of this was described by Chee et al. (2008). In staging lung cancer, stage III (locally advanced) has a better outcome than stage IV (metastatic). Until about the year 2000, this distinction was made by X-ray imaging, but in 2000 Pieterman et al. (2000) reported on the value of positron emission tomography (PET) scanning with fluoro[18]-deoxyglucose (FDG) for detecting small distant metastases. Chee et al. (2008) showed that after the introduction of PET scanning with FDG, many patients formerly graded as stage III were found to be in stage IV. As a result, the prognosis of stage IV patients was slightly improved by addition of patients with smaller stage III lesions with less obvious metastasis, and the prognosis of stage III patients was improved by removal of patients with concealed metastases.

Simple randomization can be done with a table of random numbers (Gore and Altman, 1982). For example, to divide a sample of 60 subjects into three equal-sized groups, allocate numbers 00–29 to group A, numbers 30–59 to group B, and numbers 60–89 to group C.

Then take a table of random numbers (these are usually in pairs), turn pages blindly and select a page, and then, while still not looking, put a pin point somewhere on the page. Assume this number is 75. The first subject is then allocated to group C. Then as more subjects come in take the next pair of numbers just below the first number (or just above it, or just to the right of it, but be consistent); if this is 23, that subject goes into group A, and so on. Any number between 90 and 99 is ignored. Random numbers can be generated online at http://stattrek.com/statistics/random-number-generator.aspx, http://graphpad.com/quickcalcs/randomN1.cfm, and by Excel (see http://www.gifted. uconn.edu/siegle/research/Samples/random.htm), and random number tables appear at http://academic.cengage.com/resource_uploads/downloads/0534627943_27463.pdf and http://teorica.fis.ucm.es/ft8/tablern2.pdf.

Random numbers do not have to come from a table, but can be generated by computer. Because some program has to be used to create them, these numbers are not truly random but it may take enormous effort to disprove randomness. These numbers are often known as pseudorandom numbers, and they suffice for biomedical studies. If truly random outcomes are needed, they can be based on physically unpredictable events such as radioactive decay or atmospheric noise. Such a program is available at http://www. random.org/integers/.

If the plan was to have twice as many subjects in group A as in each of the other groups, then assign numbers 00—49 to group A, 50—74 to group B, and 75—99 to group C. There is no guarantee, however, that the groups will end up with the planned numbers. Quite by chance, there might be 65 in group A, 28 in group B, and 7 in group C. This is unlikely, but nothing prevents this imbalance from occurring. If this imbalance cannot be tolerated, then restricted sampling may be done. In a trial to determine if indomethacin closes the patent ductus arteriosus in premature infants, merely allocating patients at random to indomethacin or placebo has a major disadvantage. The chances of spontaneous closure of the patent ductus arteriosus increase with increased gestational age or birth weight. Therefore, if at the end of the study there were more older infants in the indomethacin group and if this group had more closures, it would not be possible to tell if closure was due to age or treatment, even though randomization was intended to avoid this difficulty. Therefore carry out restricted (or stratified) sampling. Define homogeneous blocks by birth weight or gestational age, and then randomize each of these blocks. With two groups (indomethacin, placebo), designate blocks of 4, 6, or 8, and arrange to have each block have equal numbers of subjects. Thus if block 1 has 4 positions, patient 1 is allocated (at random) to either A or B group. The second patient is also randomized by the same method. If these two patients are randomized to A and B, then the third patient is randomized to A or B, and the fourth patient automatically goes into the other group. If the first two patients are randomized to group A, then the next two are allocated to group B. The possibilities are shown in Table 38.1 with the nonrandom allocations in bold type.

Table 38.1 Randomized blocks of 4

A,	B,	A,	B
A,	A,	B,	B
A,	B,	B,	A
B,	A,	B,	A
B,	A,	A,	B
B,	B,	A,	A

Providing that the statistician does the allocation and the investigator is unaware of the allocation, and providing the block length can be varied, there is no way that the investigator can know how the allocations are done. To avoid any possibility that the investigator may guess which patient has which agent, the blocks themselves may be changed at random from 4 to 6 to 8.

Stratified sampling has other advantages. For example, to determine if body weight and insulin resistance are associated, select at random 150 subjects and look for the association. Because exercise might be a confounding factor, subjects can be classified as no exercise outside normal activity, moderate exercise, and extreme exercise. By sampling randomly within each group, not only is there added information, but because variability will probably be smaller within an exercise group, the ability to discern differences will be improved. This is the equivalent of blocking in ANOVA.

CLINICAL TRIALS

People have tried various proposed cures from time immemorial, but Dr James Lind (1716—1794) probably performed the first controlled clinical trial. In the eighteenth century, scurvy was a devastating disease of sailors. For example, in Anson's circumnavigation of the globe from 1740 to 1744, reported in 1748, 380 out of 510 sailors died of scurvy, and in the British navy regularly about one-third of sailors died or were disabled by the disease. Lind (1753) selected 12 sailors who could not work because of scurvy. He gave two of them cider, two took elixir of vitriol, two had vinegar, two had copious drinks of seawater, two were given purgatives, and two were given fresh lemon and orange juice (one of these was the most severely affected of the 12). The two given citrus juice recovered rapidly, but the others remained ill. (Despite this demonstration, confirmed by others, it took over 30 years for the British Admiralty to order a daily ration of citrus juice for all sailors in the navy.) In the 1760s, too, John Hunter described that treating gonorrhea with (inert) bread pills produced the same cure rate as standard treatment (Palmer, 1835). It was not until 1944, however, that the MRC in Great Britain published the results of the first truly well-designed clinical trial (MRC, 1944).

There are observational studies that because of their unique nature cannot be considered without confounding issues and cannot be duplicated. Abraham Wald performed a study about aviation casualties for the Statistical Research Group that was formed just after the attack on Pearl Harbor in 1941 (Mangel and Samainago, 1984). The difficulty in that study was the absence of data from the planes that did not return. His tentative conclusions were put into practice in the Korean and Vietnam wars. Modern investigation of airline crashes, too, has to work also with incomplete data, often different for each crash, but the investigators usually manage to form a tentative conclusion and suggest possible safety measures. For example, on July 17th, 1996, TWA flight 800 crashed into the sea soon after leaving John F. Kennedy airport in New York. Despite incomplete recovery of plane fragments, the National Transport Safety Board concluded that the center wing fuel tank was empty but filled with gasoline vapor that exploded, perhaps due to overheating by the air conditioning packs that were just under the tank. This led to reconstruction of fuel systems so that this type of calamity could be avoided in the future.

Intent-to-treat is a cardinal principle of clinical trials (Peto et al., 1976, 1977). Remember that randomization is an attempt to minimize possible bias. If the subjects are randomized, then not only should known factors such as age, body weight, smoking history, presence or absence of diabetes be approximately equalized between the two (or more) groups being compared in the trial, but the hope is that factors not yet known to be important will also be equalized. Without randomizing, one group might have an excess of subjects with a factor later found to have an important influence on the outcome.

Once the groups have been randomized, each should receive its designated treatment, but this is not always possible. For example, in the large VA trial of coronary artery surgery versus medical treatment, a substantial number of patients assigned to medical treatment eventually had surgery because of deterioration of their disease, and a smaller number assigned to surgery declined operation (Peduzzi et al., 1998). How should the investigators analyze their data? The correct approach is termed the *intent-to-treat* principle (Peto et al., 1976, 1977), and this requires the investigators to record the end points (acute myocardial infarction, death) based on the original assignments. To make this clear, if a patient assigned to medical treatment had surgery and then died, that would be considered a death due to medical treatment. Now this seems intuitively wrong, because death followed surgery. However, end points based on final treatment cause a problem in that those who crossed over to surgery were not a representative group. They might have had more with diabetes, or more with a high cholesterol level, or more with obesity. If they did, then transferring to surgery might deplete the medical treatment group of its high-risk patients, and the final analysis of those who remained on medical treatment versus those who had surgery would be made on groups that were not comparable. Vickers (2009) gave a simple description of the issues involved in the intent-to-treat principle.

Of course, there is nothing to stop the investigators from analyzing subgroups that are matched, but once the randomization scheme has been broken the balance of all the other unknown factors (some of which might in the future turn out to be important) is altered in an unknown manner, and there is no longer a randomized clinical trial.

In planning a clinical trial, thought must be given to the end points. Often there is a single end point such as death or readmission to hospital, but sometimes there may be multiple end points. A trial of a method of reducing the incidence of acute myocardial infarction might have this as its primary goal, but might also examines deaths, need for coronary revascularization, and congestive heart failure as secondary end points. Examining all of these raises all the issues of multiple comparisons (Chapter 24). If the secondary end points had not been considered a priori, then some form of Bonferroni or equivalent test can be applied to keep the type-I error low. These tests are probably too conservative for planned secondary end points, and there is no generally accepted method for evaluating them (Fisher, 1999; Fisher and Moye, 1999). One approach is to divide the alpha spending function into portions dealing with the primary and secondary end points, much as the Lan and De Mets approach to partitioning alpha spending functions for interim examinations. As an example, make the alpha allocation (α_E) for the whole study 0.05, and then choose $\alpha_P = 0.02$ for the primary end point. This leaves 0.03 to be apportioned among, say, three secondary end points α_S from the formula $\alpha_s = 1 - \frac{1-\alpha_E}{1-\alpha_P}$. This value is apportioned among the three secondary end points based on $(1-\alpha_S)^3$. As an example, with three secondary end points, $\alpha_S = 1 - \frac{0.95}{0.98} = 0.0306$, and each α_S is determined from $\frac{0.0306}{3} = 0.0102$.

There is no perfect generally accepted method, but the issue of multiplicity must always be considered.

Another problem of multiple end points is that of sample size. Because clinical trials are costly in terms of time and money, the sample size is usually based on the primary end point, and may be too small for the secondary end points unless they have large effect sizes. Under these circumstances, if the primary end point is not significant and a secondary end point seems to be important but is underpowered and not significant itself, a specific trial with that end point as a goal is needed.

The results of a well-conducted clinical trial must be considered carefully, and related to the composition of the sample. At one extreme, the sample may be very homogeneous; for example, a trial of the value of a statin in reducing the risk of myocardial infarction in men between the ages of 45 and 55 years, who do not smoke, are not hypertensive or diabetic, and have no family history of coronary heart disease. If the trial shows a reduction of risk, a physician might cautiously use that treatment for subjects who match these characteristics, but can have no assurance that the treatment would help others with different characteristics. More often, the sample has subjects with different combinations of the above variables, and more caution is needed in putting the results into practice. Furthermore, a decrease in relative risk, even if significant, has to be put into context by considering attributable risk, population attributable risk, and number needed to treat (Chapter 20).

An important aspect of all clinical trials is the distinction between internal and external validity, the former referring to the success of the trial in eliminating bias, the latter to the extension of the trial results to a wider population (Rothwell, 2005). Failure of internal and external validity to agree explains why frequently a clear-cut result of a clinical trial cannot be confirmed in a larger population. Statisticians over the years have come to accept this distinction, and to be less rigid about the conclusions to be drawn from a trial. Sir Austin Bradford Hill, one of the earliest leaders in the field of Medical Statistics, changed from an unswerving reliance on figures to a more cautious approach (Horton, 2000). In the 11th edition of his book *Principles of Medical Statistics*, published in 1984 (47 years after the first edition), Hill (1984) wrote:

> *At its best such a trial shows what can be accomplished with a medicine under careful observation and certain restricted conditions. The same results will not invariably or necessarily be observed when the medicine passes into general use; but the trial has at the least provided background knowledge which the physician can adapt to the individual patient.*

Even if the trial shows, for example, that a specific treatment reduces the risk of some event, for example, a myocardial infarction, the benefit may not apply equally to all members of the group because the outcome will be influenced by sets of variables that distinguish one member of the group from another. As discussed by Dorresteijn et al. (2011), unless the group is unusually homogeneous, some subjects will benefit more than others from the new treatment, some may not benefit at all, and some may be harmed. They described methods for predicting optimal response based on the individual effects of known variables. As an example, they used the data from the Justification for the Use of Statins in Prevention (JUPITER) trial to evaluate the use of rosuvastatin in the primary prevention of cardiovascular disease. Based on Framingham and Reynolds risk scores involving gender, smoking history, blood pressure, and family history of premature coronary heart disease, they calculated the risk of cardiovascular events with and without treatment. Such a method is the antithesis of the "one size fits all" approach and would allow physicians to tailor their treatment for specific individuals. This should maximize outcomes and minimize complications and costs.

Criticism of the standard randomized clinical trial suggests that the high failure rate of these trials, and resultant waste of resources, is due in part to the "one population, one drug, one disease" strategy (Berry et al., 2015). Instead, some investigators recommend what is termed "the platform trial." These are extensions of adaptive designs (Chapter 24) that allow multiple treatments in heterogeneous populations, with changes occurring during the trial in response to intermediate outcomes.

Recently, Ebrahim et al. (2014) reexamined 37 clinical trials that were reevaluated by independent or involved investigators. The reanalyses were often done with different statistical procedures, definitions, or measurements of outcomes of interest. Thirty-five percent of the reanalyses led to interpretations that differed from those in the original article. Because details of the trial are frequently not made public, there is a potential source of error that should make us be careful about accepting the results of these trials.

Units to be studied need definition. For example, a study of the value of fluoride supplementation of toothpaste in preventing dental caries in children might assign children randomly to two groups, one to receive normal toothpaste and one to receive toothpaste with a fluoride supplement. At the end of the study, the control group might have 727 carious teeth and the treated group 207 carious teeth. What is the conclusion? The problem is that the unit is the mouth and not the individual teeth. Whatever the causes of dental caries may be, it is likely that they are similar for all the teeth in any one mouth. It may well happen that the numbers of affected children were less different in the two groups. It would be more correct to treat each child as a unit, and record how many had caries or no caries.

Animal studies incur the same risks. After placing 10 randomly selected rats in cage A and 10 others in cage B, and feeding them different supplements, what is the conclusion if the weight gain is substantially greater in cage A then cage B? The difference might be due to the supplement used, but could be due to extraneous factors. If one cage was kept in a warm quiet area, whereas the other was in a cold noisy area, quite possibly all the rats in cage A slept more than the rats in cage B, and therefore burned fewer calories. It is also possible for one or two rats in cage B to eat more than their share of food so the other rats in that cage are underfed. Here the cage is the unit. To avoid these problems, the rats should be placed in separate cages that are randomly dispersed in the room.

In addition to all the problems discussed above, clinical trials have their own problems associated with difficulties of organization and assessment. An important issue concerns outside interference with a perfectly good plan, as occurred in the early trials of the effect of oxygen therapy in premature infants. Although giving high oxygen concentrations to breathe was at one time standard because of the immature lungs of these patients, there was concern about an increase in the incidence of retrolental fibroplasia. A trial was therefore planned to compare the effect of breathing high oxygen versus lower oxygen concentrations. (In its initial application, the NIH rejected the application for funding on the basis because the referees "knew" that it was dangerous to lower oxygen concentrations for premature infants!) Appropriate randomization was carried out. Unfortunately, some of the nurses had strong opinions about the usefulness of high oxygen concentrations, and deliberately placed infants assigned to low oxygen onto high oxygen concentrations (Patz, 1957). Once again, this made interpretation of the results difficult.

Humans are particularly susceptible to suggestion. An extreme example of psychological effect has been termed the Hawthorne effect. The Hawthorne Works in Cicero, Illinois, were owned by the Western Electric Company, and manufactured a variety of consumer products including telephones, electric fans, and refrigerators. Between 1927 and 1932, Elton Mayo studied the effect of environmental influences on worker productivity. A series of changes were made: for example, increased illumination of the factory floor, removal of obstacles, decreased humidity, and increased frequency of rest periods. After each change, productivity increased. Then all the variables were returned to their original states, and once again productivity increased! The conclusion was that the increases in productivity were nonspecific and not due to the individual interventions but rather to the workers' feelings that someone was taking an interest in them. The conclusions have been challenged and debated since then, although the principle that workers perform better when they believe that people take in an interest in them still applies.

Therefore, the ideal clinical trial should make sure that everyone involved in the trial—doctors, patients, ancillary personnel, and statisticians analyzing the data—should be unaware of (blinded to) which patients are getting which treatment. Sometimes, as in comparing surgical with medical treatment of coronary artery disease, it is impossible for doctors and patients to be unaware of which group is which, but those analyzing the results should be blinded. If the patients do not know which group they are in, but the doctors know, the trial is termed a single blind. If neither doctors nor patients know which group they are in, it is a double-blind trial. Failure to randomize and conduct blinded trials may lead to bias, usually in favor of the new experimental treatment. This was the conclusion of a study by Chalmers et al. (1983) who studied controlled trials of the treatment of acute myocardial infarction and also noted that at least one prognostic variable was maldistributed in 14.0% of blinded trials, 26.7% of unblinded but randomized studies, and in 58.1% of the nonrandomized studies. Other studies have shown that investigators may try to subvert randomization in an attempt to secure what they thought was the better treatment for a given patient (Hoare, 2010; Schulz, 1995). Those trials in which randomizations been inadequately concealed tended to yield larger estimates of treatment effects (Schulz et al., 1995).

PLACEBO EFFECT

The placebo effect refers to treatment with a supposedly inert substance without the patient's knowledge. Many studies have shown that a variable, often high percentage of patients with a variety of diseases and symptoms may improve after being given the placebo (Beecher, 1955). The effect is real and presumably due to psychosomatic interactions, perhaps release of endorphins. The placebo recipients, if adequately randomized, do serve as a type of control. This is a more specific example of the complexities of human thought and emotions, and the issues were brought into focus by Kaptchuk (2003) who wrote:

> *Facts do not accumulate on the blank slates of researchers' minds and data simply do not speak for themselves.1 Good science inevitably embodies a tension between the empiricism of concrete data and the rationalism of deeply held convictions. Unbiased interpretation of data is as important as performing rigorous experiments. This evaluative process is never totally objective or completely independent of scientists' convictions or theoretical apparatus……."At the cutting edge of scientific progress, where new ideas develop, we will never escape subjectivity." 2 Interpretation can produce sound judgments or systematic error. Only hindsight will enable us to tell which has occurred.*

ALTERNATIVES TO RANDOMIZED CLINICAL TRIALS

Although randomized clinical trials are desirable, they have some disadvantages. They are usually very expensive, take a long time, and often have restricted entry criteria that make it difficult for clinicians to apply those results to patients who do not meet those criteria. Recently, Eapen et al. (2013) cited studies to show that the cost to conduct a large phase 3 or phase 4 clinical trial could exceed $400 million. Over the years, the costs of trials have been increasing and the number of trials that can be funded has consequently decreased. These authors discussed ways of reducing the costs of these important clinical trials.

To give a specific example, the ALLHAT study (**A**ntihypertensive and **L**ipid-**L**owering Treatment to Prevent **H**eart **A**ttack **T**rial), one of the largest clinical trials to date, followed over 40,000 patients with mild or moderate hypertension between 1994 and 2002 to compare the effectiveness of various treatments to reduce the blood pressure and the incidence of various cardiovascular complications (The ALLHAT, 2002; Salvetti and Ghiadoni, 2004). It cost $105 million, according to the NIH Public Affairs Department. The trial concluded, among other things, that a low-cost diuretic agent was as effective in lowering blood pressure and reducing cardiovascular complications as newer and more expensive agents. (The estimated savings to the medical system by using the cheaper agent were estimated to be $3.1 billion dollars over 10 years.) Then the question arose about what second line drug to add when the primary diuretic agent did not achieve the desired lowering of blood pressure. Another randomized clinical trial of equivalent size, cost, and duration seemed to be impractical. An alternative was provided by Magid et al. (2010) who used the electronic records of the Kaiser Permanente Health System with over 8.6 million enrolled patients to compare the results of an angiotensin blocker versus a beta-adrenergic blocker as a second blood pressure lowering treatment. Although the individual patient's physician decided treatment without any attempt at randomization, the data pool was so vast that by using sophisticated methods, the investigators were able to match for each treatment patients with similar characteristics. Although excluding confounding factors is more difficult to do by this method, it had the advantage of minimizing them by using a huge data base, producing the results in a year and a half (a fraction of the time that a prospective study would have taken), covering a much wider range of patient ages and associated conditions than a randomized trial would have covered, and did it all for only $200,000. With the proper care, an observational study of this type can lead to results as acceptable as those attained by randomized clinical trials.

Propensity Analysis

One method of allowing for differences in the covariates between two or more samples is to use propensity analysis. As summarized by D'Agostino (2007), "The propensity score is the probability that a participant is in the 'treated' group given his/her background (pretreatment) characteristics." As an example, in comparing the risks of getting pancreatic cancer in smokers and nonsmokers, it would be unethical to assign experimental subjects to these groups randomly, so we elect to compare the outcomes in the two groups observed for 15 years. Unfortunately for simple comparisons, people may become smokers because they have underlying covariates that may be the real cause of pancreatic cancer. Perhaps, for example, people who drink a lot of coffee are more likely to be smokers and to get pancreatic cancer (this was a theory once held, but never proven). Therefore, smokers and nonsmokers would differ in the proportion with the "true" underlying cause. It is to correct for this that propensity analysis was developed.

By using logistic analysis in which the outcome is treated versus nontreated, it is possible to correct for imbalances between the two groups. A simplified Love plot is shown in Figure 38.1, based on a study comparing the effect of using or not using diuretics in patients with chronic congestive heart failure (Ahmed et al., 2006).

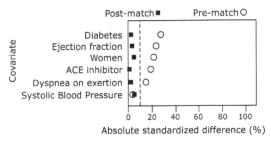

Figure 38.1 Love plot shown for covariates before and after matching. Before matching, there were often quite big differences between individual covariates. These differences almost disappeared after matching.

It is likely that carefully conducted and analyzed nonrandom studies will be used more frequently. Recently, Corrao et al. (2011) studied a cohort of 209,650 patients from Lombardy, Italy, who were treated with antihypertensive drugs between 2000 and 2001 with the goal of determining whether starting with one or two medications was better. They selected 10,688 hospitalized with cardiovascular disease, and selected three controls at random for each patient. By careful analysis, they were able to show improved results by starting with combination therapy. The huge population base allowed them to study a wide range of patient comorbidities that might not have been investigated had a smaller controlled clinical trial been done, and they did so with a fraction of the time and cost that a formal randomized clinical trial would have incurred.

REFERENCES

Ahmed, A., Husain, A., Love, T.E., et al., 2006. Heart failure, chronic diuretic use, and increase in mortality and hospitalization: an observational study using propensity score methods. Eur. Heart J. 27, 1431–1439.

Anonymous, 1948. Streptomycin treatment of pulmonary tuberculosis. Br. Med. J. 2, 769–782.

Anonymous, 1950. Treatment of pulmonary tuberculosis with streptomycin and *para*-aminosalicylic acid; a Medical Research Council investigation. Br. Med. J. 2, 1073–1085.

Anonymous, 1952. Isoniazid in pulmonary tuberculosis. Br. Med. J. 2, 764–765.

Anonymous, 2002. Major outcomes in high-risk hypertensive patients randomized to angiotensin-converting enzyme inhibitor or calcium channel blocker vs diuretic: the Antihypertensive and Lipid-Lowering Treatment to Prevent Heart Attack Trial (ALLHAT). J. Am. Med. Assoc. 288, 2981–2997.

Beecher, H.K., 1955. The powerful placebo. J. Am. Med. Assoc. 159, 1602–1606.

Berry, S.M., Connor, J.T., Lewis, R.J., 2015. The platform trial. An efficient strategy for evaluating multiple treatments. J. Am. Med. Assoc. 313, 1619–1620.

Brindle, P., Emberson, J., Lampe, F., et al., 2003. Predictive accuracy of the Framingham coronary risk score in British men: prospective cohort study. BMJ Clin. Res. Ed. 327, 1267.

Campbell, K., 1951. Intensive oxygen therapy as a possible cause of retrolental fibroplasia; a clinical approach. Med. J. Aust. 2, 48–50.

Chalmers, T.C., Celano, P., Sacks, H.S., et al., 1983. Bias in treatment assignment in controlled clinical trials. N. Engl. J. Med. 309, 1358–1361.

Chee, K.G., Nguyen, D.V., Brown, M., et al., 2008. Positron emission tomography and improved survival in patients with lung cancer: the Will Rogers phenomenon revisited. Arch. Intern. Med. 168, 1541–1549.

Corrao, G., Nicotra, F., Parodi, A., et al., 2011. Cardiovascular protection by initial and subsequent combination of antihypertensive drugs in daily life practice. Hypertension 58, 566–572.

Coulter, S.A., 2011. Heart disease and hormones. Tex. Heart Inst. J. 38, 137–141.

D'Agostino Jr., R.B., 2007. Propensity scores in cardiovascular research. Circulation 115, 2340–2343.

Dorresteijn, J.A., Visseren, F.L., Ridker, P.M., et al., 2011. Estimating treatment effects for individual patients based on the results of randomised clinical trials. BMJ Clin. Res. Ed. 343, d5888.

Eapen, Z.J., Vavalle, J.P., Granger, C.B., et al., 2013. Rescuing clinical trials in the United States and beyond: a call for action. Am. Heart J. 165, 837–847.

Ebrahim, S., Sohani, Z.N., Montoya, L., et al., 2014. Reanalyses of randomized clinical trial data. J. Am. Med. Assoc. 312, 1024–1032.

Feinstein, A.R., Sosin, D.M., Wells, C.K., 1985. The Will Rogers phenomenon: stage migration and new diagnostic techniques as a source of misleading statistics for survival in cancer. New. Engl. J. Med. 312, 1604–1608.

Feinstein, A.R., 1984. Current problems and future challenges in randomized clinical trials. Circulation 70, 767–774.

Fisher, L.D., 1999. Carvedilol and the Food and Drug Administration (FDA) approval process: the FDA paradigm and reflections on hypothesis testing. Control Clin. Trials 20, 16–39.

Fisher, L.D., Moye, L.A., 1999. Carvedilol and the Food and Drug Administration approval process: an introduction. Control Clin. Trials 20, 1–15.

Grady, D., Herrington, D., Bittner, V., et al., 2002. Cardiovascular disease outcomes during 6.8 years of hormone therapy: heart and Estrogen/progestin Replacement Study follow-up (HERS II). J. Am. Med. Assoc. 288, 49–57.

Gore, S.M., Altman, D.G., 1982. Statistics in Practice published by Devonshire, Torquay UK.

Grodstein, F., Manson, J.E., Colditz, G.A., et al., 2000. A prospective, observational study of postmenopausal hormone therapy and primary prevention of cardiovascular disease. Ann. Intern. Med. 133, 933–941.

Hannaford, P.C., Selvaraj, S., Elliott, A.M., et al., 2007. Cancer risk among users of oral contraceptives: cohort data from the Royal College of General Practitioner's oral contraception study. BMJ Clin. Res. Ed. 335, 651.

Hannaford, P.C., 2010. Investigating the link between the Pill and cancer. Signif. Virtual Med. 6–10.

Harrison, M.R., Bjordal, R.I., Langmark, F., et al., 1978. Congenital diaphragmatic hernia: the hidden mortality. J. Pediatr. Surg. 13, 227–230.

Harrison, M.R., Adzick, N.S., Nakayama, D.K., et al., 1986. Fetal diaphragmatic hernia: pathophysiology, natural history, and outcome. Clin. Obstet. Gynecol. 29, 490–501.

Harrison, M.R., Keller, R.L., Hawgood, S.B., et al., 2003. A randomized trial of fetal endoscopic tracheal occlusion for severe fetal congenital diaphragmatic hernia. N. Engl. J. Med. 349, 1916–1924.

Hill, A.B., 1984. Principles of Medical Statistics. Oxford University Press.

Hoare, Z.S.J., 2010. Randomisation: what, why and how? Significance 7, 136–138.

Horton, R., 2000. Common sense and figures: the rhetoric of validity in medicine (Bradford Hill Memorial Lecture 1999). Stat. Med. 19, 3149–3164.

Hulley, S.B., Cummings, S.R., Browner, W.S., et al., 2007. Designing Clinical Research. Williams & Wilkins, Lippincott.

Humes, E., 2000. Baby ER. Simon and Schuster.

Kaptchuk, T.J., 2003. Effect of interpretive bias on research evidence. BMJ Clin. Res. Ed. 326, 1453–1455.

Lind, J., 1753. A Treatise of the Scurvy. In Three Parts. Containing an Inquiry into the Nature, Causes and Cure, of That Disease. Together with a Critical and Chronological View of What Has Been Published on the Subject. A. Miller in the strand, Edinburgh.

Magid, D.J., Shetterly, S.M., Margolis, K.L., et al., 2010. Comparative effectiveness of angiotensin-converting enzyme inhibitors versus beta-blockers as second-line therapy for hypertension. Circ. Cardiovasc. Qual. Outcomes 3, 453–458.

Mangel, M., Samaniago, F.J., 1984. Abraham Wald's work on aircraft survivability. J. Am. Stat. Assoc. 79, 259–267.

Manson, J.E., Martin, K.A., 2001. Clinical practice. Postmenopausal hormone-replacement therapy. New. Engl. J. Med. 345, 34–40.

MRC, 1944. Clinical trial of patulin in the common cold. Lancet 2, 373–375.

Patz, A., 1957. The role of oxygen in retrolental fibroplasia. Pediatrics 19, 504–524.

Palmer, J., 1835. The Works of John Hunter. Longman, Rees, Orme, Brown and Breen.

Peduzzi, P., Kamina, A., Detre, K., 1998. Twenty-two-year follow-up in the VA Cooperative Study of Coronary Artery Bypass Surgery for Stable Angina. Am. J. Cardiol. 81, 1393–1399.

Peto, R., Pike, M.C., Armitage, P., et al., 1976. Design and analysis of randomized clinical trials requiring prolonged observation of each patient. I. Introduction and design. Br. J. Cancer 34, 585–612.

Peto, R., Pike, M.C., Armitage, P., et al., 1977. Design and analysis of randomized clinical trials requiring prolonged observation of each patient. II. Analysis and examples. Br. J. Cancer 35, 1–39.

Pieterman, R.M., Van Putten, J.W., Meuzelaar, J.J., et al., 2000. Preoperative staging of non-small-cell lung cancer with positron-emission tomography. N. Engl. J. Med. 343, 254–261.

Rothwell, P.M., 2005. External validity of randomised controlled trials: "to whom do the results of this trial apply?". Lancet 365, 82–93.

Salvetti, A., Ghiadoni, L., 2004. Guidelines for antihypertensive treatment: an update after the ALLHAT study. J. Am. Soc. Nephrol. 15 (Suppl. 1), S51–S54.

Schulz, K.F., 1995. Subverting randomization in controlled trials. JAMA 274, 1456–1458.

Schulz, K.F., Chalmers, I., Hayes, R.J., et al., 1995. Empirical evidence of bias. Dimensions of methodological quality associated with estimates of treatment effects in controlled trials. J. Am. Med. Assoc. 273, 408–412.

Schwartz, D., Flamant, R., Lellouch, J., 1980. Clinical Trials. Academic Press.

Silverman, W.A., 1980. Retrolental Fibroplasia: a Modern Parable. New York, Grune & Stratton.

The Literary Digest Poll. https://www.math.upenn.edu/~deturck/m170/wk4/lecture/case1.html.

Vickers, A.J., 2009. Why Mr Jones Got Surgery Even if He Didn't: Intention-to-Treat Analysis [Online]. Available: http://www.medscape.com/viewarticle/707140?src=mp&spon=2&uac=105072MT.

Wheatley, C.M., Dickinson, J.L., Mackey, D.A., et al., 2002. Retinopathy of prematurity: recent advances in our understanding. Br. J. Ophthalmol. 86, 696–700.

## PART 9

End Texts

ANSWERS TO PROBLEMS

CHAPTER 3

Problem 3.1

a. Interval
b. Ordinal
c. Nominal
d. Ordinal
e. Ordinal

Problem 3.2

It tells us to add up all the X values, starting with the third and ending with value before the last value.

CHAPTER 4

Problem 4.1

The two histograms should look like these: Produced from http://www.wessa.net/rwasp_varia1.wasp#output.

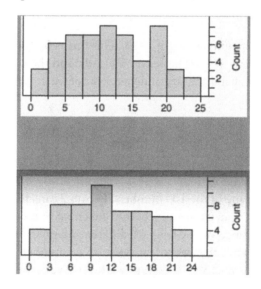

Problem 4.2

Stem and Leaf Plot:

Stem	Leaf
0	0 0 1 2 2 3 3 3 4 4
0	5 5 5 6 6 6 6 7 7 7 8 8 9 9 9
1	0 0 0 0 1 1 1 1 2 2 3 4 4
1	5 6 6 7 7 7 7 8 8 9 9 9
2	1 1 2 2
2	

Here is one plot that uses the data, produced from calculator at http://www. calculatorsoup.com/calculators/statistics/stemleaf.php. Yours may differ if you used different stems or a different calculator.

CHAPTER 5

Problem 5.1

There are 52 cards and 4 kings. Therefore the probability is $4/52 = 1/13$.

Problem 5.2

The probability of drawing a king is 1/13. This leaves 51 cards, and the probability of drawing a queen is thus 4/51. This leaves 50 cards, and the probability of drawing a jack is 4/50. These probabilities are independent of each other, so the combined probability is

$$\frac{4}{52} \times \frac{4}{51} \times \frac{4}{50} = \frac{64}{132600} = 0.0004826.$$

Problem 5.3

Person 1 can choose any of the 100 numbers. Person 2 can choose a different number in 99/100 ways. Person 3 can choose one of the remaining numbers in 98/100 ways, and so on. Therefore the chance of choosing 20 different numbers is $1 \times 0.99 \times 0.98 \times\ldots$ $0.81 = 0.1187$. Then the chances of at least two numbers being the same are $1 - 0.1187 = 0.8813$, or 88.13%. The correct answer is (e).

CHAPTER 6

Problem 6.1

The cumulative area beneath the curve for $z = -0.75$ is 0.2263
The cumulative area beneath the curve for $z = 1.5 = 0.9332$
Therefore the area between these two limits is $0.9332 - 0.2263 = 0.7069$
From http://davidmlane.com/hyperstat/z_table.html we get

HyperStat Online Home Page

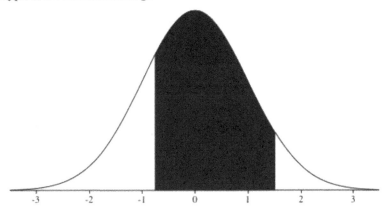

⦿ Area from a value (Use to compute p from Z)
◯ Value from an area (Use to compute Z for confidence intervals)

Specify Parameters:

Mean 0

SD   1

◯ Above 1.5

◯ Below 0.75

⦿ Between -0.75   and 1.5

◯ Outside -1.96   and 1.96

Results:
Area (probability) 0.7066

(Recalculate)

Problem 6.2

```
Skewness and Kurtosis Test

> agostino
        D'Agostino skewness test
data:  x
skew = -0.4598, z = -0.9738, p-value = 0.3302
alternative hypothesis: data have a skewness


> anscombe
        Anscombe-Glynn kurtosis test
data:  x
kurt = 7.9059, z = 3.6771, p-value = 0.0002359
alternative hypothesis: kurtosis is not equal to 3


> jarque
        Jarque-Bera Normality Test
data:  x
JB = 56.0562, p-value = 6.722e-13
alternative hypothesis: greater


> geary
[1] 0.6603605
```

The JB test shows that this is not normal. Produced from http://www.wessa.net/rwasp_skewness_kurtosis.wasp#output.

Problem 6.3

Quantile plot drawn from http://www.wessa.net/rwasp_harrell_davis.wasp#output.

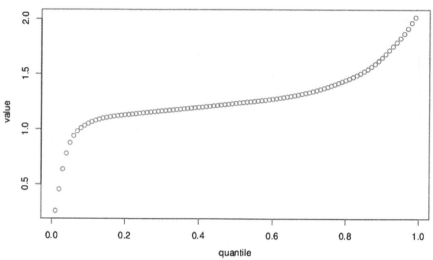

Harrell–Davis Quantiles

This is not a straight line, so that the data set is not normal. It is straight in the middle 80%, but is abnormal at each end and is asymmetrical.

CHAPTER 7

Problem 7.1

	95%	95% Range	99%	99% Range
N = 14	85.29–101.11	15.82	82.18–104.22	22.04
N = 77	90.14–96.26	6.12	88.17–97.23	9.06

Note that the limits are narrower for the larger sample sizes, and narrower for 95% limits than for 99% limits.

CHAPTER 11

Problems 11.1 and 11.2

Power	s = 0.4	s = 0.64
0.80	14	36
0.85	16	41
0.90	19	48

Sample sizes needed.

By Lehr equation for paired samples, s = 0.4 and power of 0.80, k = 8 and $N = \frac{8 \times 0.4^2}{0.3^2} = 14.2$ subjects tested before and after the intervention. If the tests were unpaired, then k − 16 and we need 28 subjects in all.

For power of 0.9, with paired samples we need $N = \frac{10.5 \times 0.4^2}{0.3^2} = 18.7$ subjects, and for unpaired subjects we need 37.

CHAPTER 12

Problem 12.1

For any one suit the chance of drawing 5 cards out of 13 is $\frac{13!}{5!8!} = 1287$. For all four suits, the chances are $4 \times 1287 = 5148$.

If this is divided by the total number of 5 card hands (2,598,960), the chances of a flush are $\frac{5148}{2598960} = 0.00198$, or about 1/505.

Problem 12.2

The possible sets are 1,2,3,4,5; 2,3,4,5,6; 3,4,5,6,7; 4,5,6,7,8; 5,6,7,8,9; 6,7,8,9,10; 7,8,9,10,J; 8,9,10,J,Q; 9,10,J,Q,K; 10,J,Q,K,Ace; the ace can rank as either a 1 or above the King. Therefore numerically there are 10 possible sequences. Each sequence represents 5 cards drawn from any of the 4 suits for a total of 4^5 hands. Therefore the total number of straights is $10 \times 4^5 = 10,240$, which represents $\frac{10240}{2598960} = 0.00394$ or about 1/254 hands.

Problem 12.3

For any suit, the number of possible sequences is 10 (remember that an Ace can be either the highest or the lowest card). There are 4 suits, therefore there are 40 straight flushes possible. In 2,598,960 possible hands, this represents 40/2,598,960 = 0.0001539, or about one in 64,974 hands.

The secret to carrying out these calculations is to set out the problem in words before calculating.

CHAPTER 13

Problem 13.1

Total number of patients = N = 16
Number of hyperreactors = X = 5
Number of nonhyperreactors = N − X = 11
Number chosen = n = 6
Number of hyperreactors chosen = 2 or 5

Calculated with http://stattrek.com/online-calculator/hypergeometric.aspx.

<table>
<tr><td colspan="2">■ Enter a value in each of the first four text boxes (the unshaded boxes).
■ Click the **Calculate** button.</td><td colspan="2">■ Enter a value in each of the first four text boxes (the unshaded boxes).
■ Click the **Calculate** button.</td></tr>
<tr><td>Population size</td><td>16</td><td colspan="2">**Note:**
One or more outputs use E-notation.</td></tr>
<tr><td>Number of successes in population</td><td>5</td><td>Population size</td><td>16</td></tr>
<tr><td>Sample size</td><td>6</td><td>Number of successes in population</td><td>5</td></tr>
<tr><td>Number of successes in sample (x)</td><td>2</td><td>Sample size</td><td>6</td></tr>
<tr><td>Hypergeometric Probability: P(X = 2)</td><td>0.412087912087912</td><td>Number of successes in sample (x)</td><td>5</td></tr>
<tr><td>Cumulative Probability: P(X < 2)</td><td>0.346153846153846</td><td>Hypergeometric Probability: P(X = 5)</td><td>0.00137362637362637</td></tr>
<tr><td>Cumulative Probability: P(X ≤ 2)</td><td>0.758241758241758</td><td>Cumulative Probability: P(X < 5)</td><td>0.998626373626373</td></tr>
<tr><td>Cumulative Probability: P(X > 2)</td><td>0.241758241758242</td><td>Cumulative Probability: P(X ≤ 5)</td><td>0.999999999999999</td></tr>
<tr><td>Cumulative Probability: P(X ≥ 2)</td><td>0.653846153846154</td><td>Cumulative Probability: P(X > 5)</td><td>9.99200722162641E-16</td></tr>
<tr><td></td><td></td><td>Cumulative Probability: P(X ≥ 5)</td><td>0.00137362637362737</td></tr>
</table>

CHAPTER 14

Problem 14.1

*	Outcome Occurred		Outcome did not Occur		Totals	
Risk Factor Present or Dx Test Positive	64	= a	216	= b	280	= r1
Risk Factor Absent or Dx Test Negative	47	= c	273	= d	320	= r2
Totals	111	= c1	489	= c2	600	= t

Confidence Level: 95   %

(Compute)

Chi-Square Tests

Type of Test	Chi Square	d.f.	p-value
Pearson Uncorrected	6.610	1	0.010
Yates Corrected	6.080	1	0.014

There is a tendency for maternal age and birth weight to be associated. If the issue is important, you should probably acquire further data. Calculations done from http://statpages.org/ctab2x2.html.

Problem 14.2

The odds ratio is $\frac{64 \times 273}{47 \times 216} = 1.72$. Some calculators, e.g., http://statpages.org/ctab2x2.html give the confidence limits for the ratio as well.

Problem 14.3

From the calculator, the total chi-square is 20.52, and $P = 0.00039$. However, this does not indicate what the association is. To find this information, perform the calculation by hand, as in the text, and examine where there are excessive or very deficient expected values.

Maternal age (year)	Birth weight (g)			Total
	<2500	2500–3000	>3000	
<20	**21** 12.025 +8.975 80.5506 *6.70*	**14** 13.65 +0.35 0.1225 *0.01*	**30** 39.375 −9.325 86.9556 *2.21*	65
20–25	**43** 39.775 +3.225 10.4006 *0.26*	**56** 45.15 +10.85 17.7225 *2.61*	**116** 130.075 −14.075 198.1056 *1.52*	215
>25	**47** 59.2 −12.2 148.84 *2.51*	**56** 67.2 −11.2 125.44 *1.87*	**217** 193.6 +23.4 547.46 *2.83*	320
Total	111	126	363	600

Observed counts in bold, chi-square in italics.
Total chi-square 20.52, 4 df, $P = 0.00039$.
As shown, the biggest chi-square value shows an excess of counts in the low birth weight babies born to mothers <20 years of age.

An online calculator that comes closest to providing this information is http://vassarstats.net/index.html.

| Select the number of rows: | 2 | 3 | 4 | 5 | 3 |
| Select the number of columns: | 2 | 3 | 4 | 5 | 3 |

Data Entry

	B_1	B_2	B_3	B_4	B_5	Totals
A_1	21	14	30	-----	-----	65
A_2	43	56	116	-----	-----	215
A_3	47	56	217	-----	-----	320
A_4	-----	-----	-----	-----	-----	-----
A_5	-----	-----	-----	-----	-----	-----
Totals	111	126	363	-----	-----	600

Reset   Calculate

Chi-Square	df	P
20.52	4	0.0004

Cramer's V =   0.1308

No message for this analysis.

Percentage Deviations

	B_1	B_2	B_3	B_4	B_5
A_1	+74.6%	+2.6%	-23.7%		
A_2	+8.1%	+24%	-10.8%		
A_3	-20.6%	-16.7%	+12.1%		
A_4					
A_5					

Percentage deviation and *standardized residual* are both measures of the degree to which an observed chi-square cell frequency differs from the value that would be expected on the basis of the null hypothesis.

For each cell, *percentage deviation* is calculated as

$$\frac{observed - expected}{expected} \times 100$$

Thus, a percentage deviation of +15% within a cell indicates that the observed frequency is 15% greater than the expected, while a percentage deviation of -15% indicates that the observed frequency is 15% smaller than the expected.

Standardized Residuals

	B_1	B_2	B_3	B_4	B_5
A_1	+2.59	+0.09	-1.49	-----	-----
A_2	+0.51	+1.61	-1.23	-----	-----
A_3	-1.59	-1.37	+1.68	-----	-----

Problem 14.4

	Outcome 1	Outcome 2	Total
Group 1	3	9	12
Group 2	7	4	11
Total	10	13	23

Fisher's exact test

The two-tailed P value equals 0.0995
The association between rows (groups) and columns (outcomes)
is considered to be not quite statistically significant.

Performed by http://www.graphpad.com/quickcalcs/contingency1.cfm. A trend, but more data are needed.

Problem 14.5

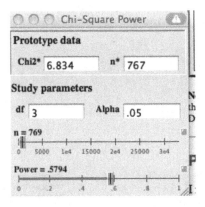

The power is relatively low. To determine the number needed for a given power, use the slider to set the power, and read the number. Determined from http://homepage. stat.uiowa.edu/~rlenth/Power/index.html.

Because of the scale the estimate is approximate, but that does not matter. In practice, you would plan for about 25–30% greater numbers to allow for dropouts and other mishaps.

CHAPTER 15

Problem 15.1

Data Entry

Cate-gory	Observed Frequency	Expected Frequency	Expected Proportion	
A	4	7.13312693	0.02476780	
B	11	14.2662538	0.04953560	
C	19	21.3993808	0.07430340	Sums:
D	31	28.5325077	0.09907120	Observed Frequencies:
E	42	35.6656346	0.12383900	288
F	50	42.7987616	0.14860681	Expected Frequencies:
G	63	49.9318885	0.17337461	256.79257
H	68	57.0650154	0.19814241	Expected Proportions:
	Reset Calculate			0.89164

Cumulative Proportions

	Observed	Expected	| O—E |	
A	0.014	0.028	0.014	
B	0.052	0.084	0.032	
C	0.118	0.167	0.049	
D	0.226	0.278	0.052	
E	0.372	0.417	0.045	
F	0.546	0.584	0.038	D_{max}
G	0.765	0.778	0.013	
H	1.0	1.0	0	0.052

Critical Values of D_{max} for n =   288

	Level of Significance (non-directional)	
	.05	.01
	0.0801	0.096

The distribution is not uniform, but more numbers would be needed to be sure. Calculated with http://vassarstats.net/ksm.html.

Problem 15.2

Frequencies-I	8	17	31	47	52	73	89	98						
Frequencies-II	4	6	19	36	44	68	93	99						

CALCULATE   CLEAR
Test Statistic 0.078101
Conclusion
No real evidence against the null hypothesis

Calculated with http://home.ubalt.edu/ntsbarsh/Business-stat/otherapplets/ks.htm.

Problem 15.3

Calculated with http://vassarstats.net/kappa.html.

Data Entry

				B						Totals
		1	2	3	4	5	6	7	8	
A	1	16	3	1	1	----	----	----	----	21
	2	3	17	2	2	----	----	----	----	24
	3	4	6	14	3	----	----	----	----	27
	4	1	1	5	16	----	----	----	----	23
	5	----	----	----	----	----	----	----	----	----
	6	----	----	----	----	----	----	----	----	----
	7	----	----	----	----	----	----	----	----	----
	8	----	----	----	----	----	----	----	----	----
Totals		24	27	22	22	----	----	----	----	95

Reset   Calculate

Unweighted Kappa

Observed Kappa		.95 Confidence Interval	
	Standard Error	Lower Limit	Upper Limit
0.5512			
Method 1	0.0646	0.4246	0.6778
Method 2	0.0645	0.4247	0.6777

0.9158	maximum possible unweighted kappa, given the observed marginal frequencies
0.6019	observed as proportion of maximum possible

Kappa with Linear Weighting

Observed Kappa	Standard Error	Lower Limit	Upper Limit
		.95 Confidence Interval	
0.6221	0.0631	0.4984	0.7458

0.9141	maximum possible linear-weighted kappa, given the observed marginal frequencies
0.6806	observed as proportion of maximum possible

Kappa with Quadratic Weighting

Observed Kappa	Standard Error	Lower Limit	Upper Limit
		.95 Confidence Interval	
0.6842	0.0903	0.5071	0.8613

0.9211	maximum possible quadratic-weighted kappa, given the observed marginal frequencies
0.7428	observed as proportion of maximum possible

CHAPTER 16

Problem 16.1

By hand:

$$P(X = 3) = \frac{50!}{3!47!}(0.07)^3(0.93)^{47} = 0.2219$$

By calculator (http://vassarstats.net/binomialX.html).

n = 100 [the number of opportunities for a head to occur]
k = 60 [the stipulated number of heads]
p = .5 [the probability that a head will occur on any particular toss]
q = .5 [the probability that a head will not occur on any particular toss]

Show Description of Methods

To proceed, enter the values for **n, k,** and **p** into the designated cells below, and then click the «Calculate» button. (The value of **q** will be calculated and entered automatically). The value entered for **p** can be either a decimal fraction such as .25 or a common fraction such as 1/4. Whenever possible, it is better to enter the common fraction rather than a rounded decimal fraction: 1/3 rather than .3333; 1/6 rather than .1667; and so forth.

n	k	p	q
50	3	0.07	0.929999999

Calculate   Reset

Parameters of binomial sampling distribution:

mean = 3.5
variance = 3.255
standard deviation = 1.8042

binomial z-ratio =   (if applicable)

P: exactly 3 out of 50	
Method 1. exact binomial calculation	0.22194674155
Method 2. approximation via normal	
Method 3. approximation via Poisson	
P: 3 or fewer out of 50	
Method 1. exact binomial calculation	0.532735302552
Method 2. approximation via normal	
Method 3. approximation via Poisson	
P: 3 or more out of 50	
Method 1. exact binomial calculation	0.689211438998
Method 2. approximation via normal	
Method 3. approximation via Poisson	

	P: 3 or fewer out of 50	
For hypothesis testing	One-Tail	Two-Tail
Method 1. exact binomial calculation	0.532735302552	1.0
Method 2. approximation via normal		
Method 3. approximation via Poisson		

By calculator http://www.stat.tamu.edu/~west/applets/binomialdemo.html.

Problem 16.2

Using the normal approximation,

p = 0.37, q = 0.63, N = 250. The 95% confidence limits are

$$0.37 \pm \left(1.96 \sqrt{\frac{0.37 \times 0.63}{200} + \frac{1}{500}} \right) = 0.37 \pm 0.0708 = 0.2992 - 0.4408.$$

By calculator http://www.graphpad.com/quickcalcs/confInterval2/.

QuickCalcs

1. Select category   2. Choose calculator   3. Enter data   **4. View results**

Confidence Intervals

Your data

Numerator = 74
Denominator = 200
Proportion (74/200) = 0.3700

Confidence intervals by modified Wald method

Agresti and Coull (The American Statistician. 52:119-126, 1998) recommend a method they term the modified Wald method. It is easy to compute by hand and is actually more accurate than the so-called "exact" method (below). Here are the results computed by the modified Wald method. (Bug in 90% and 99% CI fixed Feb 2006.)

The 90% confidence interval extends from 0.3159 to 0.4276
The 95% confidence interval extends from 0.3061 to 0.4388
The 99% confidence interval extends from 0.2875 to 0.4609

"Exact" confidence intervals

The confidence intervals below are calculated using the so-called "exact" confidence intervals, computed by the method of Clopper and Pearson (Biometrika 26:404-413, 1934), which is based on a relationship between the F distribution and the binomial distribution. The modified Wald intervals (above) may actually be more exact.

The 90% confidence interval extends from 0.3131 to 0.4298
The 95% confidence interval extends from 0.3030 to 0.4409
The 99% confidence interval extends from 0.2836 to 0.4627

Note small difference between the normal approximation and the more exact calculator method.

Problem 16.3

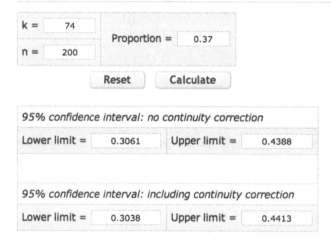

These limits are slightly different from the others and are regarded as more accurate. Calculated from http://vassarstats.net/ (under proportions).

Problem 16.4
By hand

$$P(A = 3; B = 26; C = 43; D = 9) = \frac{81!}{3!26!43!9!}0.06^3 0.37^{26} 0.41^{43} 0.16^9$$

$$= 0.0002153.$$

This is tedious and error prone, so use calculator http://stattrek.com/online-calculator/multinomial.aspx.

- First, enter the number of outcomes.
- Then, enter the probability and frequency for each outcome.
- Click the **Calculate** button.

Number of outcomes 4

Outcome	Probability	Frequency
1	0.06	3
2	0.37	26
3	0.41	43
4	0.16	9

Multinomial probability **0.00022**

CHAPTER 17

Problem 17.1

By hand

Adjusted p for the Wald limits are:

$$p = \frac{19 + 2}{113 + 4} = 0.1795$$

Therefore limits are $0.1795 \pm 1.96\sqrt{\frac{0.1795 \times 0.8205}{113}} = 0.1087 - 0.2503$

By calculator http://www.graphpad.com/quickcalcs/confInterval2/cfm.

Confidence Intervals

Your data

Numerator = 19
Denominator = 113
Proportion (19/113) = 0.1681

Confidence intervals by modified Wald method

Agresti and Coull (The American Statistician. 52:119-126, 1998) recommend a method they term the modified Wald method. It is easy to compute by hand and is actually more accurate than the so-called "exact" method (below). Here are the results computed by the modified Wald method. (Bug in 90% and 99% CI fixed Feb 2006.)

The 90% confidence interval extends from 0.1177 to 0.2341
The 95% confidence interval extends from 0.1095 to 0.2486
The 99% confidence interval extends from 0.0948 to 0.2783

"Exact" confidence intervals

The confidence intervals below are calculated using the so-called "exact" confidence intervals, computed by the method of Clopper and Pearson (Biometrika 26:404-413, 1934), which is based on a relationship between the F distribution and the binomial distribution. The modified Wald intervals (above) may actually be more exact.

The 90% confidence interval extends from 0.1130 to 0.2369
The 95% confidence interval extends from 0.1044 to 0.2501
The 99% confidence interval extends from 0.0887 to 0.2766

Problem 17.2

By calculator http://www.cct.cuhk.edu.hk/stat/proportion/Casagrande.htm.

Input		Results	
0.05			
α ⊙ one sided test (Calculate)			
○ two sided test			
β 0.20		m	1018
P_1 0.06			
P_2 0.09		N	2036
r 1			

Note:

Variables	Descriptions
α	Significance level
1-β	Power of the test
P_1	Success proportion in arm 1
P_2	Success proportion in arm 2
r	Ratio of arm 2 to arm 1
m	Sample size for arm 1
N	Total sample size for arm 1 and 2

By the Lehr equation, it is

$$n = \frac{16 \times \frac{0.06 + 0.09}{2} \times \frac{[(1 - 0.06) + (1 - 0.09)]}{2}}{(0.06 - 0.09)^2} = 1233 \text{ for each group.}$$

The calculator allows for different ratios of sample sizes.

CHAPTER 18

Problem 18.1

Although this can be done by hand, it is much easier to use the calculator http://vassarstats.net/poissonfit.html. This gives

k	Observed		Fitted Poisson	
	Frequency	Proportion	Probability	Expected Frequency
0	57	0.0218	0.01964	51.2503
1	203	0.0778	0.0772	201.4138
2	383	0.1468	0.1517	395.7782
3	525	0.2012	0.19872	518.4694
4	532	0.2039	0.19525	509.3962
5	408	0.1564	0.15346	400.3854
6	273	0.1046	0.10052	262.2525
7	139	0.0533	0.05643	147.236
8	45	0.0172	0.02772	72.3297
9	27	0.0103	0.01211	31.584
10	10	0.0038	0.00476	12.4125
11	4	0.0015	0.0017	4.4346
12	0	0	0.00056	1.4523
13	1	0.0004	0.00017	0.4391
14	1	0.0004	0.00005	0.1232
15	1	0.0004	0.00001	0.0323

Reset   Calculate

mean of observed sample =	3.88
variance of observed sample =	3.74
mean and variance of fitted Poisson distribution =	3.93

If needed, the observed and expected frequencies can be compared by a chi-square test. However, the fit to a Poisson distribution is close, and in keeping with random distribution. The easiest way to test for a Poisson distribution with the above data is to take the ratio of the variance to the mean, which is $3.88/3.74 = 1.0374$, and multiply this by the degrees of freedom. This gives chi-square $= 1.0374 \times 2609 = 2706$. From the tables this gives $P = 0.91$, so that we cannot reject the null hypothesis that the data fit a Poisson distribution.

Problem 18.2

$$d = \sqrt{2 \times 2706} - \sqrt{2 \times 2609 - 1} = 1.3375.$$

This is much less than the critical value of 1.96, so we cannot reject the null hypothesis.

Problem 18.3

By the normal approximation, the 95% limits are

$425 \pm 1.96\sqrt{425} = 384.59 - 465.41$. By using the calculator http://www.danielsoper.com/statcalc3/calc.aspx?id=86 we get

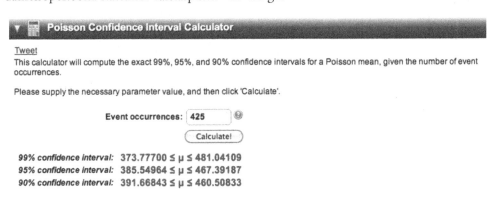

The results by the exact method are similar.

Problem 18.4

Using the above calculator, the confidence limits are

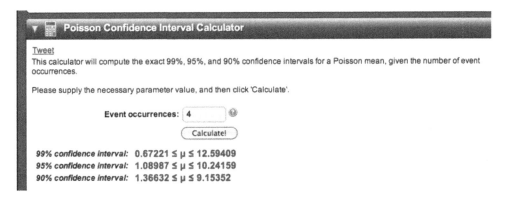

Problem 18.5

Using the calculator at http://stattrek.com/Tables/poisson.aspx, and fill in the number in the top line until an approximate probability is reached.

Poisson Distribution Calculator: Online Statistical Table

The Poisson Calculator makes it easy to compute individual and cumulative Poisson probabilities. For help in using the calculator, read the Frequently-Asked Questions or review the Sample Problems.

To learn more about the Poisson distribution, read Stat Trek's tutorial on the Poisson distribution.

- Enter a value in BOTH of the first two text boxes.
- Click the **Calculate** button.
- The Calculator will compute the Poisson and Cumulative Probabilities.

Poisson random variable (x)	6
Average rate of success	3
Poisson Probability: $P(X = 6)$	0.0504094067224622
Cumulative Probability: $P(X < 6)$	0.916082057968697
Cumulative Probability: $P(X \leq 6)$	0.966491464691159
Cumulative Probability: $P(X > 6)$	0.033508535308841
Cumulative Probability: $P(X \geq 6)$	0.083917942031303

(Calculate)

There is a 96.66% probability of getting 6 or more in the next hour.

For 32 patients in 8 h, place 24 in the second panel. The calculator gives a 95.3% chance.

CHAPTER 19

Problem 19.1

Calculating from http://stattrek.com/online-calculator/negative-binomial.aspx gives

Negative Binomial Calculator: Online Statistical Table

Use the Negative Binomial Calculator to compute probabilities, given a negative binomial experiment. For help in using the calculator, read the Frequently-Asked Questions or review the Sample Problems.

To learn more about the negative binomial distribution, see the negative binomial distribution tutorial.

- Enter a value in each of the first three text boxes (the unshaded boxes).
- Click the **Calculate** button.
- The Calculator will compute the Negative Binomial Probability.

Number of trials	30
Number of successes	8
Probability of success on a single trial	0.25
Negative binomial probability: $P(X = 8)$	0.0424824500374265

(Calculate)

CHAPTER 20

Problem 20.1

Data Entry

	Condition			
	Absent	Present	Totals	
Group 1	445	652	1097	
Group 2	794	738	1532	
Totals	1239	1390	2629	

Expected Cell Frequencies per Null Hypothesis

517	580
722	810

Calculate   Reset

	Rate	Risk Ratio	Odds	Odds Ratio	Log Odds
Group 1	0.5943		1.4652		
		1.2338		1.5763	0.4551
Group 2	0.4817		0.9295		

Rate = proportion in group with condition present
Risk Ratio = Rate[1]/Rate[2]
Odds[1] = present[1]/absent[1]
Odds[2] = present[2]/absent[2]
Odds Ratio = Odds[1]/Odds[2]
Log Odds = natural logarithm of Odds Ratio

		.95 Confidence Intervals	
	Observed	Lower Limit	Upper Limit
Risk Ratio	1.2338	1.1489	1.325
Odds Ratio	1.5763	1.3477	1.8438

	Chi-Square	
Phi	Yates	Pearson
+0.11	32.09	32.54
P	<.0001	<.0001

Chi-square is calculated only if all expected cell frequencies are equal to or greater than 5. The Yates value is corrected for continuity; the Pearson value is not. Both probability estimates are non-directional.

Fisher Exact Probability Test:

P	one-tailed	Sample size too large
	two-tailed	for the Fisher test.

Derived from http://vassarstats.net/odds2x2.html.

The confidence limits and chi-square are also provided. Because these were not samples drawn at random from a population, we cannot be sure about their representation in the population.

Problem 20.2

Using the calculator http://www.stat.ubc.ca/~rollin/stats/ssize/caco.html gives 2733 for the first set, 358 for the second set (lower because of the higher risk ratio), and 150 for the last set.

Unmatched Case/Control Studies

(To use this page, your browser must recognize JavaScript.)

Choose which calculation you desire, enter the relevant population values (as decimal fractions) for p0 (exposure in the controls) and RR (relative risk of disease associated with exposure) and, if calculating power, a sample size (assumed the same for each sample). You may also modify α (type I error rate) and the power, if relevant. After making your entries, hit the **calculate** button at the bottom.

- ⊙ Calculate Sample Size (for specified Power)
- ○ Calculate Power (for specified Sample Size)

Enter a value for p0: 0.08

Enter a value for RR: 2.7

- ○ 1 Sided Test
- ⊙ 2 Sided Test

Enter a value for α (default is .05): .05

Enter a value for desired power (default is .80): .80

The sample size (for cases and controls, separately) is: 150

(Calculate)

Problem 20.3

From http://statpages.org/ctab2x2.html we get

Observed Contingency Table

*	Outcome Occurred	Outcome did not Occur	Totals
Risk Factor Present or Dx Test Positive	53 = a	34 = b	87 = r1
Risk Factor Absent or Dx Test Negative	148 = c	165 = d	313 = r2
Totals	201 = c1	199 = c2	400 = t

Confidence Level: 95 %

Compute

Chi-Square Tests

Type of Test	Chi Square	d.f.	p-value
Pearson Uncorrected	5.063	1	0.024
Yates Corrected	4.532	1	0.033
Mantel-Haenszel	5.050	1	0.025

Odds Ratio (OR) = (a/b)/(c/d);	1.738	1.042	2.904
Relative Risk (RR) = (a/r1)/(c/r2);	1.288	1.020	1.569

Number Needed to Treat (NNT) = 1 / absolute value of DP; which = 1 / absolute value of ARR;	7.334	3.933	97.510
Absolute Risk Reduction (ARR) = c/r2 - a/r1; which = - DP	-0.136	-0.254	-0.010
Relative Risk Reduction (RRR) = ARR/(c/r2); <more info>	-0.288	-0.569	-0.020

NNT is calculated from

$$NNT = \frac{1}{\frac{53}{148} - \frac{34}{165}} = \frac{1}{0.1520} = 6.6$$

CHAPTER 21

Problem 21.1

Quantities Derived from the 2-by-2 Contingency Table	Value	95% Conf. Interval	
Odds Ratio (OR) = (a/b)/(c/d);	18.592	9.099	38.376
Relative Risk (RR) = (a/r1)/(c/r2);	16.518	8.390	33.005
Kappa	0.174	0.121	0.219
Overall Fraction Correct = (a+d)/t ; (often referred to simply as "Accuracy")	0.908	0.902	0.913
Mis-classification Rate, = 1 - Overall Fraction Correct;	0.092	0.087	0.098
Sensitivity = a/c1; (use exact Binomial confidence intervals instead of these)	0.641	0.476	0.781
Specificity = d/c2; (use exact Binomial confidence intervals instead of these)	0.912	0.909	0.915
Positive Predictive Value (PPV) = a/r1; (use exact Binomial confidence intervals instead of these)	0.118	0.087	0.144
Negative Predictive Value (NPV) = d/r2; (use exact Binomial confidence intervals instead of these)	0.993	0.990	0.996

A positive test is of little help because of the large number of false positives. On the other hand, a negative test is strongly against the diagnosis. Performed with calculator at http://statpages.org/ctab2x2.html.

Problems 21.2 and 21.3

From the same calculator we get

Positive Likelihood Ratio (+LR) = Sensitivity / (1 - Specificity);	7.315	5.247	9.182
Negative Likelihood Ratio (-LR) = (1 - Sensitivity) / Specificity;	0.393	0.239	0.577
Diagnostic Odds Ratio = (Sensitivity/(1-Sensitivity))/((1-Specificity)/Specificity);	18.592	9.099	38.376

This suggests that a positive test supports the possibility of bowel cancer.

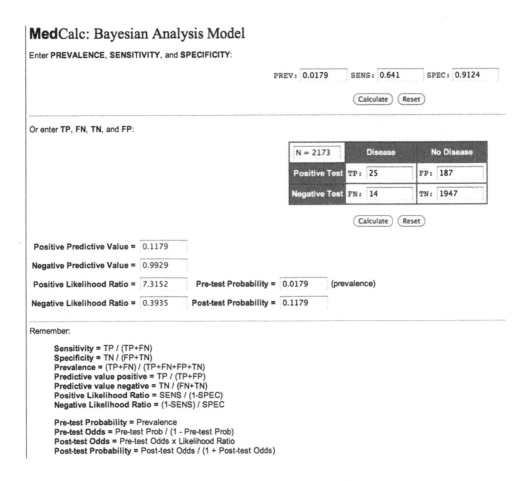

Calculated from http://www.medcalc.com/bayes.html.

CHAPTER 22

Problem 22.1

t = 4.8554, 8 degrees of freedom.

P = 0.0013.

Difference between means = 49.78, with standard error of mean 10.252.

95% confidence intervals are 26.14 to 73.42.

Conclusion: There is good reason to reject the null hypothesis, and exercise reduces peak flow rate in these subjects.

Problem 22.2

t = 1.8259 with 16 degrees of freedom.

P = 0.0866.

Difference between means = 49.78 (same as for paired test), with standard error of mean 27.263.

95% confidence intervals are −8.02 to 107.57.

The peak flow rate has been decreased, but the difference is not strongly supportive of rejecting the null hypothesis. This is due to the big increase in standard error of the mean in the unpaired versus the paired test because intersubject variability is added to the between subject variability.

Problem 22.3

Wilcoxon Signed-Rank Test Calculator

Subject	Before exercise	After exercise	Sign	Absolute value	Rank	Signed rank
1	320	297	+	23	2	2
2	235	200	+	35	3	3
3	322	220	+	102	9	9
4	376	334	+	42	4	4
5	286	210	+	76	8	8
6	254	255	−	1	1	−1
7	381	338	+	43	5	5
8	397	341	+	56	6	6
9	299	227	+	72	7	7

Obtained at http://www.socscistatistics.com/tests/signedranks/Default2.aspx.

Result Details

W value: 1

Mean Difference: 118.89

Sum of positive ranks: 44

Sum of negative ranks: 1

Z value: −2.5471 (*nb. N* too small)

Sample Size (*N*): 9

Significance Level:

0.05

Two–tailed

Result 1—Z value

The *Z* value is −2.5471. However, the size of *N* (9) is not large enough for the distribution of the Wilcoxon *W* statistic to form a normal distribution. Therefore, it is not possible to calculate an accurate p value.

Result 2—W value

The *W* value is 1. The critical value of *W* for *N* = 9 at p ≤ 0.05 is 5. Therefore, the result is significant at p ≤ 0.05.

Explanation of results

We have calculated both a *W* value and *Z* value. If the size of *N* is at least 20—see the Results Details box—then the distribution of the Wilcoxon *W* statistic tends to form a normal distribution. This means you can use the *Z* value to evaluate your hypothesis. If, on the other hand, the size of *N* is low, and particularly if it is below 10, you should use the *W* value to evaluate your hypothesis.

You should also note that if a subject's difference score is zero—that is, if a subject has the same score in both treatment conditions—then the test discards the individual from the analysis and reduces the sample size. If you have a lot of ties, this procedure will undermine the reliability of the test (and also suggests that the requirement that the data are continuous has not been met).

Problem 22.4

Before	After	Ranks before	Ranks after
235	200	5	1
254	210	6	2
286	220	8	3
299	227	10	4
320	255	11	7
322	297	12	9
376	334	16	13
381	338	17	14
397	341	18	15
		$\Sigma = 103$	$\Sigma = 68$

Based on http://www.socscistatistics.com/tests/mannwhitney/Default2.aspx.

Z ratio

The *Z* score is 1.5011. The p value is 0.13362. The result is *not* significant at p ≤ 0.05.

CHAPTER 25

Problem 25.1

I used the online calculator at http://vassarstats.net/anova1u.html because it allows you to cut and paste. The results were

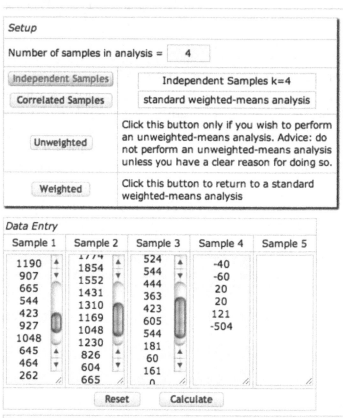

Setup
Number of samples in analysis = 4

Independent Samples	Independent Samples k=4
Correlated Samples	standard weighted-means analysis
Unweighted	Click this button only if you wish to perform an unweighted-means analysis. Advice: do not perform an unweighted-means analysis unless you have a clear reason for doing so.
Weighted	Click this button to return to a standard weighted-means analysis

Data Entry

Sample 1	Sample 2	Sample 3	Sample 4	Sample 5
1190	1774	524	-40	
907	1854	544	-60	
665	1552	444	20	
544	1431	363	20	
423	1310	423	121	
927	1169	605	-504	
1048	1048	544		
645	1230	181		
464	826	60		
262	604	161		
	665	0		

Reset   Calculate

Data Summary

	Samples					
	1	2	3	4	5	Total
N	27	17	14	6		64
ΣX	37292	31748	6670	-443		75267
Mean	1381.1852	1867.5294	476.4286	-73.8333		1176.0469
ΣX^2	89339498	98628324	4564342	274657		19280682
Variance	1455090.0	2458625.0	106658.72	48389.766		1655385.7
Std.Dev.	1206.2711	1568.0003	326.5865	219.9767		1286.6179
Std.Err.	232.147	380.2959	87.2839	89.8051		160.8272

standard weighted-means analysis					
ANOVA Summary Independent Samples k=4					
Source	SS	df	MS	F	P
Treatment [between groups]	25490448.28	3	8496816.096	6.47	0.000723
Error	78798852.57	60	1313314.209		
Ss/Bl					Graph Maker
Total	104289300.8	63			

Ss/Bl = Subjects or Blocks depending on the design.
Applicable only to correlated-samples ANOVA.

Tukey HSD Test

HSD[.05]=1241.51;
HSD[.01]=1524.63
M1 vs M2   nonsignificant
M1 vs M3   nonsignificant
M1 vs M4   P<.05
M2 vs M3   P<.05
M2 vs M4   P<.01
M3 vs M4   nonsignificant

M1 = mean of Sample 1
M2 = mean of Sample 2
and so forth.

HSD = the absolute [unsigned] difference between any two sample means required for significance at the designated level. HSD[.05] for the .05 level; HSD[.01] for the .01 level.

The figure from which these data came is

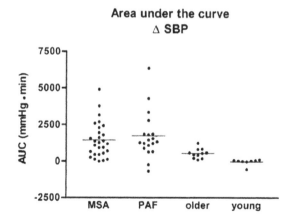

Area under the curve
Δ SBP

Problem 25.2

When the data are ranked, we get

count	Ranks for Sample			
	A	B	C	D
1	3.5	7	3.5	9
2	3.5	8	10	15
3	3.5	14	12	20
4	3.5	18.5	16	21
5	3.5		17	22
6	11		18.5	24
7	13		23	26
8			25	27

Reset   Calculate from Ranks

The mean ranks of the four samples are respectively 5.9, 11.9, 15.6, and 20.5. Then $H = 13.23$ with 3 df, and $P = 0.0042$. The conclusion is that the null hypothesis of equality of mean ranks might be rejected.

If a standard ANOVA is done on these data, $P = 0.0063$. ANOVA is relatively robust.

If we compare groups A and C by Dunn's test, then

$$Q = \frac{15.6 - 5.9}{\sqrt{\frac{27 \times 26}{12}\left(\frac{1}{7} + \frac{1}{8}\right)}} = \frac{9.7}{3.96} = 2.45.$$

The critical value for a family-wise error rate of 0.05 is a z corresponding to $\frac{0.05}{\frac{4 \times 3}{2}} = \frac{0.05}{6} = 0.0083$. The equivalent value of z is 2.638.

CHAPTER 26

Problem 26.1

I used the calculator at http://vassarstats.net/anova2u.html, and got

standard weighted-means analysis

ANOVA Summary   2rows x 3columns

Source	SS	df	MS	F	P
Rows	20.17	1	20.17	9.81	0.0058
Columns	200.33	2	100.17	48.73	<.0001
r x c	16.33	2	8.16	3.97	0.0373
Error	37	18	2.06		
Total	273.83	23			

Critical Values for the Tukey HSD Test

		HSD[.05]	HSD[.01]
Rows	2	1.23	1.68
Columns	3	1.83	2.39
Cells	6	3.23	4.02

HSD=the absolute [unsigned] difference between any two means (row means, column means, or cell means) required for significance at the designated level: HSD[.05] for the .05 level; HSD[.01] for the .01 level. The HSD test between row means can be meaningfully performed only if the row effect is significant; between column means, only if the column effect is significant; and between cell means, only if the interaction effect is significant.

Number of rows in analysis = 2
Number of columns in analysis = 3
Setup

2rows x 3columns
standard weighted-means analysis

Click this button only if you wish to perform an unweighted-means analysis. Advice: do not perform an unweighted-means analysis unless you have a clear reason for doing so.

Unweighted

Click this button to return to a standard weighted-means analysis

Weighted

Data Entry

	Col 1	Col 2	Col 3	Col 4
	4	7	10	
	5	9	12	
	6	8	11	
Row 1	5	12	9	
	6	13	12	
	6	15	13	
	4	12	10	
Row 2	4	12	13	
Row 3				
Row 4				

Reset   Calculate

The term r × c indicates the interaction.
It is good practice to put the data on a graph

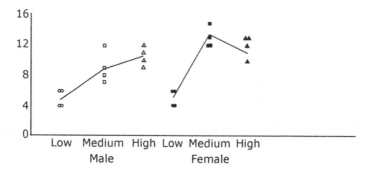

The decrease in weight gain in women on high carbohydrate content indicates the interaction.

CHAPTER 27

Problem 27.1

Draw the graph first. I used and got http://www.wessa.net/slr.wasp.

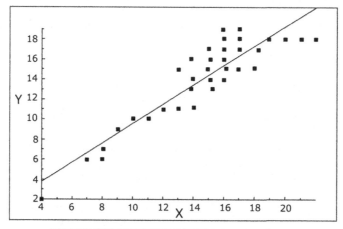

Simple Linear Regression - Ungrouped Data				
Parameter	Value	S.E.	T-STAT	Notes
Constant	2.513420			
Beta	0.850277	0.067717	12.556351	H0: beta = 0
Elasticity	0.826835	0.065850	-2.629690	H0: elast. = 1

Simple Linear Regression - Analysis of Variance			
ANOVA	DF	Sum of Squares	Mean Square
Regression	1.000000	446.250325	446.250325
Residual	33.000000	93.404026	2.830425
Total	34.000000	539.654350	15.872187
F-TEST		157.661949	

Problem 27.2

I obtained a set of residuals from http://vassarstats.net/corr_stats.html.

Data Entry

Pairs	Data Cells		Residuals
	X	Y	
1	2.098	3.98	-0.224
2	6.055	6.964	-0.652
3	6.115	7.959	0.292
4	7.134	8.036	-0.51
5	9.113	9.031	-1.221
6	10.132	10.026	-1.105
7	10.132	11.02	-0.111
8	11.091	12.015	0.057
9	11.151	13.01	1
10	11.271	14.005	1.892
11	13.129	13.852	0.137
12	13.129	15.23	1.515
13	14.029	15.995	1.504
14	14.029	15.077	0.586
15	14.149	13.929	-0.666
16	15.048	13.01	-2.36
17	15.108	14.923	-0.499
18	15.168	16.148	0.675
19	15.108	16.913	1.491
20	15.228	17.985	2.46
21	16.067	15.995	-0.253
22	16.067	15.077	-1.171
23	16.127	13.852	-2.448
24	17.146	15	-2.179
25	17.086	15.995	-1.132
26	17.086	16.99	-0.137
27	17.026	18.214	1.139
28	18.106	21.964	3.958
29	18.106	21.046	3.04
30	18.106	19.974	1.968
31	18.106	18.903	0.897
32	18.165	16.99	-1.067
33	18.165	15.995	-2.062
34	19.065	15.918	-2.915
35	19.125	16.99	-1.895

Reload Reset Calculate

and then plotted the residuals against the original X values with http://www.wessa.net/slr.wasp to get

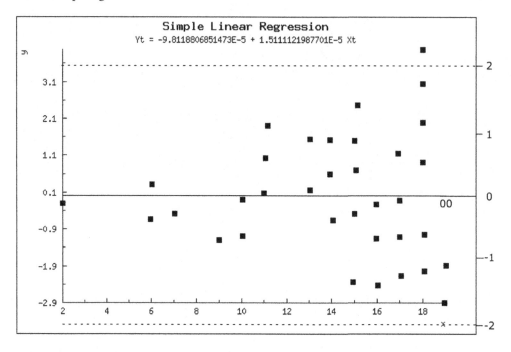

The residuals are scattered evenly above and below the line, and they show some heteroscedasticity. If we divide the Y axis by the standard deviation from regression, which is the square root of the residual mean square of $2.830425 = 1.6823$, we get a Y scale in standard deviations, as shown in the right hand vertical axis. The range from $+2$ to -2 standard deviations is shown by dashed lines. As expected, almost all the residuals fall within this range.

Problem 27.3

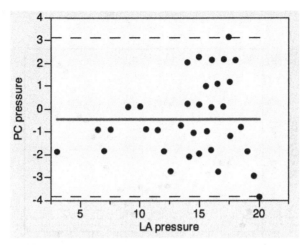

Note: heteroscedasticity

CHAPTER 29

Problem 29.1

I used http://www.easycalculation.com/statistics/correlation.php and got

	Results:
Total Numbers :	35
Correlation :	0.756186190223962

Problem 29.2

Using any of the online calculators gives:

Spearman: $r_s = 0.3935$, $P = 0.023$.

Kendall: $\tau = 0.3738$, $P = 0.13$.

There maybe slight differences among programs, depending on whether they correct for ties, and by what method they use. Any differences are likely to be negligible.

CHAPTER 31

Problem 31.1

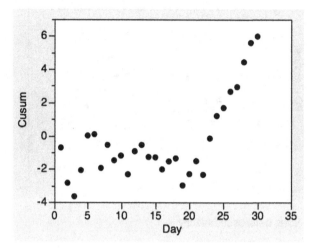

CHAPTER 35

Problem 35.1

Because the entry of data is all important, I will go over the process step by step, using https://statcom.dk/K-M_plot.php. For batch entry

1. The data must be set out as in the problem, using two separate tables and saving them as text files.
2. Open the online calculator.

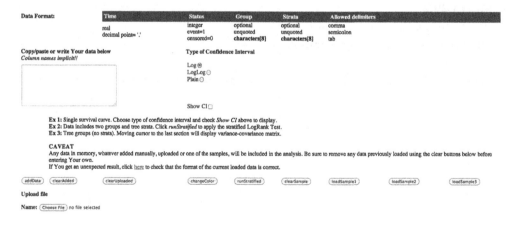

3. Select radio button loadSample 1.
4. Select radio button Choose File.
5. Select file from desktop, and select radio button uploadFile.
6. Select radio button loadSample 2.
7. Select radio button Choose File.
8. Select the second file from desktop, and select radio button uploadFile.
9. Your plot should look like this:

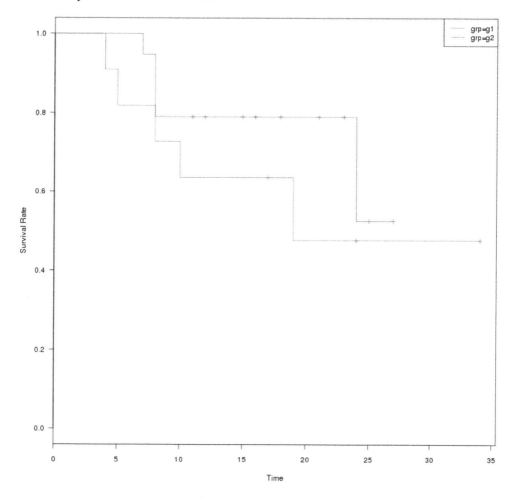

10. You may be asked to examine the plot after the first set is entered. Then continue with the second set.
11. No numbers will appear in the box. You can, if you wish, enter data subject by subject by hand.

GLOSSARY

Accuracy This describes how close the measurement is to the true value. For example, if the true cardiac output is 5 l/min (based on some gold standard), then an accurate measurement comes close to that value (e.g., 4.9 l/min), and an inaccurate one will be far from it (e.g., 3.2 l/min).

Alpha The predetermined maximum probability of obtaining a Type I error.

Alternative hypothesis If the null hypothesis (see below) is not accepted, that is, if the two parameters seem to come from different populations, then there are three alternative possibilities:

Parameter 1 $\neq$ Parameter 2

Parameter 1 $>$ Parameter 2

Parameter 1 $<$ Parameter 2

Beta The (predetermined) maximum probability of obtaining a Type II error.

Bias This indicates that an outcome differs from the correct answer in a systematic way. Unlike error (see below) the departures from the correct answer are not random.

Biased studies These occur when (intentionally or not) subjects in one group differ from subjects in another group in some meaningful way. For example, if we study the effects of a medication on blood sugar in two groups, one on the medication and one on a placebo, and if the placebo group had a large surplus of obese subjects with insulin resistance, the observations will be biased. It is more difficult to make meaningful inferences if samples are biased.

Case–control A study in which groups differing in outcome are identified and compared to determine if there are differences in possible antecedent events (causes). For example, children with and without congenital heart diseases (CHD) are compared to determine if CHD is more common if the mothers took an antidepressant drug during pregnancy.

Cohort A group with a common characteristic, such as being born in the same year, or being exposed to unhealthy atmospheric conditions.

Confidence interval The limits within which the true parameter (such as a mean) is expected to fall with a given probability when observations are sampled from a population.

Confounding If two variables are related to each other by a third factor that might or might not be known, that factor is a confounding factor. For example, an increase in the number of births in a German city parallels the increase in the number of storks nesting there. These two variables are not directly related to each other by cause and effect, but both are due to an increase in the city's population and the number of houses. Population growth is the confounder.

Correlation This describes how closely two (or more) variables are associated with each other.

Dependent variable The outcome of interest (the effect) that might change when an intervention is done.

Effect size The absolute magnitude of the difference between two (or more) parameters. The relative effect size is the absolute effect size related to the variability of the sample.

Error This has a specific meaning in statistics. It refers to variability from a parameter. Thus if the population mean weight of adult females is 50 kg, a particular member of a sample of adult females might weigh 56 kg. This difference from the parameter is termed the error, or individual deviation from the parameter. In general, errors might be due to measuring errors, random variation, or to bias. It is the function of a good experimenter to eliminate bias and try to reduce individual variability as much as possible.

Expectation This is also known as the mathematical expectation, symbolized by E. It can be regarded as the long-run average of the outcomes of many repeated experiments. More formally, it is the weighted average of all possible values of the random variable. For example, we expect intuitively that in the long run tossing a coin many times will average out as 50% heads and 50% tails. This 1:1 ratio might not apply to any one small series of tosses, but as the number of trials increases the average will approach 50% of each.

Explanatory variable See Independent variable.

Independent variable This is what is being manipulated or changed (the cause) to try and produce an effect.

Mathematical expectation See expectation.

Null hypothesis The hypothesis that two parameters (means, slopes, etc.) are so similar that they could have been sampled from the same population. Unless the parameters are identical, it is never possible to state that they could not have been sampled from two different populations, but the degree of uncertainty can be specified.

Normal An unfortunate word. In ordinary speech it implies health, or the usual state. In statistics, it implies that the distribution is compatible with a specific formula. It is a symmetrical distribution with certain properties and to avoid ambiguity is sometimes called the Gaussian or bell-shaped curve or distribution.

Overdispersion This describes a distribution, usually of counts, with a variance much greater than expected for a typical binomial or Poisson distribution. It may be due to misclassification, outliers, or clumping of data due to extraneous events (such as having high and low malaria attack rates with few intermediate values).

Parameter A quantity that describes or characterizes a population. For example, a measure of central tendency, the mean, is a parameter that gives information about where the center of the distribution is. Parameters are symbolized by Greek letters, such as μ, β, ρ, σ, and so on. This term should not be used when the term variable is meant (see Variable).

Power This is the probability of finding a true difference between parameters and is calculated as $1 - \beta$ where β is the Type II error (see below).

Precision This indicates how reproducible the measurement is. If we repeat the measurement 10 times, are the results all close together, or are they widely scattered? It is important to note that a measurement may be precise but inaccurate. If the cardiac output is 5 l/min, 10 repeated measurements of that output might range from 3.5 to 3.7 l/min; they would be very precise but inaccurate.

Probability density function If there is a random variable of the discrete type, then it is possible to calculate or determine experimentally the probability of $P(X = 0)$, $P(X = 1)$...$P(X = n)$. The probability $P(X = x)$ is sometimes called the probability density function, and symbolized by $f(x)$.

Random Randomness is a property that pertains to samples drawn from a population. To be random, each member of the sample must have an equal chance of being chosen as a member of that sample, and drawing one member should not influence the drawing of the other members of the sample.

Reexpression Finding a new scale, for example, a logarithmic or square root scale, to simplify the data analysis. There is no necessary physical or physiological connotation in selecting the reexpression. The fact that a logarithmic scale makes analysis easy does not mean that the process itself is logarithmic, although it might well be.

Regression This indicates how much a dependent variable Y changes for a unit increase in explanatory variables X_1, X_2...X_n.

Residuals Residuals are what are left over when theoretical expected values are subtracted from the actual observed values. For example, when a straight line is fitted to a series of X,Y points, the vertical differences of the observed Y values from the values of Y that lies on the line for those values of X are the residuals. Therefore Residual = Data − fitted value.

Resistant The parameter is little affected by unusually small or big measurements in the data set.

Robust This is the quality of a test that implies insensitivity to departures from the assumptions underlying the probabilistic model. For example, the *t*-test for comparing two groups of measurements is not very robust and becomes inefficient if the distributions are very asymmetrical, whereas the Mann–Whitney U test is very robust.

Scattergram Also termed scatter plot or scatter diagram. This is a two-dimensional plot that shows how two variables are related.

Significant Another unfortunate word. In ordinary speech, it implies importance. In statistics, however, it has nothing to do with importance, but rather refers to the chances of rejecting the null hypothesis incorrectly (Type I error).

Significant figures These are the digits in a number that denote the accuracy of measurement. If we describe the weight of a small animal as 50.32 g, then we are stating that the weight lies within the range 50.315–50.325 g. In this example, we are using four significant figures, in which the first three are accurate and the last has potential error.

Statistic This is similar to a parameter, except that it characterizes a sample. Statistics are written as ordinary letters, such as m, b, r, s, and so on. This is not to be confused with other uses of the word "statistic," which can be taken to mean a given value. For example, we hear the phrase: "Don't become a traffic statistic," or we talk about vital statistics, by which we mean the numbers of births, deaths, etc. that occur in a community. The context usually distinguishes these two uses.

Transformation See Reexpression.

Type I error This occurs if we reject the null hypothesis when in fact it is true. The Type I error rate is usually denoted by α. If $\alpha = 0.05$, then we reject the null hypothesis when $P < 0.05$. Usually we determine what value of α to use; it is sometimes 0.01 or 0.10, or occasionally other values.

Type II error This occurs when we accept the null hypothesis when it is false. The Type II error rate is usually denoted by β. This is determined by the difference between the parameters, the sample size, the sample distribution, and the value of α. It has to be calculated separately for each data set.

Unbiased If many samples are taken with replacement from a population, then any statistic (such as the mean) calculated from those samples will vary. On the average, however, the average sample statistic will equal the population parameter. An estimate in which the average value over all possible samples equals the population parameter is called *unbiased*.

Variable This is a number that can take on one of several values. Thus if we measure the weights of 50 adult females, each weight is a variable. Note that although parameters can also vary (e.g., the mean weight of adult females is not the same as the mean weight of adult males), the parameter is usually a distillate of all the variables and a property of all the variables in the data set.

INDEX

Note: Page numbers followed by "f", "t" or "b" indicates figures, tables and boxes respectively.

Printed in the United States
By Bookmasters